INTRODUCTION TO

Language
Development

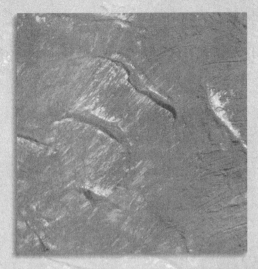

SECOND EDITION

INTRODUCTION TO

Language Development

Scott McLaughlin, PhD, CCC-SLP

Speech-Language Pathology
University of Central Oklahoma
Edmond, Oklahoma

THOMSON

DELMAR LEARNING

Australia   Canada   Mexico   Singapore   Spain   United Kingdom   United States

THOMSON

DELMAR LEARNING

Introduction to Language Development, Second Edition
Scott McLaughlin, PhD, CCC-SLP

Vice President, Health Care Business Unit:

William Brottmiller

Director of Learning Solutions:

Matthew Kane

Acquisitions Editor:

Kalen Conerly

Product Manager:

Juliet Steiner

Editorial Assistant:

Molly Belmont

Marketing Director:

Jennifer McAvey

Marketing Coordinator:

Christopher Manion

Production Director:

Carolyn Miller

Production Manager:

Barbara A. Bullock

Production Coordinator:

Thomas Heffernan

Library of Congress Cataloging-in-Publication Data

McLaughlin, Scott, 1952-
    Introduction to language development / Scott McLaughlin.—2nd ed.
        p. cm.
    Includes bibliographical references and index.
    ISBN 0-7693-0265-3
    1. Language acquisition. 2. Communication. I. Title.
    P118.M393 2007
    401'.93–dc22

                                        2005036357

NOTICE TO THE READER

To Kathy, Katie, and Conner.
In my life, I love you most of all.

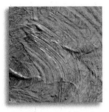

Contents

CHAPTER 10 Language Differences: Diversity and Disorders   399

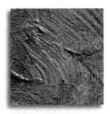

Preface

Revised and updated, *Introduction to Language Development,* 2nd edition continues to serve as an undergraduate textbook introducing readers to language development, with a balanced treatment of the different perspectives on this subject. As in the previous edition, this text presents the basic concepts and terminology associated with each of the behavioral, syntactic, semantic, and pragmatic aspects of language as they develop throughout the lifespan.

When the first edition of this book came out almost eight years ago, it was a great relief to see my labors, although they were labors of love, finally come to fruition. Anyone who has endeavored to capture any natural phenomenon between the front and back covers of a book understands what a daunting task that is. As I grappled with the challenge I had taken on, I came to admire all those who had ever written a textbook. I especially grew in respect for those who also had attempted to capture the myriad complexities and subtleties of this fascinating, multifaceted, and elusive phenomenon we call "language development."

In a broader sense, when my first edition materialized, I was also relieved to find that I had a version of language development that I could be comfortable using to teach my students this very important basic information. My goal was to provide a text that presented the essential foundational terms, concepts, theories, and observations that define our understanding of language development. I tried to do so in a way that would allow undergraduate students in the beginning stages of their studies to focus on the essential elements–biological maturation, cognitive development, linguistic patterns, behavioral principles, and social interaction. Furthermore, I attempted to help them grasp this information in an integrated manner.

My goal was to accomplish this in a "student friendly" manner. In teaching this subject for almost 15 years, I found too often that my students were overwhelmed by the multitude of "facts" accumulated through the countless research articles cited with ever-increasing density in the texts I used. While all this information is ultimately important and relevant in the larger picture, it only served to numb students' ability to grasp the full picture—they were "getting lost in the trees, trying to find the forest." Instead, I attempted to maintain a clear focus on the germinal concepts and studies that laid the foundation for this area. I believe that a beginning student in any subject area first has to understand the basic principles and processes through which we have arrived at our current understanding of the phenomenon in question. In this way, students are more likely to apply these insights in becoming the architects of more and better research as opposed to functioning as "consumers" who simply memorize facts.

Soon after the first edition published, I began receiving feedback from my students, students in other programs, and a number of instructors who were using the book. Most of this feedback was positive and encouraging. Some of it was corrective and clarifying, which gave me good reason to pursue this second edition. However, certainly the highest compliment I received came from my father-in-law, Dr. David Steen, who had taught many years in medical school. After reading the book, he said, "I can tell you wrote this to teach your students, not to impress your colleagues." To that end, I have made a number of changes, but like a physician, I made every effort to "do no harm."

Chapters 1 to 3 present basic concepts and terminology regarding the nature of human communication and its biological and interactive foundations. Chapter 4 presents the concepts and terminology of the major models of language acquisition and precedes the developmental chapters. In my view, understanding the models of language development allows students to evaluate the implications and relevance of each model to the observations presented in the later chapters that describe the development of language. The models provide a framework that students can apply in associating and understanding the information related to individual developments. Chapters 5 through 9 present language development as it evolves from infancy throughout adulthood. These chapters present the concepts and terminology that form the core of our understanding at each phase as language emerges in infants, toddlers, preschoolers, and students in their school years and beyond. Finally, Chapter 10 provides an overview of language differences— both the variations that are evident in language development due to cultural diversity and a basic introduction to those that represent disordered language development.

Literacy and language have become increasingly intertwined, especially as Speech-Language Pathologists look for treatment models that are collaborative in addressing academic concerns. In this edition, literacy information has been expanded, especially in Chapter 9. In addition, earlier chapters now include information related to the foundations of literacy— how the seeds of literacy are planted with infants, toddlers, and preschoolers. In addition, a new appendix—Appendix B—has been adapted from state-level academic goals; it has been included to provide extensive information regarding the development of specific literacy skills as they relate to academic skills throughout the grade levels.

Each developmental chapter is introduced with motor, cognitive, and social developments to "set the stage" for the developments in language during the period covered. In addition, a list of the major expected developments in language serves as a prelude to each chapter to tell the reader "what's coming" in that chapter. In my lectures, I adhere to the approach that it is important to "tell you what I'm going to tell you, then tell you, and then tell you what I told you." Therefore, the frequent section summaries and the final chapter summaries have been maintained and updated to complement these preludes.

Based on some valuable feedback from students and reviewers, I have attempted to clarify a number of sections. I have attempted to reduce redundancies where it seemed reasonable to do so. I have included a number of new tables to present difficult information and concepts more clearly. Margin notes to amplify or direct students to related information have been retained and expanded in some instances. I have retained the vignettes that preceded each chapter in the first edition. These attempts at tongue-in-cheek humor are intended to introduce each chapter with some light-hearted fun while piquing the reader's curiosity about some central concept related to each chapter.

Because different instructors take different approaches in reviewing, expanding, and testing information, each chapter still ends with a set of review questions and suggested readings. In addition, because students in the early stages sometimes find it difficult to think analytically about new information, I have included a set of practice questions at the end of each chapter. It is my hope that these multiple-choice questions require the student to understand information beyond the level of simple recognition. An Answer Key in the back of the book prompts the student to think through the nature of the information and discover the subtle distinctions that must be considered to arrive at the correct answer.

To the Student

I hope that in reading this text you discover that language development is not just a miraculous phenomenon of nature, but a complex and intricate orchestration of human abilities. Given this intriguing complexity, I encourage you to begin cultivating your ability to think analytically. Take an analytical approach to the information presented in this text and even in your own daily interactions. Identify the variables that are at work in producing the phenomenon being discussed. Analyze the subtleties that distinguish one behavior or development from another. Be sensitive to the derivations and shades of meaning embedded in the terms used to label these phenomena. In studying your text and in examining your own verbal behavior, become a true student of human communication. I think you will find it to be the most fascinating research in which you can become engaged.

One of my students wrote to me recently for encouragement and clarification. His questions were straightforward, essentially asking, "What made you become interested in this field?" I replied that in hindsight it appears that there were signs subtly leading me toward this field all along the way. However, at the time it seemed as though I literally stumbled into Speech-Language Pathology as a major. However, once I did, I instantly recognized how fascinating human communication is—and I was hooked. The subtle interplay of individuals' experiences and perspectives touches how we express ourselves and understand each other. The simplest of ideas, the most basic needs, and the most sublime emotions are all communicated through words at some level and through some modality. What seems to us to be simple words that carry straightforward ideas can convey the most subtle shades of meaning and produce minute but significant shifts in interpretation by each listener.

What appear to be individual words are actually continuous elements arranged in an infinite variety of elegant compositions. Although I am not a musical expert, I am told that the musical scales of Western civilization are generally composed of notes spanning 12 half-steps. Contemplate the breadth, depth, and variety contained in the millions of musical compositions produced by humankind—from Beethoven to the Beatles—by recombining these basic notes. Then consider that the modern dictionaries of the English language include almost 500,000 words. Although grammar dictates that these cannot be recombined in every possible way, it is still possible to think of human communication as an infinitely intricate and ever-changing symphony of our ideas, needs, and emotions. How does a child's language ability get from Chopsticks to Chopin? In short, as you begin your studies of human communication, my simplest hope is that you come to love words.

To the Instructor

My strongest motivation for writing this book and pursuing this second edition was to provide a text that is well suited to teaching. For over twenty years, I have loved teaching and especially teaching normal language development. In particular, I love the sense of accomplishment when I see "the light go on" in a student's eyes as they first grasp the sometimes very abstract concepts that have evolved around the phenomenon of language development. As an instructor, I hope you, too, revel in such moments. Further, I hope this text assists in some way as you achieve many of those moments.

I have two more levels of motivation that prompted me to write this text—that is, scholarly accuracy and paradigmatic integrity. Even as a young student in this field, it became apparent to me that there were widely disparate views on the models and theories that had been proposed to explain language development and language behavior. The two polar views, emphasizing the roles of innateness and learning in language development, were staked out in 1957 by Chomsky and Skinner. As the next two decades passed, middle-ground views began to bridge this wide gap as researchers began to recognize the important roles of cognition and social interaction. The original widely disparate views of psycholinguists and behaviorists have been gradually bridged by "interactionists" who essentially abandoned the "Which one is correct?" question and correctly moved on to asking, "How much of what does each contribute?" How much is contributed by biological, cognitive, social, and behavioral variables to the process of learning the most complex of all human behaviors?

The concern I have had for scholarly accuracy is that so many textbook treatments of the behavioral model are presented in a simplistic and sometimes inaccurate way. In fact, it seems that many textbook descriptions of the behavioral model are actually drawn directly from Chomsky's review of Skinner's *Verbal Behavior*. For example, many suggest that Skinner explained grammar through imitative learning of "word chains," a misconception contained in Chomsky's review. This is not only inaccurate–Skinner called verbal chains "intraverbals" and indicated that they have little to do with "grammar"–it ignores Skinner's far more complex treatment of "grammar," which took up three chapters in *Verbal Behavior*. Similarly, overly simplistic and inaccurate characterizations, such as suggesting that "selective reinforcement" means that caregivers must consciously decide when to reinforce their infants' speech sounds, do a disservice to our understanding and our study of such phenomena. By their nature, laboratory demonstrations of behavioral principles are "simplified"–they are simplified to isolate the principle or variable of interest from the extraneous influence of other variables. That does not mean that these same principles are not influenced by the far more complex natural environment and the subtleties of natural consequences. Skinner acknowledged this throughout *Verbal Behavior* and, in particular, in three chapters on the influence of "multiple variables."

Furthermore, my concern for scholarly accuracy in this regard is to maintain all these fundamental elements—linguistic, cognitive, social, and behavioral—in balance. Each theoretical perspective has the potential of contributing insights, and integrating those insights should result in a clearer and more complete explanation of language development. To neglect or misunderstand the contribution of any one diminishes and distorts the full picture. The analogy I give my students in this regard is as follows: Imagine the discovery of a pond in a deep dark forest in a place that had never been previously explored. To understand the history and composition of the area, three experts—a chemist, a biologist, and a physicist—are each given a sample of the pond water to analyze. When they report their results, one talks about such things as amoebae and microorganisms, one talks about oxygen levels and pH-balance, and the last one talks about neutrons, protons, and electrons. Is only one expert correct? Are the other two incorrect and contributing nothing of value? Or, are all three contributing important, relevant information based on their specialized perspective and level of analysis?

The concern for scholarly accuracy leads to my concern for the integrity of our paradigm. When we examine our actual application of scientific principles in our professional clinical practices, we may find that a "split personality" exists. As Speech-Language Pathologists, we may have been taught over the years that such concepts as reinforcement, discriminative stimuli, and stimulus generalization have no relevance to language development. However, when learning the basics of treating communication disorders, including language disorders, it is difficult to imagine any approach that cannot be couched in these same terms. Whether they are called "consequences," "contexts," or "carryover," these fundamental principles are essential to any language treatment program. In classes on normal language development, students are told that these principles are irrelevant and then in their language disorders classes they are taught how to apply them in treating disordered language development. I fear that this schism weakens the integrity of the overall paradigm we teach students. I believe that we should strive to provide students with a model in which theories are integrated and consistent with professional practices.

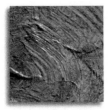

Acknowledgments

I continue to be indebted to my family and friends who inspired me—and pushed me—to write the first edition of *Introduction to Language Development* and now this second edition. I will always appreciate and admire Dr. Giri Hegde, my first true mentor, who made perhaps the most lasting philosophical impression on me and was the instigator of the first edition, simply insisting that it needed to be done. In my first edition, I failed to acknowledge a second mentor, Dr. Walter L. Cullinan, who used the Socratic teaching method so effectively during my graduate studies and caused me to refine and focus my understanding of the many concepts and controversies inherent in this subject area.

In addition, I sincerely appreciate the feedback provided by my students, students from other universities, my colleagues, colleagues from other universities, and the reviewers who so thoroughly and helpfully critiqued both my first edition and this second edition. I am being completely sincere when I invite additional feedback from anyone willing to provide it.

I must also single out Juliet Steiner of Thomson Delmar Learning. She showed infinite patience as my developmental editor as she prodded, pushed, and even provoked me into producing a much-improved version of this book. Any and all improvements that have occurred in this edition are in great measure due to her dedication to this book.

In closing, I must also express appreciation to the University of Central Oklahoma for supporting me in this project and allowing me to continue doing something that I love to do so much—teach.

The Dimensions of Human Communication

Robin's son clung tightly to a splintered board, the lone remnant from his shattered yacht. He washed ashore and collapsed on the tiny island. Later, not knowing where he was and having lost all sense of time, Robin's son slowly awoke. He felt disoriented and very alone—in spite of the smiling faces staring down at him. Robin's son tried to blink away the blur. When his eyes and head cleared, the faces he saw looked friendly. As Robin's son sat up and looked around expectantly, they spoke, but his ears somehow failed him. Robin's son shook his head. "Do you speak English?" he pleaded softly. They spoke again, and he knew he had a problem. Robin's son wondered to himself, "Would I be better prepared to handle this had I paid more attention in Miss Sintack's seventh-grade grammar class?"

This chapter addresses the following questions:

- What are the essential elements of communication?
- What roles are played by speech and language in human communication?
- What other modes of human communication have evolved?
- What is speech?
- What are the units and features of human speech?
- What is language?
- What are the important differences between speech and language?
- What are the major features of language?
- What are the major components of language?

Human communication surrounds us, defines our existence, supports our survival, describes our experience, and influences our understanding of the world around us. Our social world immerses us in speech and language from the moment we take our first breath. Even before birth, the sounds reaching the developing fetus include the mother's voice, although softened and muffled by the surrounding fluids and soft tissue.

Upon entering the world, infants are bathed in sounds—most significantly, the voices and words of their adoring family. The sounds infants hear include all those silly sounds adults are only willing to make for babies. During those early weeks and months, the sounds and words of the surrounding language are an integral part of the baby's most intimate moments, as the baby is fed, cuddled, entertained, and rocked to sleep.

During their first few years, children are immersed in the sounds and words of their language. They use them so automatically that caregivers might take this all for granted. Soon it is the intentions, insights, and humor of their child's comments, requests, and questions rather than the actual production of words and sentences that absorb their interest. The child has become a communicating, fully socialized member of their family and the surrounding community. By the time children grow into adults, language is effortlessly woven through every daily activity.

Unlike the individual in the shipwreck scenario at the opening of this chapter, most of us will never need to consciously study or analyze human communication for our continued survival. For a variety of reasons, however, many people become interested in this special and intriguing phenomenon. Some become painfully aware of its significance due to their personal circumstances. The mother whose high-risk infant may never talk or the spouse whose partner has suffered a stroke and may never speak again both understand the value of human communication. Some persons are inspired by such circumstances, and many others by their individual curiosity to pursue fields of study that closely examine human communication. These individuals might become linguists, special educators, psychologists, or speech-language pathologists.

There are three purposes to this introductory chapter: (1) to familiarize the interested beginning student with the basic aspects of human communication, including the dimensions, features, and terminology of communication, speech, and language; (2) to arouse the curiosity of the student who has yet to discover how interesting these aspects of human behavior can be; and (3) to provide a basis for the student's future study of language delay and disorders in children.

Major Dimensions of Human Communication

Throughout every day, humans busily interact in various ways. In their most important and even their most insignificant social transactions, human actions affect the behavior of those around them. Humans act in a variety of ways, including gestures, facial expressions, and talking, to influence the behavior of others. These social transactions can be analyzed into three major dimensions: communication, speech, and language.

Communication occurs in an array of natural circumstances and through a variety of means (e.g., gestures, body language). In humans, the primary means of communicating is through producing speech sounds. And, ultimately, humans communicate through language by producing meaningful arrangements of words. These three major dimensions—communication, speech, and language—are obviously closely interrelated. Ultimately, in most societies, communication takes the form of written symbols. In their most developed forms, when verbal communities rely heavily on reading and writing words to communicate, they are said to be literate societies.

Communication

In its broadest sense, communication takes place in a variety of contexts and assumes many forms. Natural forms of communication are observed in the behavior and sounds of animals. Ancient forms of human communication such as the Egyptian hieroglyphics, which date from approximately 3000 B.C., have been studied for the information they might transmit across the ages. New technology for communicating information to more people and across great distances is developing constantly. However, the most fundamental and, for many, the most intriguing form of communication is still interpersonal human communication.

Human communication can be studied from several viewpoints, including behavioral, theoretical, and linguistic perspectives. Behaviorally, communication consists of social interaction among individuals. To communicate means that our actions affect the behavior of another person or group of persons. Speech and language represent acts that affect the actions of others. On an individual basis, then, communication is a dynamic tool for influencing the behavior of others.

As a social behavior, communication is a key element in defining humans as social beings. As a species, our cumulative ability to communicate with each other creates, shares, and preserves the nature of the social interactions that make up our various cultures.

All too often we are most aware of the social significance of communication when there has been a communication breakdown. Children might throw tantrums when their needs are not understood. An uncomfortable silence occurs when two friends fail to understand each other. Major tragedies follow when emergency warning systems fail to reach people in the path of impending natural disasters. When communication fails, we appreciate its value to individuals and society at large.

From a theoretical perspective, **communication** has been defined as the process of sending and receiving messages that serve to transmit information

Major terms that are also defined separately in the margin and the glossary are printed in **bold** typeface. Related terms important to the discussion are printed in *italic* typeface. ■

communication The process of sharing ideas involving a sender who encodes a message and a receiver who decodes the message.

between persons or groups. When someone successfully transmits a message that is understood by someone else, communication has occurred. This theoretical concept has been greatly influenced by modern "mechanistic" processes for encoding and decoding messages. By analogy, communication theorists have likened human communication to the electronic transmission of messages via the telegraph or telephone. However, we must remember that we do not know precisely how the human brain functions in communication. Figure 1–1 illustrates the components of communication.

From a linguistic viewpoint, *communication* is defined as a rule-based mental system of language codes for expressing and understanding thoughts, feelings, and ideas. A **code** is a system of rules for arranging arbitrary symbols in an orderly, predictable manner that allows anyone who also knows the code to interpret the meaning.

Because the message in communication can only represent the speaker's ideas or feelings, the speaker must *encode* them into word sequences to convey them. The listener uses the same system of rules to *decode* the meaning carried by that sequence of words. Some other examples of codes we might commonly think of would be Morse code used in transmitting telegrams, the secret codes associated with military intelligence, and the codes sent from

code   The systematic, orderly nature of language that allows speakers and listeners to express and comprehend meanings.

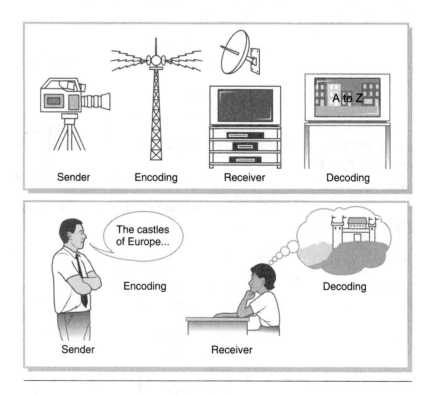

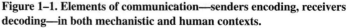

Figure 1–1. Elements of communication—senders encoding, receivers decoding—in both mechanistic and human contexts.

computers to printers. Of course, the code most relevant to our present discussion is language.

It is critical that a code is **systematic,** meaning that it must be orderly and organized. This makes the code predictable for users. As a result, beyond simply interpreting the code, listeners might be able to anticipate upcoming information or fill in missing information based on what they know about the situation and their language. For example, a listener who has heard only portions of a statement such as, *Well, when we arrived at the _____ store, we bought two bunches of _____, peeled them, and then we ate them,* would be likely to fill in the blanks with some ease.

To permit communication, a code must be shared by at least two participants. If senders (speakers) and receivers (listeners) attempt to use different codes for communicating, they will fail to exchange any information. In language, the fact that the code is shared by the many senders and receivers in a cultural group is expressed by the term **conventional.** Of course, doing something by convention means that participants all follow the same patterns or rules. If this were not the case, the result would be chaos, not communication. This might be analogous to the rules of traffic. Imagine the result if drivers all *ad libbed* while navigating through city traffic. In attempting to communicate, if speakers selected and ordered words randomly, each according to their own idiosyncratic whim, no ideas could actually be shared by anyone.

An illustration of the importance of convention in language is sometimes experienced in foreign travel. As tourists in foreign countries quickly learn when they need restroom facilities, even repeating the wrong code more loudly does not help if the listener does not know your language!

In addition to being systematic and conventional, two other key terms in the linguistic definition of communication are *symbol* and *arbitrary.* A **symbol** is an item used to represent or stand for another object, idea, or relationship. Symbols might take the form of a letter, a word, a visual form, or a gesture. We use various symbols to stand for businesses and corporations, religious beliefs, traffic regulations, and so on. Words are the symbols of language used to stand for all the things we talk about—objects, events, ideas, and relationships.

Generally, these symbols are **arbitrary,** meaning that they bear no physical resemblance to their referents. For the most part, spoken words do not sound like, nor do written words look like, the things they represent. For example, if we did not know the language, there is certainly nothing about the sound that occurs when someone says the word *chair* that would make us think of the actual item. This arbitrary nature of assigning meanings extends across all languages; the words for *chair* will sound different in every language.

There are exceptions to the arbitrary nature of words. In spoken English, and probably most languages, there are words that *do* sound like their referents: *buzz, splash, sizzle, crunch, zip,* among others. This phenomenon of words that sound like the events they represent is called **onomatopoeia.**

systematic   The regularities exhibited by speakers of a language that make occurrences in the language predictable.

conventional   The notion that language must be based on shared, customary, or implicitly agreed-on patterns of behavior.

symbol   Something (e.g., the word *chair,* whether spoken or written) that stands for or represents something else without bearing physical resemblance to it.

arbitrary   The capricious connection between words and their meanings.

onomatopoeia   Words that mimic the sounds associated with the objects or events they represent, such as *zip, splash,* or *sizzle.*

Similarly, many of the gestural signs used in sign languages and the figures used in pictographic languages appear much like the referent they are used to convey. Because they actually resemble what they represent, they are said to be *iconic*. Anyone familiar with the graphic interfaces so popular in computer programming (as in Apple's MacIntosh and Microsoft's Windows applications) is familiar with the use of icons or pictures to represent commands or program names.

Communicative Competence

All of us strive to communicate effectively in our social transactions. From the small child who wants an extra cookie to the politician who wants our votes, effective communication has probably existed as an underlying goal of human behavior since its earliest form. Philosophers, sociolinguists, and behavioral scientists have attempted to analyze the nature of effective communication.

Several researchers (Dore, 1986; Hymes, 1972; Skinner, 1957; among others) have proposed that speakers do more than just talk. Simply making sounds, saying words, or producing grammatical sentences does not make one a competent communicator. As an extreme counterexample, consider the schizophrenic patient who produces words and even grammatical sentences in an otherwise empty room. However, nobody is affected by this behavior, so it is not effective communication. At various times, we have all experienced talking with someone who does not communicate his or her thoughts clearly or appropriately. At times, young children, nervous students, and even self-absorbed instructors can be incompetent communicators. And, in all honesty, each of us would have to admit to those moments when we failed to communicate effectively.

communicative competence The ability of speakers to adjust their messages to effectively influence their listeners.

Human communication requires a speaker, a context, and a listener. However, **communicative competence** occurs only when speakers effectively influence their listeners' behaviors. Most commonly, this occurs through using language—the forms, meanings, and functions—appropriate to the speaker's status, the situational context, and the listener's needs. Competent communication must satisfy two requirements: (a) the speaker's behavior must relate to the topic or situation, and (b) the speaker's behavior must have a practical effect on the listener's behavior. As effective communicators, our language behavior must be accepted and understood by our listeners and have the desired effect on their subsequent behavior. (This changed behavior may mean only that listeners indicate they understand our meaning, not necessarily that they must agree with it.)

While sitting at the dinner table at home, the utterance, *Is the salt on the table?* normally serves to obtain the desired seasoning for the speaker. However, in a formal business dinner situation, especially with a prospective employer, most adults recognize that a more formal request, *I wonder if you would, please, pass the salt?* might be more appropriate. Although both forms are grammatically correct, the competent communicator recognizes which form produces the most desirable results under specific circumstances.

With the younger child, not all the available forms of language are yet learned. Nor are all of the subtleties of word meanings or the expectations of social situations fully appreciated yet. This often leads to some humorous situations where children are involved, so much so that many television comedies and popular comic strips are based on the results.

The essence of communicative competence is truly effective communication that goes beyond the mere production of "correct" sentences. It includes the ability to modify the grammatical forms, underlying meanings, intentional force, and the delivery style best suited to the intended message. All of these components, as well as facial expressions, gestures, and tone of voice, must be properly managed to achieve the speaker's overall goal—to effect changes in the listener's behavior.

An **agenda** refers to the logical steps toward a desired goal. Although we are usually uncomfortable admitting it, virtually all human interactions have some underlying agenda. An agenda might be as innocent as a child's attempt to obtain a cookie or as profound as a politician's attempts to change the social and political atmosphere of a nation, perhaps to become president. Speakers (children or politicians) demonstrate communicative competence when each behavior (an utterance or a campaign speech) brings their audience's behavior closer to their goal. This occurs, for example, when the caregiver attends to the child, identifies the object of interest, and then provides the desired cookie. Similarly, the electorate must recognize candidates and understand their ideas but must also vote for them. In literate societies, communicative competence extends to reading and writing. Writers must be proficient in expressing their ideas in appropriate graphophonemic form to convey ideas and emotions in a way that is appropriate to the intended audience or readers. Readers must be able to read at several levels in order to read not only the words and sentences but also to understand the ideas and intentions of the writer.

Verbal and Nonverbal Communication

Human communication can be broken down into two broad levels, verbal and nonverbal. **Verbal communication** involves the use of words as symbols to exchange ideas. In addition, verbal communication is considered *linguistic* because it generally involves the use of language systems in arranging or ordering the words. In contrast, **nonverbal communication** does not rely on the use of words; rather it conveys ideas, thoughts, or feelings through other behaviors. Table 1–1 presents the aspects of nonverbal and verbal human communication.

 A most quotable quote that the student of language might want to master to win friends and influence people was provided by Hymes (1972). *Communicative competence* was described as the child's acquisition of knowledge as to "when to speak, when not, and as what to talk about with whom, when, where, in what manner" (p. 277).

agenda The speaker's overall goal, including the steps that proceed toward that goal.

Literacy is discussed in Chapters 5, 6, 7, and extensively in Chapter 9. ■

verbal communication The use of symbols (i.e., words), whether spoken, written, or gestured by a speaker to express ideas.

nonverbal communication Conveying attitudes or ideas through gesture, facial expression, proxemics, without the use of words, whether spoken, written, or gestured.

Table 1–1. Aspects of nonverbal and verbal human communication.

Nonverbal Communication

(when behaviors communicate *without* words)
• Facial expressions (e.g., smiles, grimaces)
• Head movements (e.g., shaking, nodding)
• Eye contact (e.g., averting, rolling)
• Body language (e.g., legs crossed, arms folded)
• Gestures (e.g., beckoning, stopping)
• Proxemics (e.g., up close, distant)

Verbal Communication

(when words communicate ideas *with or without* other behaviors)

Linguistic Aspects
(when words are transmitted via . . .)

Oral-Auditory
• Spoken language

Visual-Graphic
• Written language (e.g., graphemes)
• Gestural language (e.g., American Sign Language, Signing Exact English)
• Pictographic language (e.g., Blissymbols, Rebus symbols)

Extralinguistic Aspects

(when additional aspects influence meanings)
Paralinguistic Codes (also "suprasegmental features")
(when production features are *superimposed* to affect meaning)
• Spoken language (intonation, stress, rate, rhythm, prosody)
• Written language (size, bold, underlining, punctuation)
• Gestural language (speed, effort, dimensions of movements)
Nonlinguistic Cues
(when nonverbal behaviors provide cues to *clarify* meanings)
• Facial expressions
• Eye contact
• Body language
• Gestures
• Proxemics

The linguistic aspects of verbal communication are described later in this chapter. ■

Verbal communication can be further subdivided into *oral-auditory communication* (i.e., spoken language) and *visual-graphic communication* (written, gestural, and pictographic languages). There are some 3,000 different spoken languages in the world. Beyond the written forms of these languages, there are several distinct gestural or sign languages (e.g., American Sign Language, Signing Exact English) and pictographic languages (e.g., Blissymbolics, Rebus Symbols). Again, sign languages are verbal in the sense that they involve words; however, the words are produced gesturally rather than orally. Examples of American Sign Language, Blissymbolics, and Rebus symbols are presented in Figure 1–2.

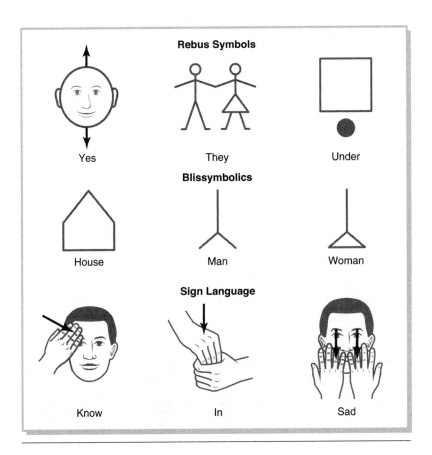

Figure 1–2. Examples of visual-graphic symbols from Rebus symbols, Blissymbolics, and American Sign Language.

Because the term *verbal* commonly refers to words or symbols in general, its meaning can become ambiguous. For example, anyone who has had experience with legal contracts knows that there is a significant difference between *oral* contracts and *written* contracts, even though both are *verbal*.

Similarly, the distinctions between oral, written, and even gestural communication should be recognized to accurately describe the form of verbal communication. For example, the distinction between oral and written communication is not necessarily clear from the term *verbal communication.* The gestural sign languages used by persons who are hearing impaired are also verbal. Hence, when discussing the modes of communication used by such individuals, professionals frequently distinguish between gestural (signed), oral (spoken), and "total" (both signed and spoken) communication.

In contrast to the more structured rule systems associated with verbal communication, nonverbal communication is much less formal or structured. Quite simply, *nonverbal communication* includes many behaviors that

Sign languages are complex, formally structured systems for communicating gesturally. These are discussed later. ∎

communicate without the associated production of words or symbols. A wink, a smile, a touch, maintaining or avoiding eye contact, even assuming a distinctive posture are all fairly universal nonverbal devices for communicating certain messages without the use of words.

Nonetheless, nonverbal communication naturally accompanies most verbal communication. Persons using sign language may use facial expression and produce gestures with greater or lesser force to supplement their verbal message. Writers, too, capitalize, underline, or italicize to do the same. And, of course, speakers use facial expression, gestures, and intonation to supplement the meaning of spoken words. When these nonverbal features accompany spoken language, they are referred to as the extralinguistic aspects of language.

Extralinguistic Aspects of Verbal Communication

Many people can be highly effective communicators through purely nonverbal means—gestures, facial expressions, body language. However, most of us are natural talkers. As we talk, we do more than simply produce strings of sounds and words. The extra nonverbal features that accompany our spoken words help to supplement or enhance the overall meaning of the entire utterance.

Linguistic aspects of communication include the production of words, phrases, and sentences according to the rules of grammar. In contrast, **extralinguistic aspects** are those nonverbal features that typically accompany the oral production of language and serve to modify, amplify, or fine-tune the actual meanings being expressed linguistically. These nonverbal features might convey attitudes, feelings, or roles that accompany the actual words of a message. They might even change the form or meaning of an utterance. In their most sophisticated application, they might even qualify or comment on the strength or adequacy of our utterances. Nonverbal extralinguistic aspects of communication include paralinguistic codes and nonlinguistic cues.

Paralinguistic Codes.   Meaning is conveyed not just by words themselves, but also by the manner in which they are produced. **Paralinguistic codes** are the melodic components of speech production that modify the meaning of the spoken message as it is produced. Paralinguistic codes include the stress, rhythm, and intonation used in producing an utterance. Although technically nonverbal, they are produced through the physical act of speech (i.e., we do not have to say actual words to produce them). The melody of speech produced by these combined factors is called **prosody**.

Because prosodic features are superimposed on utterance segments (words and phrases) as they are spoken, the term **suprasegmental devices** is also applied to them. Speakers might use these to signal their attitude or feelings regarding the message being conveyed to the listener. We all know about "the tone" with which somebody might say something. We have all heard the pleading tones of a small child in the toy store (*Puleeease, can I*

---

linguistic aspects The dimensions of grammar, semantics, and pragmatics relating to the structure, meaning, and use of language.

extralinguistic aspects The nonlinguistic elements of communication (gestures, intonation, etc.) that supplement or alter the message expressed by the words and phrases.

Linguistic aspects of communication are discussed later in this chapter. ▪

paralinguistic codes Production aspects such as prosody, intonation, rate, rhythm, and stress that accompany the spoken message to express attitude or emotion.

prosody Production features of speech, such as intonation, stress, rate, and rhythm, that provide its melodic character.

suprasegmental devices Speech production effects, including intonation, stress, and rhythm, superimposed across the linguistic segments (i.e., words and phrases) to modify their meaning.

have one?). Or the hurtful tone in a sarcastic remark, where the words say one thing, but the accompanying tone says the opposite (*Oh, your hair looks so good tonight!*).

Paralinguistic codes (or suprasegmental devices) can also modify the overall meaning of an utterance. For example, contrast the various messages conveyed by the following utterances depending on which segment is stressed (underlined) and whether the intonational contour rises (↑) or falls (↓):

Utterance	Interpretation
"Bill bought a car(↓)."	I assert that Bill did this.
"Bill bought a car(↑)."	I question that Bill did this.
"Bill bought(↑) a car."	Bill usually leases!
"Bill bought a car(↑)."	Bill usually buys trucks!

Nonlinguistic Cues.   When we speak to each other, we also communicate nonverbally through **nonlinguistic cues.** These are nonspeech behaviors that accompany the speaker's words and transmit certain cues through facial expressions, eye contact, gestures, body language, or proxemics.

Proxemics is the study of the use of proximity, closeness, or interpersonal space in communication. In other words, we can communicate subtle messages by getting closer to or farther from our listener. Four regions of proximity in communication have been identified: intimate, personal, social, and public. In most cultures, the amount of space speakers maintain between themselves and their listeners tends to be a function of how much emotional closeness is shared between them.

The combined effects of our nonlinguistic behaviors contribute to the overall message conveyed to our partner. Of course, when we smile, lean in close, and look into our listener's eyes, perhaps we send a message that our words are spoken out of a warm interest. In contrast, when we speak straight-faced, leaning back with arms folded, we send a quite different message.

Communication is a natural part of our everyday experience. It occurs in many subtle ways. We may be more aware of our verbal communication, as we hear the words that are spoken. However, we are frequently unaware of all the nonverbal elements that contribute to communication because they become so automatic.

nonlinguistic cues
Nonspeech behaviors that accompany the speaker's words and transmit certain cues through facial expressions, eye contact, gestures, body language, or proxemics.

proxemics   The study of personal space in social interactions, including interpersonal communication.

 Of course, the true significance of these nonlinguistic behaviors can vary from one culture to another. For example, although making eye contact in the mainstream American culture shows respect, doing so in Native American or Asian cultures demonstrates disrespect, especially in the case of children addressing adults.

Summary

- Communication is a behavior that makes humans social beings.
- Communication occurs when a sender transmits a message through symbols placed in a shared code that is understood by a receiver.

- Human communication relies primarily on words as symbols to represent objects, feelings, and ideas.

- Communicative competence requires that speakers apply the forms, meanings, and purposes of language in ways that are appropriate to circumstances.

- Humans use words as symbols that are spoken, written, or gestured through sign languages to communicate verbally.

- Extralinguistic aspects supplement words with nonverbal communication behaviors, such as intonation, gestures, and facial expressions.

speech   The dynamic production of speech sounds through the processes of respiration, phonation, resonation, and articulation for communication.

vocal tract   The cavities and structures above the vocal folds capable of modifying the vocal tone and airflow into distinctive speech sounds.

articulation   The modification of the vocal tone and airstream into distinctive sounds through movements of oral structures.

voice   The tone produced by vibration of the vocal folds and modified by the resonating cavities of the vocal tract.

phonation   The production of vocal tone in the physiological process of setting the approximated vocal folds into vibration with exhaled air.

resonation   The modification of the vocal tone produced through changing the shape and size of the spaces in the vocal tract.

The structures and production of speech are described in greater detail in Chapter 2. ▪

Speech

Humans use a variety of means for communication, including gestures, Morse code, and writing. However, the oldest and most prevalent means is speech. **Speech** is the physical production of sounds to communicate meaning through the neuromuscular control of the structures of the vocal tract. The **vocal tract** is composed of the larynx, pharynx, velum, tongue, teeth, lips, and the oral and nasal cavities. Speech can be separated into three basic components: articulation, voice, and fluency (or rhythm).

Articulation is the production of speech sounds through physical movement of the jaw, tongue, lips, and velum (soft palate) to change the size and shape of the vocal tract. The process of articulation produces the different sounds that we hear as the various vowels and consonants of speech.

Voice includes **phonation,** the production of sound through vibration of the vocal cords in the larynx (or "voice box"). This vocal tone is produced when air passes between the tensed vocal cords and causes them to vibrate. Phonation also carries the physical characteristics of *frequency* and *intensity.* When the voice is produced with a higher frequency of vibration in the vocal cords, listeners hear a higher *pitch,* as is typical of the female voice. When the puffs of air released in each cycle of vibration are emitted with greater intensity, listeners hear this as increased *loudness,* as when we raise our volume or shout.

The voice we hear in speech also results from **resonation,** the process of modifying the vocal tone as it passes through the vocal tract (the pharynx, oral cavity, and nasal cavity). The cavities of the vocal tract give the otherwise buzzlike vocal tone a fullness, in much the same way the resonant body of an acoustic guitar softens and mellows the vibrations of its wire-like strings.

In addition, depending on the position of the velum (or soft palate), the voice may carry a *nasal* or *nonnasal* resonance. Nasal sounds are those that also resonate in the nasal cavity (e.g., m, n, ng) because the velum is lowered; a raised velum seals off the nasal cavity during production of all nonnasal sounds (e.g., b, g, a, o).

Finally, **fluency** incorporates the *rhythm rate,* and *flow* of speech as it is produced. Rate and flow are reflected in the number of syllables we produce per second and the frequency and duration of pauses during speech. As we produce the strings of sounds for words and sentences, we must coordinate the movements for articulation and phonation. If we do so efficiently, the transitions from syllable to syllable or from word to word occur smoothly. A listener would hear the smooth flow and normal rate of speech as fluent. If instead we hesitate, repeat, and stop too frequently, the listener might consider our speech to be nonfluent.

fluency The flow of speech that is free of abnormal interruptions or disfluencies.

Speech as a Mode of Communication

As was noted previously, speech represents one of several modes for human communication. Most speakers communicate orally. Speakers can superimpose the prosodic features that contribute to extralinguistic communication. However, because most people communicate through speech, it is too easily equated with language. Of course, there are other means of communicating without producing speech sounds. For example, most of us can write, many can use sign language, and a few can even use Morse code.

Conversely, it is possible to produce speech sounds without necessarily communicating anything. Sounds produced in isolation (e.g., a prolonged /ffff/) or in nonsensical combinations (e.g., /abimi/) do not convey anything meaningful. In short, we can produce speech sounds without producing language, just as it is possible to transmit the symbols of language in ways that do not involve speech (i.e., through writing or sign language).

Ask your friends to define *speech* and you will probably hear as many different definitions as you have friends. Although they engage in speaking regularly (and, for some, excessively), your friends may only vaguely understand its nature and complexity. The *American Heritage Dictionary* (1970) defines *speech* as "the faculty or act, of expressing or describing thoughts, feelings, or perceptions by the articulation of words." Although this may serve well as a general definition, for our purposes it oversimplifies much of the process and it will be important to better understand its subtleties and complexities.

Speech as Dynamic Human Behavior

Speech is the dynamic production of sounds in the human vocal tract for verbal communication. The production of speech sounds requires precise and complex control over the *anatomical structures* of the vocal tract—the lungs, larynx, pharynx, velum, tongue, and lips. Speakers exert sophisticated neuromuscular control over these structures, rapidly and continuously changing their actions, shape, and position. Such changes modify the *aerodynamic airflow, sound sources,* and the *acoustic resonance* and produce the differences we hear as distinct speech sounds.

A more detailed discussion of the structures of the vocal tract and their role in producing the aerodynamic and acoustic aspects of speech is provided in Chapter 2. ■

Briefly, we use exhaled air as we speak. After inhaling, we bring our vocal folds together, so that the exhaled air escapes between them. This air pushes the folds back apart, then their tension brings them together again. As this cycle occurs repeatedly, they are set into vibration, creating a vocal tone. We modify this tone and the airstream by moving our jaw, lips, tongue, and soft palate. Their posturing constricts the airway, creating small apertures or openings that generate various noises—bursts and hisses—when the airflow is stopped and released or forced through these small openings. These movements are smoothly coordinated and combined into sequences of various sounds. One can barely imagine the speed and precision involved when we consider that we produce about 14 phonemes per second!

It is possible, of course, to produce a vast array of sounds through the human vocal tract—from the sublime (à la Luciano Pavarotti) to the silly (à la the "Bronx cheer"). Of all these possibilities, however, each language has adapted a limited set of sounds to be combined in forming the words of that language. For example, American English is said to involve the production of approximately 46 different speech sounds, depending on the geographic region. These sounds are produced by speakers in various combinations to produce at least 50,000 different American English words.

However, as each language has evolved, certain regularities and restrictions in these combinations occurred as well. For example, not all sounds occur in all word positions; in English, no words begin with the sound that we hear at the end of *long,* although it occurs frequently in medial and final word positions, as in *singing.*

Speech as a System of Sounds: Phonology

The hundreds of languages used by humans are produced through the production of approximately 20 to 60 different speech sounds. Although it is an oversimplification, the speech sounds used in human languages are commonly subdivided into vowels and consonants. As you were probably taught in elementary school, vowels are *open sounds*—those produced with a vocal tone resonating through a relatively open oral cavity. In contrast, consonants are *closed sounds,* produced through varying degrees of constriction or closure somewhere along the vocal tract. Consonants may or may not involve a vocal tone and are therefore referred to as *voiced* or *voiceless.* Nonetheless, the primary acoustic nature of consonants will involve some noise source.

phonology   The study of the speech sounds of languages.

Phonology is the study of the sound systems of language. In studying the individual sounds of different languages, linguists and speech scientists found that the traditional written (orthographic) letters of most languages posed a problem. There is not always a one-to-one correspondence between a symbol and a sound. For example, anyone who has watched a child learn to read American English recalls the confusion that occurs with the various ways that the *s*-sound is spelled—as in *sand, cent, scent,* and *psychology.*

To resolve this difficulty, the International Phonetic Association developed the **International Phonetic Alphabet** (IPA). The IPA represents all of the identified individual sounds of all the recognized human languages. The IPA provides a designated symbol to universally represent each speech sound, regardless of the languages in which it occurs. Some sounds occur in numerous languages whereas other sounds are restricted to very few. In using the IPA symbols, then, it is possible to transcribe the actual sounds heard into universal written symbols, regardless of the language used. The individual symbols and their sounds are presented in Table 1–2.

International Phonetic Alphabet An alphabet designed to provide universal symbols to represent all the known speech sounds used in human languages.

phone An individual instance of a speech sound production notated within brackets (i.e., [ ]).

phoneme A conceptual family of sounds whose acoustic features are similar enough to be heard as the same speech sound; notated within slashes (i.e., / /).

Phones and Phonemes. In studying the basic sound elements of language, linguists and speech scientists have classified them at two different levels, as phones and phonemes. A **phone** represents an individual production of a speech sound in a word. As discussed later, **phonemes** are groups or families of sounds that are related by their acoustic similarities.

Table 1–2. The International Phonetic Alphabet (IPA).

IPA Symbol	Examples	IPA Symbol	Examples
/p/	pat	/ʃ/	shoe
/b/	bat	/ʒ/	measure
/m/	mat	/θ/	thumb
/n/	not	/ð/	these
/ŋ/	ring	/tʃ/	chop
/d/	dog	/dʒ/	jump
/t/	tie	/v/	vent
/g/	game	/w/	water
/k/	coat	/l/	lawn
/f/	find	/j/	yes
/s/	sent	/h/	hot
/z/	zip	/r/	red
/ɑ/	ball	/ɛ/	get
/æ/	cat	/e/	take
/ɔ/	bought	/o/	over
/ə/	about	/ʊ/	book
/ʌ/	upstairs	/u/	boot
/ɪ/	insect	/ɜ^/	turtle
/i/	eat	/ɚ/	other
/eɪ/	main		
/aɪ/	dime		
/oʊ/	home		
/aʊ/	cow		
/ɔɪ/	toy		
/ɪʊ/	use		

In the IPA, phones are indicated by enclosing the appropriate symbol in brackets ([ ]). Individual productions of a speech sound vary naturally in some subtle respects. Similar to individuals' fingerprints, at some level no two phones are exactly alike, even those produced by the same speaker. If we were to analyze the acoustic patterns from the same speaker's productions of the *k*-sound "under the microscope," as through acoustic spectrograms, we would likely find that almost no two were identical in the timing and distribution of their sound energy. Figure 1–3 provides an example of a spectrogram illustrating the pattern of energy in the speech signal.

In transcribing phones, linguists use *narrow transcription*. This consists of using the IPA phonetic symbols plus various other markings (diacritics) to preserve any acoustic features that might distinguish each sound production from others. For example, the speakers of American English will tend to produce some sounds differently according to the surrounding sounds. Although these differences can be detected by the well-trained ear of a linguist, we might wonder, are they really significant to the rest of us? Not in most cases.

As an illustration, in American English the /k/ produced at the end of the word *back* can be released (where contact is made, air pressure is accumulated and released abruptly), as it might be in the phrase *I have a pain in my back*. Or, it can be unreleased (contact is made, but the tongue loses contact less abruptly, reducing the usual burst of air pressure), as it might be in *I have a back pain*. In either case, the *meaning* of the word *back* would be unchanged for the listener. Other similar variations can be observed with most speakers and many sounds, no matter which language is involved.

Speakers in all languages tend to hear certain sound productions all as versions of the same sound. **Categorical perception,** as this is called, means

categorical perception
The observation that listeners hear classes of similar sounds within a continuous range of sounds.

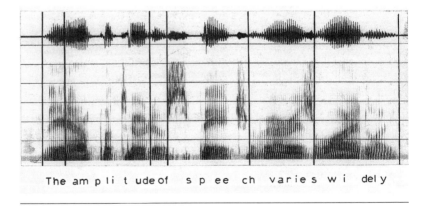

The am p li t ude of   s p ee ch   va ri e s   w i   del y

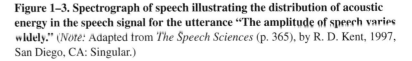

Figure 1–3. Spectrograph of speech illustrating the distribution of acoustic energy in the speech signal for the utterance "The amplitude of speech varies widely." (*Note:* Adapted from *The Speech Sciences* (p. 365), by R. D. Kent, 1997, San Diego, CA: Singular.)

that the listener tends to group variable productions of a sound together because the subtle acoustic differences are apparently insignificant. This forgiving nature of our perceptual apparatus is probably fortunate, as few of us could achieve a level of precision where every *k-*, *s-*, or *t*-sound we produce is identical to all their counterparts.

Those phones that exhibit subtle differences, but are heard as belonging to the same sound category, are called **allophones.** Taken together, the entire collection of all the individual sound productions (phones) that listeners would hear as members of the same category would be called a *phoneme.* A phoneme represents an abstract family of sounds which are all related by their similar acoustic features. Phonemes are transcribed with *broad transcription,* which uses the IPA symbols enclosed in slashes (e.g., /k/), but does not include the additional markings associated with phones. Each phoneme category disregards all the subtle, insignificant variations of the individual occurrences (the phones) that compose it.

allophones The individual sound variations that are still heard as a class of sounds.

What makes phonemes significant then? It is the fact that phonemes reflect the speakers' ability to change the words and meanings they communicate to their listeners. The significance of phonemes is demonstrated when a change in a feature of a sound changes the word that is understood by the listener. Although the variations in the /k/ in the word *back* discussed previously make no difference to the listener, a change from /k/ (with no voicing) to /g/ (with voicing) would make a difference in meaning by changing the word from *back* to *bag.*

In American English, sounds like /k/ and /g/ are phonemes because voicing is one feature that distinguishes between phonemes and, therefore, contrasts words and meanings for the listener. For example, when it is chilly, most of us ask for a *coat* rather than a *goat.* Linguists have described the features that help speakers produce these distinctions. Features or characteristics that help distinguish one phoneme from another are called **distinctive features.**

distinctive features The individual acoustic or articulatory characteristics that distinguish one class of phonemes from another.

In applying distinctive features, phonemes are notated in a binary system in which the presence or absence of a feature is indicated through pluses and minuses. Table 1–3 presents the distinctive features of English consonants described by Chomsky and Halle (1968). Each phoneme is essentially a bundle of features and can be analyzed into the features that distinguish it from other phonemes. Those phonemes that are more similar in their production will differ by fewer distinctive features (e.g., /s/ and /z/); phonemes that are more different are contrasted by more distinctive features (e.g., /m/ and /k/).

Summary

- Speech is the dynamic production of sounds for oral communication.
- The basic components of speech production are articulation, voice, and fluency.

Table 1–3. Distinctive features of English consonants.

	w	f	v	θ	ɚ	t	d	s	z	n	l	ʃ	ʒ	j	r	tʃ	dʒ	k	g	ŋ	h	p	b	m
Voiced	+	−	+	−	+	−	+	−	+	+	+	−	+	+	+	−	+	−	+	+	−	−	+	+
Consonantal	−	+	+	+	+	+	+	+	+	+	+	+	+	−	+	+	+	+	+	+	−	+	+	+
Anterior	+	+	+	+	+	+	+	+	+	+	+	−	−	−	−	−	−	−	−	−	−	+	+	+
Coronal	−	−	−	+	+	+	+	+	+	+	+	+	+	−	+	+	+	−	−	−	−	−	−	−
Continuant	+	+	+	+	+	−	−	+	+	−	+	+	+	+	+	−	−	−	−	−	+	−	−	−
High	−	−	−	−	−	−	−	−	−	−	−	+	+	+	−	+	+	+	+	+	−	−	−	−
Low	−	−	−	−	−	−	−	−	−	−	−	−	−	−	−	−	−	−	−	−	+	−	−	−
Back	+	−	−	−	−	−	−	−	−	−	−	−	−	−	−	−	−	+	+	+	−	−	−	−
Nasal	−	−	−	−	−	−	−	−	−	+	−	−	−	−	−	−	−	−	−	+	−	−	−	+
Strident	−	+	+	−	−	−	−	+	+	−	−	+	+	−	−	+	+	−	−	−	−	−	−	−
Vocalic	−	−	−	−	+	−	−	−	−	−	+	−	−	−	+	−	−	−	−	−	−	−	−	−

Note. Adapted from *The Sound Pattern of English* by N. Chomsky and M. Halle, 1968, New York: Harper & Row.

- Prosody produced in speech contributes to the extralinguistic aspect of communication.

- The vocal tract includes the structures used to produce speech—the larynx, pharynx, velum, tongue, teeth, lips, and the oral and nasal cavities.

- Phonology is the study of speech sounds.

- Speech sounds can be analyzed as individual sound productions, called phones, or as groups of similar sounds, called phonemes.

- Phonemes distinguish the meanings of words and have been classified by their unique characteristics, called distinctive features.

Language

Language is the system of arbitrary verbal symbols that speakers put in order according to a conventional code to communicate ideas and feelings or to influence the behavior of others. In communicating our ideas, the mode or manner of expression can vary from speaking to writing to gesturing. However, no matter how the message is expressed, it is the symbols of language that carry the substance of the message. Other species may naturally communicate through distinctive sounds or actions. However, these behaviors serve as signals meaning one thing, perhaps the location of food, imminent changes in weather, or the presence of a predator. These signals are thought to be primarily instinctive and lack the creativity that has developed in human language behavior.

language The system of arbitrary verbal symbols arranged in a conventional code that evolved as a social tool to communicate ideas and influence the behavior of others.

Human language, which characterizes our humanness, occurs in a variety of contexts. For those who appreciate Shakespeare, it is one medium in the arts. For those intrigued with the cultural development of humankind, it is the tracings of ancient times. For those who must communicate precise legal, scientific, or technical information, it is a fine tool to be wielded with expertise. And, for those who pass along accumulated knowledge to young children, it serves as a paintbrush for the mind. However, in the present context, language is seen as a natural phenomenon of human behavior.

Some Important Distinctions

Several aspects of speech and language can be easily confused. The ways in which we experience speech and language as speakers can cause these two phenomena to naturally overlap. In communicating from moment to moment on a daily basis, speech and language occur as seemingly automatic behaviors, in which case, we are not always conscious of their roles. Furthermore, language itself is a phenomenon that is complex and multifaceted.

It is important, therefore, to be clear about several issues that can be sources of confusion. The difference between speech and language must be appreciated. The distinction between languages and their variations, called dialects, can be vague in some cases. Finally, throughout our discussion of language, it will be important to distinguish between the notion of receptive and expressive modalities for language.

Language versus Speech.   Human communication might rely on speech as its primary medium for transmitting information. However, the nature of human communication requires that language, in some form, is involved. In short, it is possible to produce isolated speech sounds without using language. And, it is possible to transmit language apart from producing speech. The most obvious example is through writing. Some less conspicuous examples include the various forms of sign language utilized by people who are hearing impaired or the visual symbol systems incorporated in communication boards for persons who are physically handicapped.

Language versus Dialect.   Most people have at some time been aware of obvious differences in the way people talk. If the differences go beyond a specific individual's peculiarities (idiosyncratic variations) and instead are consistent within a group of speakers, those differences may constitute a dialect. A **dialect** represents a distinct variation of a major language that is spoken by an identifiable subgroup of those people using that language. Dialects might be associated with different geographical regions, socioeconomic levels, cultural differences, or ethnic subgroups. Most of the languages of the world evidence dialectal variations of the primary language. The variations might be phonological, lexical, or grammatical.

dialect   A collection of consistent or systematic variations in a major language that occur in an identifiable subgroup.

The phonological variations involve the production of individual sound segments (phonemes or syllables) in ways that differ across various groups. For example, people in the upper Midwest (e.g., Minnesota) would tell us that they sign their name with a *pen,* whereas persons in the south central plains (e.g., Oklahoma) might sound as though they would use a *pin.*

Dialectal differences can also be reflected in the lexicon or vocabulary. Due to a variety of cultural forces, some words come to mean different things in different regions of the same country. Persons from the Midwest who order a *soda* in New York City might be disappointed to find that they are served a simple glass of *pop*—no ice cream, no whipped cream, and no cherry!

Finally, people using the same major language might differ in their use of grammatical structures as well. For example, people from the upper Midwest are often guilty of dangling prepositions (*I'm going downtown. Would you like to go with?*). People from most other parts of the United States would expect this question to be punctuated with an object of the preposition (*Would you like to go with me?*) Yet the shortened form apparently sounds quite natural to the local natives of the upper Midwest. (They forget that their English teachers told them that a preposition is something you never end a sentence with.) In contrast, people in the Southwest who are standing on the street corner waiting to catch the next bus might describe their situation with the phrase, *I'm waiting on the bus.* To others this might sound as though they think they are already aboard the bus and biding their time.

Noting that someone has an accent can be either a sensitive subject or an intriguing topic for conversation. Some social situations make people self-conscious about the unfair, negative stereotypes that might be associated with these variations. However, in a culturally diverse society, such variations should be valued. They represent the variety of backgrounds and experiences that have contributed to the overall culture.

It has been suggested that with our increasingly mobile society and the proliferation of electronic media that now interconnects the various regions of the United States—radios, televisions, telephones—we will gradually sound more and more alike. Should the variety of speaking styles associated with different regions be lost and we were to all speak alike, it would certainly dull the tapestry of the American culture.

Expressive versus Receptive Language.   As we consider the major aspects of communication, it is important to distinguish between the two major modalities in which it occurs. These modalities stem from the fact that according to communication theory, there is always a sender and a receiver. As has been noted, the sender encodes the message and the listener decodes the message. This relationship is often described linguistically with the terms *expressive language* and *receptive language.* Another set of synonymous terms that correlate with these would be *production* and *comprehension.* Use of these terms referring to the processes utilized by speakers and listeners might be generally correlated in the following manner:

Speakers	*Listeners*
Encoding	Decoding
Expression	Reception
Production	Comprehension

The outgoing—incoming nature of this relationship may seem quite simple at first glance—speakers speak, listeners listen. However, the variables involved in carrying out the two tasks are quite different, especially for the young language learner. In speaking, we hypothetically formulate an idea, select the words, and produce them to convey the intended information. In contrast, in understanding, the listener must comprehend the meaning of the speaker's words. In other words, the listener must identify what caused the speaker to produce them—an inner feeling, a novel object, or notable circumstances. Listeners usually have a variety of situational clues that assist in comprehending the message.

For the young child, the familiarity of events that occur frequently (*routines*) provides predictability for the words and phrases that will be spoken in those situations. The speaker's facial expressions, gestures, and visual gaze may assist in identifying the topic of utterances. And, even the redundancy of the language itself can help the child comprehend the overall meaning of the words and phrases. For example, a mother visiting the zoo with her child might say, *Oh, look at the cuddly cubs! See the baby lions?* Where the child might have been unfamiliar with the word *cubs,* by overlapping the redundant phrase, *baby lions,* she provided her child with additional clues to interpret the potentially unfamiliar word.

The role of routines in mother-child interaction are discussed in Chapter 5. ■

Defining Language

The behavioral, linguistic, cognitive, and social interaction theories of language are discussed in greater detail in Chapter 4. ■

The modern English word *language* has derived over the centuries from the Latin word *lingua,* for "tongue." Students already exposed to coursework on speech and hearing anatomy recognize this stem word in a host of terms related to the tongue. The association of language with the tongue has an obvious and long history. In ancient times it was thought that words literally originated from the tongue (among various other less related organs). This notion is still expressed in phrases such as *speaking the native tongue, giving a tongue-lashing,* or *speaking street lingo.*

Currently, *language* can be defined from several different perspectives. The essential features of language vary according to each expert's discipline or focus. Some have focused on language as a social behavior, viewing it as a tool of sorts. Others have viewed language as one of the many behaviors learned by humans, conceiving of it as a complex ability related to our advanced intelligence. Finally, some have emphasized the structure of language, viewing it primarily as a system of mental rules.

Language as a Social Tool.   Sociolinguists (Austin, 1962; Searle, 1969) have stressed the role of language as a social tool in human interaction. They have emphasized that language does not exist separately from social interaction. According to this view, the fundamental aspects of language consist of the reasons we speak (our intentions), the situations in which we speak (the contexts), and the different ways in which we speak depending on the circumstances (the alternations).

Language as a Learned Behavior.   While also recognizing that language is a social tool, behaviorists (e.g., Skinner, 1957) have emphasized that it is a learned behavior. In this view, language is verbal behavior that is learned through social consequence. In other words, we talk because it influences the behavior of others in useful ways. The ways in which others respond to our verbal behavior provide the consequences that affect how and when we talk in the future.

Language as a System of Mental Rules.   Still others, notably psycholinguists (Berko Gleason, 2001; Bloom & Lahey, 1978; Chomsky, 1957; Hockett, 1960, among others), have emphasized the linguistic perspective, defining language as a system of mental rules. According to psycholinguists, language represents the underlying mental rules (grammar) for arranging symbols (words) to represent ideas about the world.

Linguistics: The Study of Language

A number of professionals have at least a partial interest in the study of language. Psychologists study language because a large portion of our intelligence, memory, and personality appears to be verbal in nature. Behaviorists are interested because verbal behavior comprises such a major and significant part of human behavior. Speech-language pathologists examine language because it is so vital to the communication needs of the individuals with various disabilities. Finally, linguists focus entirely on the structure of language.

Linguistics emerged as a field during the 1700s and 1800s, apparently when European scholars were exposed to Sanskrit, the language of ancient India brought back by British merchants. Having noted grammatical similarities in the Sanskrit, Greek, and Latin languages, these scholars began searching for the "mother language" that had theoretically preceded all other languages. As the field of linguistics has evolved, a number of specialized branches have appeared:

1. **Comparative linguistics** studies the variations in language that occur from one location to another.

2. **Historical linguistics** studies the differences and similarities across languages from different periods of time.

3. **Descriptive linguistics** attempts to describe the structure of individual languages.

4. **Psycholinguistics** attempts to theorize the underlying mental operations used in formulating and processing language.

5. **Sociolinguistics** attempts to describe language variations based on social and cultural variables.

6. **Developmental linguistics** attempts to describe the nature of emerging language in children's language acquisition.

As complex as language is, it is not surprising that so many specialties have evolved. Each area assumes its own unique perspective on language and researches the particular questions pertinent to that view.

Summary

- Language is an essential aspect of human social interaction and transmission of information.
- Language is the use of symbols in a shared code to convey meaning.
- Dialects are variations of a language that develop in cultural, socioeconomic, or geographic subgroups.
- Receptive and expressive language involve different processes and factors.
- Language can be defined as a social behavior, as a complex learned behavior, or as a system of mental rules.
- Linguistics, the scientific study of language, has a number of branches that study several aspects of language.

The Linguistic Aspects of Language

Linguists identify different structural components of language. The components of language occur simultaneously through the continuous stream of sounds and symbols produced as we speak. The scientific approach to studying language behavior has resulted in its artificial dissection into separate components, similar to the analysis of speech described previously.

The major linguistic aspects of language are traditionally identified as grammar (its structure), semantics (its meaning), and pragmatics (its social use). These same components have been referred to as form, content, and use, respectively (Bloom & Lahey, 1978). Table 1–4 presents the traditional and contemporary terms for the aspects of language.

Bloom and Lahey (1978) applied the term *form* to describe the structural aspects of phonology, syntax, and morphology. ▪

grammar The collection of rules that characterize the regularities or patterns of a language.

The Grammatical Aspect of Language

Grammar basically deals with the speaker's ordering of words and word parts in constructing sentences. In its most basic sense, **grammar** refers to the conventional rules for arranging the symbols of language in sequences that convey the intended meaning. According to Dever (1978), "grammar represents the patterns of behavior that occur over and over" (p. 11).

Grammar represents the regularities in our verbal behavior that have come to be considered a language. The sequences of symbols might include combinations of both "whole" words and the "parts" of words—the suffixes and prefixes of a language. As such, grammar is comprised of morphologic and syntactic elements.

Phonology was discussed previously and is frequently the focus of a separate phonetics course. The primary focus of the present discussion concentrates on grammar. ▪

Table 1–4. Linguistic aspects of language—traditional and contemporary terms.

Contemporary				Traditional
Form	- - - - -	(the structural composition of language)	- - - - -	Phonology • Phones • Phonemes Grammar • Morphology • Syntax
Content	- - - - - -	(the meanings carried by language)	- - - - - -	Semantics • Word meanings • Word relations
Use	- - - - - - -	(the purposes served by language)	- - - - - - -	Pragmatics • Functions • Alternations

The Morphologic Aspect of Grammar

Morphology is the study of minimal, meaningful units of language. Morphology deals with the form or structure of words—"whole words" and "word parts." More specifically, the minimal, meaningful units of language are **morphemes.** These are the smallest elements of language that still carry meaning. Morphemes can be composed of a single phoneme, as in the personal pronoun *I*, or a series of phonemes, as in the noun *encyclopedia*. Morphemes are considered minimal because they cannot be subdivided any further without losing their original meaning or becoming meaningless altogether.

For example, the word *chair* cannot be broken down into smaller elements without violating its original meaning. If we divide it into the elements of *ch* and *air,* we find that neither of these convey any aspect of the original meaning. The resulting isolated sound, *ch,* is meaningless. Although the remaining element, *air,* results in another recognizable word, it is unrelated to our original word. Therefore, *chair* is considered a minimal, meaningful unit of language—a morpheme.

Of course, if the situation includes more than one chair, English speakers would add the plural *-s* to the stem word to produce *chairs.* Therefore, in this context the word *chairs* can be subdivided into two smaller meaningful units—one that symbolizes the referent (the thing we sit on) and one that signals plurality (that there is more than one such referent in the situation described by the speaker).

It would be quite understandable if at first the boundaries of a morpheme seem a little elusive. Is a morpheme identical to a phoneme? Not really. Are morphemes equivalent to words? Not necessarily. Is a morpheme the same as a syllable? Not quite. So what *are* the boundaries of these minimal, meaningful units?

morphology The study of morphemes.

morpheme The minimal, meaningful units of language.

Hockett (1960) provided a comprehensive description of the 13 design features of language. Hockett described the amazing paradox of the human language—that across all the human languages a limited number of individually meaningless sounds are combined, although not in all ways, to produce hundreds of thousands of words. The meanings of these words are arbitrarily assigned and agreed upon within each language. And, further, these words are ordered by rules to express an array of ideas limited only by our human experience and creativity.

1. **A morpheme is at least one phoneme, but not all phonemes are morphemes.** For example: "I" = 1 phoneme and 1 morpheme; "w" = 1 phoneme, but not a morpheme. (The personal pronoun *I* certainly carries meaning, but the isolated sound /w/ has no significant meaning.)

2. **A morpheme is at least one syllable, but not all syllables are morphemes.** For example: "this" = 1 syllable and 1 morpheme; "catching" = 2 syllables, 2 morphemes; "envelope" = 3 syllables, 1 morpheme. (In spite of the three syllables in *envelope,* it is not capable of being subdivided, whereas *catching* includes a stem verb, *catch,* and the ending, *-ing,* which signals that the action is ongoing.)

3. **A word is at least one morpheme, but not all morphemes are words.** For example: "ball" = 1 word, 1 morpheme; "opening" = 1 word, 2 morphemes; "-ing" = 0 words, 1 morpheme. (If we understand

that the word ending -*ing* signals an ongoing action when attached to a stem word, it represents a morpheme but does not constitute a word all by itself.)

Free Morphemes.   As the preceding analysis of the word *chairs* might suggest, the morpheme "family tree" has two major branches. One aspect of morphology deals with "whole words" and the other aspect deals with "word parts." The two major types of corresponding morphemes are called free morphemes and bound morphemes. **Free morphemes** are units that can stand alone, independent of other units, and still carry meaning. Some free morphemes occur individually as words (*throw, bright, rhinoceros*) or in combination as parts of compound words (*waterfall, baseball, chairperson*). Some free morphemes essentially represent words and are therefore referred to as *lexical morphemes.* Traditionally, lexical morphemes have also been referred to as *content words.* The number of lexical morphemes or content words grows with the increase in available referents that can be expressed in a language—the available vocabulary. For example, 50 years ago the word *transistor* did not exist and no one had yet meaningfully combined the prefix *micro-* and the word *chip.*

Another subgroup of free morphemes would include those referred to as *grammatical morphemes.* These would include structures such as, *a, an, the, and, but, if, is, are, was, were,* and so forth. These are fewer in number and traditionally have also been referred to as *function* or *functor words.*

Bound Morphemes.   Bound morphemes comprise the other side of the morphological family tree. **Bound morphemes** are those morphemes that must be attached to other (free) morphemes to carry meaning. These are analogous to the word parts that have been traditionally called affixes, prefixes, suffixes, and grammatical markers. Although each type (e.g., *un-, non-, -ly, -s, -ed*) can potentially be attached to any number of free morphemes, the variety of purposes they serve within a language are limited. Bound morphemes are therefore fewer in number in contrast to the free morphemes or stem words.

Bound morphemes occur in two different types, derivational and inflectional. Table 1–5 presents the classifications of morphemes with examples. **Derivational morphemes** are defined as morphemes that serve primarily to change the grammatical class of the free morpheme to which they are attached. These are bound morphemes that *derive* a new grammatical category out of the stem word. For example, adding -*ly* to the noun *ghost* derives an adjective, *ghostly.* (As in, *The thought that a ghost might be there made the house seem ghostly.*) Of course, in addition to this example, various forms of derivational morphemes perform different operations: when -*ly* is added to an adjective (*quick*), it derives an adverb (*quickly*); adding -*ion* to a verb (*calculate*), derives a noun (*calculation*), adding -*er* to a verb (*teach*) results in a noun (*teacher*).

---

free morphemes
Morphemes that can occur independently and still carry meaning.

bound morpheme   A subclass of morphemes that are meaningless unless attached to a free morpheme; includes **derivational** and **inflectional morphemes.**

derivational morpheme
A type of bound morpheme that changes the grammatical class of the free morpheme to which it is attached (e.g., teach*er*).

Table 1–5. Classifications and examples of morphemes.

Free Morphemes		Bound Morphemes	
Lexical	**Grammatical**	**Derivational**	**Inflectional**
car	is	quick_ly_	hat_s_
boot	the	act_ion_	John'_s_
run	should	help_ful_	burn_ed_
green	and	teach_er_	play_ing_

Some derivational morphemes do not meet our definition's criterion for changing the grammatical class when they are attached to a stem word. (As anyone familiar with the English language already knows, "exceptions to the rule" sometimes seem to be the rule, not the exception!) Several prefixes such as *un-, in-, non-, dis-, a-,* and *anti-* generally negate or invert the meaning of the words to which they are attached (e.g., common vs. *un*common, correct vs. *in*correct, conformist vs. *non*conformist, order vs. *dis*order, symmetrical vs. *a*symmetrical, and communist vs. *anti*communist).

Of course, if we carry our exceptions one degree further, it illustrates that it is important to analyze each form for its end result. For example, the prefix *in-* might sometimes signal a negative connotation—we do not like to be *in*correct. However, in another context it can have quite another effect—we do like to be *in*valuable. The bottom line: Language cannot be analyzed simply by looking at the appearance of its various forms; instead these must be examined according to their effects on the meaning in the overall context.

The other major class of morphemes is inflectional morphemes. **Inflectional morphemes** are those morphemes that alter the meaning of the free morpheme to which they are attached without deriving a new grammatical category. As illustrated in Table 1–5, these occur primarily as suffixes—word endings—which inflect or modulate the stem word for plurality, possession, degree, or tense. For example, after adding the plural inflection *-s* to the noun *cat* (as in *The two cats played with each other*), *cats* is still a noun although it now carries the notion of plurality. Of course, other examples of inflectional morphemes that we are all familiar with include the *-'s* inflection for possession (*The cat's tail is furry*); the comparative (*-er*) and superlative (*-est*) inflections for degree (*My grass is green; your grass is greener; and his grass is the greenest*); and the progressive (*-ing*) and past tense (*-ed*) verb inflections (*I am painting and Bill painted yesterday*).

As we will see in later chapters, the inflectional morphemes generally appear earlier in children's language than do derivational morphemes. This would appear to be because the inflectional morphemes play the role of "fine-tuning" the more basic meanings being expressed in children's earliest simple sentences (Brown, 1973). For young children, finally adding the plural inflection *-s* to the stem word *cookie* can be a significant achievement if it actually leads to the intended result. Later, as children's

inflectional morpheme
A type of bound morpheme that inflects the word it is attached to for tense (play*ed*), plurality (cat*s*), possession (John'*s*), and degree (green*er*).

grasp of grammar is solidified and they begin to expand their vocabulary, the derivational morphemes play a more consequential role.

The Syntactic Aspect of Grammar

Morphology describes the form of words and word parts (free and bound morphemes). Words represent the individual objects, ideas, and relationships we experience. However, as speakers we must combine these words to express complex ideas or relationships in sentences.

> **syntax**   The linguistic rules that describe the relationship between word orders and the meanings they express.

Syntax describes the way in which we arrange words like "building blocks" to construct sentences that express our ideas. Syntax is that part of grammar which specifies rules for sequencing or ordering words to form phrases and sentences. Essentially, syntax deals with the rules for word order in a language. It is the order of words that conveys the relationships among the words. Syntax helps us distinguish between the newsworthiness of the newspaper headlines, "Dog Bites Man" and "Man Bites Dog."

> **declarative**   A major sentence type that makes a statement.
>
> **interrogative**   A major sentence type that asks a question.
>
> **negative**   A major sentence type that expresses denial, rejection, or nonexistence.
>
> **passive sentence**   A major sentence type in which the grammatical subject of the sentence is the passive recipient of the action in the verb.
>
> **imperative**   A major sentence type that expresses a command while omitting the sentence subject.

Sentence Types.   Most will recall the traditional sentence types they learned in English class during "grammar school." A **declarative** makes an affirmative statement (*The man is closing the window.*). An **interrogative** forms a question (*Is the man closing the window?*). A **negative** contradicts an assertion (*The man is not closing the window.*). A **passive** form indicates that the subject of the sentence is being acted on (*The window is being closed by the man.*). And an **imperative,** by omitting the subject of the sentence, imparts a commanding tone (*Close the window!*). At first glance, these examples might suggest an oversimplification of syntax—that syntax simply deals with rearranging the left-to-right order of words. Reverse *The man* and *is* and a question is formed. Insert *not* and a declarative becomes a negative. Although these observations may seem so, in truth they oversimplify the nature of syntax. Syntax involves more than the left-to-right word order. For example, compare the roles played by the word *painting* in the following sentences:

The man was painting a beautiful scene.

The man admired the beautiful painting.

The word *painting* plays the role of a verb (an action) in the first sentence, but the role of a noun (a thing) in the second sentence. Obviously, more is involved in this altered relationship than simply moving the word farther to the right. Similarly, depending on the context, the same word in precisely the same position may play two different roles. Contrast the possible underlying meanings associated with the word *ancient* in *She is an ancient history professor.* Is this a comment on her specialization or her age? Of course, the true meaning depends on the actual context. Her particular interest or her age would determine which is the correct underlying meaning.

Constituent Structures. Sentences are constructed from various elements—words, phrases, clauses. These are the **constituent structures** of a sentence. The syntax of a sentence defines the underlying roles played by the constituent structures in the sentence. From our previous example, a constituent structure might consist of a word serving as a noun (*man*), which serves as part of a noun phrase (*the man*) which furthermore might serve as the subject phrase of the overall sentence.

constituent structures
The morphemes, words, and phrases that contribute to an overall sentence structure.

Hierarchical Structure. The relationships between the constituents (words and phrases) of sentences are organized in a **hierarchical structure.** This means that the words and phrases are each related to structures at higher and lower levels. This hierarchy describes the underlying relationship within the sentence.

The hierarchical structure of sentences can be illustrated through a *sentence tree.* By referring to Figure 1–4, it is possible to see that the two phrases, *the man* and *the door,* are similar constituent structures (noun phrases), but they each relate to the verb phrase in quite different ways.

hierarchical structure
The levels of constituent structures that relate the words and phrases of a sentence to its underlying structure.

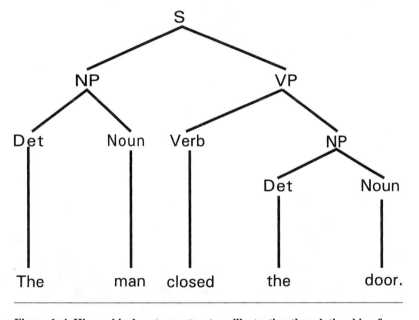

Figure 1–4. Hierarchical sentence structure illustrating the relationship of surface structures (words and phrases) to underlying levels of constituent structures. (S = Sentence, NP = Noun Phrase, VP = Verb Phrase, Det = Determiner.)

Types of Grammar

The term "grammar" has been applied by linguists in a number of ways to describe various aspects of language. Understanding these different types of grammar, with their subtle and sometime overlapping meanings, can be helpful in gaining a full appreciation for the study of language behavior.

Prescriptive versus Descriptive Grammar. This distinction might be illustrated by the contrast between "telling you how to talk" versus "describing how you talk." **Prescriptive grammar** is a set of rules that specifies how a language *should* be spoken. It refers to the notion that there is one correct way of speaking a language. This suggests that it is possible to set forth a "King's English," that is, the rules that speakers of a language must follow to be considered proper speakers of the language. The fallacy in this is obvious when we consider our own idiosyncrasies in expressing ourselves, our occasional grammatical slips, and the numerous dialects within most languages.

In contrast, the term **descriptive grammar** refers to the linguistic process of identifying and describing the regularities that occur naturally in a language. If one imagines that the man in the tongue-in-cheek scenario that opened this chapter is a linguist, his strategy in learning to communicate with his hosts would involve developing a descriptive grammar. He would do so by contrasting the utterances he hears against the situations in which they occur to identify the meaningful language patterns that reoccur predictably. As subsequent instances demonstrate the same regularities, it would become possible to reliably describe how words are arranged to produce meaningful phrases and sentences. As a linguist, he would then describe the rules that capture these observations.

Some self-appointed "guardians of the grammar," who believe that a static and rigid system of rules is desirable, forget that a language is a living, changing system. Where a prescriptive grammar prescribes what is traditionally correct, a descriptive grammar attempts to capture the current language patterns that have resulted from the social and cultural forces that influence a language.

Intuitive versus Formal Grammar. The distinction between intuitive and formal grammars might be most easily thought of as the difference between the grammar in our heads and the grammar linguists put down on paper. **Intuitive grammar** refers to the underlying knowledge speakers demonstrate by using and understanding their native language. When confronted with correct and incorrect sentences in their language, most speakers can almost instantly identify which are grammatical and which are not. Although our intuitive grammar enables us to do this almost instinctively, we may still be unable to express the specific rules that pertain to the instances that are ungrammatical.

prescriptive grammar
A collection of rules that purports to dictate correct grammatical structures to the speakers of a language.

descriptive grammar
A set of linguistic rules that describes the regularities present in a set of utterances.

intuitive grammar
Speakers' implicit, underlying knowledge of the acceptable patterns and regularities in their language.

In contrast, a **formal grammar** is the written summary of the hypothetical rules that describe the regularities in a language. Our shipwrecked friend would illustrate this process by observing, formulating, and recording the linguistic patterns (the rules) that most reliably describe the utterances that he observes in use by his hosts.

Performance versus Competence. These concepts have evolved in modern linguistics. They have been proposed to explain the observation that otherwise competent speakers of a language do occasionally produce deficient utterances. **Linguistic competence** represents speakers' idealized, underlying knowledge of their language. It refers to our hypothetical, unconscious linguistic ability. In contrast, **linguistic performance,** the actualized production of linguistic units by a speaker, refers to the reality that this idealized knowledge must be applied in actually producing language. Linguistic performance, however, will be influenced by a variety of real limitations, such as memory lapses, fatigue, illness, and distractions.

There is a paradox in the relationship between these two concepts. The linguist can only infer the nature of our underlying linguistic competence from observing our linguistic performance. It is the only available evidence. Whether spoken or written, our random slips in performance would seem to indicate a less than perfect understanding of the rules of the language. However, our slips are relatively rare and we generally recognize and correct our errors. The linguist interprets this to support the notion that our underlying knowledge is more perfect than our application of that knowledge. Nonetheless, the only evidence of our linguistic competence is our sometimes deficient performance.

Generative Grammar. This concept is central to any modern linguistic theory of language behavior. A **generative grammar** is one that is comprised of a *limited* number of rules capable of generating an *unlimited* number of acceptable sentences in a language. It is analogous to a collection of algebraic equations that have the potential to produce an infinite variety of answers as different values are plugged in for each variable.

In recognizing our own limitations, such a concept has merit. Consider the seemingly boundless variety of sentences speakers produce and understand throughout their lifetimes. Although we hesitate to admit it, our intelligence and memory capacities are limited and apparently insufficient for storing and recalling this myriad of different utterances. Given this discrepancy, linguists have proposed that our flexibility and creativity in comprehension and expression would be more economically accounted for by a generative grammar. Conceptually, then, the underlying grammar for a language merely provides all of the patterns (i.e., morpheme sequences) acceptable for expressing the possible meanings. We apply the required lexicon (vocabulary) to these patterns as we generate a seemingly endless variety of appropriate utterances.

formal grammar The collective set of written rules that describe the conventional regularities in a language.

linguistic competence Speakers' underlying, idealized knowledge of their language system.

linguistic performance Speakers' actualized production of sentences, potentially affected by memory, fatigue, and distraction.

generative grammar A grammar composed of a limited number of rules capable of generating an unlimited number of acceptable sentences in a language.

▨ Summary

- Grammar describes the structure of words and their ordering by speakers to convey meaning.

- Morphology, the study of one component of grammar, deals with the structure of morphemes, the minimal, meaningful units of language.

- Free morphemes, or words, can stand alone and still carry meaning, whereas bound morphemes, word parts, must be attached to words to be meaningful.

- Bound morphemes can derive new words by changing the grammatical class of their stem word or inflect their original meanings for plurality, tense, and so on.

- Syntax, the other component of grammar, describes the structure of sentence types such as declaratives and questions.

- The words and phrases of sentences are the constituent structures.

- The underlying hierarchical relationships among sentence constituents are illustrated in tree diagrams.

- There are various types of grammar, including prescriptive, descriptive, intuitive, formal, and generative grammars.

> To describe the area of semantics, Bloom and Lahey (1978) applied the term *content,* referring to the meanings "contained" in words and relationships between words. ▪

> **semantics**   The study of meaning in language.

The Semantic Aspect of Language

Most are probably familiar with the word *semantics.* We have all heard people say, "Exactly how are you using that word?" or "It's a matter of semantics," when there is a misunderstanding or disagreement. Such difficulties frequently arise from subtle differences in individuals' meanings for various words.

In linguistics, **semantics** is the study of meaning. Therefore, the semantic aspect of language refers to the meaning in language. Linguists view words as vessels or "containers" carrying collections of meanings and associations. These meanings may or may not combine with those carried by other words. Linguists study two dimensions of meaning in semantics, word meanings and word relations.

Word Meanings in Semantics

The first dimension of semantics is word meaning. We use words to organize our perceptions of the world. Words help us associate, categorize, and analyze our experiences. Children label the most unique, individual referents in their experience—their parents, caregivers, and siblings—with very specific words—their names. However, as children's horizons expand, they are confronted with an array of experiences and entities. These could be stored randomly as a heap of individual, unrelated events. Or, they could be stored according to some organizing scheme that helps children more efficiently recall and understand their experiences. It appears that humans have recognized that words provide a far more efficient way to store, recall, and communicate our experience of the world. For example, rather than devising a different word for every tall, leafy plant, it is far more economical in effort and memory to gather their collective features into the word *tree*.

The collection of words learned by individuals is referred to as their **vocabulary.** A related term, **lexicon,** refers to all morphemes, including words and word parts, that a speaker knows. Within a culture, word meanings change as new meanings are ascribed to old words. As noted previously, the word *chip* has evolved to a prominent status. From referring to the lowly by-product of sawmills to popular snack foods, it now refers to the powerful and valuable brain in our computers.

As a result, even as speakers are learning new words, the individual word meanings themselves may be evolving. As the meaning for a word evolves, culturally or personally, it has been characterized as a changing set of semantic features. **Semantic features** consist of the perceptual and conceptual characteristics that define the meaning contained by a word. Stated conversely, a word is a collection or bundle of semantic features. Put simply, a word is a collection of multiple associated meanings.

Furthermore, the contrasts in individual features across words reflects their different meanings. For example, the overall meaning of the word *dog* combines multiple features. It would be marked with at least the following semantic features: +*animate,* −*human,* and +*domesticated* (where + indicates the presence of a feature and − indicates absence). In comparison, the word *wolf* would be marked similarly, except for the −*domesticated* feature, which contrasts the meanings of the two words. Finally, the word *rock* would be marked −*animate,* thereby eliminating the other two features for consideration.

If the development of word meaning can be characterized as collecting and refining the relevant semantic features, it follows that this occurs as a result of successive experiences with the referent for that word. Individuals' memory of their successive experiences with the referent for a word comprises their **episodic memory** for that word. Their episodic memory is the "experiential diary" of all the episodes or experiences related to that word's meaning.

Eventually, as their overall vocabulary grows, their **semantic memory,** the collection of related words and concepts they associate with the word, also develops. By recalling other associated words and concepts their understanding of words is expanded. For example, initially children's episodic memory defines the word *doctor* strictly in terms of their individual experiences with their doctor. They know only that face and voice as representing *doctor.* As they learn related words (*sick, hospital, nurse,* and, of course, *shot!*) their understanding of the word *doctor* can also draw on the information associated with these words.

vocabulary A speaker's total accumulation of words understood or used in the language.

lexicon The total collection of words and morphemes in a language.

semantic features The perceptual features such as size, shape, color, and so on, that define a conceptual class.

episodic memory The cumulative set of experiences that make up an individual's understanding of a concept or event.

semantic memory An individual's understanding of a word's meaning, including the words and concepts they associate with that word.

Word Relations in Semantics

The second dimension of semantics is word relations. That is, how the meanings of words interact with each other. The considerations related to word relations occur at two different levels.

In the first level, we can consider the ways in which words relate to each other depending on the semantic features that make up their meanings. Selection restrictions describe why the meanings of two words are either capable or incapable of being meaningfully combined. For example, the word *rock* would not carry the +*animate* feature. Therefore, it would not usually be combined with a word that carries the +*animate* feature, such as *pet*. Normally, then, we would not expect to hear the phrase *pet rock*. However, unexpected semantic contradictions such as this are often the essence of humor (and the source of great profit, as those willing to date themselves will remember!).

Words' meanings based on their semantic features can relate to each other in other ways. Words that share the same features but are opposite in one feature are **antonyms.** Some word pairs can be *binary antonyms,* representing polar extremes that have no middle ground (e.g., live vs. dead; you cannot be "kind of dead") or they can be *gradable antonyms,* representing different gradations or points on a continuum (e.g., cool vs. warm).

Synonyms are different words that carry similar meanings (e.g., *large* and *big*), apparently because they share almost the same set of features. Note that synonyms have similar, but not identical, meanings. Each member of the pair carries a slightly different sense of the same core meaning. This becomes especially obvious in certain contexts; compare the different consequences when someone refers to "my old friend" versus "my longtime friend."

Another related way in which words overlap is referred to as **hyponymy.** Hyponyms are words that contain specific subsets of a word known as a *superordinate.* For example, the word *couch* is a hyponym of the superordinate *furniture.*

The second level of word relations involves the additional roles assumed by words through being combined with other words in a sentence. In particular, the notion of **semantic relations** describes the role each noun in a sentence has in relation to the verb in the sentence. For example, in relation to the word *hit*, *Daddy* assumes two different semantic relations in the sentences *Daddy hit the ball* as compared to *The ball hit Daddy.* In the first version *Daddy* assumes the semantic case of *agent* or *actor* (one who instigates an action), whereas in the second version *Daddy* assumes the semantic case of *dative* (an animate affected by the verb). Finally, in *I'm looking for Daddy's ball,* Daddy assumes the role of *possessor.*

The concept of semantic relations presents an intriguing illustration of how language reflects the relationships perceived and understood by speakers. By simply producing words in relation to each other we convey how we see the referents for those words relating to each other. For example, when youngsters play little league baseball, sometimes the bat hits the ball, but al-

selection restrictions Constraints on the words that can occur together because of the semantic features carried by each.

antonyms Two words whose meanings contrast due to opposite values in a single semantic feature, as in *hot* and *cold*.

synonym A word that shares the majority of its semantic features with another word having similar meaning.

hyponymy The semantic relationship in which the meaning of one word, the hyponym (e.g., *chair*), contains the meaning of another word, the superordinate (e.g., *furniture*).

semantic (or case) relations The relationships between objects, persons, and events expressed through language.

most as often the ball hits the bat. How such major events are described (i.e., the semantic relationships indicated) in the cheering that follows may depend on whether you are the youngster's caregiver.

▨ Summary

- Semantics is the study of word meanings and word relationships in language.

- The meanings of words consist of the semantic features they carry.

- The collection of all morphemes (words and morphemes) learned by speakers is their vocabulary or lexicon.

- Words relate to each other differently based on their semantic features, which might restrict whether some words can occur together.

- Words also take on different meanings as they represent different semantic roles in sentences.

The Pragmatic Aspect of Language

The pragmatic aspect of language refers to the practical use of language in social interaction. **Pragmatics** is the study of language use. The quality of *being pragmatic* may be familiar from hearing people describe themselves as "down to earth, practical, and pragmatic." Accordingly, this refers to the practical use of language for getting things done. The pragmatic aspect of language can be considered from at least three major perspectives: (1) the functions language serves in communicating speakers' intentions; (2) the alternation in language forms observed in different social contexts; and (3) the organization of language in conversational discourse.

> **pragmatics** The practical aspects of language used as a social tool, including the functions and alternations observed in social contexts.

Perhaps of the three linguistic aspects—grammar, semantics, and pragmatics—the pragmatic aspect comes closest to the heart of communication. It analyzes speakers' use of language to achieve their intended goals. Sociolinguists studying the pragmatic aspects of language de-emphasize individual words and syntactic structures. Instead, they focus on the speaker's achievement of a practical outcome through using language as a tool.

> ▨ Because in one sense sociolinguists view language as a "tool," Bloom and Lahey (1978) use the term *use* to refer to pragmatics. ▪

Functions in Pragmatics

Language serves a purpose in most any social context. Paradoxically, even the speaker who attempts to directly contradict this observation by producing a statement that is seemingly irrelevant and without purpose does so to serve the purpose of disproving this observation and thereby confirms it. Even talking to ourselves normally serves some purpose such as reassurance, reasoning, or rehearsal.

In the usual communicative context, **functions** consist of those purposes or intentions that are achieved by speakers through the use of language. The

> **functions** The pragmatic or practical purposes served by utterances.

performatives A speech act in which the utterance itself performs the intended act, such as promising, teasing, and apologizing.

speech act The concept of a unit of communication involving a speaker's intention, the linguistic form of the message conveying the intention, and the listener's interpretation of the message.

alternation The variations in linguistic structure and speaking style in response to the roles and audience in a setting.

social context The nature of a setting and the status, roles, and agendas of the speakers in that setting.

linguistic context The utterances that precede and contribute to the setting responded to by a speaker.

direct speech act A speech act in which the intention is expressed directly in the grammatical form of the utterance.

concept of language functions was introduced by Austin (1962) in his discussion of **performatives** in which the verb in certain utterances actually constitutes an act. Consider the practical impact of such utterances as, *I now pronounce you man and wife.* This idea was developed further by Searle (1969) as the concept of **speech acts,** in which all utterances are conceived as performing some act.

Linguists (Dore, 1975) have attempted to catalog the variety of speech acts performed by language, to include such practical functions as requesting, labeling, answering, repeating, and practicing. Of course, the premise that underlies any notion of pragmatics is that the meaning of any utterance is validated by its observable effects on the listener. That is, if the listener's actions fulfill the speaker's goals, the intended function of the utterance can be determined.

Alternations in Pragmatics

Speakers can achieve their goals in different ways, choosing from alternative ways of expressing the same intention. Using different words or sentence forms to achieve the same result is referred to as **alternation** (Ervin-Tripp & Mitchell-Kernan, 1977). Alternation is generally based on situational factors, such as the social and linguistic context. Linguistic context, that is, what has been said and in what way, may cause a speaker to produce one alternative form instead of another. These factors may result in the use of forms that are more or less direct, or include or omit certain information.

The same goals may be desired in different situations, yet the role of the speaker or the status of the listener may be different due to the **social context.** Social context refers to how formal or informal the situation is and the roles assumed by the individual speakers. Speakers use alternative forms based on their evaluation of listener characteristics (age, social status, racial-ethnic background, familiarity, etc.) and the degree of formality required in the situation. For example, if we feel a chilly draft due to an open window, we will use different forms to ask someone else to close the window, depending on whether we are at home with a roommate or in the office of a prospective employer.

Another factor affecting the use of different or varied forms is **linguistic context.** The information and utterances that have preceded an utterance can affect what is required in the speaker's subsequent utterance. For example, having just seen her child's lunch box on the kitchen counter and on hearing her child's question, *Where's my lunch?,* the mother's utterance *On the kitchen counter* is sufficient. However, without her child's preceding question, *on the kitchen counter* would sound quite strange; instead, additional linguistic structures would be required to convey the same information, as in *Your lunch is on the kitchen counter.*

Speech acts can be carried out through direct and indirect means, as well as in literal or nonliteral ways (Searle, 1975). A **direct speech act** achieves its end through an utterance that has only one interpretation, whereas an **indirect speech act** implies that there are several possible interpretations. For example, at the dinner table one can obtain the salt by a direct request, *Please, pass the salt.* Alternatively, requesting the salt might be softened by using indirect phrasing such as, *Is the salt on the table?* In this indirect request, the utterance can represent two potential speech acts—the explicit request to verify the presence of salt on the table or the implicit request to obtain the salt. In fact, Parker and Riley (2004) suggest that a practical test to determine the presence of an indirect speech act is to comply with the direct syntactic interpretation of the utterance. If the action seems inappropriate to the social context, then the utterance is likely to be an indirect speech act.

indirect speech act A speech act in which the speaker's intention is implied rather than expressed.

Discourse in Pragmatics

Discourse refers to an extended verbal exchange on some topic, essentially a conversation. Conversations demonstrate an organizational structure that is based on such elements as topic initiation, turn taking, topic maintenance, and repairs. Additionally, appropriate conversations adhere to standards that have been referred to as the cooperation principle (Grice, 1975).

discourse A series of verbal interchanges between speakers on a shared topic.

The cooperation principle states that in conversations each participant must: (1) include an appropriate *quantity* of information that is (2) of adequate *quality* or truthfulness and is (3) *relevant* to the established topic and (4) delivered in a *manner* that is clear and understandable. In other words, effective conversation must meet several criteria. Providing too much or too little information runs the risk of overwhelming our listeners or leaving them puzzled. The information we convey should be accurate and it should be of interest to our listeners. Finally, we should produce the information in a way that they will understand what we are communicating. We all have known some speakers who failed to adhere to these principles and, in all honesty, have probably violated them from time to time ourselves.

The elements of discourse are discussed further in Chapters 6, 7, and 9. ◼

▨ Summary

- Pragmatics is the study of the use of language as a social tool.
- Functions are the individual purposes intended by our utterances as we speak to others.
- That others frequently act on the information and requests expressed through language is the concept of speech acts.
- The social nature of language is reflected in alternation, in which speakers choose alternate ways of saying the same thing based on the situation.
- Discourse or conversation has characteristic structure including turn taking, topic maintenance, and repairs.

Chapter Summary

This chapter introduced the major components of human communication. These include the basic aspects of *communication,* our human capacity for *speech,* and the nature of *language.* These elements are intertwined as we interact verbally to influence others' behavior. In doing so successfully, we demonstrate *communicative competence,* the ability to effectively communicate using appropriate forms and meanings in various situations in both spoken and written communication. We primarily rely on *verbal communication,* using words to communicate. However, when speaking we also supplement our words with nonverbal communication by using such things as intonation, gestures, and facial expression to convey additional meanings. Communicating through writing does not allow such behaviors; the words and structures must be chosen carefully to communicate proficiently.

Speech is defined as an oral mode of communicating through the physical production of sounds. Speech includes voice, articulation, and fluency. The field of *phonology* studies the speech sounds used in language, analyzing individual sound productions, called *phones,* and groups of productions heard as similar sounds, called *phonemes.*

Language can be defined as a *social behavior,* a *learned behavior,* or a system of *mental rules* in which the symbols (words) of language are used to communicate ideas and feelings. The linguistic components of language include grammar, semantics, and pragmatics. *Grammar* is the hypothetical rule system that describes word and sentence structure and consists of morphology and syntax. *Morphology* focuses on the structure of words and word parts. The rules for ordering words to construct phrases and sentences are described by *syntax.* Linguists also study *semantics,* the meanings carried by words and how word meanings relate to each other. Finally, the social basis of language has focused attention on the *functions* or social uses of language and the *alternations,* how speakers can achieve the same goal with different utterances. In addition, *discourse* or conversation occurs when these social transactions take place between partners, taking the form of extended verbal exchanges that are organized according to certain patterns.

An underlying principle that should integrate all of the information presented in this chapter and those that follow is that humans are social creatures. Human communication is probably the best evidence of that. We communicate our needs and usually have them met by those around us. We do so through various modes—speech, gestures, writing—applied according to the conventions of language. And, although we might dismantle language into grammar, semantics, and pragmatics for the sake of analysis, the fact remains they are naturally integrated for one purpose—communication.

1. What are the three main elements in the communication process?

2. Name two synonyms each for the terms *encoding* and *decoding*.

3. What are the "considerations" a speaker must make to exhibit communicative competence?

4. What is the difference between "nonlinguistic cues" and "nonverbal communication"? How are they alike?

5. What are the similarities and differences in the ways sociolinguists, behaviorists, and linguists define *language*?

6. What are the six different branches of linguistics and what aspects of language do they study?

7. Which term in the definition of morphemes (minimal, meaningful units of language) most clearly distinguishes them from phonemes?

8. How do the major linguistic elements of language (grammar, semantics, pragmatics) relate to the concept of communicative competence?

Review Questions

To the student: You are encouraged to use the following questions to prepare for multiple-choice examinations. This exercise is not intended to simply "provide the answers to questions." Instead, it is hoped that you will use the material to develop your ability to analyze questions and choices to identify correct answers based on a critical understanding of the distinctions among the answers. Use the answer key at the end of the book to prompt your analysis of each item and to confirm the correct answer. Remember that there is a difference between recognizing the correct answer and understanding why it is the correct one.

Practice Questions

1. The rhythm, rate, and flow of speech is referred to as _____.
   a. vocal quality
   b. phonology
   c. syntax
   d. semantics
   e. fluency

2. The study of the hypothetical underlying mental operations involved in understanding and producing sentences is called _____.
   a. paralinguistics
   b. psycholinguistics
   c. nonlinguistics
   d. sociolinguistics
   e. metalinguistics

3. Which of the following is a key term that is essential to the definition of "language" (in contrast to "speech")?
   a. neuromuscular
   b. dynamic
   c. sounds
   d. symbolic
   e. resonance

4. When someone lowers his head, raises an eyebrow, and squints to indicate skepticism or doubt while talking to you, which of the following is he using?
   a. sign language
   b. gestural language
   c. nonlinguistic cues
   d. nonverbal communication
   e. suprasegmental devices

5. Sometimes, as you listen to a speaker, you react to sentences that "just don't sound quite right," but you cannot explain why. This reflects your implicit, idealized knowledge of your language or your _____.
   a. linguistic competence
   b. prescriptive grammar
   c. descriptive grammar
   d. linguistic performance
   e. intelligence

6. After being told to go to bed, a toddler responds with "No!" whereas an 8-year-old responds with "Can I wait till after I finish my homework?" These responses differ primarily in their _____.
   a. communicative intention
   b. semantic relationship
   c. pragmatic function
   d. grammatical structure
   e. dialectal influence

7. When asked to "define" what a teacher is, you recall various events and feelings you associate with your most and least favorite instructors. All your personal experiences that have been associated with the word "teacher" would represent your _____.

a. "linguistic competence" for that word
b. "metalinguistic ability" for that word
c. "episodic memory" for that word
d. "generative grammar" for that word
e. "semantic memory" for that word

8. That certain words logically "fit" together (e.g., "mommy dog") or, conversely, that other words do not "go" together (e.g., "mommy brick") in meaningful ways is described by the term _____.
   a. distinctive features
   b. semantic relations
   c. morphology
   d. selection restrictions
   e. prosodic features

9. Semantics is the study of how language units acquire meaning and most closely corresponds to the contemporary term _____.
   a. form
   b. content
   c. proxemics
   d. pragmatics
   e. none of these

10. The difference between your interpretations of the hypothetical newspaper headline "Cat chases mouse!!!" and "Mouse chases cat!!!" would primarily involve a distinction based on which aspect of language?
    a. use
    b. pragmatics
    c. syntax
    d. morphology
    e. phonology

Berninger, V. W. (2000). Development of language by hand and its connection with language by ear, mouth, and eye. *Topics in Language Disorders, 20*(4), 65–84.

Kelly, S. D., Iverson, J. M., Terranove, J., Niego, J., Hopkins, M., & Goldsmith, L. (2002). Putting language back in the body: Speech and gesture on three time frames. *Developmental Neuropsychology, 22*(1), 323–340.

Parker, F., & Riley, K. (2004). *Linguistics for non-linguists: A primer with exercises* (4th ed.). Boston: Allyn & Bacon.

Savage-Rumbaugh, S., Shanker, S. G., & Taylor, T. J. (1998). *Ape language and the human mind.* New York: Oxford University Press.

Suggested Readings

CHAPTER 2

The Structural Bases of Human Communication

Dr. and Mrs. Watson were thrilled! The excitement of this first addition to their family was beyond their wildest anticipation. Dr. Watson drove carefully as Mrs. Watson nestled herself close to this new little package of joy. She watched two shiny eyes peer out from inside the blankets. As they drove home, the proud parents silently imagined how their daughter would soon change, rapidly and dramatically. How soon would she know their faces? How soon would she know her name and understand what they were telling her? What fascinating sounds will she make as she wakes each morning? When would they hear that precious first word? And would it be "mama" or "dada"?

Later, as Mrs. Watson put things away, Dr. Watson held his new daughter tenderly, examining her tiny fingers. Could anything compare with this miracle? Perhaps the rapid development she will soon exhibit will be equally amazing. How will these next miracles unfold? Does his child start as a "blank slate," needing to learn everything she will ever do? Or does she bring some special tools to help her make her way through all the noise and confusion around her?

This chapter addresses the following questions:

- What are the basic structures of the human nervous system?
- Which major aspects of the nervous system relate primarily to our capacity for communication?
- Which anatomical structures support speech?
- Which anatomical structures provide hearing?

- How do these neurological and anatomical structures develop and mature?
- How do these developing structures give us our initial capacity for experiencing the world around us?

Probably since the time we became capable of reflecting on our own behavior, we have marveled at the miracle of human communication. At the heart of this curiosity has been the question "How much of this ability is present when we are born?" Are we the "blank slate" that the curious father pondered in the opening scenario? Perhaps we already possess all the abilities and knowledge needed and they must only "blossom" to make mature communication possible. Or do we inherit the basic tools necessary to refine our interaction with the world around us?

In the opening scenario to this chapter, the perceptive reader may have recognized the veiled reference to Dr. John B. Watson, an early 20th century psychologist. Watson was the father of "behaviorism," the extreme view that all learning comes from experience. This is the "nurture" side of the age-old nature-nurture controversy. In contrast, Descartes represented the opposite view, "nativism," or the "nature" side of this controversy. Nativists held that all knowledge and behavior was innate, or present, at birth. The modern viewpoint has struck a more balanced perspective. Our genetic history has provided certain capabilities, and our abilities develop from them as we interact with our environment.

Anyone who has had the most basic psychology course will recall the proverbial "nature versus nurture" controversy. This chapter does not attempt to settle this age-old controversy. Nor does it attempt to replace other basic texts covering anatomy of speech and hearing or child development. Instead, this chapter provides an introduction to the anatomical structures that are most significantly related to the development of human communication. They are described in very basic detail in their mature state, followed by a discussion of important aspects of their prenatal development.

Neurological Bases of Human Communication

As we consider all the tools children will use as they develop, the nervous system is vital. The developing child feels, tastes, smells, sees, and hears the surrounding world. These experiences must be sensed, collected, transmitted, analyzed, classified, and stored. In turn, the child responds by reaching, grasping, gesturing, vocalizing, and, eventually, talking.

The earliest of these actions are more reflexive and only later do they become intentional. The simplest, automatic behaviors are gradually assembled into collections of purposeful, skillful movements. We still have very little understanding of *how* this amazing learning takes place. However, we do know that an intact nervous system is necessary for normal learning. Therefore, we shall begin with a brief anatomical description of the nervous system.

The human nervous system is divided into two major systems—the central nervous system and the peripheral nervous system. The **central nervous system**—the brain and spinal cord—is viewed as the center of the human nervous system. The brain, in particular, is the central processor for incoming sensory information, mental reasoning, and outgoing motor commands. The peripheral nervous system carries these messages to and from the body. The **peripheral nervous system** extends from the brain and spinal cord outward to the body. Although there are topographical and functional differences, the two systems complement each other in carrying out the myriad of complex and fascinating behaviors we exhibit—walking, running, talking, singing, writing, and even thinking about our world and ourselves.

central nervous system The portion of the nervous system composed of the brain and spinal cord.

peripheral nervous system That part of the nervous system that conducts sensory and motor impulses between the body and the CNS.

Central Nervous System

The central nervous system (CNS) is a complex structure composed of billions of different cells. Some of these cells make up identifiable structures, such as the covering of the brain or the bodies of cell masses. Cells in certain regions perform different tasks, such as processing sensory information, generating motor commands, or simply nourishing and supporting other nerve cells.

The nervous system is said to have four major functions: (a) sensory; (b) motor; (c) integration; and (d) regulation. The sensory system helps collect sensations from the outside world and from within our bodies. The motor system generates the movement. Several systems integrate or make sense of incoming information and feedback about our movements. Finally, several systems automatically regulate our temperature, metabolism, respiration, heart rate, and other body systems.

Students should become accustomed to recognizing acronyms, such as *CNS* for central nervous system. They are used frequently for the obvious reason of economy. ▪

The Brain: An Overview

The brain, positioned at the top of the spinal cord, is the largest, most recognizable component of the entire nervous system. Of course, these two structures—the brain and spinal cord—together comprise the CNS. Figure 2–1 presents the major structures of the CNS.

The brain has three major divisions—the cerebrum, cerebellum, and brain stem. The brain is composed of a mass of **neurons,** or nerve cells, and their fibers, which are nourished by the surrounding **glial cells.** Because there are approximately 10 billion neurons and five times as many glial cells, the brain has considerable demands for life support. It requires about one fifth of the blood pumped by the heart and consumes approximately one fourth of all the oxygen used in the human body.

The billions of individual neurons make the brain a powerful processor. Individually, the neuron seems to be the picture of simplicity. Figure 2–2 illustrates the structure of a neuron. It is composed of a cell body, called the

A synonym for brain is *encephalon.* A derivative of this appears in the word *encephalitis,* which is an inflammation (-*itis*) of the brain. ▪

neuron Basic unit of the nervous system consisting of a cell body, an axon, and dendrites.

glial cells Cells that support and nourish other nerve cells in the central nervous system.

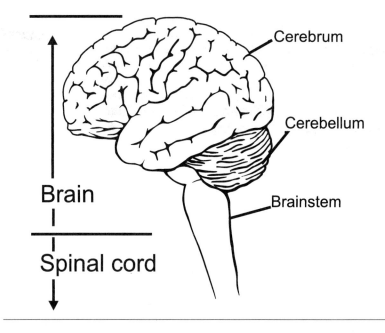

Figure 2–1. The central nervous system.

nucleus   Central element in a cell body.

axon   The single longer filament of a neuron that carries the neural impulse away from the cell body.

dendrites   Branched nerve fibers that conduct impulses toward the cell body of a neuron.

synapse   The junction or gap where neural impulses jump from the axon of one neuron to the dendrite of another.

cerebrum   The larger, most visible portion of the brain consisting of two hemispheres.

nucleus, which generates an electrochemical spark when the neuron is stimulated. The single long fiber that projects from the cell body, the **axon,** carries these neural impulses away from the cell body. The more numerous, shorter projections are called **dendrites.** Dendrites collect impulses generated in surrounding cell bodies and conduct these toward the nucleus.

The neural impulse that is generated by the cell nucleus travels the length of the axon at lightning speed. However, at the end of the axon it must jump to another cell. This juncture is called the **synapse.** Synapses pass impulses along to other dendrites and neurons, muscle fibers, or glands.

Although their electrochemical activity is microscopic, the billions of neurons in an individual's brain have a notable impact when they act together. Their interconnected activity accounts for the simplest and most complex of our abilities.

Cerebrum

The largest part of the brain is the **cerebrum.** However, it is not simply its size that makes it so exceptional. Instead, it is the intricate array of complex neural interconnections that allows the billions of brain cells to perform so efficiently. The cerebrum is responsible for our higher level abilities, including our reasoning, memory, voluntary movement, speech, language, and so forth.

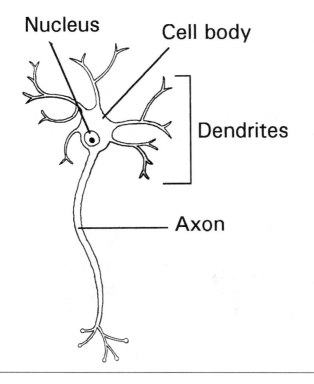

Figure 2–2. Illustration of a neuron, including the nucleus, cell body, dendrites, and axon.

The covering of the cerebrum, known as the **cortex** (from the word for "tree bark"), is composed of six layers containing billions of cells. The cortex rises and falls in convoluted folds. This greatly expands the brain's surface area and, therefore, the number of nerve cells that can be compacted into the restricted space in the cranium. The folds in the cortex create ridges and valleys. A ridge is called a **gyrus,** a valley is a **sulcus,** and a very deep sulcus is called a **fissure.** Because there are so many folds the brain has numerous *gyri* and *sulci* (plural forms). These features provide important landmarks to help us find our way around the brain's surface.

The cerebrum is made up of two major divisions: the cerebral hemispheres and the basal ganglia. These appear to have evolved from the brain structures also present in other lower species. The newer cerebral hemispheres are related to higher level, voluntary functions, whereas the older basal ganglia are responsible for integrating automatic adjustments into movements.

Cerebral Hemispheres. The cerebrum is divided into two seemingly identical halves, called **cerebral hemispheres.** Both the right and left hemispheres are further subdivided by several major fissures into regions called

cortex Outer convoluted layers of dense neurons covering the cerebral hemispheres; responsible for high mental functions.

gyrus (pl., **gyri**) The ridges or convolutions on the cortical surface of the brain.

sulcus (pl., **sulci**) The narrower, more shallow grooves that occur on the convoluted cortical surface of the brain.

fissure A deep furrow or valley in the convoluted surface of the cortex.

cerebral hemispheres The two halves of the cerebrum defined by the longitudinal fissure.

primary motor cortex
Cortical area in the precentral gyrus responsible for initiating specific, voluntary movements.

contralateral   The relationship in which cortical areas responsible for motor control and sensory reception are opposite from the body areas affected.

Broca's area   The motor speech area located in the lower region of the frontal lobe in the language dominant hemisphere.

lobes. Figure 2–3 illustrates the brain's lobes and major landmarks. The lobes are generally named for the cranial bones that overlie each region, a convention that provides a convenient way of recalling them (once the bones have been learned!).

The frontal lobe, the most anterior region in each hemisphere, contains several areas important to movement, including speech production. The **primary motor cortex,** located in the precentral gyrus, is primarily responsible for initiating specific voluntary movements. The amount of area on the motor cortex that controls the various body parts reflects the degree of precision exhibited in that part. For example, a larger area is dedicated to controlling our fingers than to our toes.

Areas controlling the body also are arranged in an inverse or upside-down manner. That is, areas controlling the legs and feet are at the top, whereas areas dedicated to the arms and trunk are midway down the motor cortex. Areas for the head and face are in the lower region, lying just above the lateral fissure. Finally, most motor control is ultimately applied to the opposite or **contralateral** side of the body.

Broca's area plays a primary role in programming the motor movements for speech production. It is strategically located just anterior to the portion of

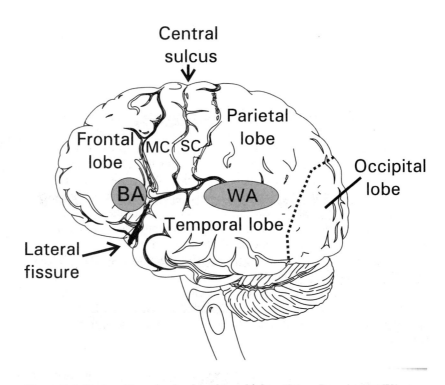

Figure 2–3. Brain with major landmarks and lobes. (BA = Broca's area; WA = Wernicke's area; MC = Motor cortex; SC = Sensory cortex.)

the motor cortex that controls the tongue and lips, usually in the dominant hemisphere, which is typically the left hemisphere for most persons.

The temporal lobe is also very important to our hearing, speech, and language. Several important areas contained in this region include the primary auditory cortex, auditory association area, and Wernicke's area. The **primary auditory cortex** is centered midway back on the superior surface of the temporal lobe. The primary auditory cortex receives neural impulses from the cochlea, the inner ear organ containing the nerve endings for hearing. This information is then shared with the surrounding cortical area, the **auditory association area,** where the significance of sounds is interpreted.

Wernicke's area, in the posterior region of the uppermost convolution in the temporal lobe, is an area of particular importance for speech and language. It plays a principal role in recognizing and interpreting incoming spoken language. Conversely, this area is also primarily involved in formulating and monitoring our own speech and language.

In the central region of the occipital lobe, the **primary visual cortex** receives neural impulses from our eyes. However, in this area we only "see" the shapes, colors, and patterns of the stimuli that our eyes are viewing. The surrounding cortex, the **visual association area,** interprets the significance or meaning of these shapes, colors, and patterns.

Finally, the parietal lobe contains the **primary sensory cortex,** located in the postcentral gyrus, just behind the central sulcus. The primary sensory cortex receives sensation (touch, temperature, pressure, pain, etc.) from the body in an arrangement that essentially mirrors the primary motor cortex. The proportional areas are somewhat different, however, because we have greater sensation in some areas that do not exhibit very sophisticated movement (e.g., our ear lobes). Just behind the primary sensory cortex is the **sensory association area,** where we interpret somesthetic sensations to identify their source.

It must be noted that the areas we study and describe separately are interconnected in many complex ways. Areas *within* each hemisphere can share information through **association fibers.** An important association fiber pathway for speech and language is the **arcuate fasciculus,** which arches from Wernicke's area forward to Broca's area. Information can be transmitted *between* the two hemispheres via **commissural fibers; the corpus callosum** represents the largest collection of these fibers. And, the fibers that allow sensory and motor impulses to travel *up and down,* to and from, the brain are called **projection fibers.** The projection fibers for motor movement comprise the **pyramidal tract.**

Watch for the subtle distinction between terms that are geographic in nature (e.g., *precentral gyrus*) as opposed to functional in nature (e.g., *primary motor cortex*). ■

Students of neuroanatomy quickly learn to become "name droppers." This is not because they are trying to impress their friends. It is simply a matter of survival! Many of the structures and regions in the brain are named after the individuals associated with their discovery. Two of the most important areas related to speech and language are named for 18th-century physicians who first described their functions. Paul Broca studied the disordered language output of an individual and then, following the man's death, performed an autopsy to identify the area apparently responsible for his disorder. Carl Wernicke, a German neurologist, similarly discovered the area that is responsible for comprehension of language (Benson & Ardilla, 1996).

primary auditory cortex Cortical area in the temporal lobe where the sensation of sound is received.

auditory association area Cortical area surrounding the primary auditory cortex in the temporal lobe; responsible for interpreting the significance of sounds.

Wernicke's area Cortical area in the posterior temporal lobe primarily responsible for interpreting oral language.

primary visual cortex Cortical area in the occipital lobe where visual sensation is received.

visual association area
The cortical area surrounding the primary visual cortex and responsible for interpreting the significance of visual stimuli.

primary sensory cortex
Cortical area in the postcentral gyrus responsible for receiving somesthetic sensations from the body.

sensory association area
The cortical areas just posterior to the sensory strip that assist in interpreting sensations.

association fibers
Cerebral nerve fibers that interconnect areas within a hemisphere.

arcuate fasciculus   The primary association fiber tract within each hemisphere; connects Wernicke's area in the temporal lobe with Broca's area in the frontal lobe of the language dominant hemisphere.

commissural fibers
Neural fibers that transmit information between the cerebral hemispheres.

corpus callosum   A major bundle of commissural fibers forming an arched body beneath the longitudinal fissure and connecting the cerebral hemispheres.

projection fibers
Neural fibers that transmit motor and sensory fibers between the cortical areas and peripheral nerves.

Basal Ganglia.   The term **basal ganglia** refers to various nuclei that are different from the surrounding areas. Although different authorities include varying collections of nuclei, those commonly listed include the **caudate nucleus** and **lenticular nucleus.** The primary role played collectively by these cell bodies is that of automatically integrating and smoothing movements. This overall role in the CNS is sometimes described by the term **extrapyramidal system.**

Considering the multitude of neural interconnections, it is difficult to imagine how any behavior or function could originate out of a single circumscribed area. Instead, recent research using computerized techniques for brain imaging has illustrated that several remote regions are often simultaneously involved in carrying out even the simplest tasks.

Cerebellum

The **cerebellum** is a major structure of the CNS and plays several important roles related to movement. Although the cerebellum does not initiate movement, it does serve a major role in coordinating movements. The cerebellum, located below the cerebrum and behind the brain stem (see Figure 2–3) is also divided into two hemispheres. Like the cerebrum, it has an outer layer of gray matter and an inner core of white matter. This explains why its name translates into "little brain."

The cerebellum receives information from other centers in the brain regarding our intended movements. It also provides **proprioception,** our sense of our body's current position. The cerebellum continuously compares our plan for a movement with the "progress reports" provided by this proprioceptive feedback. When necessary, it signals the motor cortex to adjust our movements to complete the intended action efficiently. Of course, this is critical for coordinating the rapid, repetitive, and precise movements of speech.

Brain stem

The brain stem is more than a base (or "stem") on which the brain is positioned. It contains several separate structures that house various important nerve centers. The brain stem also contains the major pathway for nerve fibers connecting the cerebral cortex and the body via the spinal cord. The brain stem includes three major divisions.

The **midbrain** is the uppermost and most narrow portion of the brain stem. It is well hidden between the hemispheres. Among other structures, it contains four swellings, called **colliculi,** that regulate various reflexes based on incoming auditory or visual stimuli.

The level of the brain stem just below the midbrain is the **pons,** easily recognized because of its rounded, bulging prominence. The pons (from the Latin word for "bridge") provides a variety of interconnections to other parts of the brain, especially the cerebellum.

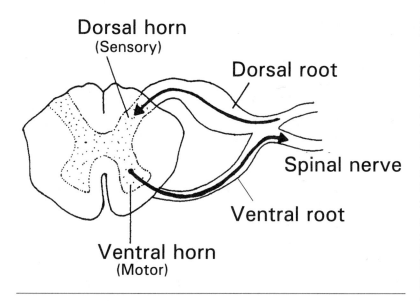

Dorsal horn
(Sensory)

Dorsal root

Spinal nerve

Ventral root

Ventral horn
(Motor)

Figure 2–4. Cross-section of the spinal cord.

pyramidal tract The tract of nerve fibers carrying motor impulses from the cortex to various levels of the spinal cord.

basal ganglia A group of large cell bodies located deep within the cerebral hemispheres whose interconnections regulate automatic background adjustments in movement.

caudate nucleus A major deep brain cell body that is part of the basal ganglia.

lenticular nucleus A cell body in the basal ganglia.

Remember, spinal *cord* is not synonymous with spinal *column*. Spinal column refers to the bony structure formed by the vertebrae. This column of rings protects the millions of fibers that form the softer spinal cord. ∎

Finally, the lowest level of the brain stem is called the **medulla oblongata,** an important structure for speech. It contains several nuclei for cranial nerves that relay neural messages for moving articulators and controlling the voice.

Spinal Cord

The **spinal cord** (see Figure 2–1) is that part of the CNS that continues out of the medulla oblongata downward through the large opening in the base of the skull, the **foramen magnum.** As such, its primary role is transmitting neural impulses up and down between the brain and most parts of the body. Spinal cord motor fibers serving different areas of the body terminate and synapse at the approximate levels for the structures they serve. Similarly, spinal cord sensory fibers bringing information to the brain synapse with incoming fibers at the appropriate levels.

A cross-section view of the spinal cord's inner core revealing two sets of horns is presented in Figure 2–4. These horns represent the different fibers passing through that part of the spinal cord. The posterior or **dorsal horns** (those closest to the back of the body) represent *sensory* projection fibers. Sensory impulses are transmitted up the fibers of the dorsal horns to the sensory cortex areas. The anterior or **ventral horns** (those closest to the interior of the body) are composed of *motor* projection fibers descending from the motor cortex.

extrapyramidal system A hypothetical system of multiple cerebral interconnections involving the basal ganglia, cortical areas, and cerebellum, which integrate background adjustments and purposeful movements.

cerebellum The lower, hindmost portion of the brain primarily responsible for coordination and balance.

proprioception   The sense of body position and orientation.

midbrain   The uppermost portion of the brain stem.

colliculi   Four paired bodies on the brain stem important for regulating visual and auditory reflexes.

pons   The middle portion of the brain stem that connects the midbrain and medulla.

medulla oblongata   Lower portion of brain stem whose fibers are continuous with the spinal cord.

spinal cord   The part of the CNS that extends below the brain stem.

foramen magnum   The large opening in the base of the skull through which the spinal cord passes to lower areas of the body.

dorsal horns   The posterior areas of the spinal cord containing nuclei for relaying incoming sensory information up the spinal cord.

ventral horns   The anterior areas of the spinal cord containing nuclei for relaying outgoing motor impulses to the body.

cranial nerves   Twelve paired bundles of peripheral nerve bundles that exit the CNS at the level of the brain stem.

spinal nerves   The peripheral nerves that exit the spinal cord.

Summary

- Although the extent of contributions is yet to be precisely determined, most agree that both our genetic makeup and our experiences contribute to our learning.
- The central nervous system includes the brain and spinal cord.
- The brain includes the cerebrum, cerebellum, and brain stem.
- The brain is composed of billions of cells that are organized to serve various purposes, including areas for speech and language.
- The billions of cells within the brain perform their tasks through the many levels of interconnection among them.
- The cerebellum is important for coordinating movements, such as those required in speech production.
- The brain stem contains many reflexive centers and nuclei for nerves serving the speech structures.

Peripheral Nervous System

The peripheral nervous system is composed of those nerves that are external to the brain and spinal cord. They extend throughout the body in an intricate network that reaches to the outermost areas, that is, the periphery of the nervous system. The peripheral nervous system includes cranial nerves, spinal nerves, and autonomic nerves.

Cranial Nerves

Cranial nerves, as the name suggests, are peripheral nerves that synapse with the CNS at the level of the brain stem and medulla oblongata. They pass through openings (*foramina*) in the base of the skull as they course to the structures they serve. As one might guess from their location within the cranium, several of these nerves are instrumental in speech and hearing. Cranial nerves have been generally named for the structures and functions they serve. Alternately, they are also numbered for the order (from top to bottom) in which they exit from the CNS.

As can be seen in Table 2–1, cranial nerves vary in serving either motor functions or sensory functions, or both. Of the 12 pairs, 7 cranial nerves are of particular importance to speech and hearing. These include cranial nerves V, VII, VIII, IX, X, XI, and XII.

Spinal Nerves

Spinal nerves synapse with the CNS along the length of the spinal cord, with their millions of fibers extending throughout the body. Spinal nerves come in pairs that connect the CNS to the neck, trunk, and limbs. Their attachments to the spinal cord are called roots. The **afferent roots** carry sensory informa-

Table 2–1. The cranial nerves, their names, functions, and potential roles in speech language.

No.	Name	Function	Potential Role in Speech-Language
I	Olfactory	Sensory: Smell	Associating smells
II	Optic	Sensory: Vision	Associating physical features
III	Oculomotor	Motor: Eye movement	Searching/tracking movement
IV	Trochlear	Motor: Eye movement	Searching/tracking movement
V	Trigeminal	Sensory: Face Motor: Jaw	Moving jaw for feeding/speech
VI	Abducens	Motor: Eye movement	Searching/tracking movements
VII	Facial	Sensory: Tongue Motor: Face	Controlling jaw and tongue; associating tastes; facial expression
VIII	Vestibular Acoustic	Sensory: Hearing and balance	Associating sound sensations, including speech
IX	Glossopharyngeal	Sensory: Tongue and pharynx	Controlling palate and pharynx for speech
X	Vagus	Sensory and Motor: Larynx, lungs, heart, esophagus, stomach	Controlling larynx for phonation
XI	Spinal Accessory	Motor: Shoulder, larynx, and pharynx	Controlling shoulders for respiration; also, larynx and pharynx in phonation
XII	Hypoglossal	Motor: Tongue movements	Controlling tongue for articulation

tion (which "affects" us) into the spinal cord, whereas the **efferent roots** carry motor impulses (which result in the intended "effects") to the body.

Some spinal nerves are motor, some are sensory, and some are both. They have been called "the final common pathway" for nerve impulses reaching the muscles of our bodies. They transmit innervation to the muscles of respiration, providing breath support for speech.

Autonomic Nerves

Finally, **autonomic nerves** provide connections for regulating major life support systems. As we adapt to changing conditions around us, the autonomic nervous system works to stabilize our vital life functions. The two parts in this system, the sympathetic and parasympathetic divisions, are said to work in an opposing manner to counterbalance each other.

The **sympathetic division** has been called our "fight or flight" system and is involved in arousing our various emotions, especially our response to fear. When alerted to an emergency, the sympathetic system increases our heart rate, blood pressure, and blood flow, among other

afferent roots The peripheral nerve bundles carrying sensory information to the ventral horns of the spinal cord.

efferent roots Nerve fiber bundles carrying motor impulses away from the spinal cord.

autonomic nerves A portion of the nervous system responsible for regulating involuntary life support systems.

sympathetic division The division of the autonomic nervous system that stimulates the body's "fight or flight" responses.

parasympathetic division The division of the autonomic nervous system that quiets and normalizes bodily functions.

reactions. In contrast, the **parasympathetic division** offsets this response by calming our body systems to their normal state and maintaining them in this condition.

The autonomic nerves do not play a significant role in speech and hearing. However, most of us have felt their effects on our speech in a tense, anxiety-provoking situation. Most of us have experienced the moist palms, dry mouth, tight throat, and shortness of breath when making an important public speech or asking for a first date.

Summary

- Cranial nerves extend from the brain stem to the structures they serve, including the structures for speech and hearing.
- Spinal nerves bring motor commands to the body and deliver sensory information from the body to the brain.
- Autonomic nerves are responsible for stabilizing basic life functions.

Anatomical Structures for Speech

In order to complete their roles, the central and peripheral nervous systems must affect the movement of structures. Of particular interest here are the structures that are used to produce speech for communication. The vital role of speech production for the child learning language normally is self-evident; for most children, the social transactions of language are mediated through speech.

Various structures contribute different functions in accomplishing the act of speech. However, as with other aspects of natural communication, their contributions must also be ultimately combined into a stream of automatic, integrated behaviors.

The Speech Mechanism

The previous section described the functions of the central and peripheral nervous systems. Especially important for present purposes is their control over our structures for speech. Of course, the nervous system with its impressive power and sophistication is only valuable for oral communication if it innervates muscles to move the structures that produce speech.

speech mechanism The anatomical structures for the production of speech sounds

The structures of speech and their functions have been collectively called the **speech mechanism.** This includes the lungs and associated structures that generate the airstream, the larynx and vocal folds that produce the vocal tone, the oral and nasal cavities that modify the resonance of the vocal tone, and, finally, the articulators that create the variety of speech sounds we produce.

The Lungs and Respiration

Our lungs are two large sponge-like structures encased within our rib cage. The primary purpose of the lungs and their associated structures is **respiration**—to move fresh air in and expel used air out of the body. The continuous, repetitive process of respiration can be broken down into two major cycles: an **inspiratory cycle** (inhalation), and the **expiratory cycle** (exhalation).

Although the primary purpose of the lungs is to serve respiration, humans (and other animals) have adapted them for communication. Speech also requires us to draw in a supply of air to use for an outgoing flow of air. The mechanics of breathing for speech are essentially the same as for respiration. The primary differences for speech relate to the duration of the cycles and our awareness of the demands to control airflow. When breathing for respiration, the inspiratory and expiratory cycles are approximately equal. However, during speech the inspiratory cycle is quicker and often deeper, whereas the expiratory cycle is more controlled and extended.

In producing speech, we restrict or valve the outward flow of air at several points along the way. The vocal folds, tongue, and lips, in particular, impede the airstream as they generate speech sounds. The respiratory muscles also play an active role in extending the duration of the expiratory cycle for speech. Additionally, as we speak louder or softer, or in longer or shorter phrases, the demands for controlling respiration change. As a result of all these factors, we are more aware of breathing for speech than we are when resting quietly in our recliner.

It should be noted that the structures of the speech mechanism are primarily intended for basic life-support functions—that is, breathing and eating. In developing our ability to communicate as humans, we have adapted these structures to be used for speech. Although we all know someone who would argue otherwise, eating and breathing are more fundamental to our survival than talking.

respiration The physiologic process of ventilating the body to inhale fresh air and exhale used air.

inspiratory cycle The respiratory phase in which air is inhaled into the lungs.

expiratory cycle The phase of respiration in which air is exhaled from the lungs.

The Larynx and Phonation

The **larynx** (or "voice box") is responsible for transforming this airstream into phonation. It is a framework of structures made of cartilage that support the major muscle of the larynx, the **thyroarytenoid muscle** (also known as the vocal folds). Figure 2–5 illustrates the laryngeal structure.

The vocal folds are attached to cartilaginous structures. Two of these can be rotated by the intrinsic muscles of the larynx. In this way, the medial edges of the vocal folds can be brought together (adducted), or separated (abducted). The space between the vocal folds is called the **glottis.** The vocal folds are illustrated in Figure 2–6.

The primary biological purpose of the larynx and vocal folds is to protect the airway below, specifically the trachea and lungs. The vocal folds close to keep foreign objects from passing through this airway into the lungs. As part of the speech mechanism, however, we have adapted the larynx to act as a valve in yet another important way.

larynx Cartilaginous and muscular framework that supports and regulates the vocal folds for phonation.

thyroarytenoid muscle (also **vocalis**) The paired muscles that contribute the bulk of the vocal folds.

glottis The source of laryngeal sound production, including the true vocal folds and the space between them.

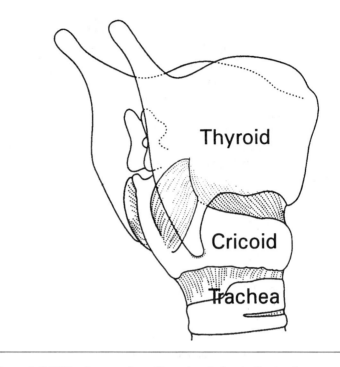

Figure 2–5. Major laryngeal cartilages in relation to the trachea.

subglottic pressure   The air pressure that occurs below the vocal folds.

For speech, the vocal folds adduct to increase the air pressure below them, the **subglottic pressure.** As this pressure increases, the folds are eventually blown open, releasing a puff of air. The elasticity of the vocal folds and the flow of air between them draws them back together, causing the subglottic pressure to rise again, reinitiating the vibratory cycle. With the vocal folds held in the adducted position, outgoing air causes this vibratory cycle to repeat with such rapidity that a vocal tone or *phonation* is produced.

Infants' ability to recognize their caregiver's voices is considered in Chapter 5. ■

The Oral/Nasal Cavities and Resonation

pharynx   Tubular cavity extending from the larynx to the oral and nasal cavities.

The spaces and structures above the vocal folds are referred to as the vocal tract. Figure 2–7 illustrates the *vocal tract,* which includes the **pharynx** (or throat), oral cavity, and nasal cavities. The unique qualities that allow us to distinguish one speaker from another are influenced by the individual physical contours of their vocal tracts. The cavities of the pharynx and mouth, and occasionally the nose, resonate and modify the sound of the basic vocal tone based on their shape and size.

nasality   Resonation of the vocal tone through the nasal cavities.

In addition to the resonant qualities contributed by the individual shape of each person's pharyngeal and oral cavities, another quality—nasality—may be present to varying degrees. **Nasality** is a resonant quality that is present to the extent that the vocal tone resonates through the nasal cavities. Of

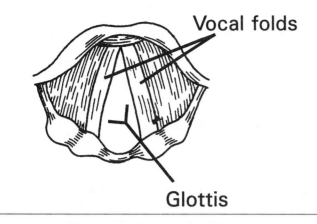

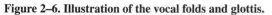

Figure 2–6. Illustration of the vocal folds and glottis.

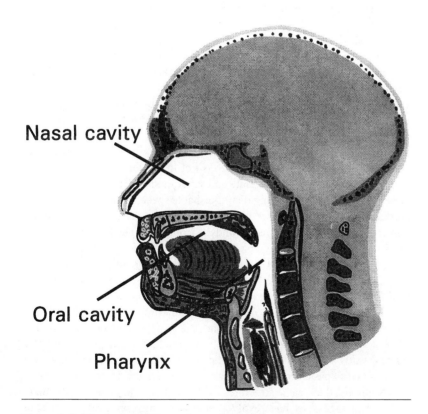

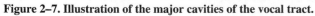

Figure 2–7. Illustration of the major cavities of the vocal tract.

course, some sounds in English (the *m, n,* and *ng* sounds) require nasality. However, most of the other sounds of English do not require nasal resonance. If a speaker exhibits nasal resonance on sounds where it is not expected, particularly on vowels, this is perceived as **hypernasality.**

To this point the speech mechanism has provided an airflow that is used to generate a laryngeal tone and this is modified by the resonating cavities that it passes through. Yet, in spite of its many qualities, all that has been produced is a tone with certain resonant qualities.

hypernasality Excess resonance in the nasal cavities during production of nonnasal speech sounds.

The Oral Structures and Articulation

The remaining structures to be considered in our discussion of the speech mechanism are the structures of articulation. In anatomy, *articulation* generally refers to the movement of a structure around a joint (e.g., the articulation of our arm at the shoulder). Even though they may not all have a joint for movement, the structures we move and reshape to produce different speech sounds are also articulators. We maneuver them to modify the vocal tone and to superimpose additional noise sources onto it. Amazingly, as listeners, we come to perceive these continuous shifts and subtle alterations in the stream of speech as distinctive segments that represent individual speech sounds.

The structures involved in articulation include the lips, tongue, teeth, jaw, and soft palate. Of course, not all of these structures are directly involved in producing each distinct sound. For example, in producing distinguishable vowel sounds, the vocal tone passes through the relatively open vocal tract. Primarily, changing the shape and position of the tongue (and the lips for sounds such as /o/ and /u/) causes the sound produced to shift from one vowel to another.

In contrast to the openness of vowels, the majority of consonant sounds involve positioning articulators to constrict the vocal tract to varying degrees. These constrictions generate and superimpose different noise sources onto the vocal tone, producing distinguishable speech sounds. For example, producing /s/ requires that we position the tongue to direct airflow through a small aperture (opening) just behind the front teeth. The hissing sound that results from this concentrated airstream is heard as the /s/ sound.

Articulators other than the tongue and lips play similar roles as well. The jaw (or *mandible*) assists in altering tongue position for vowels. The teeth articulate with other structures to provide different points of constriction for several sounds (e.g., /f/ as in *f*eet and /<δ>/ as in *th*umb). Finally, the soft palate (or *velum*) is a muscular structure draped from the posterior edge of the hard palate at the back of the mouth. The soft palate and pharyngeal walls seal off the nasal cavities for nonnasal sounds and unseal to allow sound to pass through when nasal sounds are produced.

Naturally, these same structures are present in all humans. Yet the many human languages that have evolved developed such an array of different speech sounds. There are over 100 different speech sounds in all the languages, but no one language uses all of them.

Summary

- The speech mechanism includes those structures involved in the production of speech.

- The four processes for speech include respiration, phonation, resonation, and articulation.

Anatomy and Physiology of Hearing

Most of us forget to fully appreciate the sense of hearing until we stop to cherish our favorite sounds—an orchestra, a great singer, songbirds in the morning, or the wind whispering in the trees at night. This would change immediately if we found we could no longer hear these sounds or the voices of our family and friends.

From the standpoint of learning to communicate, our ears play a role no less important than our mouths (a relationship no doubt stressed repeatedly by our caregivers). Beyond listening to others, most of us are also aware of how important it is to listen to ourselves speak to monitor the accuracy and clarity of the messages we produce.

Infants must hear the sounds, words, and phrases of the language spoken around them if they are to eventually reproduce them. As children struggle to develop all of the intricacies and subtleties of their language, their hearing provides the necessary immediate feedback. The importance of hearing to speech and language development is tragically illustrated by children with hearing impairments who must attempt to communicate without the benefit of these models and feedback.

The Ear

Many of us think of ears simply as those oddly shaped attachments on either side of our head. For some, their most important function is providing fixtures on which to hang our eyeglasses or earrings. Obviously, the ear is a far more intricate and valuable structure than this. It is composed of three major divisions—the outer ear, the middle ear, and the inner ear. Figure 2–8 illustrates the major divisions of the ear.

The Outer Ear

The most recognizable feature of the ear is the outer ear, and its most visible portion is the **auricle,** or **pinna.** This portion of the ear consists of flexible cartilage covered with skin. (Perhaps this flexibility prompted the

auricle (also **pinna**)
The outermost, visible, cartilaginous portion of the ear.

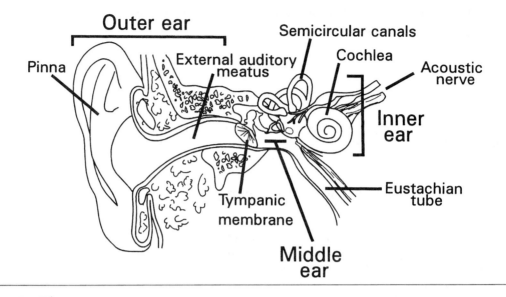

Figure 2–8. Illustration of the outer, middle, and inner ear.

idiomatic question, "Can I bend your ear?"). Functionally, its contours and funnel-shaped appearance might suggest that it would be important for collecting sounds into the ear canal, but its actual contribution in this way is minimal.

Further inward, the next major part of the outer ear is the **ear canal,** or the **external auditory meatus.** Extending through the temporal bone, this cartilaginous tube is slightly curved and generally about an inch long. Because of its shape and length, it plays an important role in resonating the sound energy that enters.

The Middle Ear

Although the outer ear provides an entrance for sound waves, the middle ear transforms them. The structures of the middle ear include the eardrum (or tympanic membrane), three tiny middle ear bones (or ossicles), and the eustachian tube. The middle ear structures work together to transform the acoustic energy of the incoming sound waves into corresponding mechanical energy. That is, their physical movements match the acoustic energy carried in the sound waves.

The **tympanic membrane** is a thin, flexible, and semitransparent membrane that separates the outer ear and middle ear. Though relatively tough, its flexibility allows it to move in and out in response to the pressure waves of incoming sounds. The mechanical movements of the tympanic membrane are transmitted to the inner ear by the **ossicles,** 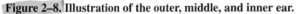 a chain of three small bones in the middle ear cavity. The ossicles include the **malleus** (which resembles

ear canal (also **external auditory meatus**) Funnel-shaped tube that conducts sound waves from the opening in the pinna to the tympanic membrane.

tympanic membrane (or **eardrum**)   The membrane that divides the outer and middle ear and receives sound waves from the environment.

ossicles   The three tiny bones of the middle ear that transmit energy from the tympanic membrane to the cochlea.

malleus   The largest, outermost bone in the ossicular chain of the middle ear and attached to the tympanic membrane.

a hammer), the **incus** (which is anvil shaped), and the **stapes** (shaped like a stirrup). The malleus is attached to the tympanic membrane, and the stapes is attached to the oval window of the inner ear.

Finally, the eustachian tube is a small duct that connects the middle ear to the pharynx. Its primary purpose is to ventilate the middle ear cavity. This equalizes the air pressure behind the tympanic membrane to optimize its flexibility and, therefore, its ability to flex with incoming sound pressure waves.

The Inner Ear

The inner ear is contained in a collection of tiny spaces within the temporal bone of the skull. The canals and cavities are fluid filled and house the extremely sensitive organs for balance and hearing. Three **semicircular canals** provide our sense of balance and equilibrium as the fluid within them moves in response to changes in body position.

The inner ear structure primarily concerned with our sense of hearing is the **cochlea.** The cochlea contains the sense organs that carry out the final transformation in hearing. It is a coiled structure, spiraled much like a snail shell (hence, its name). If one could uncoil the cochlea, it is actually a tube approximately 1.5 inches long that is subdivided lengthwise by two membranes into three tubes. All three spaces are fluid filled.

The two larger tubes within the cochlea are linked to the mechanical movements of the middle ear by tiny membrane-covered openings, the oval window and round window. Recall that the stapes is connected to the **oval window.** Because inner ear fluid is capable of moving back and forth, the round window can accommodate slower movements of the oval window as in responding to changes in middle ear pressure. However, the rapid vibratory movements associated with sound waves are too rapid to be accommodated in this way.

In responding to incoming sound, the ossicles transmit movements of the tympanic membrane to the oval window. These movements, too rapid to be accommodated by the slow shifting of inner ear fluid, are instead transmitted through the fluid to the **basilar membrane** and the **organ of Corti.** The final conversion of sound vibrations takes place in the hair cells of the organ of Corti. Depending on their frequency, the vibrations bend hair cells located along the length of the basilar membrane. This stimulates them to generate electrochemical pulses, which are then transmitted to the brain through the fibers of the *cranial nerve VIII*, or the **acoustic nerve.**

◾ Summary

- The structures for hearing include the outer, middle, and inner ears.

- In the process of hearing, sound waves pass through the outer and middle ears as mechanical energy.

---

incus The middle bone in the ossicular chain in the middle ear.

stapes The smallest and innermost ossicle in the middle ear; its contact with the oval window transmits movements to the cochlea.

semicircular canals Three fluid-filled bony loops in the inner ear that contain fluid and contribute to maintaining balance.

cochlea The portion of the inner ear that contains the sensory end organ for hearing, the organ of Corti.

oval window The resting place for the footplate of the stapes where movements of the ossicular chain are transmitted to the cochlea.

basilar membrane A membrane within the inner ear that supports the sensory end organ for hearing, the organ of Corti, along the length of the cochlea.

organ of Corti The sense organ for hearing contained in the cochlea of the inner ear.

acoustic nerve (or **cranial nerve VIII**) The eighth cranial nerve important for transmitting sound and balance sensation from the inner ear to the brain.

- The inner ear transforms the mechanical energy of sound waves into electrochemical impulses that are transmitted to the brain.

Structural Foundations for Communication

As we consider the structural bases for human communication in mature speakers, we are most aware of the contributions of the fully developed anatomical structures—the nervous system, speech mechanism, and ear. However, the seeds of human communication are sown at conception, and its structural foundations are forming long before a child's first word.

The genetic potential present at conception unfolds to form the necessary physical structures as the embryo and fetus grow. As these structures mature, they permit limited responding to the fetal environment prior to birth. Following birth, the continued maturation of these structures and interaction with the world leads to increasingly sophisticated responses.

This development continues at a rapid rate after birth. However, infants' interactions with their caregivers stimulate increasingly organized behaviors. Finally, it is becoming possible to better understand how these structures and the behaviors they control become integrated as the infant develops toward mature human communication.

Prenatal Development—an Overview

Until recent decades few details about prenatal development were understood. Recent research has made it increasingly apparent that, even during the prenatal period, the developing baby is remarkably capable of sensing and responding to the outside world.

Prenatal development occurs during two phases referred to as the *embryonic period* and the *fetal period.* The following sections present an overview of the developments occurring within each period.

The Embryonic Period—a New Beginning

The **embryonic period** applies to the interval from conception through the first 8 weeks of gestation. Once conception has occurred, the microscopic changes that follow happen rapidly but silently over the next few weeks. When the mature spermatozoa and ovum fuse together they first form a **zygote.**

Through a process called **mitotic division** the zygote repeatedly divides into an increasing number of smaller and smaller cells, becoming a **morula.** As the cells continue to divide, they form a collection of cells called a **blastocyst,** which by the end of the first week has become implanted in the mother's uterine wall. The blastocyst's outer cell mass, called the **trophoblast,** will eventually become the placenta. The inner cell mass or **embryoblast** will continue developing into the **embryo,** the fetus, and, ultimately, the neonate, or newborn. Figure 2–9 illustrates this early embryonic development.

embryonic period The period from conception through the eighth week following conception.

zygote The single cell formed at conception containing the genetic codes of both the father and mother.

mitotic division The cell division that follows conception.

morula Cluster of cells formed by the fourth or fifth day following conception.

blastocyst A fluid-filled sphere containing embryonic cells, formed by the end of the first week following conception.

trophoblast The outermost cells in the blastocyst that attach the embryo to the uterine wall and serve as the pathway for nutrients.

embryoblast The blastocyst's inner cell mass that will develop into the embryo.

embryo The fertilized egg during the first 8 weeks of development.

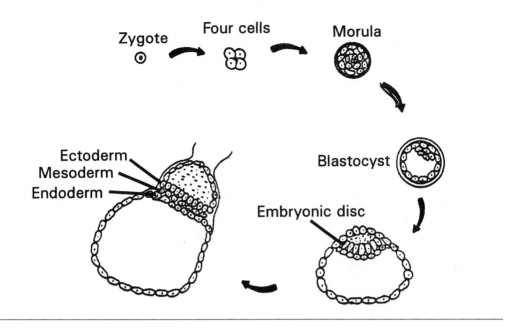

Figure 2–9. Illustration of mitotic division of the embryo.

During the third week, the mother's blood begins to circulate between the placenta and the embryo. Nutrients and oxygen in the mother's blood are passed to the embryo and, conversely, waste products are removed from the embryo to the mother through the **placental barrier.**

At the same point that the placenta is forming, several important developments occur in the embryoblast. It flattens into a form now called the **embryonic disc.** The embryonic disc forms three different cell layers. The outermost layer, called the **ectoderm,** will contribute to formation of the brain, nerves, and skin, among other structures. The **mesoderm,** the middle layer, becomes the heart, muscles, bones, tendons, several glands, blood, and blood vessels. The linings of the digestive and respiratory systems are derived from the innermost layer, the **endoderm.**

Gestation, the duration of a pregnancy, is divided into three 12-week periods called **trimesters.** From the third through the eighth week, the embryo develops the majority of important organs and organ systems (central nervous system, circulatory system, eyes, ears, and limbs). This initial 8-week period, during the first trimester, is obviously a very critical period for the embryo and the eventual development of a healthy baby. Introduction of any substances that might interfere with the normal development of these structures during this time may result in tragic birth defects. A timetable of development for major embryonic and fetal structures is summarized in Table 2–2.

placental barrier The membranous structure that allows nourishment and oxygen to pass between the mother and the embryo or fetus.

embryonic disc A cluster of cells in embryonic development at about 2 weeks following conception.

ectoderm The outermost embryonic germ layer that contributes to various organs, including the nervous system and skin.

mesoderm The middle embryonic germ layer that contributes to bones, cartilage, muscles, and blood.

Table 2–2. Approximate timetable for major developments in the embryonic and fetal periods.

	Embryonic Period (through 8th week)		Fetal period (9th week to birth)	
	Weeks 1–2	**Weeks 3–8**	**Weeks 9–24**	**Weeks 25–38**
Approximate Size	Single cell becomes a cell cluster.	Grows to 3 inches in length and 1 ounce in weight by 9th week.	Grows to 14 inches in length and 30 ounces in weight.	Measures 20 inches long and weighs 7 pounds.
Major Gestational Developments	Zygote develops into morula, blastocyst, and embryonic disc.	Maternal blood flows to placenta. Endoderm, mesoderm, and ectoderm begin differentiating.	Major growth is in length. Around 20 weeks, mother feels first movements of the fetus.	Major growth is in weight as fat develops rapidly.
Developing Foundations for Speech and Language	No specific structures forming cluster.	Weeks 3–6: CNS, heart, eyes, ears. Weeks 7–8: CNS, heart, ears, eyes, palate, and teeth.	Weeks 9–12: CNS, ears, eyes, palate, teeth. Weeks 12–24: CNS, eyes, teeth.	Continued development in CNS, eyes, teeth.

The Fetal Period—Still Growing

From the end of the eighth week until birth, the developing baby is a **fetus.** Although most basic structures had their beginnings during the embryonic period, there is still much growth that must occur for the fetus to become viable and capable of sustaining life support independently.

At the end of the first trimester, even though the major organs have begun their formation, the embryo is only 3 inches long and weighs about 1 ounce. By the end of the second trimester (approximately the sixth month of pregnancy), the fetus weighs about 30 ounces and measures approximately 14 inches in length. The eyelids of the fetus open by the 26th week and its fingernails and toenails are developed by the 28th week. The skin is thin and reddish up until the last 6 to 8 weeks of gestation when body fat develops rapidly and the fetus becomes plump and smooth. At the end of the third trimester, at the point of its impending birth, the fetus on average is about 20 inches long and weighs about 7 pounds.

endoderm The innermost embryonic germ layer that contributes to various organs, including the digestive tract and lungs.

gestation The period of embryological and fetal development from conception to birth.

trimesters Three equal intervals of approximately 3 months each in a typical pregnancy.

fetus The developing unborn child from the 10th week of gestation until birth.

Summary

- Gestation, from conception to birth, is divided into the embryonic and fetal periods.

- The first trimester, or first 3 months, of gestation is considered to be critical for development of the baby's important life systems and organs.

Prenatal Neurological Development

While the embryo, and later the fetus, quietly grows, the mother is generally unaware of its development until it attains some size, perhaps causing some discomfort. Perhaps her first indication of the baby's neurological development is the first movements.

The first kick is certainly an exciting moment but not a very direct assessment of the baby's overall development. Research has documented several important neurological developments that occur throughout gestation. The extent of neurological development prior to birth is remarkable and significant.

primitive streak A feature of the embryonic disc that generates the mesoderm, endoderm and ectoderm.

neural groove The embryonic predecessor to the neural tube.

neural folds The embryonic predecessor to the neural groove.

neural tube The embryonic predecessor to the spinal cord.

The Embryonic Brain

The brain and spinal cord begin developing in the embryo during the third week. They begin as a strip of flattened cells, the **primitive streak,** lying in a long depression called the **neural groove** on the embryo's top surface. By the end of the third week, the ridges, or **neural folds,** on either side of the neural groove approach each other and fuse together, creating the **neural tube.**

By the end of the fourth week the forerunners of the cerebral hemispheres, basal ganglia, cerebellum, and brain stem have developed. The cavities that will become the ventricles are in place by the fifth week and by the eighth week cerebrospinal fluid is circulating within them. As was noted earlier, the embryonic period is obviously a critical period and many consider the third week to be the most critical period for neural development.

The Fetal Brain

The surfaces of the cerebral hemispheres are smooth until the 20th week. With further development, their surfaces become more irregular and the beginnings of the various sulci and gyri become visible. As these features develop during the third trimester the lobes of the brain become more evident. By the end of the third trimester, at birth, it is possible to identify all of the surface features of the adult brain.

Various structures of the fetal brain develop more rapidly than others. A prominent example is the brain stem. Vital reflex centers, including the cardiac and respiratory centers, are regulated in the medulla of the brain stem. Of course, it only makes sense that the development of such basic life-supporting structures should predate birth.

Neural developments for motor control become increasingly evident throughout gestation. Spontaneous movements have been detected as early as 7.5 weeks gestation when the baby is still technically an embryo (de Vries, Visser, & Prechtl, 1982). However, the mother is usually not aware of movements until the fifth month of pregnancy when the fetus has grown substantially larger and stronger.

In spite of the presence of most adult features or landmarks at birth, the brain's development is far from complete. The most direct evidence of this is its weight. At 335 grams, it is approximately 25% of its eventual adult weight. This suggests that much more growth and maturation is left to occur during childhood.

Summary

- The nervous system's most basic predecessors are detectable in the embryo within the first month of development.

- The surface features of the brain begin to appear during the second trimester.

- Reflex centers for life support develop earlier and more rapidly than areas for motor control.

- Fetal movement has been detected much earlier than mothers would typically be capable of sensing.

Infant Neurological Development

There are several important disclaimers that should precede discussion of this topic (Haynes, 1994a–d). First, there is little confirmed knowledge that directly relates development of the human brain and the emergence of language in childhood. Several authors (Lenneberg, 1967; Locke, 1993) have provided detailed examinations of how these aspects might correlate or at least coincide. However, it has not been shown that specific neurological changes *cause* specific developments in language.

Second, what is known is difficult to specifically relate to *normal* language development. Much of our information is based on inferences drawn from studies of children with brain damage. Several researchers have explored the potential for relating disordered language development and genetic or familial patterns (Gilger, 1995; Tomblin & Buckwalter, 1994).

Third, the younger the brain, the more plastic it appears to be. In other words, it appears that different structures and portions of the brain may be capable of assuming a variety of functions if called on to do so. This raises the question as to whether certain areas of the brain are preprogrammed to handle language if, in fact, other areas are capable of also doing so, at least to some extent.

Lenneberg (1967) provided an extensive review of studies examining the developing nervous system from birth to age 2. A number of significant changes occur as indicators of the brain's maturation. These include brain weight, neuronal development, myelination, and reflex inhibition.

Brain Weight

The brain increases in weight by a remarkable 350% during the first 2 years of life. In contrast, the brain will only increase its weight by 35% during the next 10 years. Interestingly, where the major prenatal increase in brain weight comes in the lower brain stem divisions (so important to basic life support systems), the most rapid gain in the first 6 months following birth is in the cerebral hemispheres (so important to processing, storing, and retrieving information) (Love & Webb, 2001).

In regard to brain growth, Locke (1993) has noted that the ultimate size of the brain may be less important than *when* the brain grows. In our species less brain development occurs prior to birth than in most other species. Phylogenetically, this appears to relate to the time when our earliest ancestors (hominids) began to stand erect and walk. The shifting pressures on the hip and pelvis eventually reshaped and narrowed the birth canal over a period when, paradoxically, the species was generally becoming larger.

The evolutionary solution to this "obstetrical dilemma" (Washburn, 1960) was premature birth. As infants in our species became larger and our species' birth canal narrowed, only those infants born earlier would actually survive birth. The very intriguing result would be that the human infant's brain would go through its most significant development *following* birth, during the first few months of life. Significantly, this would result in an extended period of time when the infant is essentially helpless and, therefore, the focus of consistent, if not continuous, social stimulation. As Locke summarized, "One can hardly think of a developmental circumstance that would more favorably affect acquisition of complex behavior" (p. 264).

Neuronal Development

A second important characteristic of neurological maturation is in neuronal development. It is commonly thought that the human brain is so powerful because of the sheer number of neurons present. This is not necessarily so. Ironically, the lower on the phylogenetic scale a species is, the greater the density of neurons in comparison to its brain volume. (Perhaps that proverbial put-down, "He's really dense!" has some neurological basis after all!)

Accordingly, proportionate to brain volume human brains are much less densely packed with neurons than lower-order animals. Instead of the sheer number of neurons, what actually makes the human brain a more powerful processor is the density and complexity of the dendritic *interconnections* between neurons. Figure 2–10 illustrates the development of dendritic interconnections.

Significant neuronal maturation, the expansion of dendrites and axons that form a dense network of neuronal interconnections, occurs in the first 2 years of life. This directly relates to the brain's increased ability to retrieve, associate, and process information. Of particular interest is the finding that the dendrites in speech and oral motor areas of the left hemisphere, as compared to the right hemisphere, increase in number around 6 months of age, and in length at around 12 months of age (Simonds & Scheibel, 1989). As neuroimaging techniques improve there will be an increasing amount of insight into the changing neural structures that underlie developing speech. However, what seems inevitable is the recognition that structure does not drive function "down a one-way street." Instead, the brain's structural development is very likely influenced by the infant's own responses to its own activities and the environment. In other words, structure drives function, *and* function drives structure.

Myelination

The third significant development during the first 2 years of childhood is myelination. At different times during the first several years, the conducting axons throughout the nervous system develop a *myelin sheath*. This is a fatty covering that increases the efficiency of transmitting nerve impulses through such axons, much like the insulation on electrical wire improves its conducting efficiency. As myelination progresses it can serve as an index of brain maturation (Love & Webb, 2001).

At birth, the motor area of the precentral gyrus is the earliest developed area to become myelinated. This is followed quickly by the somatosensory area of the postcentral gyrus. The primary visual cortex in the occipital lobe is next to become myelinated, followed by the primary auditory cortex in the temporal lobe. The last area of the brain to evidence myelination is the mesial surfaces between the two hemispheres.

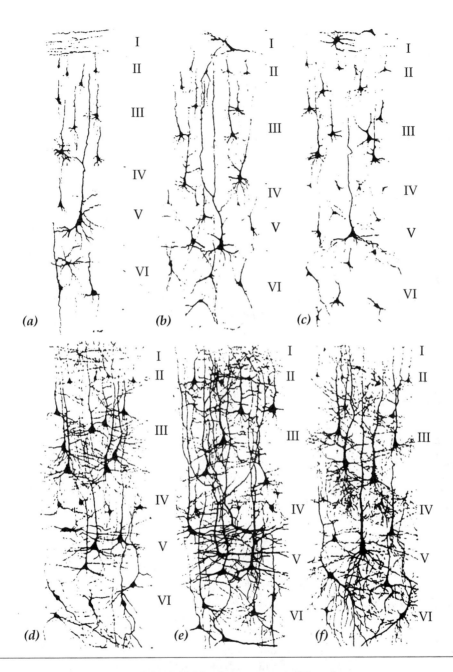

Figure 2–10. Illustration of postnatal dendritic development around Broca's area.

((a) Newborn, (b) 1 month, (c) 3 months, (d) 6 months, (e) 15 months, (f) 2 years.)

Reflex Inhibition

For the most part, the preceding indicators of CNS maturation cannot be directly observed. At best, they might be inferred from the behavioral changes that result from their occurrence. One of the key behavioral changes that parents and pediatricians monitor during the child's first several years of life is the status of reflexive behaviors.

reflexes
Preprogrammed neuromuscular responses to stimuli.

Reflexes are involuntary motor patterns that are automatically regulated in the lower divisions of the CNS (especially the brain stem or spinal cord). Most reflexes are protective in nature, helping us react quickly to survive a sometimes hazardous environment. They cause us to instinctively withdraw our hand from heat or pain, blink to avoid debris approaching our eyes, or cough and sneeze to expel irritants or obstructions from our airway. And, very important, they help us do so without having to think about it.

There are many active reflexes at birth and most of these disappear or are modified within the first 6 months of life. The presence of so many involuntary behaviors explains why newborns' motor activity appears to be a collection of random jerks, twitches, and stretches. Infants' gradual achievement of smoother, more voluntary control over motor activity is closely related to the myelination that occurs throughout the first several years. As motor axons become myelinated and more efficient in transmitting impulses to their associated muscle groups, the child's voluntary motor control improves. When myelination coincides with the rapid growth of the cerebral hemispheres, continual significant improvement in the child's motor abilities is the logical result.

Reflexes play a significant role as parents and pediatricians monitor a child's development. The absence of reflexes is obviously worrisome in its implications for the child's neurological status. Similarly, the persistence of certain reflexes might also indicate that the normal process of neurological maturation has been disturbed. Either of these indicators would indicate the child's overall development might be at risk. Further evaluation and intervention may be warranted. ■

It should be remembered that the neurological mechanisms that trigger most reflexes do not technically disappear. Instead, with myelination, the more effective control exerted by the higher cortical levels of the brain inhibits the lower level reflexive centers in the brain stem or spinal cord. However, thankfully, several lower level reflexes do continue to occur when stimulation exceeds some threshold. For example, the normal inhibition of reflexes allows us conscious choice in how and when we will move our arms. However, beyond some threshold of pain, the reflex arc at the spinal cord level instantaneously determines that we should reflexively remove our bare hand from the pan that just came out of the oven! If we had to think about it, the consequences are obvious.

specific activity reflex
A reflex that affects an individual body part.

mass activity reflex
A reflex in which the response is evidenced by the entire body.

Reflexes have been classified into two major categories—specific activity and mass activity. **Specific activity reflexes** occur when stimulation of a specific muscle group causes it to respond in an isolated manner. For example, in the palmar or hand grasp reflex, pressure on the infant's palm elicits closure of the fingers around the object. In contrast, **mass activity reflexes** are those in which the entire body reacts to stimulation of just one part of the body. See Table 2–3 for a list of neonatal reflexes. A familiar example is the Moro or startle reflex seen when a sudden, loud noise causes the baby's arms and legs to extend with a jerk followed by the hands coming together and clenching at midline. (Depending on the strength of the stimulus, a crying episode frequently follows as well.)

Table 2–3. Eliciting stimulus, behavioral response, and expected disappearance of infant reflexes.

Name	Eliciting Stimulus	Behavioral Response	Expected Disappearance
Babinski	Side of the foot is stroked, heel to toe	Toes lift and fan out	Around 1 year
Babkin	Pressure is applied to palms while lying face up	Mouth opens, eyes close, head turns straight ahead	Around 3 months
Palmar (Grasp)	Object pressed into palm	Fingers close in a grasping motion	Around 1 year
Moro (Startle)	Sudden loud noise or dropping motion	Arms extend, then return to midline; fingers grasp	Around 6 months
Rooting	Touching or stroking cheek lightly	Opens mouth and turns in direction of stroked cheek	Around 4 months
Sucking	Inserting object or nipple into mouth	Sucks object rhythmically	Around 2 months

It is assumed that reflexes are genetically transmitted within the species because they have survival value. The original purpose of many reflexes is not always readily apparent. Whatever their origins, however, we can speculate that some might be very fundamental to later language development. The palmar or hand grasp reflex provides early exploration opportunities as the infant's hand grasps various objects that it might randomly land on. The infant then continues to grip them as they are examined—usually orally. The palmar reflex might also allow infants the earliest opportunity to interact "socially" with their caregivers by instinctively "holding hands" whenever the caregiver inserts a finger into their tiny palm.

Opportunities for socialization are also prompted by the reflexive smiles exhibited by infants in response to touching the cheek or lips. Two other reflexes that may have a potential relationship to speech and language development are the sucking and swallowing reflexes. Of course, their most functional purpose is to satisfy the infant's enormous nutritional demands. Nonetheless, the possible role that sucking and swallowing play in readying the lips, jaw, tongue, and velum for later speech movements is an intriguing one.

Finally, the reflexive vocal sounds that accompany the baby's sucking, swallowing, burping, fussing, and crying are interesting in their possible link to later speech behaviors. The sounds associated with eating involve movements and contacts between the articulators, similar to those in producing consonants. Fussing and crying sounds are produced on exhalation and usually with voicing in an almost vowel-like manner.

Even when the baby is not crying, reflexive sounds that result from random uncontrolled movement of the vocal folds occur in comfortable relaxed states. Interestingly, as infants' improving control over their vocal behavior becomes more evident in increased cooing and babbling, the amount of time spent crying decreases. (Although it may be difficult to convince some parents of that, no matter how persuasive the evidence is.)

Summary

- The infant brain experiences remarkable growth and development in the months immediately following birth.
- Important indicators of the sophistication that develops rapidly in infancy are brain weight, neuron development, myelination, and reflex inhibition.
- Primitive reflexes are progressively inhibited and replaced with more voluntary, controlled behaviors.

Early Bases for Experience and Perception

Language will ultimately be based on experiencing the environment. To learn from these opportunities, the infant must possess the structures to experience, recognize, and then understand (or at least associate) events in the surrounding world. A certain amount of learning appears to occur almost instantly with the earliest experiences—even those that occur in the womb. It seems to occur with mere exposure, in the absence of any real interaction, as we normally think of it.

Prenatal learning is apparent only in capabilities demonstrated by the fetus under conditions devised by researchers. The perceptual reality of these early experiences for the fetus and newborn might otherwise remain hidden. Ultimately, these abilities may not qualify as "communication," but they help demonstrate the reality of the infant's structural foundation for learning.

Bases for Auditory Learning

Researchers have determined that auditory structures develop at a surprisingly early point in fetal development. The significance of this becomes apparent in the response of the fetus to its auditory environment.

Prenatal Auditory Development.   The importance of auditory experience to language development is obvious. What may not be as obvious is the extent of auditory experience a newborn has had prior to birth. Those expectant mothers who have received a sharp kick from their "littlest house guest" in response to a sudden loud noise would not doubt this possibility at all.

Locke (1993) provided a thorough discussion of research concerning fetal and neonatal hearing. The cochlea and auditory nerve are developed by the 24th week. Using changes in the heart rate as the fetal response, researchers have found that the fetus responds to environmental sounds as early as the 26th week of gestation. Using ultrasound technology researchers have observed reliable eye blink reflexes in response to a buzzing tone in fetuses between 28 and 36 weeks.

Prenatal Auditory Environment. The fetal structure for hearing is available early in its development, but what sounds are present to be experienced in the fetal environment? Researchers have found that the fetus is surrounded by noise from the mother's turbulent blood flow at a level of about 85 dB with the maternal pulse rising approximately 10 dB above this. What is even more intriguing is the finding that the intensity of the mother's voice is capable of exceeding these levels, especially in the frequency range where most female fundamental frequencies fall, between 200 and 250 hertz.

The fetus has the structures for hearing as well as internal and external sounds to experience much earlier than many would imagine. However, is it actually capable of "learning" anything about these sounds? One set of researchers presented speech stimuli ([babi] and [biba]) at 95 dB near the abdomens of mothers in their third trimester. They found that after presenting one stimulus a number of times, the heart rates of the fetuses slowed when the stimulus changed to the other stimulus. This change suggested that the fetuses had become familiar with or had adapted to the first stimulus, evidencing at least a basic form of learning for speech sounds.

Bases for Visual Learning

The neurological development that is occurring following birth occurs to a great extent in response to stimulation. The visual sense is a significant source of this stimulation.

Visual Acuity. It is widely known that at birth newborns arrive with at least some limited visual acuity and they develop rapidly thereafter. At birth infants can focus approximately 20 centimeters (almost 8 inches) away from their face. Interestingly, this is the approximate distance to the caregiver's face when the infant is held in the usual position for feeding. By 4 months of age the infant is capable of visual focus that approaches that of an adult (Haynes, White, & Held, 1965).

Acuity is also evident in their ability to discriminate simple geometric shapes. They prefer moving objects with contrasting contours and areas of light and dark. And, fittingly, they appear to favor humanlike faces over inanimate objects. For example, the infant attends closely to geometric shapes arranged to mimic a human face but pays little attention when the same shapes are arranged randomly.

Visual Tracking. During the first month of life infants become capable of detecting and tracking objects in motion by moving their heads. They appear to perform more favorably when the object is large with highly visible contrasting features and also makes a noise (Lane & Molyneaux, 1992). By

3 months of age infants are able to track moving objects with eye movements alone, independent of any head movement.

Learning through Other Senses

Research has properly focused on the visual and auditory modalities of the developing infant. These are the two primary channels through which the infant initially receives meaningful stimulation. The other major sensory modalities—olfactory, tactile, and gustatory—are certainly available but effectively limited by the infant's immature motor control. A variety of sights and sounds can impose themselves on the infant's experience from anywhere in the immediate surroundings. In contrast, smelling, touching, and tasting will rely for some time on caregivers to bring such stimuli sufficiently close for the infant to experience. Nonetheless these probably play some minimal role and deserve mention.

The tactile sense (or touch) is considered to consist of four types of sensations received by nerve receptors in the skin. These sensations—touch, cold, warmth, and pain—are present in infants but mature only as myelination progresses in the somatosensory area of the brain. As mentioned before, the infant's experience with tactile senses are limited to the sensations made immediately available to the infant. However, it is interesting to consider the areas that have been found to be most sensitive on the newborn. These are, from most to least sensitive, the face, especially the areas around the lips, eyes, and nose; the hands; the bottoms of the feet; and the abdominal area (Lane & Molyneaux, 1992). Given the obvious importance of the rooting and sucking reflexes, the strategic importance of sensitivity around the mouth is logical.

The gustatory sense (or taste) is perhaps the earliest sensation experienced by the infant. (Many caregivers will claim that it is the only sensation their baby experiences when not sleeping.) Research has shown that infants are capable of discriminating sweetness and saltiness in solutions fed to them. Eating also involves the tactile sense as the texture and consistency of food can affect our enjoyment of it. However, the gustatory sense is probably most closely linked to the sense of smell, with taste sensations being greatly affected by the associated smells. Of course, many aspects of infants' relationship with their caregivers will be influenced by the emotions associated with eating. Nursing sessions are the first and closest social occasions for the infant and, for most families, sharing meals together continues to be a basic element of family life.

The olfactory system is closely integrated with the limbic lobe or rhinencephalon, which means "nose brain." ■

The human olfactory sense (or smell) is very sensitive, although we probably do not rely on it as much as we once did in our species' history. The structures that deal with smell are also thought to be involved in mediating emotion and motivation. A variety of emotional responses have been attributed to the limbic lobe, including pleasure, satiation, guilt, alertness, and excitement (Love & Webb, 2001).

The powerful connection between the sense of smell and the various emotions apparently begins very early in life (Locke, 2001). Infants have been found to distinguish among smells and even to exhibit the characteristic facial expressions adults associate with them. Very young breast-feeding infants have been shown to distinguish their mother's smell from other women using olfactory cues only. Of course, it is not insignificant that the emotions of pleasure and satiation from nursing would be so closely associated with the smell and, most likely, the voice of the infant's caregiver.

There are probably a myriad of other associated smells and emotions that continue to build strong emotional attachments between children and their caregivers. Most of us can easily conjure up many memories of past holidays when we smell the foods that we traditionally eat on those occasions.

Summary

- Research has determined that structures for experiencing external stimuli develop remarkably early in gestation.

- Research has suggested the potential for prenatal auditory learning due to the development of auditory structures and the availability of sounds in the fetal environment.

- Infants are also exposed to a wealth of visual stimuli and appear to have the visual abilities to learn from them soon after their birth.

Chapter Summary

This chapter has presented basic information about the anatomical structures related to speech, language, and hearing. This provided the foundation for appreciating the role these structures may play as they develop in the embryo, fetus, and infant long before true communication can occur.

As does any human behavior, communication relies on biological structures. Principal among these are the nervous system, the speech mechanism, and the ear. The *central nervous system* is comprised of the *brain* and *spinal cord*. The *peripheral nervous system* consists of *cranial nerves, spinal nerves,* and *autonomic nerves*. Through complex interconnections at various levels, called *synapses,* the billions of *neurons* and nerve fibers of these systems provide the potential for the most basic and complex human activities and learning.

The potential for these biological systems and the behaviors they support are present from conception and may develop sooner than most imagine. The prenatal development of the *embryo,* and later, the *fetus* is called *gestation*. Critical organ systems for life support develop early but are soon followed by development of the brain and other structures for learning.

These important structural developments and the related learning continue throughout infancy and beyond.

Infants enter the world with underlying systems that prepare them for exploration and rapid learning. Initially, these systems respond primarily to the world with *reflexive behavior.* However, with maturation and experience, infants are increasingly capable of controlling these systems for attending and responding to available auditory, visual, olfactory, tactile, and gustatory stimuli. In other words, they learn about their worlds at an ever-increasing rate.

Review Questions

1. How do the central and peripheral nervous systems differ?

2. What are the main functions associated with the cerebrum, basal ganglia, cerebellum, and brain stem?

3. How do the structures of the speech mechanism contribute to the production of speech?

4. Describe the structures that transfer and transform sound in the process of hearing.

5. In what two ways is the process of gestation divided into periods?

6. Characterize the differences seen in the neurological development of the embryo in contrast to the fetus.

7. Describe the developments that illustrate the significance of maturation in the infant's nervous system.

8. What stimuli is the infant prepared to respond to just prior to and following birth?

Practice Questions

To the student: You are encouraged to use the following questions to prepare for multiple-choice examinations. This exercise is not intended to simply "provide the answers to questions." Instead, it is hoped that you will use the material to develop your ability to analyze questions and choices to identify correct answers based on a critical understanding of the distinctions among the answers. Use the answer key at the end of the book to prompt your analysis of each item and to confirm the correct answer. Remember that there is a difference between recognizing the correct answer and understanding why it is the correct one.

1. A neuron includes a cell body, a nucleus, an axon, and dendrites. Which of the following would *not* be an accurate characterization?
   a. the cell body is the "processor"
   b. the axon is the "transmitter"
   c. the dendrites are the "collectors"
   d. cell bodies outnumber axons
   e. dendrites outnumber axons

2. Damage in the precentral gyrus in the left hemisphere would be evidenced by _____ .
   a. visual deficits in the right eye
   b. visual deficits in the left eye
   c. paralysis on the left side of the body
   d. paralysis on the right side of the body
   e. paralysis in the lower half of the body

3. The vocal tone or phonation produced for speech is the result of _____ .
   a. increased subglottic pressure
   b. adduction of the vocal folds
   c. increased air pressure above the vocal folds
   d. a and b
   e. b and c

4. Several physicians in the 1800s discovered areas of the brain that appear to be integrally involved in speech and language. These areas and their functions include _____ .
   a. Broca's area, which is involved in programming the motor movements for producing speech
   b. Wernicke's area, which is involved in recognizing and interpreting incoming language
   c. Wernicke's area, which is involved in formulating and monitoring our own speech and language as we produce it
   d. a and b
   e. a, b, and c

5. Which of the following structures or systems would be least involved in the production and/or comprehension of speech and language?
   a. autonomic nerves
   b. cranial nerves
   c. cerebellum
   d. spinal nerves
   e. cerebrum

6. Which of the following sequences accurately represents the sequence of development following fertilization of the ovum?
   a. zygote, blastocyst, morula, embryonic disc
   b. zygote, morula, blastocyst, embryonic disc

    c. embryoblast, embryonic disc, morula, zygote

    d. zygote, morula, embryonic disc, blastocyst

    e. embryonic disc, zygote, morula, blastocyst

7. According to most sources, when does the fetal period generally occur?

    a. it extends from conception through the eighth week

    b. it extends from the ninth week to birth

    c. it overlaps all three trimesters

    d. a and c

    e. b and c

8. Which of the following does *not* occur as the infant's neurological system develops?

    a. reflexes become more frequent and pervasive

    b. brain weight increases

    c. dendritic interconnections between neurons become denser

    d. myelination forms along neural pathways

    e. none of the above is accurate

9. Infantile reflexes _____ .

    a. can be characterized as "mass activity" or "specific activity"

    b. can be characterized as providing survival mechanisms

    c. generally diminish over the first 2 years of life

    d. provide the bases for later voluntary behaviors

    e. all of the above are true

10. Which of the following sensory experiences is the most "ready" at birth and will play the most significant role in language development?

    a. vision

    b. auditory

    c. olfactory

    d. gustatory

    e. tactile

Suggested Readings

Caplan, D. (2001). Functional neuroimaging studies of syntactic processing. *Journal of Psycholinguistic Research, 30,* 297–320.

Frederici, A. D. (2001). Syntactic, prosodic, and semantic processes in the brain: Evidence from event-related neuroimaging. *Journal of Psycholinguistic Research, 30,* 237–250.

Green, J. R., Moore, C. A., & Reilly, K. J. (2002). The sequential development of jaw and lip control for speech. *Journal of Speech, Language, and Hearing Research, 45,* 66–79.

Hickok, G. (2001). Functional anatomy of speech perception and speech production: Psycholinguistic implications. *Journal of Psycholinguistic Research, 30,* 225–235.

CHAPTER 3

The Interactive Bases of Human Communication

Mr. Babbles was deep in thought as he pushed the broom along that morning. The hospital hall was particularly quiet with just a few nurses working on records at the maternity ward station. Further down the hall, he stopped outside the nursery window. Soft light escaped from the room beyond, illuminating the rows of basins with small bundles wrapped in clean blankets. He remembered the sweet smell of his first child's head as he gave her a bottle each morning. Her tiny hand wrapped around his large finger, her eyes searched and found his, and then they smiled.

A small sound—a whimper—came from inside. Someone was stirring. Which one? The whimper became a cry, a quivering, effortful call for attention. His youngest daughter was already grown, but this sound still pulled his heartstrings. Still, no one came looking for this small voice. He waited, watching for someone to react to this plaintive call. First a shadow, then a silhouette appeared in the doorway. She moved silently and quickly to attend to this morning's first distress call. A reassured, peaceful grandfather moved quietly down the hall, smiling as he pushed his broom along the shiny floor.

This chapter addresses the following questions:

- What motivates infants to attend to the behaviors of those around them?
- What is the basis for attachment between infants and their caregivers?
- How do infants initiate social interaction with their caregivers?
- What behaviors do caregivers exhibit as they engage their infant's attention and interaction?

- How do children's understanding of experiences grow out of their interactions?

- How do our interactions with the people around us affect the way we come to understand our world?

- What basic learning principles explain how our behaviors change as we interact with the world and people around us?

We will adopt the term *caregiver* because children are raised in many different circumstances. ▪

This chapter discusses the basic foundations for language learning. Understanding how infants interact with, understand, and regulate their environment even before language emerges is important to understanding the information presented in later chapters. ▪

The previous chapter described infants' biological or structural foundations for communication. Even though the basic neurological, auditory, and oral structures are in place at birth, these may not be fully matured for some time. Yet, infants do not passively wait for language to begin its evolution. In fact, their very nature does not allow them to be passive. Their sensory capacities are designed to respond to certain aspects of the environment and their motor capacities provide behaviors that will draw the attention of their caregivers.

It is customary to expect children's first words to occur around their first birthday. Although this momentous first word may wait for approximately a year, every day during that year, infants are pushed along toward it. Infants are impelled by their own changing biological structures. Every day, maturing sensory and motor systems give them new capacities. Every day, as these capacities expand, so do the expectations of those around them. The nurturing behaviors of caregivers change daily with their infant's developing abilities. In turn, each infant's capacities expand in response to the challenges posed by their caregivers, pushing them along toward the most complex social behavior, language.

We may never be able to truly answer the most basic question, "Why do children behave as they do in learning language?" However, we have observed the results of certain interactions and organized those observations at several levels. The infant's development has been viewed from the standpoint of *social* interaction. Certain behaviors, whether random or intentional, function as tools for infants or their caregivers to engage the other as a social partner. Infants' development has also been described in terms of their *cognitive* development. As infants experience the world, it becomes apparent in their behavior that they recall and relate certain aspects of those experiences. Finally, many have regarded infants' development as the evolution of an increasingly efficient *behavioral* repertoire. As they interact within their own social marketplace, the accumulated outcomes of their transactions alter both the likelihood and the form of future actions.

No matter the appeal of any one theory or classification, we must bear in mind that as infants are nurtured, all three domains interact with each other. And, all three are continuously influenced by infants' changing biological capacities. In this chapter we address the social, cognitive, and behavioral factors that interact in a nurturing environment to promote language development.

Social Principles of Learning

Due to the timetable for our species' gestation, the relationship between caregivers and infants is a nurturing one for a relatively long period. Although these interactions may begin as one sided, they evolve into an intense partnership that forms the basis for infants' future social interactions.

The Motivation to Speak

Before any real notion of communication emerges, infants merely possess a fragmented collection of undeveloped capacities evidenced only by random, unintentional behaviors. With their immature senses, infants hear sounds, experience hunger and pain, and react to familiar faces and voices. With only unrefined motor responses available, they move their limbs and change facial expressions reflexively. They gaze only in directions that their meager head control allows and produce a limited selection of random vocal sounds.

Initially, infants do not relate the chaotic sensory experiences impinging on them and their own poorly controlled motor activity. However, as they gradually begin to control their experiences through their own behavior, the seeds of communication are sown. But what, then, prompts this to occur?

As Locke (1993) pointed out, many traditional descriptions of language development assume that the child is naturally interested in language. He pointed out that if this premise is accepted *carte blanche,* then all that researchers need to do is simply enumerate the ages at which various language structures are mastered. However, it is unlikely that at the outset infants are even aware of communication, much less "interested" in language. What they are more likely interested in are the events that provide their most basic needs—food, warmth, sleep, comfort. It would seem that the primary motivation for the infant is to cause the familiar moving mouths, soothing voices, and expressive eyes that accompany this attention to reappear. No matter how simple, the behaviors that result in such outcomes most frequently and reliably will become the early building blocks of social interaction. The infant's interest in language is "primed and nurtured by faces that smile and eyes that attend" (Locke, 1993, p. 142).

To begin this examination of the infant's underlying motivation to communicate, we must appreciate a more fundamental concept—the basis of early nurturing social interaction. **Social interaction** occurs when the behaviors of two individuals mutually influence the subsequent behaviors of the other. Each individual's subsequent behavior is linked to the other's preceding behaviors. The influence exerted might be to direct or distract attention, prompt or facilitate action, even to halt or inhibit action on the part of the other.

It is likely that caregivers are the only participants who are cognizant of any agenda in the earliest interactions. Only caregivers realize that their activities are intended to lead to well-nourished, clean, happy infants (or even for present purposes, a peaceful, sleeping baby).

A more detailed description of the evolution of actual communication behaviors of infants follows in Chapter 5. ∎

social interaction
Successive interchanges between at least two persons in which the behavior of one affects the other.

These earliest forms of caregiving may not technically qualify as "social interactions." Among the many species, human infants are perhaps the most helpless offspring and are dependent on their caregivers' nurturing for a greater proportion of their life span. Human infants will rely on caregivers to tend to their basic biological needs—feeding, diapering, bathing, sleep, safety, and medical concerns—for months and years.

No less important is the need for social stimulation— cuddling, talking, and playing. Whether or not these are instinctive nurturing behaviors, they represent the caregiver's early bids for social exchanges with the infant. Eventually, infants' developing capacities will permit them to go beyond this more passive level of attachment, becoming active partners who contribute more and more in the caregiver-infant interactions.

Caregiver-Infant Attachment

attachment The development of recognition and expectations for interaction between caregivers and infants.

dyad Two individuals interacting as a unit; for example, a caregiver and child.

Attachment refers to the close, nurturing, long-term relationship that develops between the caregiver and the infant. This would imply that the two individuals recognize one another, readily interpret the other's behaviors, and have come to depend on the other's participation to meet certain needs through their interaction. In other words, the two individuals develop an interdependence that defines them as partners or a **dyad.** These needs will certainly become quite complex. However, initially these needs might be primarily emotional for the caregiver and biological for the infant.

Attachment is probably best considered to be a two-way street and there are as many different routes as there are infant-caregiver dyads. Most paths are smooth, some paths are bumpy, and almost all take many unexpected turns along the way by the time the child becomes self-sufficient. Infants and their caregivers contribute different behaviors to the process. At the same time, the individual members within each pair can vary widely in what they contribute.

Infants vary in their temperament—their levels of arousal, irritability, activity, as well as their sleeping, eating, and crying patterns. Most caregivers would not be surprised to find that researchers have identified different patterns of temperament in infants (Westby, 1994b). Infants who maintain more regular schedules, accept changes more readily, and are less upset by discomfort have been described as *easy* (by researchers and caregivers alike). Those who are almost as easy going but draw back from new situations have been labeled *slow-to-warm-up*. Finally, those babies who exhibit less typical routines and express their reactions to the most insignificant disruptions more strongly and negatively have been called *difficult* (again, by researchers and caregivers alike).

On the other side, caregivers also contribute dynamics stemming from their emotional and experiential makeup. The emotional part of being a nurturing adult may be at least partly instinctive, but most would agree that we also learned many of our specific nurturing behaviors and attitudes from the way we were raised. This process underlies many of the best child-rearing traditions families hand down from one generation to the next. However, we should also be aware that this process can also result in cycles that are vicious and destructive. The neglect and abuse, hate, and prejudice that some children suffer through is too often repeated with their own children.

Almost without exception, anyone who has experienced the arrival of his or her first child will agree with the truism, "Your life will never be the same again." Caregivers' adjustment to this tumultuous event is based on a variety of factors including their career obligations, their communication styles, their memories of childhood, and their perception of each other's roles (Lane & Molyneaux, 1992).

There is also a "chemistry" or interaction between the caregiver and infant. Researchers have found that differences in an infant's temperament can influence the caregiver's behaviors toward the infant. Infants who are more frequently alert and more active seem to elicit the most consistent nurturing from their caregivers (Breitmayer & Ricciuti, 1988). On the other hand, more irritable, fearful, or temperamental infants might also have a negative impact on the attachment process. Although some parents might interpret their baby's fussing as attempts at communicating its needs, other parents react with annoyance when the infant makes such demands (Lane & Molyneaux, 1992).

As students and professionals dealing with caregivers and children, it is important to be aware of potentially harmful circumstances. Whenever neglect or abuse of a child is suspected, there is a legal obligation to report it to authorities. Perhaps it is even more critical to anticipate the circumstances that might provoke a caregiver to harm a child. Poor parenting skills, financial or emotional stress, and chemical dependency are all "red flags." Caregivers in high-risk situations should be offered support and appropriate community resources. Even in the most ideal circumstances, being a caregiver is a truly difficult job.

Overall, it would be ideal if nature would arrange a "good fit" for each child's optimal development (Westby, 1994b). It would be desirable if more difficult infants could somehow be raised by caregivers who have greater patience and insight with children. In reality, although we know this cannot always happen, the vast majority of child-caregiver dyads actually exhibit impressive flexibility, patience, and accommodation. These qualities allow for their initial attachment, laying the foundation for their long-term relationship. A number of capacities and behaviors have been examined for the role they may play in forming this attachment. The ways in which these behaviors might contribute to attachment might be divided into two major components—recognition and interaction.

Recognition between Caregivers and Infants

Perhaps the most basic requirement for attachment is **recognition,** the ability of two individuals to attend to and recognize each other's presence, as distinguished from that of others. Historically, the literature in this regard has labeled the 2- to 3-month period following birth as the "undiscriminating social responsiveness" phase (Shulman, 1994, p. 68). This suggests that

recognition The perceptual process of identifying a stimulus as having been experienced previously; the ability of individuals to attend to and identify a particular person's presence.

the newborns are initially incapable of recognizing their caregivers at any level. This may have been a reasonable assumption given what is known about the infant's immature visual and auditory systems. However, it may be that researchers had not yet discovered a means for infants to signal their recognition of significant persons, especially their biological mothers.

Recent research has found that infants are capable of signaling recognition when allowed to use an available response mode to do so. For example, very young infants might express a "preference" by learning to produce different sucking patterns that selectively expose them to certain stimuli. In fact, through such means infants have demonstrated that they can recognize their mother's odor, voice, and face.

Recognition of Olfactory Cues.   Infants have the ability to recognize their mother through their sense of smell. Infants who breast-feed have been found to discriminate between their mother and other women strictly on the basis of their odor. (The ladies who participated would all probably prefer the term "fragrance.") Interestingly, this recognition of olfactory cues goes both ways. It has also been found that 2 days after birth mothers can discriminate their own infant from other 2-day-old infants on the basis of smell. Research in human olfactory cues suggests that a mother's odor is more chemically similar to her infant than is that of other women. This might be as a result of their shared genetic makeup; that is, they very likely have similar body chemistries which might be detectable through olfaction (Locke, 1993).

It takes very little to recognize the strong role of smell in our emotions. So many emotions are stirred by the smell of our child's head, our loved one's favorite fragrance, or our favorite home-cooked meal. Research suggests that we begin to establish these connections very early.

The significance of smells in emotional attachment has been described in neurological terms as well. Cortical areas responsible for integrating smell with emotional arousal have been referred to as the *emotional brain.* The same connections integrate smell with basic vegetative functions, in particular feeding (Bhatnagar & Andy, 1995). This neurological relationship suggests that infants' physical closeness to their caregivers while feeding ensures that caregivers' olfactory cues are closely associated with this nurturing experience.

Recognition of Vocal Cues.   Infants also have been shown to recognize their mother's voice almost immediately following birth with seemingly little exposure to it (DeCasper & Fifer, 1980). One-day-old infants have learned to suck at faster or slower rates to "choose" whether they would hear recordings of their mother's voice as opposed to another adult female. It is instructive to note that the early versions of the mothers' voices had been filtered to sound as they would when transmitted through the uterine wall. Therefore, these infants' initial recognition abilities were based on substantial experience, even though it was *in utero.* Nonetheless, these results suggest the possibility that infants are capable at some level of perceiving their mother's presence, at least when given the auditory cues present in her voice.

On the other side of this dyad, it has been suggested that mothers are able to recognize their infant's cry within 48 hours following birth. In fact, in maternity wards where six mothers and their babies shared the same space, after just the third night, mothers were awakened only by the cry of their own baby (Formby, 1967). (Some would suggest this is an ability that few fathers develop with just one baby in the house for a year!)

Recognition of Facial Cues.   The importance of the caregiver's face in establishing attachment cannot be overestimated. It is the first and most available source for reflecting emotional affect. Of even greater consequence is the fact that it is also the source of the mother's voice. (Of course, this is obvious to us, but maybe not so to the infant.) The fact that this already familiar voice emanates from her face makes it that much more intriguing from the very start. Furthermore, the mother's face is consistently associated with satisfying the infant's most basic need, nourishment. During feedings (even for those who are bottle-fed) the mother's face is strategically located at the optimal distance and position, given the infant's visual acuity and abilities.

As mentioned in the previous chapter, researchers have found that infants pay more attention to stylized stimuli using geometric shapes to approximate the human face than stimuli incorporating the same geometric shapes scrambled to bear no such resemblance.

Of greater relevance to attachment are findings that infants evidence a visual preference for their mother's faces within the first several days following birth (Locke, 1993). As Locke pointed out, this remarkable facility would at first seem to be almost instinctive. The infant has had precious little time to study its mother's face as it has spent most of those first few days sleeping. Furthermore, even when awake, its visual acuity is supposedly limited. Locke, among others, speculates that the explanation for this rapid learning may come from the fact that the infant's first exposure to the mother's face is most likely associated with her voice, a stimulus that is already familiar from the infant's intrauterine experiences. This might be further supported by the observation that infants' preference for their mothers' faces is even stronger when her voice is also available (Field, Cohen, Garcia, & Greenberg, 1984).

By the time infants are 7 months, they will begin to associate particular faces with voices, fixing their gaze on the appropriate photograph when exposed to a recording of each parent's voice (Spelke & Owsley, 1979). Finally, it is not surprising that on the other side of this "two-way street" the caregivers, from a very early point, quite readily distinguish the facial features of their infant from other infants (Porter, Boyle, Hardister, & Balogh, 1989). This should be somewhat reassuring to those nervous first-time fathers who worry that "babies all look alike." It seems that when it's yours, the facial features are so important you memorize them instantly!

Interaction between Caregivers and Infants

Infants' recognition of and attachment to their primary caregivers sets the stage for true social interactions to emerge. As if adults' infatuation with their baby is not enough, the infant's biological and emotional needs will certainly prompt plenty of opportunities for social contact. Even though caregivers' talking to their infant is essentially one sided, it will likely accompany most interactions, as caregivers seem compelled to narrate most every activity.

Although adults are not consciously "teaching" speech and language to their child through their narration, their facial and vocal behaviors are an integral part of every interaction. As Locke described it, "The facial and vocal movements produced by people who are talking are the currency of social transactions" (Locke, 1993, p. 104). Furthermore, it is a currency that compounds in value. Because infants recognize the faces and voices that are a central part of every interaction, they take on increasing importance. So much so that the infant naturally attends to every movement and sound emanating from them. It is as though they cannot get enough of these smiling faces, expressive eyes, and moving mouths.

With repeated exposures during the everyday routines of eating, dressing, diapering, bathing, and cuddling, infants' behavior gradually becomes intertwined with those of nurturing adults. Finally, as infants begin to anticipate adult nurturing behaviors, their own behaviors begin to interact with and influence the adults' nurturing routines. Out of these nurturing routines, the beginnings of social interaction are, in fact, nurtured.

The early foundations of this process include physical, vocal, emotional, and visual components that occur on both sides of the caregiver-infant dyad. The process eventually culminates in more outward demonstrations of social interaction in which the adult and infant experience mutual interest in a shared object or activity and even reproduce each other's behaviors.

Physical Contact.   Touch is a primary avenue for emotional communication. Close proximity helps the caregiver understand the infant's level of excitement, comfort, pleasure, and displeasure. Through physical contact, infants' levels of activity, tension, or calmness are directly transmitted to caregivers. Infants' moods and physical states are conveyed to receptive adults by their fidgety wriggling or their relaxed calmness. These signals allow caregivers to adjust the manner in which they hold their infant or to consider their infant's other physical needs (e.g., hunger, warmth). Conversely, the infant is apparently capable of perceiving similar cues from their caregivers. Most have seen an otherwise calm baby squirm in the arms of a nervous, uncomfortable adult.

Physical contact between infants and caregivers is as necessary as breathing. In the most basic sense, infants would not survive without it. Infants' survival needs must be met through the intervention of caregivers.

This is virtually impossible to do without establishing some level of physical contact. Caregivers must be in close proximity to provide for their infant's every biological need. Feeding, bathing, diapering, and quieting infants are all definitely hands-on tasks. The required proximity, that is, the closeness that is part of these tasks, brings the caregiver's voice and face into the infant's immediate experience.

Although all of the infant's needs met through physical contact are important, perhaps feeding occurs with the greatest frequency and urgency. For most caregiver-infant dyads, early feeding sessions provide the most consistent form of physical contact. Generally, whether the infant is breast-fed or bottle-fed, it will be held against the caregiver's body in a way that allows the two to conform to each other's shape. While in this contact, the infant simultaneously experiences the relief of hunger with the closeness, warmth, and rhythmical breathing of its caregiver. For the caregiver, this provides the opportunity to hold, examine, and view the infant closely while experiencing a sense of satisfaction in providing for its needs.

Infants' sensory and motor capacities will be limited for some time. However, feeding, the most natural connection with caregivers, provides the perfect platform for social interaction to evolve. The process of providing nourishment is a vital mechanism for nurturing social interaction. (Fortunately, at this stage of life, there's no such thing as a "drive thru.")

Infant Vocalization and Motherese. The production of vocal sounds from either partner provides another critical basis for the development of interaction. These exchanges may not be true communication for some time, but if social interaction is demonstrated when the behavior of one partner influences the behavior of the other, then this form of interaction qualifies as social from a very early point.

The beginnings of social interaction may be found in the infant's earliest reflexive cry vocalizations. The infant's overall internal state is reflected in the vocalizations it produces. The different physical states of the infant—hunger, pain, general discomfort—are the stimuli that trigger the basic primitive reflex of crying. This reflexive activity generally includes a tensing of the infant's muscles, visually evident in its tensed limbs, clenched fists, and facial grimacing. This tension also becomes audible as a cry when the baby forces air through the tensed vocal folds.

The characteristics and significance of infant vocalizations are discussed in Chapter 5. ■

Although unintentional, the infant's cries have a demonstrable effect on the caregiver's behavior. Just as we have always assumed, researchers have found that most infant cries are followed by a responsive caregiver's action. Caregivers' responses to infant cries may teach infants the most fundamental lesson about communication—the vocal behavior of one individual can influence the behavior of another.

Here again, it is important to recognize that cultures differ. In some societies, infant cries are not treated as pleas for attention. In other cultures, infants are attended to so continuously that they rarely need to cry.

Following birth, the infant's cries reportedly differentiate to signal different causes. Researchers have identified four basic cries in infants—the birth cry, hunger cry, pain cry, and anger cry (Wolff, 1969). More important, research suggests that mothers can discriminate among certain cries and the basic needs that might underlie them. It has even been speculated that by 2 months of age infants might cry deliberately to gain the attention of their caregivers (Lane & Molyneaux, 1992). Whether or not it is a conscious ploy, the influence of infants' crying over their caregivers' behavior is an almost universal form of early social interaction.

With maturation, crying becomes less reflexive and the associated breathing patterns more closely resemble those that will eventually accompany speech. It has been speculated that the inhibition of the cry reflex is evidence of both infants' neurological maturation and their responsiveness to their caregivers' vocalizations. Caregivers' speech has been closely associated with other nurturing activities (e.g., feeding). As caregivers talk soothingly to comfort their crying infant, the infants may associate this sound with pleasant circumstances and find it consoling. It is difficult to cry and listen at the same time, so infants suppress their cry in order to hear their caregiver's voice. Again, infants' responding to their partner's voice in this way may represent yet another seed of social interaction.

The characteristics and role of *motherese* in language learning is discussed further in Chapters 5 and 6. ▪

On the other side of the dyad, caregivers not only respond to the crying, cooing, babbling, and even burping, but they also adjust their speech patterns in response to their partner's abilities. These adjustments result in a phenomenon referred to as *motherese,* or more traditionally, as **baby talk.** Caregivers (as well as most older children and adults) tend to shorten and simplify their utterances, exaggerate their prosody and enunciation, vary their rate, and use more pronounced facial expressions while talking to infants. These characteristics of motherese appear to highlight the adult's speech and frequently elicit infants' attention. Research suggests that infants attend more closely to such vocal patterns and are more likely to respond with vocalizations themselves (Owens, 2005).

baby talk   Characteristic speech patterns, including shorter phrases and exaggerated intonation, used when talking to infants.

Eye Contact and Eye Gaze.   When it comes to human communication, "The eyes have it!" Of course, it is actually the "ayes" giving an affirming vote that prompts this phrase. Nonetheless, our eyes have an intriguing role in human communication. The mainstream American culture requires that we look each other in the eye to determine the truth value of what is said. We raise an eyebrow of disapproval and squint our skepticism through doubting eyelids. Anyone who appreciates the art of flirting knows that it would just not be the same without eye contact. Research has even shown that speechreading is more efficient when facial activity including the eyes is available to supplement the speaker's mouth. Locke (1993) has even suggested that their role in communication should earn for our eyes the status of "full-fledged members of the 'articulatory' system" (p. 55).

Infants also find the eyes a source of intrigue from a very early time. Infants as young as 3 to 11 weeks old evidence a preference for looking at the eyes and the nearby borders of the face (Haith, Bergman, & Moore, 1977). This was the case even when the face was talking, when one would expect the associated mouth movements to be of greater interest. Complementing this phenomenon on the other side of the dyad, mothers have reported a greater sense of emotional fulfillment while feeding an infant if eye contact is established (Klaus & Kennell, 1976).

When infants combine eye contact with a smile, there is the sense of the first true **social smile.** By the middle of the second month they are able to engage their partners in long intervals of eye contact (Wolff, 1963). Infants fixate their stare with bright, widened eyes—and they usually win such "staring contests" hands down. On the other side of the dyad, watchful caregivers are typically looking at their infants when they establish eye contact. The caregiver is then usually drawn to respond by coming closer, vocalizing, and initiating play with the infant.

social smile A smile in response to another person's presence or behavior.

Infants' use of their eyes to influence caregiver behavior has been categorized by researchers into different patterns (Owens, 2005). In **mutual gaze,** infants are thought to be signaling increased interest in the person with whom they are sharing eye contact. A second pattern, called **gaze coupling,** follows an alternating pattern of eye contact much like that seen in later conversations. Finally, in using **deictic gaze,** infants effectively point with their eyes at objects that intrigue them. Caregivers can follow the infant's line of sight to find the object of apparent interest. Conversely, the infant may also follow the caregiver's gaze, shifting back and forth between the caregiver's face and the object of their attention. These behaviors may appear as early as 2 months and increase rapidly by 8 months (Locke, 1993).

mutual gaze Shared eye contact with a partner to signal attention.

gaze coupling A gaze pattern in which caregivers and infants maintain eye contact in long, alternating intervals.

deictic gaze A gaze pattern in which visual focus on an object directs a partner's attention to that object.

Deictic gaze introduces a third dimension to infants' interaction with their caregivers, creating a triad. By visually including an object in their interaction, the adult and infant then share its associated words and actions.

Joint Attention.   A basic requirement in social interaction is **joint attention**—whether both partners share attention to the same topic. This aspect has been an important area of research in examining the social interaction between caregivers and their infants. Two forms of joint attention that have been of interest are joint reference and joint action.

joint attention Shared attention on a context by partners.

Joint reference is established when an object becomes the focus of shared attention between partners. When caregivers talk to their infants, it is frequently **referential** in nature. That is, it is said that caregivers' behaviors refer or "point" to some object. Furthermore, the things they talk about are most often in the immediate present—the "here and now." These characteristics provide the basic elements for a conversation—two partners and a topic available to both. Caregivers frequently exhibit any of several behaviors to establish their infant's attention on the item they are describing to the infant (Bruner, 1977).

joint reference Establishing an object as the shared topic of communication.

referential Behaving in ways that identify a stimulus as the topic for communication.

joint actions   Actions shared by partners that result in their mutual or shared attention.

■ The behaviors associated with establishing joint reference and joint action are discussed in greater detail in Chapter 5. ■

Turn taking   The alternation of speaking and listening behaviors in a conversation.

Bruner (1977) has also stressed the importance of **joint actions,** familiar routines that join the infant and caregiver in shared activity. These joint actions evolve out of the most basic activities shared by the infant-caregiver dyad—feeding, bathing, diapering—and evolve into true social games.

These joint actions are critical to infants' development of language. Because of their inherent nature as *routines,* these shared events provide repeated, familiar contexts in which a limited set of words are used to refer to a very predictable sequence of actions. Underlying all this is the fact that these interactions typically occur in the most pleasant circumstances, strengthening the attachment between caregivers and infants.

Turn Taking.   A major aspect of social interaction is **turn taking,** the alternating contributions of speakers and listeners. Turn taking is an essential skill for later communication as partners sharing ideas must take turns speaking and listening. When infants and caregivers alternate in contributing to a sequence of behaviors, no matter how subtle, they are laying an important foundation for later communication. This seems to evolve out of the various aspects of recognition, attachment, and social interaction.

Researchers trace the beginnings of turn taking back to the earliest feeding sessions. In these early interactions, caregivers and infants engage in a distinctive pattern in which the caregiver attempts to adapt to the infant's feeding pattern. What evolves is a dialogue of sorts in which the infant sucks for an interval, then pauses. The mother, in turn, responds to this pause by jiggling the baby or the nipple to stimulate the infant's feeding again.

The alternation of turns seen in feeding sessions is also evident later in the infant's responses to the caregiver's vocalizations and play behaviors. As noted in describing joint actions, infants soon learn the routine and how to fill their turn. Infants are more likely to vocalize following vocalization by the caregiver. The turn taking by the infant and caregiver in these interactions is so much like the behavior of mature conversational partners they have been called *protoconversations* (Bateson, 1971).

Imitation.   The old adage says that "imitation is the highest form of flattery." This probably describes a critical dynamic in the infant-caregiver relationship. The caregiver is present from the beginning in the infant's most vital experiences—feeding, cuddling, diapering. The caregiver's facial expressions, gestures, vocal intonation, and speech are intimately associated with these events. Although the infant is not yet conscious of this, there are few others whose behaviors will be so important to emulate.

■ Imitation is not always intentional, even later in life. It is always interesting to hear your friends say, "Oh my gosh, I sound just like my mother!" ■

There are numerous questions surrounding research in this area. Nonetheless, it has been found that within hours of birth, infants are capable of reproducing facial gestures such as tongue protrusion, mouth opening, and lip protrusion (Meltzoff & Moore, 1977). Kuhl and Meltzoff (1982) found that very young infants vocalized in synchronized response to a woman's face, producing rhythmical series of vowels. It was later found that

90% of the vocalizations that were speechlike could be categorized by adult listeners. Later development of infants' phonetic inventories has been found to increasingly reflect the repertoires of their caregivers. This phenomenon, called *phonetic drift,* is why babies of French parents sound increasingly French and babies of American parents sound increasingly American.

The underlying mechanism for imitation is essentially unknown. However, beyond the obvious prerequisite biological capacity to reproduce the behavior in question, it appears to have its roots in the notion that reproducing events that have strong positive associations is in itself rewarding. Reinforcing the social nature of imitation, several researchers have found that infants appear most inclined to "talk" to faces and especially if those faces are talking to them (Locke, 1993).

Cultural Differences in Caregiver-Infant Interactions

The preceding information should all be interpreted with some caution. Much of the research with regard to infant-caregiver interaction has been carried out in the mainstream American culture. There are very likely significant differences among the different cultural and socioeconomic groups within the American population, and certainly differences exist in other cultures around the world (Westby, 1994b).

For example, it has been found that some African American families do not perceive their infants as communicative and are less likely to respond to their cries and vocalizations. Lower socioeconomic status mothers are generally less responsive to their infants' vocalizations and they are less likely to use questions.

Tribes in New Guinea do not reduce the complexity of their language to their children, and Samoans are generally less responsive to their children's utterances (Westby, 1994b). Even the amount of infant crying might vary according to the culture. In more primitive cultures, infants carried with the mother throughout the day may be more frequently attended to and have less need to cry. In fact the very notion of a singly important caregiver may not apply in cultures that rely on extended family members to raise the children.

Every student of human behavior (and, we all are) should remember that "my way is not necessarily the right way." Children all over the world learn to talk and communicate, so considerable variation and latitude in these social interactions must support language development.

Summary

- Infants' motivation to communicate may grow out of the nurturing social interactions that reliably follow their early random or reflexive behaviors.

- Infants attend to and quickly learn to recognize olfactory, facial, and vocal cues associated with their caregivers.

- Through daily nurturing interactions, caregivers and infants share physical contact, distinctive vocalization, and speech patterns while establishing joint attention on topics in the here and now.

- Although cultures may vary, the nurturing interactions that occur through the infant-caregiver dyad facilitates recognition and social interaction between infants and caregivers.

Cognitive Principles of Learning

cognition The mental processes related to organizing and understanding experience.

A natural result of the nurturing infants receive is the movement, handling, and stimulation they experience. As infants learn to respond to these experiences in predictable ways, it suggests the evolution of cognition. **Cognition,** understanding our experiences through mental processes such as perception, recall, and reasoning, provides an important element for the development of language.

Piaget's Origins of Intelligence

Jean Piaget, born in Switzerland in 1896, was a child prodigy who had his first scientific article published when he was just 11 years old. His early interest was biology, but this was later broadened to include philosophy and logic. In particular, he became intrigued with the field of *epistemology,* the study of the origins of knowledge. These two fields, biology and epistemology, eventually combined in their influence on Piaget's studies of cognition.

While assisting in the development of standardized intelligence tests at the Binet Laboratory in Paris, France, Piaget had ample opportunity to interact with children. In this work with children, Piaget became fascinated with the *incorrect* answers of younger children to test questions. In these responses he recognized that younger children did not simply know *quantitatively* less than older children. Instead, their incorrect responses reflected a *qualitatively* different thought process (Ginsburg & Opper, 1969).

Subsequently, Piaget spent his years developing his concept of how intelligence evolves. In describing intelligence as a special case of biological adaptation, Piaget characterized cognition as "one kind of biological achievement, which allows the individual to interact effectively with the environment" (Ginsburg & Opper, 1969, p. 14). In his view, the two domains—biology and cognition—inherently interact as the individual organism changes its behavior in response to its changing experiences. Viewed in this way, intelligence was not a fixed, predetermined quantity, but an evolving process that changes with physical maturation and experience (Ginsburg & Opper, 1969).

In Piaget's view, our inherited biological structures define the form and limits of our intelligence. For example, creatures that have evolved with less-developed vocal tracts will not develop articulate speech or verbal intelligence as we know it. Piaget also suggested that the influence of inherited biological structures on infants' behavior, in the form of reflexes, is greatest in the days immediately following birth. Infants eventually modify these reflexes in response to their experiences and maturing neurological system. Within this framework, Piaget made extensive observations and kept detailed records of children's developing cognitive abilities (Ginsburg & Opper, 1969).

The Nature of Intelligence

To Piaget, intelligence was not a static quantity, but a dynamic process. Piaget proposed three major cognitive principles that are fundamental to the development of intelligence—equilibrium, organization, and adaptation.

According to Piaget, the driving force behind our developing cognition is **equilibrium.** This concept generally refers to the need for balance between forces, whether biological, physical, or psychological. Cognitively, when children are confronted with an unfamiliar experience, the equilibrium between this novelty and their understanding of the environment is disturbed. The mismatch or disequilibrium must then be resolved to regain the balance between the children's understanding and experience of their environment.

equilibrium The goal of adaptive processes in cognition in which new information is assimilated or accommodated.

As Piaget characterized the nature of intelligence, another central concept was **organization.** As organisms evolve, their biological systems (e.g., respiratory and circulatory systems) organize and interact more effectively for improved survival. As our understanding of the world evolves, we also organize physical systems and cognitive responses to interact with the environment more effectively. For example, in order to explore, the first mechanism available to the infant is *grasping.* It will be recalled (from Chapter 2) that this behavior is initially mediated by the primitive palmar reflex; when an object is placed in infants' palms, their fingers reflexively close around it. Of course, this limits exploration to just those items placed in their palm or those that the hand haphazardly lands on.

organization The cognitive process of structuring patterns of interaction to deal more effectively with the environment.

As infants develop better voluntary control over their arms, they can organize *limb extending* with *grasping* to independently explore items within their reach. Of course, the primary structure for experiencing the world to this point has been the infant's mouth. (Remember, all they do is eat and sleep and . . .). So, of course, to examine items further they automatically begin *mouthing* them. Eventually, they will organize additional elements for more effective exploration by obtaining objects through *pointing.* Ultimately, by organizing motor and verbal responses, they can add even more sophisticated means of exploring, as in *asking* with an outstretched pointer finger, "What's in that big box on the top shelf, Daddy?"

According to Piaget, individuals organize behaviors into an identifiable pattern called a **scheme.** These organized patterns, or *schemata,* are not static but are continuously modified in response to changing biological structures and experiences. In a similar way, as children collect experiences through

scheme Organized patterns of responding to stimuli.

adaptation   The
cognitive process of
organizing new
experiences to achieve
equilibrium in one's
understanding of the
world.

assimilation   A process
of cognitive adaptation in
which new experiences
are organized into existing
schemes.

accommodation   A
process of cognitive
adaptation that modifies
an existing scheme in
response to new
experiences.

the various schemes, they are assembled and organized into cognitive structures. Children develop cognitive structures that represent organized information about all of their experiences with sensations, movement, sounds, locations, people, objects, and speech, among others.

Just as infants' schemes evolve with new experiences, so will their cognitive structures, their organized understanding of a changing environment. The process of modifying our understanding of a changing environment, our cognitive structures, is called **adaptation.** In reality, the environment may be changing less and our biological and behavioral capabilities to experience it are changing more. Nonetheless, to reestablish equilibrium, the individual must adapt to new experiences. Piaget described two major processes for this adaptation: assimilation and accommodation. **Assimilation** refers to the individual's tendency to deal with new experiences in terms of currently available cognitive structures. **Accommodation** is a complementary process in which the individual changes existing structures or develops new ones to deal with new experiences.

To illustrate, a toddler who has just learned to label the family's Boston terrier as a "Doggie" might easily assimilate the Chihuahua next door without having to change the underlying cognitive structure. However, the Great Dane across the street will not fit. To accommodate this new experience, the toddler must modify his cognitive structure for *doggie*. The child may also later try to assimilate the first experience of a cat by calling it a "doggie." Most likely, the family will intervene by providing a new label, saying "No, it's a *kitty*." Although the new label (*kitty*) may accelerate the process, the child must also find a way to adapt to this mismatch—it is furry and four-legged with a tail, but it does not bark, wag its tail, or lick your hand. To accommodate this new experience, a new cognitive structure must be created that organizes the new features for *kitty*.

Obviously, this is a simplified illustration. The underlying processes as the child proceeds through the myriad of experiences life offers are far more subtle and complex.

Stages of Intelligence

Because Piaget viewed intelligence as a continuous process of biological and cognitive adaptation, he eventually described the stages in its development. As with any stage model, Piaget's stages are characterizations of the broad, overlapping periods that seemed to reflect changes in the nature of intelligence.

Piaget described four broad stages of cognitive development: sensorimotor, preoperational, concrete operational, and formal operational. The stages occur in a progression, because an individual must master the features of one to progress to the next. The major features of Piaget's stages are presented in Table 3–1. Although all four are described briefly, we will later examine the sensorimotor period more extensively due to its obvious relationship to the cognitive developments in infancy.

Table 3–1. Piaget's stages of cognitive development.

Sensorimotor (0–2 yrs.)	Preoperational (2–7 yrs.)	Concrete Operational (7–11 yrs.)	Formal Operational (11-Adult)
Infants and toddlers:	Preschoolers:	Young students:	Adolescents and adults:
Initially rely on reflexive actions.	Initially use words to represent broad categorizations.	Develop ability to consider more than one dimension in problem solving.	Demonstrate ability to categorize abstract classes and relationships.
Repeat interesting actions (primary circular reaction).	Begin categorizing objects through direct paired comparisons.	Reason flexibly by mentally reversing processes.	Demonstrate ability to reason flexibly and verbally through complex problems.
Combine existing schemes with new stimuli (secondary circular reactions).	Gradually refine word meanings.	Begin mentally categorizing objects without direct comparisons.	Demonstrate ability to reason through hypothesis testing.
Imitate actions they already perform.	Perceive situations from their perspective only (egocentric thought).		
Imitate new actions not previously performed.	Focus on one dimension in problem solving.		
Demonstrate intention to influence behavior of others (means-end).			
Actively search for missing objects or persons (object permanence).			
Play with objects flexibly (symbolic play).			

Sensorimotor. Piaget named the period from birth to 2 years the sensori-motor period. As this name implies, a major task for infants is to gain greater control over integrating their sensory and motor systems. At birth, infants are served only by their reflexes, responding to most events or sensations with little or no voluntary control. However, eventually as these reflexes become differentiated, infants exhibit increased voluntary motor control. A second major feature of this period is the maturation in infants' ability to mentally represent reality. As they progress through this period, they show sustained interest in novel events. Infants attempt to cause novel events to reoccur and imitate the behaviors of others, eventually when they are no longer present. Infants search for interesting objects that have disappeared. In all of these developments, infants demonstrate their emerging recognition that the environment has a reality that is outside of their own.

Preoperational.   Piaget's second period in the development of intelligence is the preoperational period, from 2 to 7 years of age. During this period children become better able to represent the environment's reality through symbolic behavior. They make major headway in developing language. Children exhibit problem-solving skills and begin the process of categorizing and sorting the world. In spite of all this development, children continue to see the world only from their own (*egocentric*) point of view.

Concrete Operations.   The third period, from 7 to 11 years, is referred to as the concrete operational period. This period is characterized by the child's improved ability to use reasoning, especially in relation to more concrete relationships, such as size, mass, or volume. Classification of their experiences of the world becomes more organized and hierarchical and they continue to develop the ability to see things from the perspective of others, a process called *decentration*.

Formal Operations.   Finally, during the fourth period, 11 years of age and beyond, individuals become capable of formal operations involving abstract reasoning, hypothetical ("what if"), and deductive thought processes. In addition, they become even more flexible in modifying their perspective to consider the viewpoints of others.

Sensorimotor Foundations for Language

Of the available cognitive models, Piaget's has clearly received the majority of attention in the literature addressing language development. In particular, several aspects of the sensorimotor period have attracted the attention of language researchers. This appears to be the case because, logically speaking, it seems likely that these dimensions would be closely related to the emergence of language in the infant and toddler. However, research intended to verify their contributions is still in the early stages. A number of different relationships among these aspects and language, or altogether different theoretical perspectives, could eventually emerge (Highnam, 1994). Yet, for the present, the following Piagetian sensorimotor principles seem to be the central topics of current research in cognitive interactions and language.

Imitation.   Piaget recognized the value of imitation. He considered it a critical means for infants to expand their interactions with the environment. Imitation technically involves the recognition of the existence of the behavior of others and the ability to mentally translate that behavior into one's own actions to reproduce it.

Infants appear to imitate various facial expressions and gestures at a very early point. They imitate the actions that have occurred with objects to seemingly represent the object. In the infant's babbling and later vocal play, we hear the sounds and intonational contours of adult speech.

In previous discussion, imitation was also discussed in the context of social interaction. However, Piaget considered the earliest forms of imitation to be more cognitive in nature, stemming from infants' tendency to reproduce their own interesting behaviors ("primary circular reactions"). Piaget considered younger infants to be incapable of distinguishing between events stemming from their own behavior and that of others. In this case, early instances that seemed to be vocal imitation, where infants reproduce series of sounds from a model, may actually result from the infants' perception that the sounds originated from themselves. The following notes by Piaget (Ginsburg & Opper, 1969, p. 40) describe some of the earliest developments he noted:

> At 0;1(21) [zero years, one month, and 21 days], Lucienne spontaneously uttered the sound rra, but did not react at once when I reproduced it. At 0;1;(24), however, when I made a prolonged aa, she twice uttered a similar sound, although she had been silent for a quarter of an hour.
> At 0;1(25) she was watching me while I said "a ha, ha, rra," etc, I noticed certain movements of her mouth, movements not of suction but of vocalization.
> At 0;3(5) I noted a differentiation in the sounds of her laughter. I imitated them. She reacted by reproducing them quite clearly, but only when she had already uttered them immediately before.

Later the infant demonstrates *selective imitation,* which more clearly reproduces certain aspects of other's behavior, and *deferred imitation,* in which the model is no longer present. Regardless of its origins or the age of its true occurrence, Piaget recognized the importance of imitation in expanding children's repertoire of behaviors for interacting with the environment. Imitation in language learning has continued to be an important source of some controversy.

The issue of imitation is discussed again in some detail in Chapters 4, 6, and 8.

Means-End.   Attaining a desired goal through purposeful action is what Piaget characterized as **means-end** schemata. As their social interactions evolve, infants' opportunities to recognize the reality of their external world also increase. The interaction brings to their attention the fact that the world contains important people (family and significant others), interesting objects, and events. As children increasingly understand that these experiences can *re*occur, repeated interaction with these people, objects, and events becomes the goals of their behavior.

means-end Cognitive ability to apply a scheme or behavior pattern to achieve a desired goal.

A simple example of means-end behavior would include infants pulling their blanket (the means) toward themselves to reach a favorite toy (the end) positioned on it. Many researchers have related this kind of behavior, the use of tools, to the eventual use of gestures and words (Highnam, 1994). In the same way that infants learn that different objects can serve as tools to obtain a desired object, they later learn that gestures, vocalizations, and eventually words serve as very effective tools when directed to an interested and willing caregiver. Overall, researchers have found strong relationships between children's means-end abilities and the development of communication and language skills (Highnam, 1994).

Object Permanence.   Object permanence is the concept that the physical world has an existence beyond our immediate experience. That is, things exist whether or not we can see them. When we leave our car out of view in a parking lot, we know that it still exists. (Even if it is no longer there when we return, we know it still exists!) The fact that a language symbol can refer to people, events, objects, and relationships among them indicates that these exist in some form, even when they are absent. Such a statement seems so simple and yet is as paradoxical as Descartes's rational proof of his own reality, *Cogito, ergo sum* ("I think, therefore I am").

According to Piaget, the reality of the external world is something that only gradually emerges for the infant. For young infants, the objects they experience exist only in their mind. When they are no longer part of their immediate experience, the objects no longer exist to them. Infants demonstrate this when we simply cover an object that is currently the focus of their attention. Although it is only hidden by a towel and would be revealed by simply removing the towel, infants at this stage behave as if it has vanished into thin air. Additional experience with things that disappear and reappear allows infants to gradually recognize that objects continue to exist even when they cannot be seen.

Piaget and many others reasoned that the development of object permanence is fundamental to language. Because the nature of language is to represent the world through symbols, it seems logical that the infant must first recognize the separate existence of the things that language represents. If objects outside of our immediate experience no longer existed, we would not be able to refer to them with language. In fact, there would be no need to as we would not talk about something that does not exist.

In spite of its logical importance, much of the research with regard to object permanence has been conflicting (Highnam, 1994). It may be an important underlying concept whose initial appearance is prerequisite to language, but whose subsequent development does not otherwise correlate with the further development of language.

Symbolic Function.   The ability to allow one thing to represent another thing is what Piaget called **symbolic function.** Symbolism is the essence of language. The words of language stand for the things they refer to. Even the relationships between words represent the relationships between their referents.

symbolic function   The cognitive process of using symbols to represent actual objects or events.

Piaget placed the symbolic function in his second stage, the preoperational stage of intelligence, where children will make the greatest progress in using language. However, the symbolic function certainly has its roots in the sensorimotor period and may actually emerge before the child enters the preoperational period.

In the beginning of the sensorimotor period, the infant has a view of the world that is *egocentric* and closely tied to its *concrete* reality. The infant's view of the world is called egocentric because infants do not have a concept of themselves as existing separately from the world around them. Their earliest experiences are simply a part of them because they are incapable of conceiving of anything beyond their own experience. Infants' behavior is *concrete* because they are only capable of acknowledging those things that are physically present. Younger infants imitated only behaviors that were present and physically available, perhaps without even distinguishing the model's actions from their own.

By the end of the sensorimotor period, infants have begun to represent the world in a more *conceptual* way. This shows itself in their imitation, gestures, play, and, ultimately, in their words. The ability to delay imitation indicates that they can mentally represent the model's original behavior and then reproduce it some time later. Where earlier demands for feeding were tied to the physical presence of a bottle, they can later point to its usual location (the refrigerator) and reproduce appropriate gestures and vocalizations to signal their requests. Earlier play was tied more directly to the actual function of objects. Pushing a toy car, rolling a ball, combing a doll's hair with a toy comb are all examples of earlier *functional play*. Later, when children use a wooden block for a car, turn a ball into a spaceship, or pretend to comb a doll's hair with a ruler, they are demonstrating *symbolic play*, in which one thing is used to represent another. Casby (2003) described eight levels of symbolic play previously described by Piaget that extend from the sensorimotor period into the preoperational period. These primarily vary based on the extent to which the child projects actions onto objects or another person and the extent to which the child combines sequences of action schemes. These are summarized in Table 3–2.

Although there are still many questions regarding the relationship of symbolic function to language, it appears to be a relationship worth examining (Owens, 2005; Patterson & Westby, 1994). What form do the mental symbols take? Are they visual images, auditory traces, sensorimotor patterns, or verbal stimuli? We might speculate that they are different for different individuals. Perhaps persons who are hearing impaired operate with visual symbols. Perhaps younger children manipulate symbols that are

 It is important to recognize the difference between a *symbol* and a *sign;* sources vary on how they define these terms. For the present discussion, a *symbol* is a stimulus that stands for a referent *without bearing any physical resemblance to it.* In contrast, a sign stands for something *by sharing some physical resemblance with it.*

For example, some "road signs" are technically "symbols." Those red octagonal "signs" with four white letters spelling STOP bear no direct resemblance to the behavior they prompt. In contrast, those yellow triangular signs with a figurative truck on a sloped line do bear some physical similarity to what they represent—"hill ahead." The latter, therefore, is truly a road *sign.*

Table 3–2. Piaget's developmental levels of symbolic play.

Level	Age	Description	Example
IA	18 mos.	**Projection of schemes into new objects** Applying familiar actions they have used themselves to other people or objects	After playing "pretend to sleep" for some time, the child puts teddy bears and dolls to bed to pretend they are sleeping.
IB	18 mos.	**Projection of imitative schemes onto new objects** Imitating the action of others with objects that are not typical play items.	Pretending to use a needle and thread to sew or pretending to read a newspaper.
IIA	24 mos.	**Simple identification of one object with another** Pretending that one object is another and using it in that way.	Pretending to use a seashell to drink water or a block to brush a doll's hair.
IIB	24 mos.	**Identification of one body with another person or object** Pretending to be another person, animal, or object.	Pretending to be a dog or a car.
IIIA	3–4 yrs.	**Simple combinations** Assembling the details of a situation that have been previously reproduced only in isolation.	Instead of only brushing a doll's hair, the child washes, dresses, and grooms the doll.
IIIB	3–4 yrs.	**Compensatory combinations** Attempting to correct reality through resolving a disappointment.	Having been disallowed to play in water, the child immediately pretends to pour and splash nonexistent water.
IIIC	3–4 yrs.	**Liquidating combinations** Attempting to correct reality through play, only at a later time.	Having been deprived of playing in water, the child pretends to play in water later that day.
IIID	3–4 yrs.	**Anticipatory combinations** Anticipating possible outcomes and adapting play actions for each.	While describing an earlier situation, the child injects an imaginary event or consequence.

Note. Adapted from "The Development of Play in Infants, Toddlers, and Young Children," by M. W. Casby, 2003, *Communication Disorders Quarterly, 24*(4), pp. 163–173.

closely tied to associated sensorimotor patterns. Eventually, do most children who can hear think verbally through the words and phrases that represent what they are thinking about?

Cognition and Language

Interest in the development of language has prompted a classic "chicken and egg" controversy. Which comes first, thought or language? This question, with philosophical implications for the nature of intelligence and the origins of language, has been considered by psychologists and linguists.

Four major perspectives have evolved representing a range of possible relationships between cognition and language (Owens, 2005). One viewpoint would hold that the two domains develop and function entirely *independent* of each other. The three remaining possibilities would assert that cognition and language are *interdependent;* that is, they influence each other in one of several ways. Figure 3–1 illustrates these potential relationships.

Independent Theory. Paradoxical as it may seem, one possible relationship between cognition and language is that there is no relationship. Some have held that the two domains develop and function separately. Perhaps the strongest proponent of this viewpoint is Noam Chomsky.

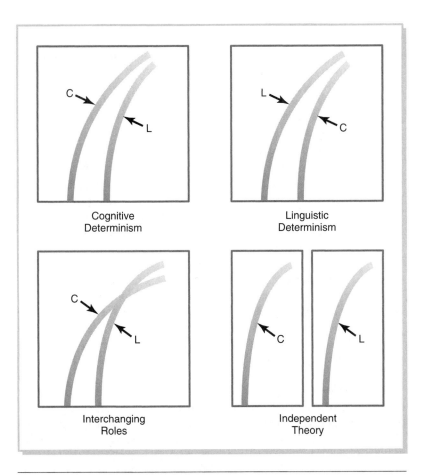

Figure 3–1. Illustrations of the possible relationships between the development of cognition (C) and language (L).

Chomsky's overall theory of language acquisition associated with this viewpoint is described more completely in Chapter 4. ▪

Chomsky has maintained that language is an innate "mental organ" that does not rely on intellect or experience for development any more than our eyes or heart. Chomsky has asserted that language develops at a time when the child is not capable of "complex intellectual achievements" (1968, p. 37).

Cognitive Determinism.   In contrast to Chomsky's position, others have asserted that cognition does play an influential role in the development of language. This school of thought, primarily based on the work of Jean Piaget (Ginsburg & Opper, 1969), would contend that cognition determines the course of language. Language is secondary to thought and serves to express thought. Therefore, language must rely first on the development of certain prerequisite cognitive abilities. According to this view, such developments as object permanence, means-end, and the symbolic function are the underlying cognitive processes that guide the child's development of language.

Linguistic Determinism.   A third viewpoint, described by Benjamin Whorf (1956), asserts that language is the dominant force influencing thought. Also known as the Whorf hypothesis, this position holds that the language that is available to an individual limits or expands his or her potential thought processes.

For example, people in some more primitive cultures have a limited number of color names. One African tribe reportedly uses only two color names, one for the blue-green spectrum and another for the yellow-red spectrum. The number of color names found at the cosmetics counter in an American department store would stand in stark contrast to this. Conversely, although most Eskimos have a number of names for snow, most of us (even avid skiers) probably get by with three or four (e.g., *new, powder, pack*).

The Whorf hypothesis suggests that these differences in available vocabulary limit or expand the ability of individuals in these cultures to perceive and express these phenomena.

Some might suggest that this hypothesis speaks less to the beginnings of language than to the cultural influences on language. Culturally, the differences in available words for colors or snow, for example, might only reflect different histories of economic and survival consequences. Perhaps perceiving and communicating fine differences in color fashions and snow types have been important enough in certain cultures to prompt the evolution of the necessary words to communicate those differences.

Interchanging Roles.   The fourth variation on the roles of language and cognition comes from the work of Vygotsky (1934/1962). According to Vygotsky, language and cognition initially develop on separate tracks. In the younger child, thought does not require language and early language is not based on thought. Thought is nonverbal, perhaps being composed of visual and auditory imagery. Conversely, early words do not represent the child's thought; from the child's viewpoint, early words are an essential part of the object with which they are associated. It is as though the sight and feel of the object plus the child's motions and word are all integrated into the experience of the object itself.

However, according to Vygotsky, at approximately 2 years of age the two domains converge, intertwine, and become interdependent. Beyond this point, children increasingly use language as a tool for thought, using a word in their repertoire to reason through cognitive problems. Conversely, at other times, the child's language is spurred on by cognitive developments in which discovering a new relationship leads to learning the words to express it. Each domain bootstraps on developments in the other to progress further as they interchange roles.

Comments.   It is probably not possible to determine that any one of these viewpoints is exclusively correct. Language and thought are both complex phenomena, influenced by a myriad of subtle, underlying factors. However, it is apparent to most that cognition at some level is intrinsically intertwined with language development. Children's awareness of themselves and understanding of their world is what they talk about. And, in turn, as they talk about themselves and the world with others, their understanding grows.

Summary

- Cognition, how we understand our experiences, has been viewed as a major factor in language development.

- Piaget viewed cognition as a dynamic process of adapting to our environment by achieving equilibrium between how we understand and experience the world.

- In adapting to our environment, we organize behaviors into schemes, or patterns of behavior, and subsequently assimilate or accommodate new experiences.

- Of Piaget's four stages of intelligence, the developments of the sensorimotor period appear to provide some foundations for language development.

- Several possible relationships between cognition and language development have been proposed by researchers.

Information Processing and Perception in Cognition

Beyond Piaget's theory of intelligence, there are other cognitive models relevant to language development. Several are still evolving (Highnam, 1994). Although Piaget's model related to general cognitive abilities and understanding of our experiences, others have attempted to analyze information processing and perception in language development.

Information Processing

information processing
The hypothetical concept of mental stages or processes that organize and access information.

Information processing theories are cognitive models that describe the hypothetical stages or components individuals use to manage incoming stimuli. It can be assumed that in managing incoming stimuli, individuals (including infants) must process them at various levels, such as sensation, discrimination, and association. Over the years, information processing models have evolved to include different components and have proposed various configurations (Nelson, 1993).

Specific definitions of the perceptual processes involved, such as sensation and discrimination, are given later in this section. ∎

The earliest models were based on *serial bottom-up* information processing. In this view, stimuli are processed through a series of successive stages, beginning with lower level stages, such as sensation, and passing through to higher levels, such as association. Later, *parallel bottom-up-top-down* processing models acknowledged that the higher levels of processing might influence the processing that occurred at lower levels. For example, information available at a higher level, such as established associations between stimuli, might influence how incoming stimuli are processed at lower levels, such as perception. More recently, *interactive* models have acknowledged individuals as active participants in that their experiences, intentions, and expectations might influence their processing. In addition, these models have attempted to include the relative influence of the context.

As it turns out, even current information processing models have failed to provide a broad understanding of language learning (Nelson, 1993). For the most part, this is because they speculate on processes that, although they certainly occur, are still inaccessible. We understand much about the anatomy and physiology of the brain but very little about *how* it actually processes information. In this regard, the brain continues to be the proverbial "black box."

Perception

perception   Process of attending to, identifying, and interpreting stimuli.

Information processing models do not directly correlate with neurological structure; that is, very few attempt to assign particular processes to specific areas or structures of the brain. Nonetheless, we know that **perception,** the recognition and interpretation of incoming stimuli, does occur as we experience the world. Understanding the basic perceptual processes, regardless of their neurological basis or their theoretical role, is valuable.

Myklebust's (1964) classic model provided an initial description of the auditory perceptual processes children might experience while learning language. Based on the premise that language is based on experience, his hierarchy begins at a level called *concreteness,* which refers to the fact that all experience is based on physical phenomena—objects, people, actions, and their relationships. The hierarchy culminates at the level of *abstraction,* the highest level for understanding the relationships that organize our experiences. What follows is a selection of the intervening stages that represent the basic perceptual processes for experiencing and understanding incoming stimuli.

Sensation, the awareness that a stimulus is present although not yet identified, is the entry level for perception. When the physical world provides stimuli that our sense organs can detect, we experience sensation. Developmentally, newborns are bombarded by sensations from the noisy, colorful, warm, fuzzy world around them. Perception, the next level, occurs when a received stimulus is identified, selected, and organized. Identification implies "recognition" at its lowest level—only the notion that a stimulus is similar to one experienced previously. Developmentally, infants might indicate through some physiological response that they perceive two stimuli as similar (e.g., two presentations of a speech sound) but are obviously not yet able to name them in any way (e.g., "the 'p' sound").

At a higher level, **imagery,** a partial or entire stimulus is recalled in its absence. It is important to note that, in contrast to the previous two levels, imagery does not require the stimulus to be present. By definition, the stimulus is either physically absent or at least plays no immediate role in the image being recalled. As adults we recall visual images of favorite places, auditory images of favorite music, or our parents' voices. For developing infants, the opportunity to restimulate themselves may come from their perceptual capacity for imagery. It seems possible that certain stimulus events, once experienced and stored, replay themselves through imagery at various times.

At the level of **symbolization,** an auditory, visual, or gestural stimulus is used to represent the original referent. This is in contrast to imagery, where at least a part of the original stimulus is recalled. Developmentally, symbolization closely correlates with Piaget's symbolic function. After children recognize that things exist beyond their immediate experience, they can begin to represent them with a symbol. Therefore, this is the first level at which the true words can occur.

The level of **conceptualization** is where experiences and objects are categorized, indicating that they are perceived as sharing some significant feature or relationship. For children and adults, using a word to label a new referent beyond the original one experienced for a word indicates that they perceive some similarity between them. The similarity for a given category may be rather loose at first. A child may label both a cat and dog as "doggie" and call all adult females "mommy." Although incorrect by adult standards, these attempts illustrate the child's conceptualization of these stimuli.

Developmentally, conceptualization may have its genesis in some of the earliest motor behaviors exhibited by very young infants. For example, Piaget suggested that when young infants apply the same motor scheme to seemingly different objects (e.g., shaking them), they may be signaling that they perceive a basic conceptual similarity between them.

Abstraction is the ability to perceive selected or isolated aspects of an object, event, or person. This ability permits understanding relationships that exist in isolated but similar features shared by objects, events, or persons. For example, colors exist only as a physical feature (light waves) reflected by the many objects in which we appreciate them. Red does not exist separately from apples, roses, crayons, and so forth. Yet we are able to

sensation The initial stage of perception in which sense organs are affected by a physical stimulus.

imagery A perceptual level in which at least part of a stimulus is recalled.

Infant speech perception is discussed in detail in Chapter 5. ■

symbolization The perceptual ability to identify the symbolic representation of objects or events with words.

conceptualization The perceptual level at which stimuli are responded to as a class or concept based on some similarity.

The verbal behavior that provides early evidence of conceptualization, *overextensions,* is described in Chapter 6. ■

abstraction The ability to perceive relationships among isolated aspects of objects, events, or persons.

respond to or abstract red as a feature separate from those objects. On a higher level of abstractness, there are no physically concrete examples to represent *love, justice, charity,* and so forth. Instead, we each abstract these according to the relationships we perceive in the behaviors of people.

Developmentally, children must progress through the previous perceptual levels to attain the level of abstraction. This level of interpreting experiences occurs well beyond the time when the foundations of language are being established in infancy.

▨ Summary

- Perception, the ways in which we manage incoming stimuli, has been analyzed in specific stages or components.

- The relationship of these perceptual processes to language has been hypothesized in various theories of information processing.

Behavioral Principles of Learning

The word "behavior" appears frequently in most discussions of language development. It appears in various terms, including *vocal behavior, verbal behavior, gestural behavior, social behavior,* and *language behavior,* among others. It is easy to recognize from this that if we did not *behave* outwardly in some manner, communication could not occur and language would not exist in the sense that humans know it.

Chapter 2 describes the biological structures for speech, hearing, and language. The preceding sections of this chapter have described the underlying social motivation and the cognitive capacities that contribute to the child's learning of language. However, the biological, social, and cognitive components must ultimately be reflected in the child's behavior for language to emerge.

Among those who study language development, some may emphasize the importance of one component over the others. Some might focus on the biological structures, others on the social interactions, and still others on the cognitive processes. However, each of these factors is inseparable from the total process of learning language. In language, the individual must have the need to communicate to others, have the ideas to communicate to them, and be endowed with the biological structures to do so. However, as simple as that may seem, it is invaluable to appreciate that when the individual learns to actively integrate all of these elements, the observable result can be the most fascinating of human behaviors—language.

Types of Learning—Classical and Operant

Historically, two general types of learning have been described—**classical (or respondent) conditioning** and **operant** (or **instrumental**) condition-

classical (or **respondent**) **conditioning**   A model of learning in which a neutral stimulus (e.g., a bell) associated with an unconditioned stimulus (e.g., food) subsequently elicits conditioned responses similar to the unconditioned response (e.g., salivation).

operant   A group of behaviors that operate on the environment and are affected by the consequences that follow their occurrence.

operant (or **instrumental**) **conditioning**   A learning model in which behaviors that act on the environment are affected by the consequences that follow their occurrence.

ing. A number of writers have applied these to the learning of verbal behavior in various ways.

Classical Conditioning

Classical conditioning occurs when a stimulus that does not normally elicit a particular reflex or emotion comes to do so after it has been paired with a stimulus that does naturally elicit that reflex or emotion. The classical conditioning model is illustrated in Figure 3–2. The *conditioned stimulus* (CS) acquires this capability only after being associated with the *unconditioned stimulus* (US). Because the reflexive or emotional response to the unconditioned stimulus does not have to be learned, it is called an *unconditioned response* (UR). However, the response to the CS occurs only after it has been paired with the US a number of times and is, therefore, termed the *conditioned response* (CR).

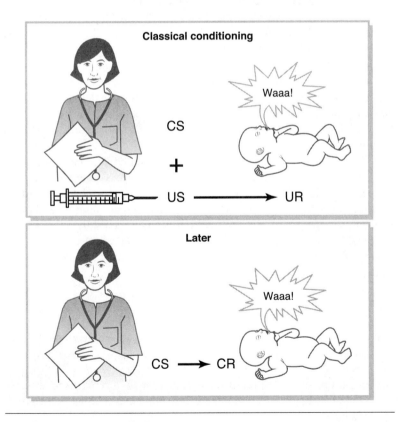

Figure 3–2. Illustration of the classical conditioning model of learning.
(CS = conditioned stimulus, US = unconditioned stimulus, UR = unconditioned response, CR = conditioned response.)

Most students will recall Pavlov's experiment from their basic psychology course. Pavlov paired meat powder (the US) and a bell (the CS) to condition a dog to salivate in response to the bell. The bell was *associated* with the meat powder, which caused the dog to salivate when it heard the bell. Pavlov demonstrated that a reflexive behavior (salivation) was capable of being classically conditioned to occur in response to an otherwise neutral stimulus through association. It should be noted that not all reflexes can be so conditioned (e.g., the patellar or knee-jerk reflex). Therefore, many refer to those behaviors that can be influenced by classical conditioning as *respondents* (Bijou & Baer, 1961).

Operant Conditioning

Operant conditioning, in contrast to classical conditioning, is based on conditioning voluntary behaviors that operate (have an effect) on the environment. A collection of such behaviors are called an operant. The behaviors that make up an operant occur under similar circumstances and are affected similarly by the consequences that follow. For example, a collection of behaviors we might call "greetings" (*Hello! How are you? Good morning!*) tend to occur when we first see someone each day and they do so because in the past the various versions have been followed typically by a friendly response. Consequences that predictably follow a behavior are **contingent.** Furthermore, if the consequences of a behavior enhance the likelihood that similar behaviors occur under like circumstances, then that behavior has been reinforced. The relationships in the operant model are illustrated in Figure 3–3.

> **contingent** A conditional or interdependent relationship between stimuli.

The basic demonstration of operant conditioning, of course, would be B. F. Skinner's numerous experiments with pigeons. Skinner arranged for the pecking behavior of hungry pigeons to be followed by food delivered according to various requirements. In doing this, Skinner found that the frequency and strength of pigeons' pecking behavior could be influenced in predictable ways. Because the class of behaviors (pecking) was capable of being operantly conditioned by the consequences that followed, it is considered an **operant behavior.**

> **operant behavior** Behavior that is influenced by the consequences it produces.

Classical versus Operant Conditioning

Several important contrasts exist between the two types of learning. In classical conditioning the critical link is in the pairing or association of two stimuli, hence it is occasionally referred to as a *stimulus-stimulus* (S-S) model. In contrast, operant conditioning focuses on behavior that occurs in response to or follows a stimulus and is, therefore, known as a *stimulus-response* (S-R) model.

Perhaps the most important contrast between the two types of learning, however, is in the types of behaviors they influence. Classical conditioning

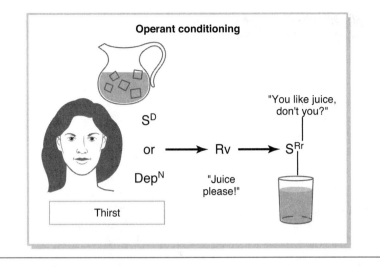

Figure 3–3. Illustration of the operant conditioning model of learning. (S^D = discriminative stimulus, Dep^N = deprivation state, Rv = verbal response, S^{Rr} = reinforcing stimulus, where R = primary and r = secondary reinforcers.)

is generally viewed as affecting reflexive or autonomic responses—more specifically, respondent behavior. Respondent behaviors are *elicited* by a stimulus that precedes them and are not influenced by any stimuli or events that follow them. For example, the pupillary reflex of the eye is elicited automatically and consistently by a bright light; it will not be altered by any rewards or punishments that we might cause to follow.

In contrast, operant conditioning influences voluntary responses. In addition, operant behaviors are *evoked* by stimuli. That is, stimuli that have been present when a behavior was reinforced will signal that reinforcement may be available again. This simply increases the probability that the behavior will reoccur; the behavior does not *have to* occur, as a knee-jerk reflex must in response to a well-placed tap on the knee.

By its nature, human communication is generally intentional and voluntary behavior. If language serves human communication, then it, too, is volitional in nature. Therefore, classical conditioning would be the *wrong* model to apply to language behavior (Winokur, 1976). It would be more appropriate, then, to concentrate our consideration on the operant model.

Summary

- Behavioral scientists have described two general types of human learning, which differ in the classes of behavior that are influenced.

- Classical conditioning primarily affects reflexive or autonomic responses which come to be elicited by associated stimuli.

- Operant conditioning influences voluntary behaviors which are strengthened by their consequences; that is, depending on the consequences that follow, they are made more or less likely to occur in future similar circumstances.

Skinner's Model of Operant Behavior

Considered by most to be the father of modern behaviorism, B. F. Skinner published a number of books that laid its foundation. These include *The Behavior of Organisms* (1938), *Science and Human Behavior* (1953), *Contingencies of Reinforcement: A Theoretical Analysis* (1969), and *About Behaviorism* (1974). In 1957, he also published his analysis of human language, *Verbal Behavior.*

 It is interesting to note that Piaget and Skinner had similar beginnings in their career paths. Like Piaget before him, Skinner's initial interest was in the biological nature of digestion and central nervous system functions. A chance event in these studies in which an automatic pigeon feeder malfunctioned over one weekend piqued his interest in the effect of consequences on behavioral patterns. We owe much to Piaget's mollusks and Skinner's pigeons for inspiring their studies of human development and behavior.

In the operant model described by Skinner, the scientist is committed to a *natural science account* of behavior. This restricts the scientist to considering only predictable relationships among observable variables. The primary variables that the behavioral scientist is interested in are the responses, stimuli, and consequences related to behavior. Skinner's behaviorism does not deny the role of genetic, biological, and neurological variables that serve as a foundation for operant learning. In fact, Skinner has stated that behaviors are caused by two sets of variables: biological and environmental. His experimental analysis concentrated on environmental variables. This only delineates the boundaries of the behaviorist's domain (Skinner, 1974).

Responses and Operants

response induction The behavioral process in which there is a tendency for responses different from the original to occur.

The spread of responses to new but similar circumstances—*stimulus generalization*—is discussed later. ▪

In the context of human learning, *behavior* would generally refer to the various actions of individuals. A *response* is a specific action occurring in a given situation. If that response is effective, a natural behavioral process called response induction may occur. In **response induction,** responses that are similar to the reinforced response tend to occur in future similar circumstances.

With additional learning, a collection of responses evolves, all related by their historical link to similar situations. This class of responses related to similar circumstances and effects is called an *operant.* This process of response induction and the spread of responses to similar circumstances (stimulus generalization, discussed later) illustrate our amazing capacity to learn. No one questions that humans are incredibly fast learners, but when does that learning begin?

The infant exhibits a broad repertoire of available behaviors at birth. However, the earliest behaviors are primarily reflexive in nature. These involve specific automatic movements of particular structures—the eyelids, tongue, lips, fingers—or more general movements of the limbs, torso, or head and neck. Although many infant behaviors may be very precise, they are controlled by a neurological system that is immature and incapable of carrying out specific intentional movements. On the other hand, some of the research discussed previously in this chapter has suggested that infants can alter certain behaviors (their eye gaze and the pattern and rate of sucking) to obtain different outcomes (hearing their mother's voice or seeing her face).

Maturation of the infant's biological systems (neurological, motor, auditory, visual, etc.) provides the expanding potential for responses of greater variety and sophistication. The developing child's behaviors become increasingly differentiated into many variations of previous behaviors. They become increasingly voluntary, occurring more selectively in response to certain circumstances. And, finally, they become integrated into complex sequences of behaviors as the child masters the task of coordinating the various systems and structures.

This behavioral elaboration probably does not truly represent the spontaneous creation of new, previously nonexistent behaviors. Just as infants are born with every muscle fiber that will ever develop and strengthen, we can also conceive of the *potential* for every adult behavior being present in the infant's behavioral repertoire. With nutrition and exercise, each muscle fiber matures. Through interaction with the world around them, the multitude of potential behaviors slowly evolves (Bijou & Baer, 1965).

This gradual evolution of behavior, **shaping,** occurs when responses that successively approximate some final form of behavior are differentially reinforced. The behavioral process of shaping has been clearly demonstrated under both experimental and clinical conditions. Although it is more difficult to analyze the process under everyday circumstances, close observation tells us it is a very natural phenomenon nonetheless.

shaping The gradual modification of a behavior as reinforcement follows variations that progressively approximate a final form of the behavior.

Setting Events

Circumstances that set the stage for human behavior are **setting events.** Humans interact in circumstances defined by the people, objects, events, locations, and motivations associated with those circumstances. For infants and caregivers, nurturing interactions occur naturally in circumstances that become familiar and routine setting events for the behaviors of both.

setting events The collection of stimuli present in a setting that are capable of influencing behavior.

Deprivation States. A deprivation state (Dep^N) occurs when a stimulus that has otherwise been available is withheld. Because people tend to act in certain ways when deprived of something they have come to expect, a deprivation state is the same as a motivational state. A deprivation state can become a setting event for a behavior that occurs and is reinforced during the deprivation. We typically think of food and water as the kind of stimuli that create a deprivation (motivation) state when withheld. Although the corresponding inner states of *hunger* and *thirst* cannot be observed directly, we can still document the deprivation state by measuring the length of time food or water have been unavailable. In this regard, animal researchers are very precise as a matter of practice; caregivers are less exacting but typically just as conscious of these states and the behaviors they occasion.

The natural cycles of metabolism and caregivers' philosophies regarding schedules probably play the biggest roles in setting up deprivation states. Besides food and water, other early stimuli that, when withheld, create states of deprivation include warmth and social contact. As the child grows and becomes accustomed to additional stimuli (a favorite toy, book, record, the car on Saturday night, etc.), these, too, become potential contributors to deprivation states when they become unavailable for certain periods.

Discriminative Stimuli.   To the extent that our senses allow us to experience them, every physical event can be considered a *stimulus*. However, we certainly do not overtly act on every stimulus that impinges on our senses. To do so would be exhausting, if not physically impossible. In other words, many stimuli remain just that—stimuli to which we are otherwise unresponsive.

Our experiences may cause other stimuli to become significant to us. If they are *salient* or conspicuous, we tend to respond to those stimuli under most circumstances. If our responses are effective in that transaction, then we will be prone to behave that way under similar circumstances in the future. Stimuli that are frequently present when certain behaviors are reinforced and subsequently set the stage for similar behaviors to occur again are referred to as **discriminative stimuli** (S^D).

discriminative stimulus (S^D)   A stimulus that has been often present when a response has been reinforced and comes to influence the likelihood of that response occurring.

From one perspective, the ability to discriminate among stimuli (i.e., respond differently to different stimuli) is invaluable. Infants soon learn that not every object that finds its way into their mouth warrants a nursing response. As the ability to inhibit reflexive behavior improves, they may continue to explore nonnutritional objects orally. However, the true sucking response occurs more selectively, only when the mother's (or the bottle's) nipple is presented. In addition, the infant soon becomes familiar with all of the surrounding stimuli that accompany those times when nursing behavior has been fulfilling. Very young infants, when quite hungry, exhibit sucking behavior immediately upon hearing their mother's voice, detecting her fragrance, or seeing her face.

It is obvious that, for survival sake, the infant's responding must be selective in order to economize its efforts. There is little point in using the energy that goes into sucking behavior unless it provides nutrition. However, we know that infants continue to suck on various non-nutritive items—our fingers, their fingers, pacifiers, and so on. This sucking becomes differentiated and takes on different qualities but occurs nonetheless. Eventually, the less similar the item is to the nutritive nipple, the less genuine the sucking behavior is, until perhaps only the most similar of items (a pacifier or a thumb) prompts a sucking response.

Stimulus Generalization. The process of discrimination permits us to respond specifically and appropriately to the world around us. From another perspective, however, if we were only capable of discrimination, it would mean that a response to every new stimulus must be learned individually.

Children might learn the word *ball* in response to their first such toy, let us say, a large, blue, felt-covered one. If discrimination were the only behavioral process at work, they would then have to relearn this word for every other sphere that is of a different size, color, or texture. Instead, the process of discrimination is offset by a process called stimulus generalization.

In **stimulus generalization,** other stimuli, to the extent that they resemble the original stimulus, come to evoke the behavior the original stimulus evoked. In the current example, stimulus generalization would cause children to label other round objects they had never seen before. Stimulus generalization allows learning to be much more efficient than it would otherwise. The ability of humans to so easily form concepts and categories through recognizing even subtle, underlying similarities suggests that we are excellent at it!

stimulus generalization
The behavioral process in which old responses occur to new stimuli.

The counterbalancing of these two processes, stimulus discrimination and stimulus generalization, is critical in creating behavior appropriate to the various new and seemingly unfamiliar circumstances that confront us. Although as young children we said "Hello!" to everyone we met, we eventually learned not to. Instead, we greet people according to the various factors that we have learned to discriminate. These signal when a greeting is appropriate and will be met with approval in some form even in new situations, and when it will not. Influenced by discrimination alone, we would have to be prodded in meeting anyone for the first time to say, "Hello!" (or some such greeting). With unchecked generalization, we would say, "Hello!" to every new face, no matter what the circumstances or the consequences.

Consequences: Reinforcement and Punishment

The consequences of behavior are the third critical element in the operant model. The significance of a behavior (its meaning) is essentially defined by how it *operates* on the environment. This is reflected in the consequences that follow it. A most elegant example in human language can be seen in the significance of a simple question. The true meaning of *Is the salt on the table?* is best defined by observing the situation and the outcome. If the table is being set, a verbal confirmation ("Yes") is a satisfactory outcome; if dinner has been served and the gravy is bland, it may not be. The consequences described by Skinner in the operant model are of two types, reinforcement and punishment.

reinforcement
Procedures that result in increased response strength through contingent presentation or withdrawal of stimuli.

reinforcer   Any stimulus presented contingently that increases the frequency or strength of a response.

positive reinforcer   A stimulus that when presented contingent on a response increases the likelihood of that response; compare **negative reinforcement.**

negative reinforcement
A procedure that increases the frequency of a behavior by removing an aversive stimulus contingent on each occurrence.

punishment   The contingent presentation of an aversive stimulus that results in a decrease in the probability of a response.

Type I punishment   The procedure of delivering a stimulus contingent on a behavior that results in its decrease.

Type II punishment
The procedure of removing a stimulus contingent on a behavior that results in its decrease.

primary reinforcers
Stimuli that have reinforcing potential due to their survival value.

Reinforcement.   **Reinforcement** occurs when a stimulus event—an object or action—that follows a behavior increases the likelihood that that behavior will occur in similar circumstances in the future. Any stimulus event that has this effect of increasing the future probability of a behavior is a **reinforcer.** Reinforcement can occur in two general ways, by presenting or removing a stimulus event. If *presenting* a stimulus event causes an increase in responding, it would be called a **positive reinforcer.** In contrast, if *removing* (or "negating") a stimulus event results in increased responding it would be referred to as **negative reinforcement.**

Punishment.   The other form of consequence that Skinner described is punishment. As the converse of reinforcement, **punishment** occurs when the stimulus event that follows a behavior results in a decrease in the future likelihood of that behavior under similar circumstances. There are analogous positive and negative versions of punishment as well. **Type I punishment,** like positive reinforcement, relies on the presentation or delivery of some stimulus event that decreases the frequency of a response. If caregivers' uttering *No!* actually decreases the probability their infants reach for fragile items, it is a Type I punisher. In contrast, **Type II punishment** occurs when a stimulus event is removed to weaken a response. Caregivers who remove a fussy child from a situation (time-out) or remove treats from the child's food tray (response cost) following disruptive behavior are using Type II punishers.

Primary and Secondary Reinforcers.   A second distinction that can be made among consequences is whether they involve primary or secondary stimuli. **Primary reinforcers** are stimuli that do not require a learning history to achieve their reinforcing potential. They are generally said to have "survival value." Obvious examples would include food, water, and warmth. In contrast, **secondary reinforcers** acquire their reinforcing potential through association with primary reinforcers. In other words, they require a learning history and are, therefore, sometimes referred to as **conditioned reinforcers.** The affection and approval of our loved ones is a very powerful conditioned reinforcer. If a conditioned reinforcer has been associated with a wide variety of other reinforcers, it may become a **generalized conditioned reinforcer.** Money is probably the most universally recognized form of generalized conditioned reinforcers. Stimuli employed in punishment would be distinguished similarly.

Natural Consequences.   A critical distinction that is often overlooked when discussing reinforcement and punishment is the reality of *natural consequences.* Much of the research to define the basic principles of learning—discrimination, generalization, reinforcement, punishment, and so on—has been done in laboratory settings. However artificial this might seem, this is necessary for experimental control. Eliminating the influence of extraneous or unrelated variables allows the researcher to precisely define the nature of the variable being investigated. Natural environments are simply too complex and unpredictable to permit this.

This distinction is frequently missed when researchers look for consequences—reinforcers and punishers—related to language development. The stimulus events that truly become reinforcing (or punishing) go well beyond delivery of food items and the stereotypical phrases, *Good boy!* or *Good girl!*

Primary reinforcers do play a fundamental role in the nurturing interactions between caregivers and infants. From the beginning, the caregiver's presence, fragrance, facial expressions, voice, and so forth are part of the infant's experiences. These are immediately and consistently associated with potent primary reinforcers, including the food, warmth, and cuddling provided by nurturing caregivers.

As a result of this history, perhaps the most powerful reinforcer that emerges is the natural consequence of *attention.* Attention can take various forms throughout a child's development, including basic caregiving activities, eye contact, smiles, proximity, and vocalizations (e.g., "motherese").

Eventually the caregiver's responses to the child's speech attempts with actions and verbal responses, even if inaccurate, constitutes reinforcement. Ultimately, the child will become even more discerning when the extent to which the caregiver responds appropriately indicates how much attention they are giving (*No, more* cookies! or *Dad, I said I needed a 20, not a 5!*).

Genetic Endowment and Individual Learning. An individual's behavior comes from two identifiable histories—their species' genetic history and their individual learning history (Skinner, 1974). Fundamentally, genetic endowment determines the structures and biologically based behaviors that are vital to the individual's survival. Genetically endowed behaviors occur in a species because the environment has historically imposed consequences that affected the survival of certain members of that species. Over the generations, those individuals who interact most effectively with their environment ultimately contribute more to their species' future gene pool. Over the evolution of a species then, environmental consequences in the form of survival and procreation serve as "feedback" for genetic "responses"—the potential resulting from genetic variations and mutations. Those characteristics that contribute to survival will survive genetically and be expressed more frequently within that species. In terms of individual biological makeup, these genetic features determine the types of stimuli that are most salient to members of that species. That is, the genetic history has shaped a species to be more receptive to certain stimuli, both from a perceptual sense and from the standpoint of reinforcement.

In individuals, genetically built-in reflexive behaviors occur without regard to immediate feedback from the environment. Those reflexes critical to survival will continue to do so. However, as biological structures mature, the

secondary reinforcers Stimuli that obtain their reinforcing potential through association with primary reinforcers.

conditioned reinforcers Stimuli that take on reinforcing properties as a result of their association with a known reinforcer.

generalized conditioned reinforcer Stimulus that obtains its reinforcing potential from association with a variety of other reinforcing stimuli.

individual experiences the potential for a wider range of voluntary behavior. Many of these behaviors produce interesting and useful results. For a developing child, the consequences of interacting with the environment stimulate biological maturation, which furthers the evolution of individual behaviors. And, ultimately, consequences influence which behaviors endure and which do not.

Early Operants: Stimuli, Responses, and Reinforcers

A number of authors have attempted to identify the operants that are most likely to evolve out of the infant's early experiences. Kantor (1959a, 1959b) analyzed child development as the interaction between infants' biological makeup, their behavior, and the environment's responses to changes in both. Bijou and Baer (1961, 1965) later elaborated on this conceptualization. As discussed before, the number of available stimuli, responses, and opportunities for interaction are probably countless. Nonetheless, an initial inventory of those that might be most significant may be instructive.

Bijou and Baer categorized the stimuli experienced most intimately and consistently by the infant as *specific stimulus events*. These naturally fall into basic categories that correlate with the senses. For the most part, visual, auditory, tactile, gustatory (taste), and olfactory stimuli comprise persons' experience of their external world.

The specific stimuli commonly experienced by infants include the sensations associated with caregiving. The caregiver's face, voice, and possibly smell become discriminative stimuli that precede and accompany the presentation of positive reinforcers—food, water, warmth. The caregiver would also become discriminative for negative reinforcement in removing aversive stimuli—wet or soiled diapers, open safety pins. It is of no small consequence that human infants spend the largest proportion of their life span being dependent on the adult for their care, or that most caregivers talk to their infants throughout the course of providing that care.

An increasing number of useful responses become available to the infant. Motor responses demonstrated in grasping objects, extending their legs, waving their arms, and turning their heads from side to side. Perhaps the single most important infant response is vocalization. With limited dexterity and virtually no mobility, they rely entirely on vocalization to establish contact with those around them.

The earliest vocalizations are reflexive cry vocalizations. Research has suggested that when caregivers respond to crying, infants learn to use it as a tool for attracting attention (Lane & Molyneaux, 1992; Locke, 1993). Eventually, infants learn that the noncrying sounds they make—the cooing and babbling—draw others into their proximity. And, those others often engage in taking turns making additional similar sounds. But why would this be of any significance to the infant?

It was noted previously that infants have a strong preference for hearing their caregiver's voice. As we have just described, the caregiver's voice and the sounds that accompany it are consistently associated with the presentation of food and warmth, or, conversely, the removal of discomfort. In other words, the caregiver's proximity, face, voice, and sounds have been consistently associated with primary reinforcement (both positive and negative), making them very powerful conditioned reinforcers. Later, as the variety of reinforcers expands (to toys, allowances, bikes, and cars), the caregiver's attention, voice, and speech become potentially powerful generalized conditioned reinforcers.

This potent relationship between caregivers' attention (whether in the form of physical contact, eye contact, or speech) and infants' behavior may be the observable evidence of attachment. Further, ongoing changes in infants' behavior may well illustrate the coupling of social, cognitive, and behavioral influences in their daily interactions.

Summary

- Skinner's model of operant conditioning provides a framework for analyzing the influence of setting events and the consequences that follow operant behaviors.

- The association of caregivers with primary reinforcers through nurturing interactions between caregivers and infants provides a natural mechanism for establishing various caregiver behaviors as potent generalized reinforcers.

- Many infant behaviors are shaped into increasingly complex behaviors through natural caregiving routines that provide predictable setting events as stimuli for responses that are attended to by caregivers.

Chapter Summary

This chapter has described the interactive foundations for language that are established from birth. Infants' earliest nurturing interactions with the world are significant in establishing the social, cognitive, and behavioral dynamics that will motivate language learning. Early *attachment* in caregiver-infant *dyads,* facilitated by their shared *recognition* and *social interaction,* provides the basis for the countless transactions that will comprise *social behavior.*

These social interactions provide the context for infants' continuing experiences and their cognitive understanding of the world. Throughout Piaget's *sensorimotor stage,* infants exhibit *schemes,* or behavior patterns, that change as infants *adapt* to the environment through *assimilating* or *accommodating* new experiences. Many researchers are interested in the influence of *imitation, means-end* behavior, object permanence, and *symbolic function* on language development, as suggested by Piaget's work.

Finally, the behavioral dynamics that evolve between infants and caregivers come full circle. Both *classical conditioning* and *operant conditioning* probably occur within infant-caregiver interactions; however, the influence of operant conditioning appears to be of central importance to language development. The natural nurturing interactions (or routines) between caregivers and infants provide consistent *setting events.* Within these setting events, caregivers' attention is consistently associated with *primary reinforcers* and established very early as an important *secondary reinforcer.* As infant behaviors reinforced by caregiver attention become more complex behaviors through *shaping,* they prompt even greater expectations on the part of caregivers.

Ultimately, we must remember that developments in all three areas—social, cognitive, and behavioral—are coupled to maturing biological systems that provide the expanding potential for each.

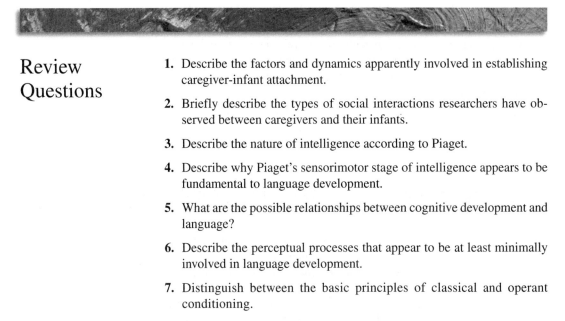

Review Questions

1. Describe the factors and dynamics apparently involved in establishing caregiver-infant attachment.

2. Briefly describe the types of social interactions researchers have observed between caregivers and their infants.

3. Describe the nature of intelligence according to Piaget.

4. Describe why Piaget's sensorimotor stage of intelligence appears to be fundamental to language development.

5. What are the possible relationships between cognitive development and language?

6. Describe the perceptual processes that appear to be at least minimally involved in language development.

7. Distinguish between the basic principles of classical and operant conditioning.

8. Describe how the influence of early caregiver-infant interactions on language development might be analyzed within an operant conditioning framework.

To the student: You are encouraged to use the following questions to prepare for multiple-choice examinations. This exercise is not intended to simply "provide the answers to questions." Instead, it is hoped that you will use the material to develop your ability to analyze questions and choices to identify correct answers based on a critical understanding of the distinctions among the answers. Use the answer key at the end of the book to prompt your analysis of each item and to confirm the correct answer. Remember that there is a difference between recognizing the correct answer and understanding why it is the correct one.

Practice Questions

1. Which of the following would *not* be necessary for the development of human social attachment?
   a. that two individuals "recognize" each other
   b. that two individuals are capable of influencing each other's behaviors
   c. that two individuals have appearances that are distinctively similar (i.e., they resemble each other)
   d. that two individuals come to depend on each other
   e. all of these are necessary

2. In infants, deictic gaze occurs _____ .
   a. when the infant avoids eye contact
   b. when the infant gazes into the mother's eyes
   c. when the mother shakes an item in front of the infant to focus his or her attention on it
   d. when the infant's gaze directs the mother's attention to an object of apparent interest
   e. only after the first word has developed

3. Which of the following does Whorf's "linguistic determinism" suggest?
   a. cognition influences the development and content of language
   b. language influences the development of cognition
   c. people who have only two words for the food groups will tend to "see" or categorize food in that way
   d. a and c
   e. b and c

4. In Myklebust's hierarchy of experience, which of the following levels are "stimulus bound" (i.e., they can only occur if the stimulus is physically present)?
   a. abstraction and conceptualization
   b. imagery and symbolization
   c. perception and imagery
   d. sensation and perception
   e. all of these

5. Which of the following statements is true regarding infant vocalizations within the first few weeks?
   a. infants' earliest vocalizations begin as responses to physiological stimuli
   b. infants' earliest vocalizations are reflexive in nature
   c. infants' earliest vocalizations are not conscious attempts to communicate
   d. infants' earliest cry vocalizations evolve into different cries that many mothers can distinguish
   e. all of these are true

6. Which of the following is *not* a characteristic of motherese?
   a. simpler utterances
   b. exaggerated facial expressions
   c. variable rate
   d. longer utterances
   e. exaggerated prosody

7. Negative reinforcement and Type II punishment are similar in that _____ .
   a. both decrease the frequency of behaviors
   b. both increase the frequency of behaviors
   c. both involve presenting stimuli
   d. both involve removing stimuli
   e. both are elements of classical conditioning

8. "Assimilation" in Piaget's theory of cognition refers to _____ .
   a. modifying existing cognitive structures or schemes to "fit in" new stimuli that do not fit available schemes or concepts
   b. the ability to assume a color and configuration that matches one's environment
   c. using available schemes to incorporate or "fit in" new stimuli experienced in one's environment
   d. higher level cognitive functioning that occurs only in the "formal operational" period
   e. being able to assume your listener's perspective

9. In an operant analysis, the mother's smile, praise, and hug at the end of each "game," especially after the infant "plays along," are probably _____ .
   a. negative reinforcers
   b. conditioned reflexive responses
   c. unconditioned stimuli
   d. conditioned stimuli
   e. secondary reinforcers

10. Symbolic play would be best illustrated by _____ .
    a. an infant bringing his rattle to his mouth
    b. a child using a wood block as though it was a car, and then as a table, and then as a building
    c. a child pushing a toy car back and forth on a table
    d. an infant babbling various English consonants
    e. the Moro reflex

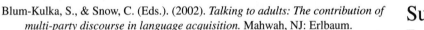

Blum-Kulka, S., & Snow, C. (Eds.). (2002). *Talking to adults: The contribution of multi-party discourse in language acquisition.* Mahwah, NJ: Erlbaum.

Casby, M. W. (2003). The development of play in infants, toddlers, and young children. *Communication Disorders Quarterly, 24* (4) 163–173.

Tamis-LeMonda, C. S., Chen, L. A., & Bornstein, M. H. (1998). Mothers' knowledge about children's play and language development: Short-term stability and interrelations. *Developmental Psychology, 34* (1), 115–124.

Suggested
Readings

CHAPTER 4

Models of Language Development

Grandma Leo climbed the dark, winding staircase with her usual determination. She loved to end her day by climbing as close to the stars as her little house would allow. Her late husband built this little house with a special watchtower, a place where she could get above all the noise and worry of the day. With the telescopes he made for her, she studied the night sky. Each pinpoint of light took her far away from her earthly worries. Her husband gave her more than a house with a view to the sky. Their time together also gave her a passionate curiosity about her world. As her curiosity became more intense, and even taxing to him, he would laugh heartily and exclaim, "She's quite a gal, that Leo!"

She started out wondering about the stars that she could see. Soon, she was pondering what was there between them and beyond them. What was out there that she could not see? With her husband she had wondered how far away they were and how long it took for their light to reach her. And, if they fell to earth, would the larger stars fall faster?

She would find such peace in her reflections, but occasionally she was interrupted by the loud chatter of small children who should have been asleep in their beds. They would run and chase down below her lookout. So many children playing and hiding, laughing and shouting, directing and complaining in the dark. Incessantly arguing about rules and steps and winners! She wondered what made children talk so much? What made children talk at all? So many others before her have probably puzzled over these same questions. She would find it exasperating if it were not for the joyous energy and remarkable wisdom in their words. Instead, her curiosity would simply turn back to earth and the phenomenon she heard as each child negotiated the next turn of events.

This chapter addresses the following questions:

- What is the study of language development based on?
- What are the basic goals of science?
- What are the basic attitudes of science?
- What are the basic questions that science has attempted to answer regarding language development?
- What models have been proposed to explain language development?
- What impact has each model had on our understanding of language development?
- How are these models different and how are they similar?
- How can the individual contributions of each model be integrated into a comprehensive understanding of language development?

The fictional vignette used to open this chapter (with apologies to Galileo) was intended to introduce two points. First, people probably have been curious about language development for hundreds, if not thousands, of years. Second, this curiosity has inspired research that has brought us to our current, although still incomplete, understanding of language development.

Too often we think of "scientific research" as being concerned only with the most compelling phenomena—curing disease, predicting earthquakes and tornadoes, dissecting the atom, understanding the universe, and so on. Perhaps because we generally speak so often and with so little effort, many of us fail to appreciate the miracle of nature that language represents. However, many others have taken interest in language and its development.

Over the centuries, philosophers, psychologists, linguists, sociologists, and researchers from various disciplines have attempted explanations of language development. Given that each specialty views the world from a different perspective, the resulting explanations can be quite varied. This chapter introduces those models of language development that are most significant, based on their historical prominence and their current role in research.

Central Questions and Issues

Our questions about language development arise from more than idle interest. As a defining characteristic of our social behavior as human beings, understanding our language behavior is central to understanding our own nature. In addition, the fact that some children may not achieve their potential due to deficient language development makes it imperative that we seek to understand the factors related to normal language development.

Science and Research in Language Development

Science is a special way of asking and answering questions to gain an objective understanding of the world. Science deals with explaining natural events and relationships, such as language development in human behavior.

Goals of a Science of Language Development

Science is driven by several different forces. Two basic forces are our natural curiosity about how the world works and our practical hope to make it work better for us (Hegde, 1996). The curiosity that drives science has the overall goal of *explaining* natural phenomenon. Therefore, a major goal for the science of language development is to explain it. A **scientific explanation** of an event is achieved when its causes are experimentally demonstrated. That is, the elements that appear to be related to an event have been systematically manipulated to determine which ones cause it to occur and which do not. Historically, our curiosity regarding language development has focused on variables such as genetic inheritance, neurological factors, adult models, and imitation, to name just a few.

The other goal, **technical application,** goes beyond curiosity in *applying* knowledge for practical solutions to real problems. Researchers apply new information to develop better technology to develop new medical procedures, new pharmaceutical products, more efficient energy generation, safer automobiles, and so on. Professionals concerned with language development in children similarly evaluate new, more effective approaches to evaluate and improve children's language skills.

There are several subgoals that precede the explanation of a phenomenon (Bachrach, 1972). These include at least: (a) understanding; (b) prediction; and (c) control. Appreciating these goals will be important as we evaluate the state of our knowledge in language development.

Understanding. The first step in achieving a scientific explanation of a phenomenon is **understanding,** identifying the nature and causes of an event. In doing so careful, repeated observations are needed to describe the phenomenon. This process allows researchers to understand which variables are related to its occurrence.

Researchers have made great strides in understanding language development by observing and analyzing it from different perspectives (i.e., behaviorally, grammatically, semantically, pragmatically). Earlier research efforts focused on describing language behaviors typical of different age levels. Recently, researchers have focused on the nature of social interactions related to language development.

Prediction. Understanding a phenomenon leads to prediction. **Prediction** of the occurrence or nonoccurrence of an event is based on understanding which variables reliably precede it. With regard to normal language

science A body of principles and attitudes that attempts to objectively understand natural phenomena.

scientific explanation Identification and verification of the variables that cause an event to occur.

technical application The goal of applied science in which knowledge results in technology that is helpful to society.

understanding The process of decoding meaning from an encoded message, as in comprehending the significance of words and sentences.

prediction The scientific goal of identifying the variables that reliably precede a phenomenon.

development, researchers have identified biological, cognitive, social, and behavioral variables that make normal development likely. Conversely, detecting risk factors such as hearing loss, genetic syndromes, neurological damage, and so forth may lead professionals to predict potential communication problems for a child. Such predictive factors permit early intervention and the potential to change the course of events for that child.

Control.   The level most consistent with a scientific explanation and the ultimate outcome for a scientist is control. **Control** refers to the scientist's ability to influence whether an event will or will not occur by manipulating the variables. Through experimentation, researchers identify the variables that control a phenomenon (i.e., its causal variables), which also achieves a scientific explanation of that phenomenon.

Professionals concerned with language disorders have achieved an admirable level of control as demonstrated in language treatment. Through various procedures, clinicians control or influence a child's development of effective communication. There could be nothing more rewarding than the feeling that one can make a difference in a child's future.

Scientific Dispositions

That science is a special way of asking and answering questions suggests that it is a collection of "attitudes" about knowledge. Scientists are disposed to explaining the world with caution and honesty. This aspect of science can be characterized as a set of scientific dispositions (Bachrach, 1972; Hegde, 1996).

Science looks for lawful (i.e., consistent, predictable) relationships among events. **Scientific determinism** is a fundamental belief that *events do not occur capriciously or haphazardly,* without some identifiable cause. Language researchers believe that there are real causes—biological structures, social interactions, cognitive development, behavioral principles—that explain language development.

In science there are no heroes, superstars, or gurus. There are experts or authorities, individuals who have extensive experience in a given area. However, **scientific objectivity** prevails in science, meaning that only objective evidence can be considered, even if it conflicts with "expert opinion." *In science, data prevail, not experts.* In language development research, there are many individuals who are deserving of great admiration for their efforts. But we should not allow their stature to influence our evaluation of the facts surrounding language development.

Perhaps the most difficult thing for an "expert" to say is, "I don't know." There seems to be implied pressure on professionals to know everything! However, the simple phrase, "We don't know," illustrates the **scientific restraint** that scientists and professionals must display. When it comes to explaining our world, *it is better to go without an explanation than to settle*

---

control   A scientific goal in which scientists seek to influence whether or not a phenomenon occurs.

scientific determinism The belief that all events have causes.

Determinism would be the antithesis of superstition. ■

scientific objectivity The belief that data and evidence are more important than authorities or opinions.

Perhaps Joe Friday of the classic television show *Dragnet* stated this one best: "The facts ma'am, just the facts." ■

for an inadequate one. The history of research in language development has had an interesting history that may illustrate this caution.

The universe can appear to be a very complex puzzle. Such enormous complexity might seem to require very complex scientific explanations. However, **scientific elegance** asserts that the best explanations are those that capture complex phenomena with the fewest laws. Sometimes referred to as *Occam's Razor* (after the 12th-century English scholar, William of Occam), this disposition states that *the simplest theory is the best theory.* Language is a very complex phenomenon, but an elegant model would require a minimum of principles to capture all of its complexities, irregularities, subtleties, and peculiarities.

Summary

- Science, its methods and dispositions, plays a fundamental role in understanding language development.

- Through basic research, science addresses our curiosity about language development and through applied research, science addresses the needs of children with language disorders.

- Scientific dispositions require us to approach data and theories with caution and objectivity.

Models of Language and Language Learning

As stated previously, different disciplines have taken interest in language and its development. Each has contributed concepts and models that fit its particular perspective—its precepts, beliefs, and methods.

The Basic Question

The basic question underlying the research in language development is "How does the child get from point A to point B?" Point A and point B have also been referred to as the *initial state* (no grammar) and the *final state* (adult grammar) (Parker & Riley, 2004). As simple as this question sounds, it is the heart of the issue—how does the child progress from no recognizable language to using competent language in a matter of a few years?

Answering this question has been approached in two general ways. The pivotal word seems to be "how." Some take the perspective of *describing* how a child develops language. Operating from this viewpoint, the chronological sequence in language development (i.e., which skills are learned by what age) has been extensively researched. However, such chronologies are essentially based on the passage of time. This is not a precise variable because "getting older" combines a myriad of other variables—including maturation, new experiences, and additional interactions.

scientific restraint   The willingness to wait for objective, scientifically supported explanations.

scientific elegance   The belief that the best scientific explanation is the most economical explanation.

It seems that we would have learned this lesson well enough from Copernicus and Columbus. ◼

Perhaps the most widely recognized example of scientific elegance is $E = mc^2$, Einstein's expression of the relationship between mass and energy. That such a simple equation captures the complex behavior of the universe is the epitome of scientific elegance. ◼

In all fairness, much of the developmental research has been done to generate data that would lead to a theory. The reasoning being that if a theory "fits" our observations, it might, therefore, explain language development. ∎

The term *model* is being used in preference to *theory.* This is because several of the explanations discussed were not proposed in the usual sense of a formal theory with hypotheses to be confirmed or refuted. ∎

nativism   The philosophical perspective that certain knowledge and abilities are innate.

mentalism   A philosophical perspective that emphasizes that knowledge derives from the organization of the mind.

structuralism   A philosophical perspective that emphasizes that the structure and organization of language reflects the inherent nature of the mind.

empiricism   The philosophical view that experience is the source of learning and knowledge.

behaviorism   A philosophical perspective on learning and behavior that emphasizes observable behaviors and their effects.

Others have approached this basic question with the goal of *explaining* how a child develops language. That is, focusing on the actual mechanisms or processes that cause the child to develop language. These proposed explanations have included learning principles, mental structures, cognitive processes, and social factors.

The former approach, describing the sequence of development, has provided the normative information contained in the chapters beyond this one. The latter approach, explaining the mechanisms or process that cause language to develop, is the subject of this chapter.

The Philosophical Spectrum

Those who have been interested in language and its development represent a broad range of disciplines. Accordingly, the proposed models span a broad spectrum of philosophies. The "-ism's" that result can be initially confusing. However, mastering them and their associated concepts is helpful in learning the related theories.

Essentially, the polar extremes on this spectrum represent the age-old "nature versus nurture" controversy. At one extreme of the spectrum is a school of thought called **nativism.** In its most fundamental sense, this philosophical position would hold that children are born knowing *all* that they will ever know about language; this knowledge merely "blossoms" as they mature biologically. Language develops because it is part of each child's genetic *nature* (Parker & Riley, 2004).

This perspective is also associated with the psychological school called mentalism or structuralism. **Mentalism** is associated with the belief that knowledge primarily derives from inborn mental processes. **Structuralism** emphasizes the structure (as opposed to the function) of language. Noam Chomsky exemplifies this psycholinguistic school of thought in language.

At the other end of the spectrum is a school of thought called **empiricism.** The most fundamental version of empiricism would hold that children are born with *none* of the knowledge they will eventually obtain. Genetics provides the basic tools—the biological structures and neurological capacity for learning. Given these, however, children's language abilities develop primarily from experience with their environment. Language develops because experiences provided by the environment *nurture* it. The psychological school corresponding to this perspective is **behaviorism,** which assumes that knowledge is the primary result of our behavior and its consequences. Most would associate B. F. Skinner with this school of thought.

Historically, and somewhat arguably, B. F. Skinner's behaviorism, known as *radical behaviorism,* is described as an extreme polar position that opposes nativism. It is true that Skinner did not subscribe to the notion of innate knowledge of language structures that simply unfold in language development. However, radical behaviorism does not hold that biological (neurophysiological and genetic) factors do not influence behaviors. As described in the next section, radical behaviorism proposes that behaviors, including language, are caused by both biological and environmental variables (Skinner, 1986, 1990). Skinner's and Chomsky's positions contrast mostly in terms of the roles of innate mechanisms and environmental variables.

 Remarkably, the two landmark books that initially staked out polar positions on this spectrum were published in 1957: Skinner's *Verbal Behavior* and Chomsky's *Syntactic Structures.*

As Table 4–1 illustrates, these polar positions contrast in a number of ways, including the contributions of learning principles, mental structures, cognitive processes, and social factors. Few researchers hold rigidly to either of these most extreme polar positions today. It is generally agreed that the most complete model probably lies somewhere between these extremes. The issue is rarely posed anymore as "nature *versus* nurture," but instead, "how much of each?" The middle ground positions, called **interactionism,** ask what is the nature of the interaction between children's genetic makeup and their experiences that results in language learning? In one case, *cognitive interactionists* emphasize the child's interaction with the environment in ways that foster cognitive structures that support language. On the other hand, *social interactionists* emphasize the role of interacting with people in social transactions that facilitate language.

interactionism A philosophical perspective that emphasizes the mutual influence of cognitive processes or social contexts on language development.

The Operant Model: Skinner's *Verbal Behavior*

Skinner published his operant analysis of human verbal behavior as "an exercise in interpretation" (p. 11) in 1957. It has been subsequently summarized by MacCorquodale (1969, 1970) and Winokur (1976).

Skinner's model was "not theoretical in the usual sense" and made "no appeal to hypothetical explanatory entities" (1957, p. 12). He instead emphasized "an orderly arrangement of well-known facts, in accordance with a formulation of behavior derived from an experimental analysis of a more rigorous sort" (1957, p. 11). In other words, he was extending well-documented principles of behavior in general to *verbal* behavior based on extensive observation and analysis of people's talking (a widely available phenomenon).

Skinner considered language as a part of human behavior. Therefore, his general conceptualization of behavior applies to language as well. He believed that behaviors are shaped and maintained by two kinds of variables: biological and environmental (Skinner, 1986, 1990). Biological variables determine the nature of species and the environmental variables determine the behaviors of individual members of the species. His *functional analysis* focused on environmental variables that affect behaviors, mainly because that was the domain of his interest and research.

Because language does not exist except for the behavior of humans, Skinner's extension of behavioral principles to language seems reasonable.

 Some have misinterpreted the notion of "prediction and control" in an onerous, Orwellian way. It has been implied that Skinner was conspiring to control our behavior in ways like those described in George Orwell's *1984*. This was not the case. Instead, his hope was that we should understand our behavior well enough to change it for the better. The influence that language professionals exert in successfully treating disordered language is an example of control that would thoroughly please Skinner.

Table 4–1. Philosophical spectrum and associated characteristics of language models.

Characteristics	Philosophical Roots			
	Empiricism	Social Interactionism	Cognitive Interactionism	Nativism
Language model	Operant Model	Pragmatic Model	Cognitive Model	Structural Model
Associated concepts	Behaviorism	Sociolinguistics	Semantics	Psycholinguistics
Unit of analysis	Verbal operants	Speech acts	Case relations	Syntactic structures
Primary factors in language development	Caregiver models and feedback, imitation, and natural consequences of effective communication.	Effects of intentions expressed in caregiver-child social interactions.	Cognitive development provides meanings that are expressed through language form.	Innate language acquisition device processes language input to derive underlying rules and transformations for the generative grammar.

His ultimate scientific goals were both basic and applied: "the prediction and control of verbal behavior" and "immediate technological applications" (1957, p. 12).

Skinner's definition of verbal behavior as "behavior reinforced through the mediation of other persons" (1957, p. 14) emphasizes its social nature. Furthermore, this definition includes a broad range of human communication behaviors such as writing, typing, gestures, and even pointing, if it alters the behavior of others (e.g., using the pointer finger for the proverbial *They went thataway!*). However, the primary focus of his model was on *vocal* verbal behavior—spoken language.

Although the model was based on basic behavioral principles, Skinner admitted that "it would be foolish to underestimate the difficulty of this subject matter" (1957, p. 3). He acknowledged that "verbal behavior is usually the effect of *multiple causes*" (1957, p. 10), including past experiences, listeners, and variables both present and remote. Nonetheless, as complex as language is to describe, Occam's Razor would still require us to pare our explanation down to the fewest principles and factors necessary.

Basic Elements of the Operant Model

To understand the subtleties of any model of language, it is important to become familiar with its basic elements. Understanding the following aspects of Skinner's model is an important starting point.

The Unit of Analysis.   Traditional accounts of language have focused on formal structures such as words, phrases, or sentences as the unit of interest. However, if we analyze verbal behavior as a social behavior, we must focus on its effect on the listener. For example, the utterance *Is the salt on the table?* can be formally analyzed as 16 phonemes, or as six morphemes, or as a yes-no question. However, this does not clarify it as an *occurrence* of verbal behavior—why would someone say this? As verbal behavior, it must be analyzed in terms of the circumstances in which it occurred and the effects it subsequently had. If uttered while setting the table, it might characteristically prompt someone to retrieve the salt shaker. If spoken during the meal with the salt already present, it might prompt someone to pass it. In the present context, it even serves the purposes of providing the reader with "food for thought," if you will.

In a broad sense, then, our unit of analysis is an utterance for which the setting events and effects can be identified. More technically, Skinner's model refers to the concept of responses and operants. A **response** is an instance or occurrence of a behavior (e.g., the greeting you may have used today, *Hello! How are you?*), whereas *operants* are a kind of behavior (social greetings—smiles, nods, waves, stereotyped phrases, etc.). Operants might be thought of as a group or family of responses that are related according to when and why they occur.

Skinner's original text is 478 pages long and obviously quite detailed in its presentation. Readers may find "readers digest" versions by MacCorquodale (1969) and Winokur (1976) to be helpful in gaining an initial grasp of this model. ■

Direct quotes from Skinner's formulation are used extensively. Historically, this model has been frequently paraphrased and simplified. In some cases this has led to inaccuracies. ■

response   A reaction to a stimulus.

response strength
Indicated through the frequency, probability, or intensity of responses.

probability   A behavioral concept indicating response strength.

Other aspects regarding the unit of verbal behavior that should be appreciated include the strength and probability of responses. **Response strength,** the production effects evident in a response, is influenced by present circumstances and past experience, and might be gauged by its *audibility* (a whisper vs. a shout), its *speed* (e.g., *I'm starving! Squeat!*—as in, "Let's go eat"), or *repetition* (*No! No! No! You can't have one!*).

Probability, or the likelihood of a given behavior, is a very subtle aspect. It also derives from the present and past circumstances. Where the probability of a *specific* response form may be nearly impossible to project, the type or class of (operant) behavior should be. When our path crosses with someone else for the first time each day, there is a strong probability that we will produce a greeting response, even though the specific form may not be predictable.

The relative probability of specific responses reflects that verbal behavior does not usually occur as automatic or reflexive behavior. Even when you slam your finger in the car door, various factors may influence whether you say anything and, if you do, what. However, most have had the experience of knowing someone so well that we can predict precisely what they will say in a given situation.

The concepts of responses and operants, setting events, and consequences are discussed in greater detail in Chapter 3. ■

Conditions and Consequences.   Skinner analyzed verbal behavior as a function of its controlling variables. That is, certain verbal responses are more likely as a function of the relevant conditions and consequences, past and present. The conditions include the deprivation states or stimuli that make up the setting event for a response. When we smell food cooking, it sets the occasion for any of a number of related responses. Depending on how hungry we are and the context, we may or may not speak. And, if we do, what we say might vary from *What's cookin', Ma?* to *I am so pleased you invited me to your dinner party. What is that delicious aroma?*

Because verbal behavior is socially mediated the consequences or effects that follow speaking are a critical element. Speaking may result in primary positive reinforcement (e.g., food or water) or primary negative reinforcement (e.g., someone's boot heel lifted from our toe). However, it is important to note that the consequences, especially reinforcing consequences, are frequently far more subtle and transient than these. If we only spoke when we wanted something tangible, it would be a very utilitarian and boring existence. Instead, we are reinforced in our interactions by obtaining useful or entertaining information or sometimes by simply alleviating an awkward silence. (How many times in modern history has the word *weather* been uttered on an elevator?)

The contingent relationship between child utterances and caregivers' *expansions* and *extensions* is discussed in greater detail in Chapter 6. ■

Children apparently find the attention that usually follows their verbal behavior to be very reinforcing. Much of this attention may be nonverbal in nature. However, most significantly it may take the form of caregiver comments that are related to the same setting events (extensions) or corrective feedback related to the child's utterance (expansions) (Moerk, 1994).

Interlocking Verbal Paradigm.   Finally, an important aspect of Skinner's analysis, which further underscores the social nature of verbal behavior, is the **interlocking verbal behavior paradigm.** This illustrates that in social verbal behavior, each partner plays an alternating role in most verbal exchanges. Additionally, the way in which utterances can serve as both discriminative and reinforcing stimuli is made apparent. In the example illustrated in Figure 4–1, each speaker's utterances serve alternately and simultaneously as verbal responses (Rv), setting events (S^D), or as reinforcement (S^{Rr}) following the other's utterances.

> **interlocking verbal behavior paradigm**
> Skinner's model illustrating the interactive nature of verbal exchanges between speaking partners.

Primary Verbal Operants

A **verbal operant** is a disposition or tendency to respond verbally to a certain state of affairs (or setting event) in a certain way because of past reinforcement (Winokur, 1976). In simpler terms, we tend to say certain things in certain circumstances because similar responses in similar situations have been effective in the past. Skinner classified verbal behaviors according to the relationship between their antecedents (or setting events) and the responses that are likely because of past reinforcement. This contingency is the defining relationship for each basic type of verbal behavior. Table 4–2 defines the primary verbal operants.

> **verbal operant**   A group of responses that share a history of occurring under similar circumstances and resulting in similar consequences.

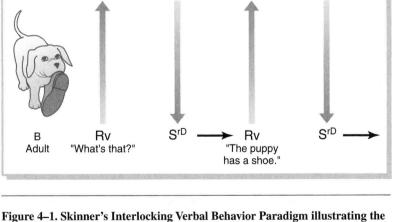

Figure 4–1. Skinner's Interlocking Verbal Behavior Paradigm illustrating the interconnection between utterances exchanged by a caregiver (speaker B) and child (speaker A). (S^{rD} = Reinforcing and discriminative stimulus, Rv = Verbal response.)

Table 4–2. Definitions and variables related to primary verbal operants.

Verbal Operant	Definition	Setting Event ($S^D \rightarrow$)	Verbal Response ($Rv \rightarrow$)	Consequence (S^{rR})
Mand (Traditional terms: command, demand, request)	Verbal behavior that specifies its reinforcer in response to deprivation states or aversive states	Deprivation states: hunger, thirst, loneliness, etc. Aversive states: pain, cold, etc.	Reflexive cries, vocalizations, words, direct requests, indirect requests, etc.	Providing the specified reinforcer—food, water, cuddling, object, action, or attention
Echoic (Traditional terms: imitation, echo)	Verbal behavior that reproduces acoustic properties of another's verbal behavior	Another speaker's utterance, which may or may not include a prompt (mand) to repeat	Reproduction of the acoustic properties of the other's utterance, either entirely or in part	Attention, feedback, and verbal responses based on approximation to the model
Tact (Traditional terms: name, label)	Verbal behavior that corresponds to other's responses to events, persons, objects, or relationships	Objects, persons, events, or relationships, which can occur in isolation or in clusters	Utterances that correspond to those exhibited by others in similar circumstances	Attention, feedback, and related verbal responses based on accurately corresponding to the circumstances
Extended Tact (Traditional terms: overextension, simile, metaphor, idiom, etc.)	Verbal behavior that occurs in response to stimuli other than the original stimuli due to stimulus generalization	Objects, persons, events, or relationships similar to another original stimulus	Generalization of verbal responses that convey similarity between setting events	Attention, feedback, and related verbal responses based on usefulness of the relationship
Intraverbal (Traditional terms: counting, reciting adage, tongue twister, etc.)	Verbal behavior that is influenced by the speaker's own prior verbal behavior	Words, phrases, sounds as they are produced in fixed orders or clusters	Subsequent words, phrases, sounds that have historically followed those that preceded them	Effects of successfully producing expected orders or associations
Textual (Traditional term: reading)	Verbal behavior in response to written or printed stimuli	Printed or handwritten text or any form of printed symbolic material	Production of the "name" of each stimulus	Access to information or stimulation through others' verbal behavior in their absence

Mands. A **mand** is a verbal operant whose setting event is a deprivation state or an aversive stimulus and whose verbal response specifies its reinforcer. The essence of a mand is requesting. It may be helpful to recognize that the term *mand* was derived from related traditional terms such as *demand* and *command.*

When responding to deprivation states such as hunger or thirst we mand exactly what will relieve our condition. We are most likely to behave that way if we recognize that the reinforcer is available and there is a cooperative listener. However, in the most severe deprivation states (e.g., our fourth day in the desert) we are likely to begin manding regardless of the availability of reinforcement or a listener (*Water! Water!*).

Some might ask why listeners cooperate with mands. Listeners comply because generally others have done so for them and they may want the speaker's assistance in the future. However, their cooperation is not a simple knee-jerk reflex. Prior history with the speaker may have taught them that the favor will never be returned. Or present circumstances may present a danger if they should comply (*Mommy, can I play with Daddy's gun?*).

It is notable that Skinner began his analysis with the mand. It is likely that this is the first verbal operant to evolve in the infant. Hunger pangs accompany the deprivation state that naturally develops between feedings. These internal stimuli prompt a physiological, **reflexive cry.** The normally attentive caregiver recognizes this cry (or at least anticipates it based on their feeding schedule) and then provides a feeding. Although unintentional, the foundation for manding has been laid.

What usually occurs with the continued interaction between caregivers and infants is that the topography or form of the mands become increasingly conventional, which makes the delivery of reinforcers more timely. Any parent who has experienced the frustration of being unable to understand what their crying child needs knows how important this progress is.

Later, as manding progresses, the nature of the required reinforcer might also become more sophisticated. The persistent toddler constantly asking *Wassat?* (What's that?) or the child asking *Why?* might truly be asking for labels or explanations. Or they may simply be vying for continued attention.

Echoics. An **echoic** is a verbal operant in which the setting event is another's verbal behavior that is reproduced by the speaker's verbal response. In other words, someone else's speech is the setting stimulus and the speaker is reinforced contingent upon accurate reproduction of that speech. Again, Skinner used the term *echoic,* although not truly a neologism, to avoid all the connotations of the more traditional term *imitation.*

The analysis suggests many circumstances in which echoic verbal behavior is useful. We echo other's verbal behavior when instructed to do so (*Repeat after me, I . . . do solemnly swear . . .*). Echoics are useful to adults to restimulate ourselves or hear something again (*Okay, you said, "Turn*

mand A primary verbal operant that occurs in response to a deprivation state or aversive stimulus and specifies its reinforcer; the behavioral equivalent of commanding, demanding, or requesting.

It should be noted that Skinner did not propose his model as an explanation for language development. Nonetheless, because of the universality of the learning principles involved, many have found it easy to make the extension to language development. ■

Skinner used *neologisms* ("new words") for most of his classifications to avoid confusion with the more traditional terms. ■

echoic A primary verbal operant whose reinforcement is contingent on reproducing the acoustic characteristics of others' speech; the behavioral equivalent of imitation.

right at the third stoplight, then . . ."). And, sometimes we find echoic behavior to be useful in delaying punishment. This is also known as "buying time," as when the unprepared student responds to the professor's impromptu question by repeating most of it, *Ah, yes, the three main factors that caused the United States to delay its entry into the European theater in World War II were . . .*

Echoic behavior is reinforced for a variety of reasons. Usually it signals attention, understanding, or agreement by the person who has echoed our verbal behavior. Additionally, caregivers reinforce children's echoics (Adult: *No, that's a dog.* Child: *Dog.* Adult: *That's right!*) because there is a remote sense of security when our children are later able to reliably tell us about their experiences.

Echoic behavior (or imitation) has been generally accepted as a primary means for children to learn the vocabulary of their language. Caregivers produce words they want their child to know and praise the child for a reasonable reproduction. However, the roles of echoic behavior in phonological and grammatical development have been more controversial.

 The theories and research dealing specifically with phonological development in infants are discussed in greater detail in Chapter 5. ∎

Some have proposed that infant's babbling exhibits *phonetic drift,* in that it increasingly contains consonants similar to the adult language around them. Further, some have suggested that this might be the earliest precursor to echoic behavior (Mowrer, 1960). In this process, infant sound productions that more closely approximate sounds made by caregivers would be *self-reinforcing* for the infant due to their association with the caregiver. The infant becomes more likely to produce those sounds again as opposed to unfamiliar ones.

In terms of an applied technology, the clinical application of echoic behavior is widely observed in treating language disorders. Regardless of the philosophical orientation, most procedures rely on immediate, delayed, or partial imitation to establish desired language skills.

Contrary to a common misconception, this formulation does *not* suggest that the caregiver is consciously involved in attempting to selectively reinforce individual sounds. (What caregiver has the time or energy?) Further, it is interesting to consider that, according to Piaget, infants' earlier egocentric view of their world might not permit them to even distinguish who produced a given sound. It simply is a sound they hear that is also associated with their most significant reinforcing experiences.

It should be noted that echoic behavior may also reproduce only selected elements (sounds, words, phrases) or other aspects of production such as pitch, rate, inflection. As adults, our speech may gradually reflect more of a new region's accent the longer we live there. In the nonsensical strings of infants' jargon, we are certain we hear the intonational contours of commands, questions, and even scolding. Finally, the role of echoic behavior in grammatical development has been well documented in the form of *selective imitation* (Owens, 2005), in which children echo a portion of the adult's preceding utterance (Father to Wife: *Do you know where my hat is?* Toddler: *Where hat is?*).

Tacts. **Tacts** are verbal operants whose setting event is an event, object, or relationship. The traditional term that correlates to tacting would be *naming.* Tacts are descriptions, comments, and verbal responses that "contact" the environment. Tacts are produced in response to actions, objects, people, attributes, spatial relations, and so on. Skinner adapted the neologism *tact* to convey that this verbal behavior benefits the listener "by extending his contact with the environment" (1957, p. 85).

The reinforcement for a tact is contingent on a conventional correspondence between the setting event and that tact. In other words, to be reinforced the response must resemble what others in that verbal community would say under similar circumstances for them to be useful.

The underlying principles that affect tacting are complex. First, there must be a correspondence or match between the verbal response and the referent to reinforce the speaker. Yet, some variance is permitted in some cases. The correspondence between the tact and the setting event might be *distorted* (*Oh, you have some dust on your dress. Let me brush it off*). This is, coincidentally, the essence of "tact" (as in diplomacy). If the speaker is younger, we tolerate less correspondence. The 1-year-old's *duse* might be initially accepted for milk (after all, it is moo-juice, right?). However, as adults, if there is no match between the tact and the actual state of affairs (*This car is like new!*), it is called a "sales pitch" or more accurately, a lie.

The motivation for reinforcing tacts may seem elusive. Hypothetically, the listener could ask, "What's in it for me?" It is more apparent when we consider the usefulness of being in contact with the world through another's verbal behavior (*Hey, your headlights are on!*). And, of course, the interest and attention that caregivers have for their children is rewarded in hearing where they have been, what they have seen, and what they have been doing.

Extended Tacts. The simplest notion of a pure tact is the ability to produce a label for something because we have a learning history with it. However, this poses the problem that we continue to confront a myriad of individual objects, events, and relationships with which we have had no experience. In spite of this, we are typically not speechless. Two processes, stimulus generalization and discrimination, rescue us from our dilemma and actually result in some very useful and highly complex forms of verbal behavior.

Stimulus generalization allows us to respond to stimuli other than those involved in the original learning. This behavioral process is based on some similarity between the new stimulus and the original stimulus. An instance of verbal behavior in which a tact occurs in response to stimuli other than the original one represents an **extended tact.**

Tacts might be extended to new stimuli based on simple stimulus generalization. That is, new stimuli differ in some ways, but are still similar enough to cause the tact to occur. When we see a foreign-built automobile we have never seen before, we are still able to call it a *car* without any

tacts A primary verbal operant that occurs in response to an object, event, or relationship and the form of the response exhibits a conventional correspondence to others' responses; the behavioral equivalent of naming, describing, or labeling.

The notion that language must be "conventional" is discussed as part of defining language in Chapter 1. ■

extended tact A primary verbal operant in which responses to stimuli other than the original stimuli occur due to stimulus generalization; the behavioral equivalent of figurative language.

The traditional term for this overgeneralization—*overextensions*—is also discussed in Chapter 6. ∎

This behavioral process corresponds well with the perceptual process of *abstraction* described in Chapter 3. ∎

additional tutoring. Children do not have to see every dog in the world to know what to call the present one. Stimulus generalization makes for very efficient learning and humans are good generalizers.

Another form of generalization is based on stimulus clusters. Many complex stimuli are actually clusters of stimuli. Various complex stimuli may share features, parts, or relationships. Stimulus generalization then allows the tact for one to be extended to the other. This results in some of our most colorful verbal behaviors, such as *similes* (*She's as light as a feather*), *metaphors* (*He's a bull in a china shop*), and *idioms* (*Who spilled the beans?*).

Extended tacts also explain why we can talk about missing items. Because stimuli cluster, responses have also come under control of those stimuli that accompany the expected stimulus. If we walk into a theater and there are no seats, we are still able to say the word *seat,* as in *There are no seats!* All the other characteristics are still there to support that response. However, under normal circumstances in that same familiar theater, we are not likely to utter *There are no Senators!* as they are not an expected accompaniment to our theater-going experience.

Stimulus generalization does allow for great economy in learning. Carried to an extreme, language could be very simple—everything we saw could be called by the first word we learned. Children give us a small glimpse of such a world when every furry, four-legged animal is called *goggy!* Life could get very confusing. Fortunately, generalization is offset by discrimination. With appropriate feedback from those around us, we learn to extend our tacts only in so far as it is useful to our listeners. As caregivers respond to children's generalizations differentially (i.e., reinforcing only the appropriate ones), only those responses that are relevant and useful endure in those circumstances and become a discriminated response class.

intraverbal   A primary verbal operant in which a speaker's verbal behavior is influenced by his or her own prior verbal behavior; the behavioral equivalent of chains as in recitation, alliteration, tongue twisters, and clichés.

Intraverbals.   An **intraverbal** is a verbal operant for which the setting event is prior verbal behavior. There is not a direct source of control or influence beyond a preceding verbal stimulus. The prior verbal behavior may come from others or from speakers themselves. This makes intraverbals a unique class of verbal behavior in that speakers' own verbal behavior can be the exclusive cause of their subsequent verbal behavior.

Intraverbals result in many of the social responses we make to others, as in *How are you? I'm fine.* In actuality, we can be miserably ill and still say what we always say because the connection between these responses is so thoroughly conditioned. Intraverbal control also accounts for what is called "word associations," as in *sea . . . food, new . . . car,* and *foot . . . ball.* The way we link such words is affected by the number of times these words have been associated and reinforced for a given speaker. (My wife would have been more likely to respond with *shore, house,* and *wear,* respectively, to the previous stimuli.)

chaining   A behavioral process in which responses are learned as fixed sequences in which each response leads to a subsequent response.

Perhaps the most prevalent example of intraverbals is a phenomenon called **chaining.** In chaining, the preceding sequence of verbal behaviors serves as the setting event for the responses that follow. Among the most common examples would be counting (*one, two, . . .*), recitations (*I pledge allegiance . . .*), and adages (*You buttered your bread, now . . .*).

An important distinction must be noted: chaining is *not* the source of grammatical behavior in Skinner's model. It does allow us to recite Lincoln's grammatical behavior, in the form of the Gettysburg Address, to please our seventh grade history teacher. That this misconception has been reprinted so often is especially bewildering in light of the entire section—three chapters—Skinner used to present his analysis of grammatical behavior (as autoclitic behavior, discussed below).

Textuals. It has been pointed out previously that verbal behavior is not restricted to spoken language. A verbal operant that occurs in response to written or printed stimuli is called a **textual.** Obviously, the traditional term most closely related to textual behavior is *reading.* However, it must be remembered that the stimuli might involve more than letters and words, including other visual stimuli as Blissymbols or Rebus symbols.

textual A primary verbal operant that occurs in response to written, printed, or graphic stimuli; the behavioral equivalent of reading.

Secondary Verbal Behavior: Autoclitics

First a confession and then a brief caveat. A confession is in order because many of the preceding sample utterances (in italics) used to illustrate the primary verbal operants were composed of word sequences. In their purest sense, the primary operants might occur in a more isolated manner—the mand *water* to satisfy our thirst, the tact *bird* in response to a winged creature, and so on. The preceding examples used word order (sentences) to place the primary verbal operants in more familiar contexts.

Now the caveat: Autoclitic behavior is perhaps the most subtle part of Skinner's model, which might explain why it is so often overlooked or misunderstood. Patience and an open mind will be valuable assets as we consider it.

The primary verbal operants (mands, tacts, echoics, and intraverbals) effectively make some simple isolated responses available to the speaker. However, for the most part we produce "strings" of responses. We commonly refer to the "stream of speech" and "lines of print." Furthermore, the words are arranged and rearranged in special ways. And yet, the world does not present itself in a single stream of experiences, and the events and objects mentioned in our speech are not lined up from left to right. In other words, we must wonder how our verbal responses come to be arranged in particular sequences. The quick and easy answer would be "Because we use grammar!" However, this is circular reasoning. "Grammar is the name of an effect, and not a cause" (Winokur, 1976, p. 128). It describes the results of how we behave verbally.

Skinner conceived of two levels of behavior to deal with these "special arrangements of responses" (1957, p. 313). The lower level provides the "building blocks" of verbal behavior (primary verbal operants) and the upper

Formal theories on reading and literacy are discussed in Chapter 10. ■

level manipulates these behaviors and, in so doing, comments on the relationships among them. This ordering is described by Winokur (1976) as "talking about talking" (p. 129).

The upper level of behavior is the source of autoclitic behavior. An **autoclitic** is defined as a tact whose setting event is the speaker's available verbal behavior and whose form will vary according to the relationships among the setting events for that verbal behavior. It is the secondary behavior that orders responses to indicate how each relates to the others. Autoclitics are verbal operants that come closest to the traditional notion of "grammar." The forms of autoclitic behavior include autoclitic orders, autoclitic words, and autoclitic tags.

Figure 4–2 presents a simple illustration of autoclitic ordering. The basic tacts are available to name the objects (*baby, chair*) and the relationship between them (*on*). Ordering these tacts comments on their relationship to each other. If this ordering is reinforced, then the order itself becomes an available response in similar circumstances in the future (through stimulus generalization). Skinner referred to these available ordering responses as *autoclitic frames*. This overall conceptualization fits well with an overview of language development, in which children learn their first words and then begin attempting to combine them to express the relationships between the objects or events they are perceiving.

autoclitic   A secondary verbal operant in which a conventional form (a tag, word, or order) comments on the relationships among the primary verbal operants; the behavioral equivalent to syntax and grammar.

 A qualification is called for with regard to word order. It tends to receive a great deal of attention, because English relies so heavily on word order to convey different meanings. In all fairness, some languages do not, and instead rely primarily on tags (inflections) to mark which words are the subject, object, indirect object, and so on. Japanese and Russian, in particular, are two prime examples of this.

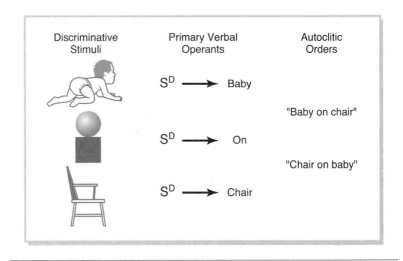

Figure 4–2. Illustration of autoclitic ordering of primary verbal operants (tacts). (S^D = Discriminative stimulus.)

Again, it has been a misconception that Skinner represented grammar as a "chain." A further misconception is that Skinner suggested that a child must experience and be reinforced for every possible variant of such "chains" (*girl on chair, book on chair,* etc.) to produce those utterances subsequently. Instead, the processes of stimulus generalization and response induction describe our ability to very rapidly apply this autoclitic frame to a variety of similar circumstances, arranging the relevant responses for each.

Other autoclitic elements include *autoclitic words* and *tags.* Autoclitic words include responses that we traditionally refer to as grammatical or function words (*is, was, not, this, that,* etc.). When properly inserted these convey assertion (*He is tall*), negation (*She is not tall*), and so forth. Similarly, autoclitic tags include what we traditionally call bound morphemes (*-ing, -ed, -s, -'s,* etc.). Finally, other autoclitic processes (primarily phrases) allow the speaker to comment on the reasons for the ensuing verbal behavior (*Mom told me to tell you that . . .*), its source (*The President said that . . .*) or its strength (*I think that . . .* versus *I am certain that . . .*).

Just as with primary tacts, the speaker must order responses in a conventional way to accurately comment on the relationships among the primary stimuli. If we do not, we may distort, omit, or deceive. Listeners do not reinforce us in those instances. For dishonest people, the extrinsic reinforcers gained in doing so apparently outweigh the approval of their listeners.

Children's autoclitic behavior that *accurately* comments on relationships is valuable to caregivers. Consider Figure 4–2 again. Should a child produce the wrong order (*chair on baby*) in relating a baby brother's situation in another room, the caregiver would be frantic. After rushing to examine the actual situation, the caregiver would be relieved. However, the caregiver might also adamantly repeat the proper order in hopes of avoiding such confusion in the future. In shaping autoclitic behavior in children, caregivers normally attribute inaccuracy to their child's developing language until it is clear that the expected autoclitic behaviors have been mastered; after that, it is lying.

Supplementary Variables

The variables discussed previously, such as deprivation states and setting events, are primary variables in that they give the speaker something to talk about. However, this is not always sufficient to produce verbal behavior. Other factors, called **supplementary variables,** strengthen or increase the likelihood that speakers will talk or even influence which of the available responses is produced.

supplementary variables Those stimuli, such as audiences, that additionally influence the likelihood of certain verbal behaviors.

Audiences. The social nature of this model naturally emphasizes the importance of the listener. In the previous interlocking verbal episodes (manding, tacting, etc.), the listener's role is linked to the speaker primarily as reinforcement mediator. (Of course, speakers and listeners alternate in their

audience Persons whose presence may set the occasion for an address or naming response, influence whether an utterance occurs, or influence the form of the utterances that do occur.

roles.) When listeners exert other influences on the verbal episode their role is referred to as an **audience.**

The audience can serve as the sole sufficient stimulus that sets the occasion for a specific response. When this occurs the verbal response is an *address,* as in *Bill, Madam President, Your Honor,* and so on. An audience can serve as a *response strengthener,* influencing *whether* we say something because someone is there. If the audience influences *what* we say, their role can be that of *response selector.* Of the many responses available when we slam our finger in a car door, certain ones are less likely depending on who is within earshot. The audience is a supplementary variable when it acts to strengthen or select responses.

Multiple Causation.   Finally, it is important to recognize, as Skinner did, that our verbal behavior is a phenomenon of great complexity. Skinner expressed this as two facts that must be dealt with: "(1) the strength of a single response may be, and usually is, a function of more than one variable and (2) a single variable usually affects more than one response" (1957, p. 227). At any one point in time, there is a host of factors that converge to influence us. At any moment, those with stronger conditioning histories or those that are more salient may determine which responses we produce. Suffice it to say, there is not sufficient space here to discuss the subtlety and complexity addressed in Skinner's three chapters analyzing the various effects of multiple causation.

Assessment of the Operant Model

The operant model described by Skinner has been the topic of much discussion. Its criticisms have come primarily from those who view language from an altogether different perspective. This is not entirely surprising; however, several misconceptions have persisted in the literature.

Limitations.   Skinner's model has been reviewed by several individuals (MacCorquodale, 1969, 1970; Morris, 1958). However, most criticisms appear to trace back to Chomsky's (1959) review of *Verbal Behavior.* The criticisms most relevant to language development generally relate to the model's treatment of reinforcement, imitation, and grammatical behavior. However, some have questioned whether Chomsky's criticisms represent the model's shortcomings or Chomsky's unfortunate misconceptions about it (MacCorquodale, 1969).

Chomsky asserted that there is no evidence that "slow and careful" reinforcement applied with "meticulous care" is necessary for acquiring language (Chomsky, 1959, pp. 39, 42, 43). Actually, as MacCorquodale (1970) pointed out, Skinner's model never required "slow," "careful," or "meticulous" reinforcement; in fact, those are Chomsky's words, not Skinner's. Nonetheless, Brown and Hanlon (1970) examined parents' praise of their children's utterances and found that very few instances were based on grammatical correctness. Instead, they primarily praised semantic accuracy (*That's right, it's a kitty*), suggesting that reinforcement has a minimal influence on children's grammatical behavior.

However, suggesting that overt, conscientious, and selective parental praise is the only source of reinforcement in children's verbal interactions is perhaps too narrow. Natural consequences, as in whether or not the child's utterance achieves the desired outcome, is a more likely reinforcer. Admittedly, this is difficult to evaluate because children do not always protest their parents' inaccurate interpretations. When misunderstood, they may acquiesce and change their utterance the next time.

Preschoolers' responses to adults' requests for clarification are discussed in more detail in Chapter 7. ■

Additionally, there is the potential influence of continued attention when children's utterances are acknowledged and understood. Ask any caregiver: there is probably no more powerful reinforcer for children than attention. And, finally, the role of self-reinforcement when children reproduce the verbal behaviors of their significant others has not been fully considered.

The second limitation asserts that imitation is of little use to the child learning language because adult speech provides such a deficient model. Adult-to-adult speech contains too many broken words, incomplete sentences, hesitations, and so forth. It was also noted that adults would not provide models for child utterances, such as *I runned*.

Verbal forms of signaling attention and providing corrective feedback—*expansions, extensions,* and *adult imitations*—are described in Chapter 6. ■

At the time of Chomsky's review, there had been little research regarding the nature of *adult-to-child* speech. As it turns out, adults greatly adjust their language to children (as in "motherese"), providing simplified models that are frequently repeated. They also unconsciously use consequating behaviors (Owens, 2005) that, in turn, prompt the child to imitate the adult's grammatically progressive models.

In Skinner's model, the explanation of utterances such as *I runned* in children's language would not rely on imitation. Utterances such as this stem from learning an autoclitic frame that overgeneralizes. These are eventually discriminated in reverting to the correct version *I ran*.

Finally, many critiques of Skinner's model allude to Chomsky's supposition that Skinner explained grammar through left-to-right chaining—the notion that each word in our sentences has been conditioned to follow the preceding word. This, of course, suggests that children (and adults) have heard, imitated, and been reinforced for every sentence in their repertoire. Obviously, verbal behavior is far more creative than this would permit. Skinner did *not* propose that chaining was the mechanism underlying grammatical behavior

Children's (and all speakers') ability to create (or "generate") a seemingly infinite variety of novel, yet grammatical, utterances is explained by Skinner primarily through autoclitic behavior. It is the result of learning basic elements—that is, words and phrases—and then learning to arrange them in autoclitic frames. These frames generalize to express new, but similar, circumstances. These behavioral processes result in new, "creative" responses that are useful to listeners because they correspond to relationships in the setting event and conform to accepted conventions.

Perhaps the model's most significant shortcoming is the limited descriptive range of its classifications. For example, to describe an utterance as a tact provides information about the circumstances of its occurrence and its consequences. However, whether it was in response to an object, action, attribute, or a relationship is not immediately clear. At least for professionals dealing clinically with specific utterances on a day-to-day basis, more specific terms (nouns, verbs, adjectives, prepositions, etc.) are often needed to describe the actual forms being observed in research or trained through intervention.

Contributions. Three closely related contributions of Skinner's model are apparent. First, its fundamental view of language as a social behavior has influenced pragmatic and sociolinguistic perspectives on language behavior. The functional units within the operant model correspond well with the communicative functions emphasized by pragmatics. However, the operant model also explains the source of meaning (the contingent relationship between stimuli and responses) and word order (autoclitic behavior).

Second, the social bases of the operant model emphasized the importance of interactions with the environment, especially in terms of relationships within setting events, caregiver models and feedback, imitation, and consequences. These aspects continue to be explored by behavioral scientists and sociolinguists alike.

Finally, the elements of the operant model have formed the basis of a technology of intervention for disordered language. It is difficult to conceive of a treatment procedure, no matter what it might be called, that does not provide a context (stimulus setting) to facilitate (evoke) some response that is followed by some functional outcome (consequences) (McLaughlin & Cullinan, 1981).

Summary

- The operant model was proposed by Skinner in 1957 as a functional analysis of verbal behavior as a social behavior.

- Primary verbal operants are classified based on their specific effects on others and are analyzed in terms of their setting events and consequences.

- Secondary behavior, in the form of autoclitic behaviors, acts on primary verbal operants to arrange them according to the relationships among them.

Structural Models: Chomsky's Syntactic Theories

Chomsky's formulations of language and language learning are at the opposite end of Skinner's on the philosophical spectrum. As a psycholinguistic model, Chomsky's focus was on the structure of language and the structure of the mind.

A disclaimer is in order: There is the natural tendency to contrast Chomsky's and Skinner's models. We should be careful not to prematurely throw either baby out with the proverbial bath water. To say that either viewpoint is completely wrong or completely right serves little purpose. It would be akin to saying that in analyzing a sample of swamp water, a chemist's conclusions are completely wrong and the biologist's completely right. They will obviously approach the task at different levels, using different terminology.

In this regard, Skinner, the behaviorist, restricted himself to observable relationships among objects, events and behavior. Chomsky, the linguist and philosopher, chose to speculate on the underlying natures of language and the mind. Both have many intriguing ideas to offer. Chomsky's transformational generative grammar (TGG) created a veritable revolution in linguistics. He has since embellished on it with government-binding theory.

Transformational Generative Grammar

The title of Chomsky's landmark book, *Syntactic Structures* (1957), stated its focus clearly. Chomsky's view that language structure reflects the structure of the human mind has emerged further since then (1965, 1981). Chomsky believes that language itself has structure that reveals its special status among human mental capacities. This underlying structure must explain how we are able to *generate* and *transform* an infinite variety of acceptable sentences, given our limited mental capacity. Chomsky's theory about the underlying organizational structure of language became known as **transformational generative grammar** (TGG). Two concepts fundamental to understanding TGG are *linguistic universals* and the *language acquisition device*.

transformational generative grammar   A linguistic theory proposing that universal rules generate underlying structures that may be transformed by rules to derive the specific sentence forms of each language.

Linguistic Universals.   Chomsky proposed that in spite of the diversity across individual languages, all human language is based on several shared principles, *linguistic universals.* For example, all languages include simple active declarative sentence forms and a means of negating them. Furthermore, sentences in all languages must include a subject and a predicate. (This prompts the proverbial chicken-egg question—perhaps all languages include these because humans learned to talk, and people, objects, and events are present in all environments?) Chomsky and his associates enumerated a number of universals that encompassed phonological and syntactic features common to all languages.

Ultimately, these features universal to all human languages suggested to Chomsky that language is an innate, species-specific capacity of humans. Lenneberg (1967) proposed a number of assertions supporting this biological foundation: First, that the onset of language in children coincided with other physiologic correlates; namely, their first step. Second, that development of language follows a fixed sequence; that is, all children learn language in the same order. Third, that language cannot be suppressed in humans; even those with limited mental capacities develop language at some level. And, fourth, that language cannot be taught to subhuman species.

Research since Lenneberg's writing might place some qualifications on the biological foundations. For example, there is more variation in children's sequences of language development than was recognized at the time. Also, animal researchers continue to find that other high-level primates (especially chimpanzees) exhibit impressive symbolic abilities. Meanwhile, we have yet to break the code barrier with dolphins and porpoises. Their apparent intelligence and the wide range of sounds they produce and perceive makes their potential for communication especially intriguing.

language acquisition device   The hypothetical innate mental structure that allows the child to process incoming language and derive a generative grammar.

McNeill (1970) later achieved "gender equity" by proposing a language acquisition system—that is, a LAS to complement Chomsky's LAD. ∎

Language Acquisition Device.   Language is exceedingly complex and yet seemingly acquired without effort by children. Furthermore, they do so even with limited and deficient input from adults. This contrast suggested a special biological feature to Chomsky. If language is an innate capacity unique to humans, then the human brain must be specially structured for processing language.

Chomsky proposed the **language acquisition device** (LAD) as a concept to represent this special innate organization of the human brain. In spite of the word *device,* there is no suggestion of an identifiable physical structure in the brain. The "structure" is in the special organization of the human brain—the unique way in which it might be "pre-wired" for processing language.

The LAD might be conceived of as the proverbial "black box." Not much is known about the device itself—its physical makeup, its organization, even its existence are all hypothetical. Nonetheless, psycholinguists such as Chomsky have speculated on the nature of its operation. Figure 4–3 illustrates the concept of the LAD.

Basically, the LAD receives linguistic input and extracts from it a generative grammar. The child's LAD operates much like a linguist decoding an unfamiliar language. The data received include any samples of linguistic information within earshot—the *corpus of speech.* The LAD extracts regularities from these samples and then forms hypotheses about them. As further samples are received, these regularities either reoccur and are confirmed as rules of the grammar, or they are contradicted and eliminated. Through this process children extract all the rules of grammar for the language around them. An important distinction to note is that the LAD requires *only* input to be activated. No additional interaction (i.e., feedback or correction) is necessary for the LAD to derive a generative grammar for the language.

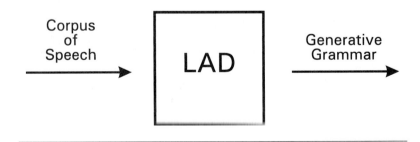

Figure 4–3. Schematic of Chomsky's language acquisition device (LAD).

The Components of TGG

Chomsky's model hypothesized mental processes and structures at several levels which allow humans to comprehend and generate an infinite variety of sentences.

Deep and Surface Structures. Chomsky's transformational generative grammar is based on a two-level model. The **deep structure** is a hypothetical mental construct proposed to represent the basic meanings and relationships underlying a speaker's sentence. The **surface structure** is the actualized production of a sentence expressing those meanings and relationships. Figure 4–4 illustrates the hypothetical relationship between deep and surface structure.

> **deep structure** The underlying structure of a sentence generated by the phrase structure rules.
>
> **surface structure** The actualized production of a sentence by a speaker.

The direction of the process between the surface and deep structures depends on the operation. To produce a sentence, the underlying thought begins at the level of the deep structure ("deep within the mind") and must be converted to and produced as surface structure (the words that "surface" to carry that idea). Conversely, to comprehend someone else's sentence, the listener must process the surface structure heard to derive the meanings and relationships in the underlying deep structure. There are two related components involved in these mental processes: a generative component and a transformational component.

> The concepts of *surface structure* and *deep structure* correlate closely with *linguistic performance* and *linguistic competence* discussed in Chapter 1. ∎

The Generative Component. **Phrase structure rules** *generate* the underlying deep structure of sentences, based on the speaker's generative grammar. To produce a sentence (a surface structure) the speaker begins with an idea. (Yes, some of us start talking without one, but we will operate

> **phrase structure rules** The underlying universal rules that generate the basic syntactic relationships in the deep structure of a sentence.

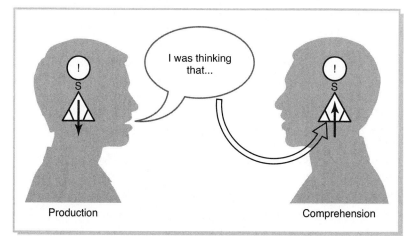

Figure 4–4. Illustration of the bidirectional nature of production and comprehension. (! = idea, thought, etc.; S = sentence deep structure.)

under normal circumstances here.) The speaker's idea is just the "germ" of a sentence. There are no words; just a thought without linguistic form. To be expressed, this thought must be converted into linguistic form. To accomplish this the speaker applies phrase structure rules to generate the elements of a sentence that will express that thought. This is not a conscious activity; the linguistic knowledge is implicit and the processes are intuitive. Also, because the underlying linguistic relationships are universal, phrase structure rules are also considered to be universal.

Chomsky viewed the phrase structure rules as analogous to the rules of algebra. These permit expression of an infinite number of outcomes (meanings) through values (phrase structures) related through a given formula (syntax). Given the formula $X = A + B$, we can plug in infinite combinations of values for A and B and arrive at an infinite variety of Xs. In addition, we can add underlying relationships to the formula, as in "where A = (3n) and B = 3 + 12n." (Don't ask me to solve this!) For a speaker, given the underlying rules (formulas) of his or her generative grammar, the speaker plugs in the words to produce an infinite variety of acceptable sentences.

Phrase structure rules follow these same principles while generating statements of the relationships in a sentence and relating each level of a sentence to the other levels. Figure 4–5 is an illustration of a "sentence tree." The elements in each level, including the spoken words of the sentence, are all called *constituents*. Each constituent is related hierarchically to the constituents immediately above and below it. Therefore, in the tree the immediate constituents of the first noun phrase (NP) are a determiner (Det) and noun (N). In turn, their immediate constituents are *the* and *horse,* and so on.

The upper portion of Figure 4–5 presents the phrase structure rules that would generate this sentence tree. Remember that these phrase structure rules describe the underlying patterns for this sentence; other sentences could be shorter, requiring fewer rules, or longer, requiring more. In addition, the underlying structure of sentences can be more complex.

The Transformational Component.   Chomsky hypothesized that deep structures are universally *simple active declarative* (SAD) in form. That is, they contain only one *subject + predicate* relationship (simple), the subject is carrying out the verb (active), and it is not an interrogative, passive, negative, or imperative construction (making it a declarative). Such a sentence might be, *The boy is kicking the ball.*

Of course, not all sentences we produce are SAD. The same basic relationships might be expressed in several forms. For example, consider the following variations of this sentence:

> *The boy is not kicking the ball.*
>
> *The ball is being kicked by the boy.*
>
> *Is the boy kicking the ball?*

In spite of their varying forms, we still recognize the same basic relationships (a young male acting on a sphere with his foot) carried in each,

A mnemonic device to help remember this might go something like, "All deep structures are SADLY ACTIVE, I DECLARE!" ■

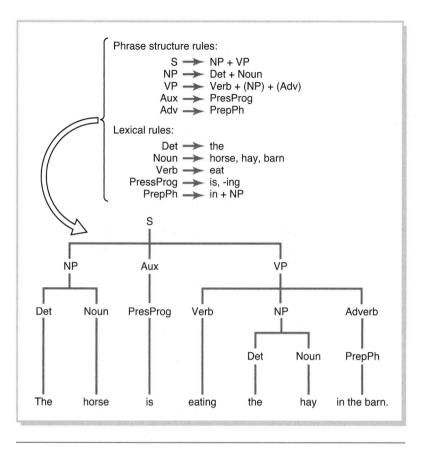

Phrase structure rules:

$$S \longrightarrow NP + VP$$
$$NP \longrightarrow Det + Noun$$
$$VP \longrightarrow Verb + (NP) + (Adv)$$
$$Aux \longrightarrow PresProg$$
$$Adv \longrightarrow PrepPh$$

Lexical rules:

$$Det \longrightarrow the$$
$$Noun \longrightarrow horse, hay, barn$$
$$Verb \longrightarrow eat$$
$$PressProg \longrightarrow is, -ing$$
$$PrepPh \longrightarrow in + NP$$

Figure 4–5. Illustration of underlying phrase structure rules, sentence tree, and the resulting utterance. ($\Rightarrow$ = "is realized as," S = Sentence, NP = Noun phrase, VP = Verb phrase, Aux = Auxiliary, Adv = Adverb, PresProg = Present progressive, PrepPh = Prepositional phrase.)

which were also present in the original SAD form of this sentence. This suggests that these variations were created by transforming the underlying SAD of the deep structure while preserving the original basic relationships.

Chomsky accounted for this relatedness among such sentences by proposing the hypothetical mental construct called transformational rules. **Transformational rules** operate to alter the basic syntactic structures generated in the deep structure. Transformational rules describe the underlying mental operations speakers apply to transform a SAD construction into such variations as interrogative, negative, passive, or imperative constructions.

There are two types of transformational rules. **Elementary operations** alter a single deep structure, whereas **generalized operations** operate across more than one deep structure to create compound or complex constructions. The operations these describe are assumed to be available (i.e., universal) in

Preschoolers' mastery of the basic sentence types is discussed in Chapter 8. ■

transformational rules The linguistic rules applied in each language to transform underlying sentence structure into the varying surface structures produced in each language.

elementary operations
Transformational rules that are applied to a single deep structure, such as addition, deletion, transposition, and substitution.

generalized operations
Transformational rules that are applied across more than one deep structure to create complex or compound sentences.

conjoining   The linguistic process of linking two independent clauses into a single sentence structure.

embedding   The linguistic process of inserting a subordinate clause into an independent main clause.

all languages. However, each language applies them differently. As a result, for example, the surface structure of questions may not be similar across languages.

Elementary operations include addition, deletion, transposition, and substitution. For example, to transform the SAD form of *The boy is kicking the ball* into a negative form, the speaker "tags" the underlying deep structure for negation (T_{NEG}). In English, this calls for the operation of *addition,* which inserts *not* into the surface structure, *The boy is not kicking the ball.* Table 4–3 provides definitions of elementary transformations and Figure 4–6 illustrates typical ways in which these operations might be applied to create basic variations of a sentence.

Generalized transformations operate to combine elements of two underlying deep structures. The two generalized operations, **conjoining** and **embedding,** result in single surface structures with at least two predicates. The process of conjoining inserts a conjunction to connect the two deep structures. This results in a *compound sentence.* In these, both predicates may be expressed, as in the sentence, *John walked and Mary laughed.* Figure 4–7 illustrates this application of a generalized transformation. In other instances, if the underlying predicates are redundant, (i.e., both subjects performed the same action) the two separate actions are implied through a compound subject, as in *John and Mary walked.*

In embedding, elements of one deep structure are inserted within the other. The simplest example is in the case of adjective modifiers used in noun phrase elaboration. For example, the seemingly simple sentence, *The big dog barked,* is actually composed of two underlying deep structures, *The dog is big* and *The dog barked.* Other complex constructions relating more than one proposition in a single sentence include such forms as relative clauses (*I like the cat that has stripes*) and noun phrase complements (*I think I want this one*).

The discussion and examples given provide a very basic introduction to transformational generative grammar. As complicated as most languages

Table 4–3. Types and examples of elementary transformations.

Transformation	Operation	Example
Addition	Adds an element	This is fun. (SAD) This is [not] fun. (Negative)
Deletion	Deletes an element	You close the door. (SAD) [~~You~~] close the door. (Imperative)
Transposition	Rearranges elements	He is laughing. (SAD) [Is he] laughing? (Yes/No Question)
Substitution	Substitutes an element	The girl is reading. (SAD) [She] is reading. (Pronominal)

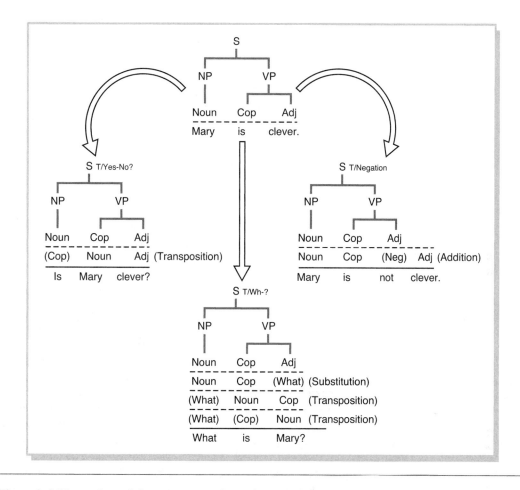

Figure 4–6. Illustrations of elementary transformations applied to a basic sentence to generate varied sentence structures. (S = Sentence, NP = Noun phrase, VP = Verb phrase, Cop = Copula verb, Adj = Adjective.)

are, one can appreciate that the intricacies of transformational generative grammar can not be explained or illustrated in a few pages. Recently, Chomsky elaborated on these concepts further yet.

Government-Binding Theory

In government-binding (GB) theory, Chomsky (1981) made a number of revisions in an attempt to address several issues that were not adequately accounted for in TGG. Concerns with the diversity of languages, peculiarities and exceptions within languages, and the overall learnability of language for children.

The newer GB theory still presumes an innate, biologically given predisposition to learn language. The grammar proposed by GB theory is still

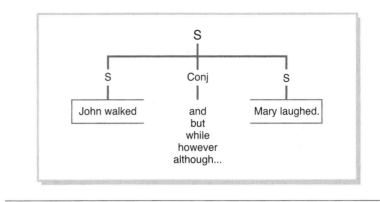

Figure 4–7. Illustration of a generalized transformation applied to conjoin two simple sentences into a compound sentence. (S = Deep structure, Conj = Conjunction.)

an internalized generative grammar that is universal and capable of being derived from limited exposure to language. The *universal grammar* of GB theory is comprised of a set of constraints on the structure of languages. These constraints describe what mechanisms are permissible in a language, even though specific languages may accomplish them in different ways.

There are four levels in the universal grammar of GB theory. The first level, **D-structures** (deep structures), includes sentence structure rules and the speaker's lexicon (words). The second level, **S-structures,** relates closely to the concept of surface structures (in TGG) with the exception that they are abstract, not actualized as in TGG. **Phonetic form rules** constitute the third level and the abstract phonological component. The fourth level, **logical form rules,** describes the abstract process of interpreting sentences, especially ambiguous or confusing sentences. In addition to the two additional levels, there are six subtheories in GB theory that describe the various constraints and influences that syntactic and semantic considerations exert on various structures such as noun phrases, pronominals, and relative clauses.

Assessment of TGG

Figuratively speaking, Chomsky's *Syntactic Structures* was the other "shot heard round the world" in 1957. Published the same year as Skinner's *Verbal Behavior,* it had a revolutionary impact on linguistics and has been thoroughly analyzed and discussed.

Limitations.   The criticisms that have been posed against TGG refer to its lack of comprehensiveness, its predictiveness, and its limited potential to *explain* language development.

D-structures   A component within government-binding theory that contains the sentence structure rules and the lexicon.

S-structures   A component of government-binding theory that occurs just prior to the production of the surface structure.

phonetic form rules A component of government-binding theory that generates an abstract characterization of sounds.

logical form rules The component of government-binding theory dealing with the logical aspect of sentences.

One of the immediate criticisms of TGG regarded its one-dimensional view of language. The account focuses entirely on the syntactic structure of language. It severely neglects the phonological, semantic, or pragmatic aspects of language. The contexts in which speakers talk, the purposes their utterances serve, as well as real human communication as a social behavior are effectively omitted.

The theory made many predictions about the course of language development based on its indexing of grammatical complexity. Although these predictions hold true with children in general, the theory did not account for the many individual variations found by researchers since its publication (Bloom & Lahey, 1978).

Finally, perhaps the most criticized component of the theory was the innate language acquisition device. Very few (not even Skinner) would suggest that the human brain contributes nothing to language learning. However, a "black box" with no real form, structure, or location does little to actually *explain* the process or dynamics of learning language.

Many of the assumptions made to support the LAD have fallen away (Bohannon & Warren-Luebecker, 1985). There is research to suggest that parents do tutor their language learners, responding differently to grammatical and ungrammatical utterances. The assertion that language develops rapidly and effortlessly at a very early age has been continually revised, extending the age of language mastery into adolescence and even adulthood for more subtle features. Additionally, the notion that children deduce the rules based on a severely limited sample must be questioned (Chapman et al., 1992). It has been estimated that a typical child has spoken 10 to 20 million words and listened to 20 to 40 million words by age 4 (Wagner, 1985)! Finally, research in primate communication abilities suggests that humans may simply represent the high range of symbolic ability.

Another criticism has involved the characterization of children as active versus passive language learners. In TGG, the child is essentially a passive location for the LAD, which merely needs language input to process. Researchers have instead found that children are active communicators interacting with adults who intuitively provide them with well adapted models, feedback, and consequences.

Additionally, in terms of scientific control and the prospect of an applied technology, the notion of a LAD that is unaffected by feedback would make the efforts of the best language clinicians futile.

Chomsky's government-binding theory addresses several limitations of TGG in considering phonological and semantic aspects of language. However, it has not developed a large base of research yet and its influence in clinical applications is not yet apparent. As a result, its overall contributions are difficult to assess at this point. The major concern that should be noted is its immensely expanded complexity over TGG—four levels and six subtheories! Those who look for scientific elegance might already be reaching for Occam's Razor!

In terms of Skinner's operant model $S^D \rightarrow Rv \rightarrow S^{Rr}$, it could be said that Chomsky's TGG primarily addressed the "Rv" component. ∎

Recall the role of Occam's Razor in achieving scientific elegance, described earlier in this chapter. ■

Contributions.   Remember, a proper caution about "throwing the baby out with the bath water" was given at the outset of this section. Chomsky's TGG theory has had a significant impact in linguistics with many "spin-off" contributions to other fields, including psychology and speech-language pathology.

Chomsky's TGG created a revolution in linguistics. It prompted renewed interest in understanding the psychological process of understanding sentences. The concepts of deep and surface structures illustrated the hypothetical concept of underlying manipulation of language behaviors.

TGG provided new insights into the structure of language. For example, the notion of transformational rules as a "map" of the underlying mental operations of generating and comprehending sentences has been useful in indexing the relative complexity of language. Listeners generally comprehend sentences with fewer transformations more quickly.

Similarly, this concept fits the overall picture of language development; that is, sentences involving more transformational operations are generally produced and understood by children later than simpler ones. Further, the ability of TGG to describe the underlying relatedness of language structures suggests training strategies. Understanding the nature of developing sentence elements, as illustrated by TGG, is often helpful in manipulating language structures as they are trained clinically. This, combined with its retention of mostly traditional syntactic terms (e.g., nouns, verbs), makes it a precise *descriptive* model.

Paying attention to the patterns of language behavior described by TGG has the potential to suggest research questions in verbal behavior. Skinner's primary verbal operants and autoclitic behavior have been compared to Chomsky's phrase structure rules and transformational rules, respectively, and found to be very analogous concepts. They differ primarily in their terminology and level of analysis (Moerk, 1992b; Segal, 1977). For example, Skinner's autoclitic behavior refers to the speaker's autoclitic arrangement of primary verbal operants to express relationships in the stimulus setting, according to the conventional patterns of the verbal community. Chomsky, alternately, mapped the hypothetical mental process of arranging behavior in terms of underlying movements of sentence elements according to the rules of a TGG, which reflect conventional patterns of the language.

Summary

- Chomsky proposed transformation generative grammar (TGG) in 1957 as a theory of the mental processes for understanding and formulating sentences.

- Two fundamental assumptions of TGG included the existence of linguistic universals and the innate, species-specific nature of language.

- Chomsky proposed the language acquisition device (LAD) as the hypothetical, innate mental structure that allows children to develop language in a seemingly effortless manner.

- TGG proposed a two-level model based on the underlying deep structure of a sentence which is ultimately produced or actualized as surface structure.

- In TGG, phrase structure rules generate the basic syntactic relationships in the deep structure and transformational rules transform this into other sentence forms prior to being produced.

The Semantic Model: Fillmore's Case Grammar

It is the nature of science to progress in response to past attempts—both successes and failures. For linguistics, Chomsky's transformational generative grammar theory provided a stepping stone. It fostered appreciation for the concept of a generative grammar and the underlying complexity of language.

On the other hand, there were those who responded to its shortcomings. For example, Chomsky asserted that the syntax of the deep structure was all that was needed to interpret a sentence, even an ambiguous one. Consider the sentence *They are baking potatoes,* which can be interpreted either of two ways. It might refer to the ongoing activity of several cooks or, it could refer to the best use for certain potatoes (baking versus boiling). According to TGG, this ambiguity would be resolved by analyzing the two different deep structures.

Others (Chafe, 1970; Fillmore, 1968; Katz & Fodor, 1963) disagreed with this notion, suggesting that meaning was better understood at a semantic level. They emphasized that semantic concepts—meanings—exist separately from the syntax of language. Meaning is in the relationships among events and objects in the environment. Words and word orders merely encode those relationships symbolically.

From this perspective, then, the previous ambiguous sentence about potatoes is a problem of distinguishing between two possible environmental contexts. There *are* two different syntactic deep structures, as Chomsky asserted; that is the essence of ambiguity. However, resolving the ambiguity comes from identifying which context prompted the original statement. In other words, knowing the situation allows the listener to select the relevant deep structure for interpretation. Figure 4–8 illustrates the relationship of ambiguous sentences and their contexts.

Shortcomings such as this and a general belief that meaning requires greater consideration in any formulation of language prompted new semantic models. Fillmore's case grammar theory has played a principal role in this area of child language.

Case Grammar Theory

The basis of case grammar is meaning. The semantic aspect of language assists us in "making sense" of sentences. The meanings of words and how words relate to each other affects our understanding of sentences. Some words, because of their underlying meanings, cannot go together in spite of the grammatical

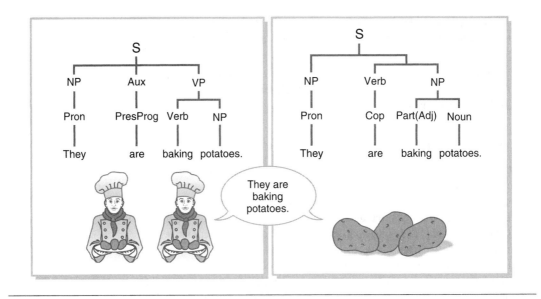

Figure 4–8. Illustration of the relationship of an ambiguous sentence to deep structures and setting events.
(S = Sentence, NP = Noun phrase, VP = Verb phrase, Aux = Auxiliary verb, Pron = Pronoun, PresProg = Present progressive, Cop = Copula verb, Part [Adj] = Participle, or a verb acting as an adjective.)

roles they fill. For example, we can say, *The girl washed the car,* but we cannot logically substitute *tree* for *girl.* Even though they are both nouns, the tree differs in the semantic features that permit the girl to play the role she does in this sentence. Specifically, the girl can execute the verb, the tree cannot. How the nouns in a sentence relate to its verb is the essence of Fillmore's case grammar.

case grammar A generative grammar that emphasizes the cases or semantic roles assumed by nouns in relationship to the verb of a sentence.

Case grammar is a psycholinguistic generative grammar in which meaning defines the fundamental relationships in a sentence. A *semantic relation* (or *case relation*) specifies the semantic role played by a noun in relation to the verb in a given sentence. Table 4–4 presents the universal semantic relations outlined by Fillmore.

The categorical unit, the noun phrase in this relationship, also carries the potential for modifiers as well as an optional preposition. In our previous example, the noun phrases (*The girl, the car*) could have carried modifiers (*tall, young,* and *old, blue,* etc.). Had a noun phrase for location been included, it would have likely carried a preposition (<u>in</u> *the driveway*).

Case grammar does not replace the syntactic level; it takes precedence over it. In other words, the semantic deep structure of the sentence is generated before its syntactic form. Although the concept of deep structure was retained in case grammar, its composition is different from TGG.

Students should be forewarned that several different classification schemes exist. Although many of the same relationships are included in all, the specific names for them can vary. ∎

Modality and Propositions

In case grammar the underlying deep structure is composed of a modality and a proposition. The **modality** refers to a collection of markers signaling

Table 4–4. Fillmore's universal semantic case relations.

Semantic Case	Definition	Example
Agentive	The initiator of the action indicated by the verb.	*Mary* baked a cake.
Dative	The animate affected by the action or state indicated by the verb.	Bill gave *Mary* a present.
Experiencer	The animate who experiences an event or internal state.	*Mary* felt the cool breeze.
Factitive	An object or being that results from the action indicated by the verb.	Bill assembled the *toy*.
Instrumental	The object used in the action indicated by the verb.	Bill tightened the bolt with a *wrench*.
Locative	The location of the action or state indicated by the verb.	Mary's car is in the *garage*.
Objective	The object or being affected by the action indicated by the verb.	Bill painted the *house*.

the eventual syntactic form the sentence will take. The modality indicates such aspects as the tense and sentence type of the intended sentence. The **proposition** is a set of semantic relations that specify the relationships between the nouns of the sentence and its verb. These relationships constitute the overall meaning of the sentence. Figure 4–9 illustrates the relationship of sentence modality, propositions, and case relations in sentence deep structure according to case grammar.

modality The component of deep structure in case grammar that carries the tense and sentence type.

proposition The set of semantic relations that specify the relationships between the nouns of the sentence and its verb.

An important distinction to appreciate involves word order. Case grammar does not dictate word order; syntax continues to be the domain of TGG. This is not an insignificant distinction, especially as we examine languages other than English. Brown (1973) provided an insightful analysis of this distinction in English and Japanese. Where English relies heavily on linear (left-to-right) word order to indicate semantic relations, Japanese depends heavily on "tags" (called particles or postpositions) attached to each noun to indicate its semantic role. Brown (1973, pp. 9–11) analyzed this contrast in typical productions of the sentence, *Mr. Smith cut the rope with a knife,* in both languages:

Mr. Smith		**cut**		**the rope**		**with a knife.**
(agent)		(action)		(object)		(instrument)

Sumisu-san	**wa**	**nao**	**o**	**naifu**	**de**	**kirimashita.**
(Smith-Mr.)	(agent)	(rope)	(object)	(knife)	(instrument)	(cut)
						(action)

There are possible variations of the English version. For example, the passive word order would have been, *The rope was cut by Mr. Smith with a*

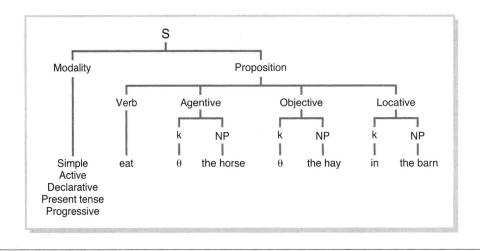

Figure 4–9. Illustration of sentence deep structure according to case grammar. (k = preposition marker, T = null, NP = Noun phrase.)

knife. In English, we would focus on the word order to interpret the underlying relationships. (This is even more apparent in reversible relationships, as in *The girl was kissed by the boy.*) However, the Japanese word order can vary far more than this and still be properly interpreted. Their secret is in the "tags" *wa, o,* and *de.* These mark the semantic agent, object, and instrument, no matter in what order they occur. In summary, although most semantic relations are considered universal, the grammatical devices (word orders, grammatical words, and grammatical tags) for encoding them might vary substantially across languages.

Observations such as this reinforced the notion for Brown and others that semantics takes precedence over syntax—that meaning precedes form. The meanings are universally available in the environment and then speakers acquire the forms to signal the meanings in their language.

Impact on Child Language Research

In fairness to Fillmore, his was a general semantic theory. It was not his intention to explain child language development. Others found the concept of case grammar useful in their research in child language development. ■

The emergence of semantic theories such as case grammar changed more than just the prevailing perspective of language in general. It altered the theoretical model of language development. This new perspective significantly influenced procedures in child language research and introduced new considerations in treating children with disordered language.

Impact on Theories of Language Development.   The natural insight from a semantically based grammar is that cognition might play a significant role in language development. Previously, Chomsky's syntax-only TGG with its LAD had minimized the influence of cognition in language development. The LAD only required linguistic input; the child need not interact with the environment in any way.

In contrast, semanticists emphasized that the meanings expressed by children rely on their perception and understanding of the world. Children do not simply deduce word orders (syntax) and then look for occasions to apply them; instead, they recognize relationships as they interact with their environment and then attempt to express those relationships to their audiences. From this perspective, children's language reveals their cognitive development.

That children's language development reflects their cognitive development is a theoretical concept referred to as **cognitive determinism**— cognition determines language (Bloom, 1973). A related term, *cognitive interactionism,* implies that language also emerges out of interaction between a child's available linguistic forms and the cognitive problems to which the child applies them. The resulting language reflects the child's cognitive solution, no matter how limited (Brown, 1973).

Researchers have found that children demonstrate certain cognitive abilities at the approximate time a corresponding language behavior emerges (Clark, 1973a). For example, children begin to express basic reflexive relations (appearance, disappearance, nonexistence), producing a word for a missing object at about the time that they demonstrate the concept of object permanence. Similar relationships have been found between developing language and related cognitive abilities. However, it must be remembered that correlation is not the same as causation; because two events occur at about the same time does not necessarily mean that one caused the other.

Impact on Research Procedures.   The premise of the semantic school of thought, that meaning precedes form (Bloom & Lahey, 1978), altered researchers' methods in two major ways. It became necessary to alter the way in which utterances were classified and to expand the scope of data collected in studying children's language.

It had been the practice for researchers to apply the prevailing syntactic analysis to children's utterances. However, it became apparent to Bloom (1970) that applying the rules of adult grammar to describing children's utterances was inadequate. Bloom's illustration of this involved a now classic quote from Kathryn, one of her subjects: *Mommy sock.*

This utterance occurred two times that were notable in Kathryn's language sample. A syntax-only analysis would have classified both occurrences as *Noun + Noun.* However, Bloom recognized that the two situations that prompted this same utterance form were actually different. One instance involved possession (Kathryn retrieving her mother's sock), whereas the other indicated action (a comment on Mommy dressing Kathryn). Obviously, *Noun + Noun* failed to capture this very important difference. Semantically, the underlying relationships were *Possessor + Entity* and *Agent + Object.* Researchers began coding utterances semantically to preserve the underlying semantic relations that prompted them.

cognitive determinism
A philosophy that emphasizes the primary role played by cognition in determining the acquisition of language.

 Cognitive determinism is discussed in Chapter 3. ■

Compare case frame rules and semantic-syntactic rules with Skinner's autoclitic frames. The concept of expressing relationships through word order is present in all three. ■

method of rich interpretation Process of analyzing children's utterances while considering the linguistic and nonlinguistic context.

Compare the method of rich interpretation and a behavioral analysis of the contingent relationship between setting events and verbal operants. ■

One-word utterances and early word combinations were assigned semantic relations according to their apparent relationships. The significance of expressing semantic relationships through consistent word orders prompted researchers to refer to the orders as *case frame rules* (Brown, 1973) and *semantic-syntactic rules* (Bloom & Lahey, 1978).

The other change in method was actually necessitated by this shift in focus. Bloom noted that fully understanding the meaning of children's utterances would be more easily accomplished if the linguistic and nonlinguistic contexts were analyzed. In other words, utterances that preceded the child's utterance and the actions, objects, events, gestures, and facial expressions that accompanied it were preserved in the transcripts. This became known as the **method of rich interpretation.** (It is instructive to note that a premature acceptance of a syntax-only theory delayed linguists' "discovery" of a technique caregivers resorted to long ago, especially when confronted with a tantrum.)

Assessment of the Semantic Model

The semantic model was not intended to replace Chomsky's syntactic model. As it generated increased attention during the 1970s, the semantic model expanded the psycholinguistic perspective of language. As a result, it has been generally viewed as a complementary model.

Limitations.   Most researchers judge that although cognition is a major component in language development, it cannot explain it entirely. Correlating a cognitive ability with a seemingly relevant language behavior does not mean that the one caused the other. The strongest statement that seems reasonable is that cognitive abilities seem generally related to language development and certain cognitive skills may even be prerequisite to the development of language structures that express them.

A semantic model faces some problems with reliability and objectivity. Several classification systems have evolved (Bloom, 1973; Brown, 1973); variations across them may affect the reliability (consistency) of data. However, the larger difficulty comes from the nature of the analysis. There is a measure of subjectivity ("mind reading") in classifying utterances. Whether the child's word order reflects the intended meaning and, if it did, whether the partner's interpretation was accurate might not be immediately apparent, even with the method of rich interpretation.

With each additional rule system the definition of scientific elegance is stretched a little further. Stacking syntax on top of semantics suggests speakers must operate sequentially through two different rule systems to express themselves or comprehend others. Once again, although both rule systems provide detailed *descriptions* of language, Occam's Razor might question the lack of economy in such a two-tiered explanation.

Finally, our basic question of explaining (as opposed to describing) *how* children develop language has prompted researchers to continue looking for the catalysts in this process. A semantic-based case grammar excludes a very dynamic element—the child's daily social and communicative transactions. Case grammar describes the importance of the relationships expressed by the child, but neglects the purposes in expressing them—communication!

Contributions. Consideration of semantics in language and language development expanded the generative model of language. Linking syntactic devices to meaning put speakers back in contact with the relationships that prompt them to talk.

Placing the semantic model in the context of the operant model suggests that it accounts for two of the three major components of the operant model (i.e., $S^D \rightarrow (Rv)$. Semantic relations classify meanings; meaning is based on the relationship between S^Ds and their corresponding responses, the Rv. ■

The research indicates that the same early semantic relations tend to occur across languages. In addition, it appears that children tend to rely on similar word orders to express these relations, no matter which language is spoken (Brown, 1973; Slobin, 1985).

This shift in focus prompted additional research into children's cognitive abilities for both language and in general. This has enhanced our ability to fine-tune the contexts in which children learn, whether in an educational or clinical setting. Improved understanding of children's cognitive abilities has reinforced careful consideration of providing appropriate contexts ("stimulus support") when training language in children and adults.

■ Summary

- The semantic model analyzes sentences in terms of case grammar, in which meaning is carried in the relationships between each noun and the verb in a sentence.

- The semantic model focused language development research on the influence of cognition on language development.

- In applying the method of rich interpretation, researchers recognized the importance of considering the context to determine meaning of children's utterances.

The Pragmatic Model: Searle's Speech Acts Theory

Semantic models of language (e.g., Fillmore's case grammar) expanded the theoretical framework of language. It pushed linguists a step further, beyond the structure of sentences to consider the meanings and relationships they express. However, to many researchers, there was one major element still missing—human communication.

For these individuals, communication remained as the most fundamental reason for the existence of human language. In this view, there is no practical reason for syntax to exist or for meaning to be expressed other than for the purpose of communicating some goal or intention. Therefore, these researchers were interested in the pragmatics of language.

It would even be reasonable to state that the validity of the syntactic and semantic elements of language rely on a pragmatic analysis. In other words, the only means we have to determine the true interpretation of the structure or meaning of an utterance is to evaluate its effect on the listener. If we observe a speaker in a hypothetical foreign land who says what seems the equivalent of "Go jump off a bridge" to each passerby, but without fail they check their watch and tell him the time, then what is the true meaning of the utterance? There are many such utterances (e.g, idioms, indirect requests) that function in ways that conflict with purely structural analysis.

Those linguists who emphasize the pragmatic use of language to communicate in social contexts are called *sociolinguists*. The field of sociolinguistics has analyzed several basic elements of pragmatics. First, the *function* of language refers to its various uses as a practical tool for accomplishing goals through social means (through the help of others). The second aspect, *alternation,* refers to the differences in styles, lexicon, and organization that occur across social contexts. These sociolinguistic aspects of language, among others, have been most often analyzed within the context of the speech acts theory.

Speech Acts Theory

Published in 1962, the title of John Austin's book, *How to Do Things with Words,* stated its basic premise very succinctly. Austin's work was subsequently elaborated on by Searle (1969) and has become referred to as the speech acts theory. In this formulation, the unit of analysis returned to a somewhat broader framework, not unlike Skinner's model. The unit, a *speech act,* is defined as any act of oral communication, which might range from a grunt (*Hmph!*) of disapproval, to a president's State of the Union address to "sell" the legislative agenda for the coming year.

The name "speech act" was designed to indicate that an utterance can have the same impact as an action. To request water from a willing listener has the same effect as the *act* of walking to the kitchen yourself. Some speech acts called *performatives* are said to execute (perform) the act that they state. For example, when we express an apology (*I'm sorry to be late*), there is an implied action that is carried out by the words themselves. The real impact words can have in a performative is more clearly illustrated by all the social, emotional, and legal ramifications of the statement, *By the authority vested in me, I now pronounce you husband and wife.*

The Basic Elements of Speech Acts

Speech acts have been analyzed into several basic elements. These concepts clarify their functioning in communicative contexts and its overlap with the semantic and structural aspects of language.

propositional force The linguistic meanings expressed by the words and phrases of a speech act.

The Forces of Speech Acts.   The first two dimensions of a speech act to consider are its propositional force and its illocutionary force. The **propositional force** of a speech act comes closest to the semantic relations contained in utterances. In a sense, it is the "literal" meaning as the speech act is stated. However, the propositional force of the speech act does not necessarily predict its effect. The **illocutionary force** is the speaker's intended effect in making the statement. In the kitchen, utterances such as *Is the salt on the table?* or *Are those cookies as good as they smell?* are speech acts whose propositional force (literal meaning) is different from their illocutionary force (intended effect). The intentions conveyed with the speech acts classified by Searle (1969) are presented in Table 4–5.

The Components of Speech Acts.   The parts of a speech act are not distinguishable in the sense that parts of a sentence are. Nonetheless, speech acts are thought of as being composed of three major components. The words and propositions are the **locutionary** component of speech acts; for example, the words spoken as stated previously are the locutionary component of those speech acts. The speaker's intention is the **illocutionary** component of speech acts; the previous utterances were probably *intended* to request the food items mentioned. Finally, the listener's interpretation of the speech act represents the **perlocutionary** component; listeners' interpretations are primarily determined through the effect the speech act has on their behavior. In the case of inaccurate interpretations, speakers may abandon their intention (illocution), or change their wording (locution), and hope for a more favorable interpretation (perlocution).

It should be noted, again, that sociolinguists did not propose that speech acts theory would replace either of the rule systems for syntax or semantics. Instead, the rule system governing functions and alternations was intended to work in conjunction with those for generating meanings and structures in language.

Impact on Child Language Research

The primary impact of the sociolinguistic perspective on child language has been its inclusion of the communicative partner. It is the partner's interpretation

illocutionary force
Speakers' dispositions or attitudes toward their utterances.

Locution derives from the Latin word for "to speak," as in *circumlocution,* which means to express something in a "round about way." ∎

locutionary The component of speech acts that includes the words and propositional content used by speakers to convey their intentions.

illocutionary The component of a speech act that includes the outcome or effect intended by a speaker.

perlocutionary The component of speech consisting of the listener's interpretation.

Table 4–5. Searle's speech acts and their intentions.

Speech Act	Intention
Representatives	Utterances intended to describe persons, objects, events, or relationships (e.g., *It's a pretty day*).
Directives	Utterances intended to influence others to do something (e.g., *Come here!*).
Commissives	Utterances intended to commit the speaker to a future action (e.g., *I'll be there, if you need me*).
Expressives	Utterances intended to convey feelings or inner states (e.g., *I could eat a horse!*).
Declarations	Utterances intended to alter circumstances (e.g., *With the power vested in me, I pronounce you husband and wife*).

and subsequent action that defines the utterance as a speech act. As such, sociolinguistic research expanded the focus beyond just the structure of utterances and the meanings they encode to include the outcome of the speech act. Current social formulations, accordingly, emphasize the effect of caregiver-child interactions on language development. The resulting models are sometimes referred to as *social interactionist* theories.

Bruner (1977) characterized the "social commerce" in caregiver-infant interactions as a catalyst for language development. From this perspective, sociolinguistic research focused on learning through social interaction in the earliest caregiver-infant transactions carried out in the context of nurturing routines.

Sociolinguists have classified the specific nature of the various transactions in several ways; however, they generally focused on the intent apparent in each. Halliday's (1975) classification scheme, known as *communicative functions,* resulted from observing his infant son's development. Dore (1974) developed a classification system for functions that are executed primarily through gestures with the possible addition of a characteristic vocalization (the pointing + grunting technique). Dore classified these prelinguistic behaviors as **primitive speech acts** (PSAs). For example, these included labeling, repeating, answering, requesting actions, requesting answers, calling, greeting, protesting, and practicing.

The sociolinguistic model also focused on the social context. Researchers proposed that several types of contexts might be fundamental to language development. Turn-taking behaviors appear in rudimentary form in the feeding behaviors of caregivers and infants. They later become part of *game playing* (e.g., pat-a-cake, peek-a-boo) and caregiving *routines* (e.g., bathing, feeding, diapering). Early turn-taking behaviors may eventually contribute to discourse (conversation) skills.

Another aspect of social contexts studied by sociolinguists included the development of *joint attention*. In these interactions, the caregiver and baby interact while they simultaneously engage in some action or attend to some referent. The context, whether a recurring event or an unchanging object, provides for simultaneous attention and the social basis for their interaction.

The individual features of Halliday's and Dore's classifications for functions are described in Chapter 5. ∎

primitive speech acts
Dore's classification of intentions expressed by infants and toddlers through characteristic gestures and vocalizations.

Assessment of the Pragmatic Model

The pragmatic perspective received increasing attention during the 1980s. The sociolinguistic themes in language learning have continued to generate important research on infant- and child-caregiver interactions across several disciplines.

Limitations.   The sociolinguistic account of language presents a shortcoming shared by several other models. It too emphasizes one aspect of language behavior to the omission, or at least neglect, of the other aspects. There is no specific accounting for the development of linguistic structure (syntax) or relational and lexical meanings (semantics). These rule systems are assumed to evolve due to the dynamics of social communication. If the pragmatic rules of communicating in a social context become the basic underlying component of language, is it added to the syntactic and semantic rule systems? If so, this becomes an even more cumbersome and unwieldy explanation for language behavior.

Another very practical shortcoming is that the sociolinguistic model is so recent in its evolution. As a result, there are still some inconsistencies in its classification schemes. There is still a lack of research on its basic assertions, although the base of research, especially in caregiver-infant interactions and child directed speech, is growing and enlightening.

Contributions.   The major contribution of the speech acts theory and the sociolinguistic model in general is significant. This model once again expanded the scope of the inquiry to include the final element—listener outcomes. Syntactic models focused on the form of the utterance. Semantic models emphasized the relationship of the utterance to the context. And, ultimately, the pragmatic model has reminded us of the reason for the utterance in the first place—the purposes, functions, or consequences of communicating with others.

The impact of sociolinguistics has been seen in clinical applications as well. The sociolinguistic model has emphasized the role of context and consequence in normal language development. Because application should follow theory, professionals treating individuals with disordered language have become more cognizant of including these aspects of natural communication in treatment programs.

Finally, the sociolinguistic model has prompted a flurry of naturalistic research. Researchers are looking more closely at the interactions of caregivers and their children as they develop language. As a result, we are developing a better understanding of what children use language for, how adults modify their input, the influence of contexts and outcomes, and the considerable amount of experience that is generated by the countless exchanges as children develop their language abilities.

Finally, in terms of the operant model, $(S^D \rightarrow Rv \rightarrow S^{Rr})$, the third element has been addressed. What pragmatics might call *feedback* or *outcomes* is analogous to the operant model's consequation (S^{Rr}). ∎

Other Interaction Models

Semanticists examined the interaction between cognition and language. The pragmatic perspective of sociolinguists concentrated on the influence of human interaction in social contexts on language. Several recent models also have examined interaction among the syntactic, semantic, and pragmatic aspects of language. In addition, these models view the process of language development as social interaction for the purpose of learning about the physical and social world.

Chapman's Process ("Child Talk") Model.   Chapman et al. (1992) recently emphasized a *process* approach to language development. Their goal was to develop a model of "language production that accounted for everyday conversation in all its diversity" (p. 3). This developmental process model, called "Child Talk," is intended to address "the process by which a child decides to talk, finds something to say, a way to say it, and with more or less success, says it" (p. 4).

In the classical account of language development the linguistic components operate as self-contained modules or rule systems. According to Chapman et al. (1992), this is inadequate for explaining more naturalistic occurrences of child language. Strong evidence of context-specific language production suggests that the earliest language learning is based on "specific, episodic knowledge." This means that children's language behavior is an integral part of their understanding of each situation, how others behave in that situation, and how they can behave effectively in that situation.

Children's earliest knowledge of language is less linguistic (the rules of syntax, phonology, and semantics) and more representational. Children's language is used to represent their knowledge "of the world's speakers, actions, events, situations, feelings, and goals" (p. 12). Linguistic knowledge evolves, but not as a distinct, autonomous component. It evolves as one aspect of the child's overall development of world knowledge "of how to plan and carry out goal-directed action" (p. 13).

In the Child Talk model, the knowledge of how to talk is related to the processes of comprehension or production. It is integrated with world knowledge and stored in memory in multiple ways. Child Talk is automatized by repeated use and generalized across situations that share words. Utterance frames are generalized based on experiences that share similarities across several dimensions.

Whole Language Theory.   A model that has expressed similar rejection of classical accounts of language is the Whole Language Theory. Its name emphasizes a holistic, as opposed to fragmented, view of language. Kamhi (1992, p. 57) stated that a basic tenet of the holistic perspective is that "the properties of the parts can be understood only from the dynamics of the whole." In other words, this model would emphasize understanding the dynamic reasons for which language exists to appreciate its elements.

Whole Language is just one application of holism, a version that happens to relate to child language. In Whole Language, language is based on **world knowledge,** the entirety of information gained from the child's experiences with others, objects, events, and settings in life (Milosky, 1990). A preliminary aspect of obtaining world knowledge is developing event knowledge. **Event knowledge** is the child's representation of familiar routines. These events (feeding, bathing, etc.) have distinct structure and contexts that remain fairly constant. This allows the child to represent them through *scripts,* predictable sequences of actions and words.

The most common format in which Whole Language has been discussed is in teaching reading. In this approach, reading is viewed as being fundamentally based on spoken language. There are three basic tenets of language learning from the Whole Language perspective (Sawyer, 1991).

world knowledge An individual's understanding of the world based on his or her accumulated experiences and memory.

event knowledge The child's accumulation of experiences in familiar routines.

First, children learn language in contexts that are saturated with models. Second, because children use language to actively seek outcomes they desire, language learning is self-directed by each child. And, caregivers and adults facilitate language learning by providing carefully tuned models and responding appropriately to children's communication attempts. The effectiveness of Whole Language as a teaching approach has not been documented and has been a source of some controversy.

Assessment of Child Talk and Whole Language.   The primary reservation with regard to these models is that they are relative newcomers as models of language development. There has been limited time to define their basic tenets in experimental terms and develop the appropriate research models to evaluate their potential to explain language development. The primary contribution made by both models is their emphasis on reintegrating language into its entirety and placing it back in the realm of behavior that seeks to operate effectively in the world.

New models often reinvigorate our search for answers, but it may tempt us to forget where we have been. As Kamhi (1992) points out, these recent models remind us to focus on such considerations as "the purposes and functions of language, the culture and values of the individual, and the contexts of communication" (p. 59). However, he continues, "one must have knowledge about which language forms are appropriate for which functions, in which contexts" (p. 59). In looking for the explanations for language development, we must exercise caution so as to not "throw the baby out with the bath water."

Summary

- Sociolinguists shifted the research focus to the effects and variations of language in social contexts.

- Speech acts theory analyzed communication into locutionary, illocutionary, and perlocutionary components.

- Interaction and routines within the infant-caregiver dyad have received increased attention as important factors in the development of language.

- Other models also emphasizing interaction have evolved recently, although their full impact is not yet apparent.

Overview of Language Development Models

If we look at the wealth of relevant literature generated over the past four decades, it is obvious that the search for an explanation of language and its development has proceeded with vigor. Generally speaking, within linguistics the perspective has shifted from a primarily syntactic (transformational generative grammar) view in the 1960s to a semantic model (case grammar) in the 1970s, followed by an emphasis on pragmatics (speech acts) in the

1980s. Through these shifts, researchers have successively focused on the forms, the meanings, and, most recently, effects of language.

It would appear that the next stage might be to integrate these perspectives. Just as we might reassemble a device that was disassembled out of curiosity, perhaps the time has come to reintegrate the elements of communication back into its natural state—human communication. Interestingly, the theoretical shifts described before have carried the question full circle back to a formulation that includes the basic variables of Skinner's operant model. From this perspective, verbal behaviors ("structure") are analyzed in relation to their setting events ("meaning") and their effects on others ("functions"). An integrated model will explain language development in the context of the genetic and social dynamics that caused language to evolve in all of its human dimensions (spoken, gestural, written, etc.) in a scientifically elegant manner (Skinner, 1986).

Chapter Summary

Language pervades our experience; in so many ways we experience it as a natural outlet for personal feelings and creative energy. It is easy to forget that, as a natural phenomenon, language behavior is also a proper subject for scientific inquiry. *Science* asks and answers questions in objective ways to satisfy our basic curiosity and to apply knowledge to improve the human condition. Through scientific explanations, we hope to *understand, predict,* and *control* phenomena that affect us.

Four prominent theories or models to explain language development have been proposed over the past four decades. The theories span a range of philosophical perspectives from *nativism* to *empiricism.* The *operant model* focused on verbal behavior as a social behavior that has identifiable effects. The *structural model* hypothesized the underlying structural organization of language itself and the innate structure of the human mind. Those who emphasized meaning as more basic than structure in language proposed the *semantic model* as an expansion of the structural model. Most recently, the *pragmatic model* has returned emphasis to the nature of social interactions and the effects of language in human communication.

Review Questions

1. What two purposes do researchers hope to serve in applying scientific research to normal language development?

2. Describe accomplishments in research that would illustrate achievement of understanding, prediction, and control in the context of language development.

3. How are primary verbal operants classified?

4. What is the relationship between primary verbal operants and autoclitic behaviors?

5. How would reinforcement and shaping occur through the natural consequences in interactions between caregivers and their infants and children?

6. Describe the two levels used to process or generate sentences according to transformational generative grammar.

7. What role is played by transformational rules in transformational generative grammar?

8. Describe the hypothetical mechanism for language development proposed in association with TGG.

9. What are the two main components of a sentence according to case grammar?

10. In case grammar, which relationships within a sentence carry the meanings that comprise the sentence?

11. Describe what semanticists meant when they stressed that meaning takes precedence over form in language.

12. What is the significance of the term "method of rich interpretation"?

13. Describe the two basic elements of the pragmatic model.

14. Describe the unit that is analyzed by the pragmatic model.

15. Describe the three components of a speech act.

16. In what ways are the pragmatic and operant models similar in their view of language development?

Practice Questions

To the student: You are encouraged to use the following questions to prepare for multiple-choice examinations. This exercise is not intended to simply "provide the answers to questions." Instead, it is hoped that you will use the material to develop your ability to analyze questions and choices to identify correct answers based on a critical understanding of the distinctions among the answers. Use the answer key at the end of the book to prompt your analysis of each item and to confirm the correct answer. Remember that there is a difference between recognizing the correct answer and understanding why it is the correct one.

1. According to the transformational generative grammar, the "data" that the child's LAD (or LAS) has available to it to process are characterized as _____ .
   a. only the intentions and purposes of the adults in his environment
   b. only adult utterances that are the best examples of the standard grammar of that language
   c. all of the utterances, including those that are deficient, that occur "within earshot" of the child
   d. a complete, transformational generative grammar
   e. models, tutorials, and reinforcing praise provided by parents

2. While his mother is washing the dishes, a young child pulls at her slacks and repeats urgently, "cookie, cookie, cookie." She reaches in the cookie jar and passes him a cookie. He quiets and begins to eat. His utterance most likely represents _____ .
   a. a mand
   b. a tact
   c. an echoic
   d. an extended tact
   e. an intraverbal

3. According to transformational generative grammar, if *no* "transformational operations" are applied to the deep structure, which of the following would actually occur as the surface structure?
   a. Is Bill washing the car?
   b. Bill is not washing the car.
   c. Bill is washing the car.
   d. The car is being washed by Bill.
   e. The was car Bill by washed not.

4. Which of the following pairs of individuals would generally agree most closely on the underlying social nature of language?
   a. Skinner and Chomsky
   b. Fillmore and Chomsky
   c. Searle and Skinner
   d. Chomsky and Searle
   e. Fillmore and Skinner

5. In the sentence, "Bob polished his old Buick in the garage," the noun "Buick" represents _____ .
   a. the agentive case
   b. the factitive case

   c. the locative case

   d. the dative case

   e. the objective case

6. According to Searle's speech acts theory, the effect that a speech act has on the listener, as demonstrated by the listener's subsequent action, represents its _____ .
   a. locutionary component
   b. illocutionary component
   c. case relations
   d. perlocutionary component
   e. none of these

7. Sociolinguists have stressed that _____ .
   a. mastering syntax is the most fundamental motivation behind language learning
   b. the LAD is the sole determinant of language development
   c. the use of language to communicate and fulfill needs is the central driving force behind the learning of language
   d. reinforcement, in any form, plays no role in language learning from their perspective
   e. all of these are true

8. Something that "sets the occasion" for a response because previous similar responses in its presence have been reinforced is a _____ .
   a. reinforcing stimulus
   b. phrase structure rule
   c. discriminative stimulus
   d. punishing stimulus
   e. suprasegmental

9. The notion of "syntax" is most closely correlated with Skinner's _____ .
   a. manding behavior
   b. autoclitic behavior
   c. tacting behavior
   d. echoic behavior
   e. nonverbal behavior

10. The "semantic revolution" that followed Fillmore's semantic model _____ .
    a. portrayed children as first recognizing meanings/relationships and then learning the forms used to express them
    b. suggested that cognitive development is fundamental to language development
    c. resulted in the view that children were not simply learning "N+V syntactic word orders," but were expressing perceived semantic relationships in using consistent word orders
    d. might be simply summed up by "meaning precedes form"
    e. all of these are true

Suggested Readings

Chomsky, N. (1965). *Aspects of the theory of syntax.* Cambridge: MIT Press.

Corballis, M. (2002). *From hand to mouth: The origin of language.* Princeton, NJ: Princeton University Press.

Fillmore, C. (1968). The case for case. In E. Bach & R. Harmas (Eds.), *Universals in linguistic theory.* New York: Holt, Rhinehart, & Wilson.

Kuhl, P. K. (2000). A new view of language acquisition. *Proceedings of the National Academy of Science, 97*(22), 11850–11857.

Segal, E. V. (1977). Toward a coherent psychology of language. In W. K. Honig & J. E. R. Staddon (Eds.), *Handbook of operant conditioning* (pp. 628–653). Englewood Cliffs, NJ: Prentice-Hall.

Skinner, B. F. (1957). *Verbal behavior.* New York: Appleton-Century-Crofts.

CHAPTER 5

The Beginnings— Infant Communication

The small group had wandered some distance from their village. Their ancestors had warned them about the strange people living beyond the giant forest. Perhaps they had gone too far, but this particular day they had experienced such good fortune in gathering plump, sweet berries. In fact, they had been scolding one another for eating too many as they picked them. After such a long absence, it would be especially important to return with a good supply to show for their efforts.

As they consumed more berries they became increasingly thirsty. Thirst soon became an urgent issue. With few words and many gestures, they decided to head toward "laj bon"—the lost stream. They traveled quietly with a measure of apprehension. The stream was called "lost" because once the people beyond the forest began using it, no one from their tribe had ever returned to it. As they approached the water, they heard a strange sound. A gurgling, bubbling sound. At first it sounded like the stream itself, but as they drew closer they noticed a large round basket lodged against a rock in the babbling brook. Over the rim they could see two small hands. It was a "tiny one!" (They had no word for infant.) This tiny one made so many noises.

As they retrieved the basket and withdrew the tiny one, a note fell to the ground unnoticed. In a language alien to them nonetheless, it read, "Please, take care of my baby! He is 9 months old." As they carried this tiny one back to their village, they discussed a name for him. As they walked he continued to produce a stream of noises different from any of their tiny ones who rode in their mothers' slings all day. As they approached their village, they determined that his name should be Ilo Kushinari, which translates as "Look who is talking."

This chapter addresses the following questions:

- Which motor, cognitive, and social developments contribute to infants' communication behaviors?

- How do infants' auditory abilities contribute to the development of speech behavior?

- What traditional milestones of speech behavior are achieved by infants prior to the first words?

- What infant behaviors prompt the interactions that lead to communication?

- How do caregivers interact with infants to establish and facilitate communication?

- How do infants adapt their behaviors to influence those around them?

Several decades ago this chapter may not have existed in a text on language development. The prevailing view for many years had been that language does not begin until the first word has occurred. The traditional "rule of thumb" for the first word places its occurrence around the first birthday. Therefore, the first year of life was thought to precede true language development.

According to the *American Heritage Dictionary* (1970), the word *infant* is derived from the Latin "enfant" meaning "one unable to speak." Traditional accounts typically acknowledged the development of infant vocal behaviors (cooing, babbling, vocal play, etc.) and presumed that they were somehow related to the eventual form of speech. However, beyond this, there was little recognition that the first year of life was directly related to language development.

Subsequently, researchers and the prevailing models of language expanded their scope of interest from the forms of language to its meanings and, finally, to the functions of language. This latest development resulted in a surge of information regarding the interactions of infants and caregivers from birth through the first year. As research focused on the pragmatic functions of language, it provided the framework to analyze communication behavior.

In this chapter, it will become apparent that there is a continual evolution of infant and caregiver behaviors throughout the first year. However, infants' evolution can no longer be viewed as going from *no* communication toward the *onset* of communication; communication, at some level, is *present from birth.* The repertoire of behaviors available to infants, their emerging control over them, and the ability to interact effectively is evolving from the beginning *as a result of* communicating with those around them (Locke, 1993).

In fact, the custom of organizing information in chapters is an unfortunate one. It obscures the continual evolution of our communication behavior throughout the life span. ■

Development in Related Domains

Language does not develop in isolation as a separate system of behavior with special status. The behaviors that eventually evolve into recognizable language behavior are supported by the child's whole development in the motor, cognitive, and social domains.

Each domain—motor, cognitive, and social—builds on development in the others. Although our focus is on language, it is important to view the entire process and to understand how these related domains set the stage for language to evolve.

The first year is an eventful one. So many changes occur so rapidly in all the domains: motor, cognitive, and social. The changes in these systems do more than precede language. These changes continuously channel infants' evolution toward true language. What follows is a brief summary of the highlights that characterize developments in each area throughout the first year (Lane & Molyneaux, 1992; Owens, 2005; Shulman, 1994). These selected highlights can only provide a glimpse of the myriad of significant developments that occur so rapidly. However, it is hoped they will provide a backdrop against which the evolution of language makes sense.

Motor Developments

Motor development arises from biological maturation of the nervous and skeletal muscle systems and each individual's experiences in coordinating their use. Infants generally progress from random, involuntary movement to more controlled, volitional actions. The following developments are evident throughout the first year:

- Motor control begins developing from the head down following birth.
- Visual acuity is best within 8 inches from birth until around 1 month.
- Achieves visual focus around 2 months.
- Reaches for and grasps objects around 3 months.
- Establishes head control around 4 months.
- Sits up with slight support around 5 months.
- Jaw control for chewing improves; grasps and transfers objects with both hands around 6 months.
- Crawls and pulls self to standing around 7 months.
- Manipulates objects and explores with index finger around 8 months.
- Stands briefly without support and rolls into and out of sitting position around 9 months.

Children do not develop at precisely the same rate. To emphasize this, the developmental ages are stated as approximations, as in "around 6 months." ∎

- Makes stepping movements; holds and drinks from cup around 10 months.
- Takes first independent step around 11 months.
- Walks with one hand held; picks up objects with thumb-finger apposition around 12 months.

Cognitive Developments

Cognitive development describes the process of experiencing and understanding the world. Infants' cognitive abilities develop with accumulated experience with objects, people, and events. These developments are illustrated by the following characteristics during an infant's first year:

- Visually prefers movement and contrasting visual patterns following birth.
- Demonstrates regard for caregiver's face and nearby objects around 1 month.
- Recognizes caregiver's face and anticipates objects' appearance around 2 months.
- Visually searches for sources of sound around 3 months.
- Localizes sound sources; stares at place from which object was dropped around 4 months.
- Recognizes familiar objects; explores objects through mouthing and touching around 5 months.
- Enjoys dropping and picking up objects; shakes toys to make noise around 6 months.
- Imitates complex behaviors already achieved when able to view own performance around 7 months.
- Prefers novel and relatively complex toys; unwraps wrapped objects around 8 months.
- Uncovers hidden object if observes act of hiding; imitates familiar actions around 9 months.
- Points to body parts on request; attains goal with trial-and-error approach around 10 months.
- Recognizes own name when called; imitates increasingly around 11 months.
- Uses common objects appropriately; imitates movements not already in repertoire around 12 months.

Social Developments

Social development is evidenced in increasingly sophisticated interactions with others. Infants become increasingly attached to their caregivers and eventually more responsive. The following developments throughout an infant's first year contribute to this process:

- Quiets to soft, high-pitched voices; smiles reflexively following birth.
- Establishes eye contact with caregiver; quiets to gentle touching, holding, rocking around 1 month.
- Excites when sees people; exhibits unselective spontaneous smile around 2 months.
- Visually discriminates different people and things; exhibits selective "social" smile around 3 months.
- Prefers smiling face versus angry face; anticipates being lifted around 4 months.
- Distinguishes family members from strangers; reacts differently to smiling and scolding around 5 months.
- Prefers people games ("peek-a-boo"); focuses on speaker's mouth more than speaker's eyes around 6 months.
- Enjoys bath time as play time; exhibits "teasing" as beginning of humor around 7 months.
- Cries for mother out of attachment; reaches for and touches other babies around 8 months.
- Shouts for attention; "performs" for family around 9 months.
- Indicates wants by gesturing; gives toy on request around 10 months.
- Seeks approval; attempts modifying caregiver's goal around 11 months.
- Expresses people preferences; exhibits different emotions (e.g., jealousy, affections, sympathy) around 12 months.

Language Expectations

During infants' first year, a number of foundational behaviors will emerge. Initially, these behaviors are primarily physiological in nature. That is, they are "built in" through the infants' reflexive capabilities for reacting to stimuli. Later in this period, the elements in these behaviors come under increasing voluntary control—reflexive behaviors are inhibited and their voluntary counterparts are gradually exhibited in more selective and socialized contexts. The following overview is intended to provide an initial picture of the overall developments expected during this period:

- Infants will produce a variety of unintentional, undifferentiated motor and vocal behaviors that reflect the reflexive responses of an immature nervous system.
- Infants will localize, attend to, and eventually respond to familiar sounds in their environment (e.g., voices, household sounds, pet sounds).

- Infants will produce sounds that are initially undifferentiated and unrecognizable and will increasingly become recognizable as approximations of fully developed speech sounds.
- Infants will produce gestures and accompanying speech sounds that become increasingly intentional as part of turn-taking and game-playing interactions with caregivers.
- Specific words spoken by others, especially names, will become signals for infants to localize and search for familiar people, pets, toys, and so on.
- Consistent gestures and stereotypical vocalizations will come to be used as "tools" to obtain objects, attention, and interaction.
- Infants will become familiar with books as objects of exploration and interaction displayed to them by their caregivers.

The Prelinguistic Foundations for Language

Infants eventually recognize much of what they hear and gain more control over their speech structures. Even though they may be alert to hearing a familiar word or produce a string of sounds that are almost recognizable, these abilities are still prelinguistic; that is, they precede true language. Nonetheless, they represent the seeds of conventional language behaviors.

Researchers have attempted to describe and understand the capacities available to infants long before their first word will occur. This includes their ability to hear differences among speech sounds and to produce sounds that appear to lead to speech.

Infant Speech Perception

It does not take a rocket scientist to see that, beyond scholarly curiosity, the classic "nature versus nurture" controversy was driving much of this research. ▪

Researchers have been interested in infants' readiness to attend to, select, store, and recognize the significant sounds they hear in the speech stream. Researchers have developed several innovative procedures to investigate infants' ability to distinguish among the sounds present in speech. The issue that has intrigued researchers is whether infants are able from birth to discriminate the important differences that contrast classes of speech sounds (voicing, place, manner of production) or whether this ability requires experience.

The two most commonly reported procedures differ in their response modes. One uses infants' sucking response and the second utilizes infants' visual behavior. The first method, *nonnutritive sucking* (NNS), is also called the *high-amplitude suck* (HAS) paradigm. This technique is used frequently with younger infants, although it has not proven reliable with infants younger than 1 month old. In this procedure, infants suck on a pacifier-type nipple connected by tubing to a device that measures the fluctuations in air pressure caused by their sucking. In this way, the frequency and strength of infants' sucking can be recorded.

It has been found that infants will learn to suck the nonnutritive nipple when it is followed by a novel auditory stimulus (e.g., the syllable /da/). When this stimulus is no longer novel, infants' sucking is no longer reinforced by it and the sucking response diminishes. When the rate of sucking slows to a criterion level, the stimulus is changed (e.g., to the syllable /ta/). If infants are capable of discriminating the difference, the new stimulus is again novel and reinforcing, resulting in increased sucking.

The other procedure, *visually reinforced infant speech discrimination* (VRISD), relies on conditioning infants to anticipate a change in their visual field when they perceive a similar change in the sound stimulus (e.g., from /da/ to /ta/). First, a sound stimulus is repeated while toys are visible in front of the infant. When the sound stimulus is changed, a visually reinforcing toy (e.g., a drum-playing bear) appears to one side. This eventually conditions the infant to anticipate the visually reinforcing toy when a change in sounds is detected. The infant's discrimination of contrasting sounds is inferred from the occurrence of searching responses following sound changes.

Through these and similar procedures, newborns have demonstrated remarkable auditory abilities. Infants just 16 hours old have evidenced a quieting response in preference to recordings of their own cry (to which they obviously have had limited exposure) versus those of other infants (Martin & Clark, 1982). One-day-old infants have learned to suck at rates to "select" recordings of their mother's voice as opposed to that of another adult female. Of course, here again they have had very limited time to hear their mother's voice following birth. Although in some studies infants have not demonstrated a preference for their own cry, it has been found that within hours of birth, infants exhibit vocal suppression or a quieting response when exposed to cry stimuli (Riccillo and Watterson, 1984). This response has implications for infants' attending behaviors and their ability to interact with their environment. As your third-grade teacher probably told you, "You can't listen if you're talking"—or in this case, crying.

Responses that indicate preference for their mother's voice could reflect both prenatal and postnatal auditory learning, because the mother's voice has been internally transmitted to the fetus prior to birth. In fact, in early sessions of this research infants preferred a version of their mother's voice that had been filtered to sound much like it would have in the womb. In later sessions, infants preferred their mother's voice in its normal state, reflecting their most recent experience of it (DeCasper & Fifer, 1980).

Researchers have also found that infants' impressive auditory abilities extend beyond recognizing the broader acoustic characteristics of cries and voices. Infants within the first few months following birth are capable of discriminating a number of consonant pair contrasts (e.g., /ma/ from /pa/, /pa/ from /ba/, and /ba/ from /ga/), vowel pairs (e.g., /a/ from /i/, /i/ from /u/), and changes in intonation and stress across bisyllables (e.g., ['baba] versus [ba'ba]) (Jusczyk, 1992). These contrasts represent differences that are not only acoustically subtle, but also linguistically significant; that is, they contrast different words and meanings.

Our understanding of *categorical perception,* the ability to hear groups of sounds based on very fine differences, had been established with adult listeners. Researchers have shown that mature speakers do not detect small changes *within* a consonant category. For example, in listening to the syllable /ba/, in spite of small differences in the delay of voicing for the vowel following /b/ ("voice onset time"), we hear the various productions all as /b/. However, at some point, the delay crosses a perceptual boundary and results in the perception of another category of sounds, for example /p/.

Because adults would have had extensive experience responding to such contrasts (/p/ versus /b/), these findings were illuminating, but not necessarily surprising. However, the presence of these abilities in young infants, with seemingly limited experience, certainly seemed remarkable. This, in fact, caused some researchers to propose that human infants are born with specialized neural structures, making them innately prewired for detecting the acoustic boundaries between different speech categories (Eimas, 1974).

Eimas (1974) proposed innate Linguistic Feature Detectors, analogous to Chomsky's LAD, to account for this phonetic ability. ∎

With further research, however, a number of other findings emerged that qualified speculations about infants' specialized perceptual readiness. Although the abilities that had been demonstrated were impressive, the contrasts tested represented only a small sample of the contrasts and syllabic contexts that are possible, given the number of available variables (i.e., different consonants, vowels, syllable positions, etc.).

Eventually, research revealed that infants are not initially capable of detecting a number of other contrasting consonants such as /sa/ from /za/, and /fa/ from /ta/ (Eilers & Minifie, 1975), or syllable sequences (Trehub, 1973). Discrimination for some contrasts does not emerge until the second half of the first year. Furthermore, given what is known about the fetal acoustic environment, it may be that the fetus may have been exposed to speech and its intonational variations. Finally, researchers have found that rhesus monkeys (Morse & Snowden, 1975; Waters & Wilson, 1976) and chinchillas (Kuhl & Miller, 1975) are also capable of discriminating the voiced-voiceless contrast in speech sounds.

Locke (1993) discussed many of the issues that must be resolved before a final model of infant speech perception emerges. It must be recognized that if there are any specialized neural structures, they may receive more prenatal experience than we have previously appreciated. Furthermore, it appears that such auditory abilities may not be unique to humans (Kuhl, 1989); they may be present in a broad range of mammals. Initially, the contrasts that are most efficiently detected by these structures may have been merely acoustic, and only later were they adapted by humans to signaling linguistic contrasts, that is, different words.

In view of these considerations, Locke (1993) and others have suggested that it may be valid to reverse the innateness reasoning. Perhaps these acoustic contrasts only became relevant or useful in human speech because humans (like other primates or mammalians) evolved with the biological capacities to detect them. Certain contrasts became functional in speech only because they were perceptible to us and affected communication. In fact, there are contrasts that infants are capable of detecting that will not be significant to them as adult speakers (Trehub, 1976). If certain contrasts are not present in the language environment, communicating effectively does not rely on responding differently to them. The capability to perceive them will diminish whereas others are maintained. This selection process reflects the influence of the interaction of our biological capacity with the language environment and the practical value in responding effectively to the language spoken to us (Kuhl, 1991).

Summary

- Researchers have developed experimental procedures to study infants' **speech discrimination** abilities.

- Newborn infants can recognize their own cry, their mother's voice, and they can perceive a number of significant speech sound categories.

- Adults' categorization of sounds that differ equally along some dimension is called categorical perception.

- Infants' ability to detect phoneme categories does not extend to all speech sound contrasts and similar abilities are exhibited in several other mammals.

- The extent to which infants' speech perception abilities are innate or require experience with speech sounds is not clear at this time.

speech discrimination
The ability to distinguish meaningful differences between speech sounds.

Prelinguistic Development of Speech

Regardless of the underlying auditory capabilities possessed by infants, their development of speech sounds has been well documented. A number of researchers have carefully observed and classified the sounds produced by infants at their various stages of development.

Traditionally, infants' development toward speech and language was viewed simply as progression toward the proverbial "first word." Because the traditional view emphasized that these behaviors preceded true language, they are considered to be *prelinguistic*.

Developmental Milestones in Infant Speech

Certain behaviors have been traditionally associated with the time lines in which their development would be expected. These time lines, called "milestones," gauge infants' progress during that first year along the road to language. Table 5–1 presents the traditional milestones of prelinguistic development. The behaviors included as milestones for prelinguistic developmental focus on the various sounds produced by infants, based on the notion that this is a period of practicing sounds prior to "real speech."

Table 5–1. Traditional milestones in infant prelinguistic development.

Age Range (Approx.)	Prelinguistic Behaviors
0–1 mo.	Birth cry, vegetative sounds
1–4 mos.	Cooing
4–6 mos.	Marginal babbling
6–8 mos.	Vocal play, reduplicated, and nonreduplicated babbling
8–12 mos.	Echolalia
9–12 mos.	Jargon

Several disclaimers regarding the milestones are in order. First, the behaviors included are labeled with terms that are familiar to most; however, some unintended connotations carried by these traditional terms may be misleading. Second, the ages noted for each period are fairly conventional, but sources may vary somewhat. Finally, as with any outline of developmental progression, the ages are approximate; individual infants can vary substantially in their rate of development and there will most likely be an overlapping of periods.

More information about the significance of infant cries is presented later in this chapter. ∎

vegetative sounds Infant oral sounds (e.g., clicks, burps) associated with feeding and digestion.

quasi-resonant nuclei Early infant oral sounds that are not as resonant as mature vowel sounds.

cooing Infant sound productions in the first few months that are vowel-like and associated with comfortable states.

marginal babbling Infant sound productions with a variety of vowels and consonant-like productions that approximate syllables.

Birth to 4 Weeks: Crying/Vegetative Sounds. The first sounds noted during the period immediately following birth are cries, vegetative sounds, and early pleasure sounds. The reflexive cry is assumed to be physiologically based starting with the first breath and later in reaction to internal stimuli such as pain and hunger. Oral **vegetative sounds** (lip and tongue clicks, burps, coughs) are associated with feeding and digesting. Finally, noncrying sounds occur when infants are in a pleasurable state. Some of these sighlike sounds, called **quasi-resonant nuclei (QRN),** are almost vowel like (hence, the prefix *quasi-*) but are not as fully resonant as vowel sounds will be eventually (Oller, 1978).

One to Four Months: Cooing. The second milestone behavior, cooing, is thought to appear around 4 weeks of age. **Cooing** is described as sound productions that are more vowel like in nature, typically with an /u/ — /oo/ quality. As the name of this vocal behavior suggests, this vocalic sound may be preceded by velar or uvular sounds that are almost a /k/ or /g/ in their consonantal quality. Traditionally, it has been believed that infants are most likely to emit these sounds in comfortable, pleasurable states. This often occurs in face-to-face interactions with their caregivers.

Four to Six Months: Marginal Babbling. This period has been portrayed as containing perhaps the most significant developments for later speech. During this time, infants begin to exhibit **marginal babbling,** described as the production of a variety of vowel-like sounds with occasional vocal tract closure, which together approximate simple consonant-vowel (CV) syllables, as in /ba/, or vowel-consonant (VC) syllables, as in /ab/ (Oller, 1978). In addition to including sounds that approach consonants, infants' vowels resonate more fully. These resulting tones are referred to as **fully resonant nuclei (FRN).** The pitch and duration of these vowel sounds can be quite variable.

Initially, there are fewer consonants produced in this period. In shifting from the back sounds associated with cooing, the early consonants of babbling tend to be front and middle sounds, including the labial (/p/, /b/) and alveolar sounds (/t/, /d/). With developing motor control in the front structures of the mouth, labial sounds become most prevalent by the end of this period.

There is generally an expansion in the variety of consonants, vowels, and their combinations as time goes on. Infants' earlier sounds also tend to be predominately stop-plosives; the all-or-none production of stop-plosives (e.g., /p, b, t, d, k, g/) is considered physically simpler than the fine control required to form and maintain the smaller apertures or openings for fricatives (e.g., /f/, /ð/), affricates (e.g., /tʃ/, /d₃/), and sibilants (e.g., /s/, /z/, /ʃ/).

Six to Eight Months: Vocal Play. As infants gradually exhibit a greater variety of sounds, it has been traditionally suggested that infants are "playfully" experimenting with different combinations. Whether infants are consciously experimenting or the sounds are randomly produced as they attempt to control the vocal tract is not entirely clear, but the repertoire of infants' sounds expands conspicuously from 6 to 8 months.

The traditional term for this period, **vocal play,** refers to the longer strings of syllables that expand out of marginal babbling as infants continue to "play" with sounds. In total, there are three phases of babbling. In the previous period, marginal babbling, infants were producing single CV or VC syllables. During the present period, vocal play, their babbling passes through two more phases—reduplicated and nonreduplicated babbling.

In **reduplicated babbling,** the syllable is duplicated in strings of repetitive syllables. For example, where /da/ might have occurred in marginal babbling, this syllable would be repeated as /da-da-da-da/ in reduplicated babbling.

During the final phase of babbling, called **nonreduplicated babbling** or **variegated babbling,** the strings of syllables are more varied. The consonants and vowels may change from one syllable to the next within the same string, as in /gabida/. Often the effect for the listener is even closer approximations to the character of true words—a greater mix of consonants in multisyllabic forms.

Eight to Twelve Months: Echolalia. By the time infants are 8 months old much has changed. A maturing neurological system and a wealth of experience listening to and producing sounds have brought infants ever closer

fully resonant nuclei Infant sound productions that more closely approximate mature vowels.

The debate over the relationship of babbling to later speech is covered later. ■

vocal play Infant sound productions exhibiting longer strings of varied syllables.

reduplicated babbling Babbling in which a syllable is repeated in strings, as in *dadada*.

nonreduplicated babbling (also **variegated babbling**) Babbling that consists of strings of varied syllables.

The *echoic* described by Skinner may have its roots in the babbling period, but it becomes especially recognizable at this stage. ■

echolalia Infants' sound production that appears to immediately imitate the speech around them.

to true speech. The term for the behavior that emerges in this period, **echolalia,** refers to infants' relatively immediate reproduction (i.e., imitation) of speech heard in the immediate environment.

The derivations of the word echolalia describe this behavior quite aptly: *echo,* meaning to reverberate, and *lalia,* referring to speech. Although infants may not be imitating in a meaningful way, the phonemic sequence, syllable structure, and intonational contours in the speech of those nearby are reproduced accurately enough to give one that impression.

Nine to Twelve Months: Jargon.   The final phase of the prelinguistic stage may actually overlap with and extend into the onset of true language—the first meaningful words. **Jargon** consists of strings of syllables produced with stress and intonation that mimic real speech. Infants' vocalizations may sound much like an adult's statement, command, or question. Nakazima (1962) found that infants as young as 8 months appear to imitate the intonation of adult utterances.

jargon Infant sound production consisting of syllable strings produced with adultlike intonation.

 Skinner (1957) suggested that intonation may be a fundamental form of autoclitic behavior. The intonational contour superimposed on the utterance "comments" on the relationships in the utterance. ■

Several researchers have suggested that infants are using intonation to signal diverse meanings or functions such as commanding, stating, requesting, and protesting (Sachs, 1985). Those who have spent any time with infants in this period have found themselves stopping to think, "Did you really *say* something?" Jargon appears to be a natural final step in the progression from crying to cooing to babbling to speech.

Summary

- Speech sounds produced by infants are considered prelinguistic because they precede true language.

- Infants' sound productions develop at relatively predictable times called milestones.

An interesting analogy is seen in the adult use of the term *jargon.* Those who have immersed themselves in an entirely new area of study, whether it was computers, genealogy, electronics, or macramé, have experienced jargon. Confronted with an entirely new set of terms and phrases peculiar to the new topic, it might seem that the instructor is somehow speaking a foreign language that just *sounds* like English!

- Infants' earlier sound productions appear to be reflexive or vegetative, with reflexive crying and cooing reflecting their state of discomfort or comfort.

- Later sound productions, such as babbling and vocal play, appear to result from infants' experimentation with greater control over the oral structures.

- As the end of the first year nears, infants exhibit echolalia, in which their sound productions appear to reproduce segments from the speech of those around them.

- As the first year ends, infants produce jargon, which approximates the intonational contours of mature phrasing.

The Phonological Nature of Babbling

As nonsensical as the term *babbling* might sound, it has been a source of scientific curiosity and controversy for some time. Anyone who seriously contemplates the roots of human speech and language must consider the intriguing similarities and differences between babbling and later speech.

Some have judged that the two phenomena are distinctly different and unrelated. Others claim that the seeds of later speech sounds are found in infants' earlier vocalizations. As a result of this controversy and our natural curiosity, a number of researchers have explored the nature of babbling.

Most instructors realize they have had students who would offer them as evidence of the direct link between babbling and speech. ▪

Babbling: Composition and Characteristics

In evaluating the composition of babbling it should be recognized that the task of identifying highly variable sounds produced by infants with no identifiable context is an especially difficult one (Stockman, Woods, & Tishman, 1981; Winitz, 1969). Frequently sounds may only approximate adult phoneme categories, perhaps falling somewhere between several. This is compounded by the fact that infants' sound productions are not attempts at naming any specific referent, which might otherwise provide a clue as to which phoneme had occurred. Finally, these difficulties are compounded by the fact that infants develop rapidly and variably.

Given these qualifications, it is still possible to characterize the composition of infants' babbling, at least, as a group. An early study by Irwin (1947) had suggested that with regard to *place of production* the first sounds in babbling tended to be back sounds (e.g., /k, g, h/). More recently, however, researchers have tended to identify front (/b/ and /p/) and middle (e.g., /t, d, θ, n, s, z/) sounds as the most prevalent (Kent & Bauer, 1985; Locke, 1983; Oller, Wieman, Doyle, & Ross, 1976).

As described by Winitz (1969), interest in infant sounds probably has a long history.

In 1877, Darwin published one of the earliest studies of infant vocalizations. However, the true trailblazer was Orvis C. Irwin. During the 1940s, without the benefit of sound recording equipment (not to mention video-recording), Irwin led a landmark research project to study infant vocalizations. Irwin and his associates transcribed and analyzed samples of speech sound productions of 95 infants during their first 2 1/2 years of life.

This discrepancy may result from the difficulty in transcribing the phonemic categories reliably. Another possible source of variation is in the broad chronological boundaries of babbling. For example, Oller et al. (1976) studied infants 6 months and older. Kent and Bauer (1985) studied the sound inventory of infants 1 year of age. In contrast, Irwin's infants were studied from birth to 2½ years of age. The age group Irwin designated as representative of the onset of babbling was 5 to 6 months old. The back sounds present in Irwin's younger infants may have been remnants of the cooing stage which just preceded. Nonetheless, it is generally reported that the sounds most characteristic of the entire period of babbling are predominately front and middle sounds.

From the standpoint of *manner of production,* babbling consists primarily of plosive sounds (e.g., /b, p, t, d/) in the initial and medial positions of syllables and fricatives (e.g., /s, z, θ/) in the final position. In terms of *syllable position,* most early consonants occur in medial position (VCV), as in /aba/. However, initial position (CV) consonants, as in /ba/, eventually increase to achieve a balance between the positions. The less frequent final position (VC) consonants, as in /ap/, are most often voiceless in nature.

The range and variety of sounds produced in babbling appear to increase steadily, although different rates have been observed. Infants of parents with higher levels of education demonstrate a greater variety of phoneme types, beginning at approximately 7 or 8 months of age (Irwin, 1948). In contrast, no significant differences have been found between male and female infants or infants from different racial groups (Irwin, 1952). By 1 year of age, a core group of sounds (/h, d, b, m, t, g, w, n, k/) comprise over 80% of the consonants present in the babbling of infants from homes in which American English is spoken.

Babbling: Discontinuity versus Continuity

discontinuity hypothesis
The phonological theory that the sounds in babbling and eventual speech are unrelated.

As noted before, the relationship between babbling and later speech has been a source of controversy. Some have held that babbling bears no direct relationship to speech, a theory referred to as the **discontinuity hypothesis** (Jakobson, 1941/1968). It was inferred that the two may be distinct because babbling is "playful" and speech is "purposeful." Those who subscribed to the discontinuity hypothesis also asserted that after infants produce a wide range of sounds in babbling, there is a brief period of decreased babbling before true speech begins abruptly with a limited number of sounds. Finally, the discontinuity perspective asserted a biological foundation to babbling. According to this view, regardless of their language environment, infants generally exhibit the same sounds in babbling, in what could be called *universal babbling,* because they are human (Lane & Molyneaux, 1992).

continuity hypothesis
The phonological theory that the sounds of babbling evolve into the sounds of speech.

In contrast, the opposing view, the **continuity hypothesis** holds that babbling gradually approximates the language in infants' environments. This continuity position proposes that each infant's repertoire of sounds is gradually shaped toward the surrounding language. Sounds that infants experience in their surrounding language persist and are produced in greater proportion. Conversely, sounds that do not occur in the surrounding language will gradually diminish in frequency. The effect of this process, in which infants sound increasingly like the speakers around them, has been referred to as *phonetic drift.*

Although the actual state of affairs may include aspects of both perspectives, the overall results most strongly support the continuity hypothesis. As the discontinuity hypothesis suggests, researchers have found the early sounds in marginal babbling are relatively uniform (i.e., universal) across languages. That is, regardless of their language environment, infants initially have the physical capacity to produce sounds from any of the human languages; obviously, not every infant will produce every sound. This capability to produce a range of speech sounds reflects the biological early influence of maturing articulatory and neural structures. The universal nature of this early vocal behavior is illustrated by the finding that adult speakers from different language backgrounds have difficulty identifying the native language environments of younger infants based on their early babbling. However, adults are more successful identifying the native language of older infants as their babbling approximates the sound sequences and intonational contours of their language environment (deBoysson-Bardies, Sagart, & Durand, 1984).

It has been found that infants' babbling eventually includes proportionately more sounds related to the language to which they are exposed (Cruttendon, 1970). Furthermore, the order in which later speech sounds are mastered is reflected in their relative frequency in earlier babbling (Menyuk, 1977; Oller & Eilers, 1982). Some have also observed that the reduplicated syllables of babbling may emerge as early words for infants (Oller et al., 1976). Overall, it appears that younger infants display a generic sampling of those sounds their immature vocal apparatus is capable of producing. With further maturation of their articulatory and auditory capacities, the influence of the surrounding language becomes increasingly apparent.

The influence of experience is further illustrated in the babbling of deaf infants compared to hearing infants. Although some early differences have been noted, the importance of experiencing speech sounds, produced by others and themselves, becomes especially apparent during the second half of the first year. While the hearing infant's overall vocalizations continue to increase, the deaf infant's begin to decrease. Whereas the normal infant's repertoire of consonants increases with age, the range of babbled consonants decreases with age in deaf children (Oller, Eilers, Bull, & Carney, 1985; Stocl-Gammon & Otomo, 1986).

These differences support the view that the ability to produce sounds from the surrounding language requires experience using the articulators *combined* with auditory feedback. But the question remained, what causes infants who hear normally to integrate these capabilities as they sound more and more like those around them?

One early attempt to explain the continuity observed in phonetic drift was proposed by Mowrer (1952). Briefly, Mowrer's hypothesis, called the Autism Theory, proposed that infant sound productions are essentially operant behavior, capable of being influenced by their consequences. This hypothesis suggests that the caregiver's vocalizations become secondary reinforcers for infants as a result of being associated with primary reinforcement during feedings and other caregiving interactions. The more infants' sounds approximate their caregiver's sounds, the more infants' sounds become self-reinforcing through this association. This manner of reinforcement, therefore, is both automatic and selective—those sounds produced by infants that more closely resemble their mother's instantly reinforce infants' production of them.

The nature of reinforcement in child behavior is introduced in Chapter 3. ■

It should be noted that the mechanism for selective reinforcement in Mowrer's formulation has been frequently misunderstood. Contrary to what some have suggested, the caregiver is *not* consciously attempting to selectively reinforce specific sounds. Caregivers generally have more to worry about than determining whether a given sound is in their language and then attempting to promptly reinforce it. In fact, in this formulation the caregiver is not reinforcing infant sounds at all, except indirectly. The potential for self-reinforcement occurs through the natural association of the tender, loving care (primary reinforcers) caregivers provide with the concurrent speech sounds they produce (which become a secondary reinforcer). As infants' sounds more closely approximate their caregiver's, the more likely it is that those sounds will be self-reinforcing.

Operant influence of infant vocalizations has been demonstrated in a number of studies. Researchers have generally used social reinforcers in the form of adult attention (a smile, a touch, and "tsk-tsk-tsk" sounds). Presenting this social stimulus immediately following infant vocalizations has increased their frequency (Rheingold, Gewirtz, & Ross, 1959; Todd & Palmer, 1968; Wahler, 1969; Weisberg, 1963). As limitations, these studies utilized younger infants and did not address their ability to differentiate vocalizations (which they were probably not yet biologically capable of anyway).

Vocal response differentiation in infants has been demonstrated (Routh, 1969). Three groups of infants received selective reinforcement following production of consonant-like sounds in one group, vowel-like sounds in the second, or for any vocalization in the third group. Each group exhibited a significant increase in the response category reinforced in that group.

As our understanding of babbling has progressed, it has become increasingly apparent that babbling does bear a significant relationship to speech. The influence of biological maturation is self-evident in infants' developing control of oral and vocal structures. However, it is also obvious that infants' vocal behavior is strongly influenced by their language environment. From crying to cooing to babbling, infants' vocal behavior is intertwined with caregivers' responses. Only recently has the extent of social interaction prompted by infants' vocalizations been fully recognized. Furthermore, the coupling of infants' developing vocal behavior, cognitive understanding, and social interaction carries the partnership between infants and caregivers closer to true communication (Stark, Bernstein, & Demorest, 1993).

Summary

- Place of production in infant babbling has been found to be predominately front and middle sounds.
- In terms of manner of production, plosive sounds are most prevalent in infants' babbling.

- Most consonants in babbling occur in medial position (VCV) productions earlier, but shift to initial position (CV) consonants.

- Those who view infant sound productions as being unrelated to later speech subscribe to the discontinuity hypothesis.

- Those who subscribe to the continuity hypothesis hold that with experience, infant sound productions gradually approximate and eventually become part of mature speech.

- Research has illustrated the influence of the language environment as infants' sound productions mature, strongly supporting the continuity hypothesis.

Infant and Caregiver Communication

The interaction between infants and their caregivers lays so many foundations for later learning. Infants' most basic social, emotional, and cognitive development arises out of the earliest experiences with their caregiver.

The transactions between infants and their caregivers consist of more than caregiving. Caregivers negotiate through the hundreds of daily caregiving activities every day. Caregiver responses to infant behaviors and infants' reactions to them form the origins of communication.

Investigating Infant Communication

Researchers have increasingly recognized the communicative significance of interactions between the infant and caregiver. In contrast to the traditional view that infants are merely "practicing" making sounds, waiting passively for their first word so language could begin, researchers now recognize the different levels of communication occurring throughout infants' first year of life.

The increased attention to communication in the first year of life and its role in laying the foundation for language resulted in a flurry of related research activity over the last several decades. To fully appreciate the fruits of this work, however, it is important to recall the goals of such research, the nature of the phenomenon being studied, and the methods that are available.

The goals of this research include attempts at describing: (a) the significance of infant and caregiver behaviors in natural communication at each level of prelinguistic development; (b) the mutual influence of infant and caregiver behaviors on later development of mature language; and (c) the extent to which infant behaviors of interest appear to be based on biological structures and experience.

The phenomenon itself—infant behavior—is elusive, transitory, and variable. Infants are notoriously unpredictable in their sleeping patterns, alertness, responsiveness, temperament, and so on. They are easily influenced by the most subtle stimuli affecting the familiarity of the setting and participants. A behavior of interest may be exhibited consistently or infrequently due to some mysterious cue. This leaves the researcher attempting to differentiate between behaviors that may be an important skill or an irrelevant fluke.

Beyond these concerns, researchers must make a number of practical considerations concerning the methods applied in their investigations. Researchers must decide whether the data will be collected in naturalistic observations or through more structured experimental manipulations. Naturalistic observations may provide a broader range of behaviors that are more ecologically valid, meaning that they occur naturally in the infant's daily interactions. In contrast, experimental procedures may allow the experimenter to evoke behaviors that infants are capable of, but might not otherwise exhibit in their normal daily routines.

Another consideration is the means for recording observations. With the increased appreciation of the role of context, it has become critical to record the setting and events that accompany significant behaviors. In the past, researchers could rely on the time-honored method of taking written notes to preserve the contextual information that seemed relevant to each behavior. However, more recently, electronic video recording equipment has become widely available and increasingly affordable.

Researchers must also make basic, practical decisions regarding the number of infants to be studied and the time span of the observations. Studying fewer infants may permit a more intensive, detailed analysis of their development, but the ability to generalize any findings may be limited. On the other hand, observing similar behaviors in a greater number of infants would increase the overall significance of that behavior as a research finding.

In a related decision, the researcher must also consider the advantages and disadvantages of longitudinal as opposed to cross-sectional studies. A study using a **longitudinal research design** would observe the same infants over an extended period of time. This perhaps provides better insight into the continuity of infants' overall development, but runs the risk that some infants will drop out of the study due to illness or family relocation.

Research based on a **cross-sectional research design** collects data simultaneously from separate groups of infants who represent the different developmental ages of interest. The obvious advantage is time efficiency; that is, the researcher does not need to wait for the infants to mature. However, the continuity in observing the overall development of individual infants is lost.

Still other researchers may elect to focus on certain behaviors by using individual infants in experimental designs. Interest in how infant behaviors might be influenced by certain factors have been addressed through **single-subject experimental designs.** For example, as noted before, a number of researchers have investigated whether the frequency of certain infant vocalizations or sounds can be increased by the events that follow their production. Using individual infants, researchers establish a baseline, or the usual frequency of a randomly produced sound. Then, an additional factor, such

longitudinal research design   Research design that follows the continuous development of its subjects.

cross-sectional research design   Research design in which groups of subjects at different ages are used to simulate changes related to chronological development.

single-subject experimental designs   Research design in which an individual subject serves as his or her own control.

as reinforcement (a taped sample of the caregiver's voice), is presented following productions of that sound during one interval and not presented during the next interval. Any changes in the frequency of that sound is monitored. Such research designs allow researchers to change the frequency of specific behaviors and isolate factors that might influence them. However, until such experiments are repeated, the limited number of subjects involved limits how much the researcher can conclude about all infants.

Certainly, studying the development of infants would seem to be a fascinating and appealing assignment with plenty of pleasant and entertaining moments. On the other hand, it also demands a great deal of planning, discipline, objectivity, and flexibility.

Summary

- Interest in pragmatic aspects of communication has prompted research into infant-caregiver interactions.

- Researchers have attempted to identify the infant and caregiver behaviors that contribute to development of communication.

- Research with infants is especially difficult due to their rapidly changing physical and emotional state and rapid overall development.

- Researchers can study overall development from a long-term perspective in longitudinal designs, from a broader perspective in cross-sectional designs, or by focusing on specific behaviors in individual infants in single-subject experimental designs.

Prelinguistic Communication

Even before the production of the first word, communication between infants and caregivers is occurring—at some level. Although infants have not yet produced their first words, the evolution of communication throughout infants' first 12 months has been correlated with the pragmatic elements of speech acts outlined by Searle and Austin (Bates, 1976). Accordingly, the three stages are referred to as the perlocutionary, illocutionary, and locutionary stages.

These pragmatic elements are present in an individual instance of a mature speech act. The speaker first has an intention (illocution) that is expressed in an utterance (locution) and subsequently interpreted by a listener (perlocution). However, the sequence of the these elements is somewhat altered in the phases of communication development during infancy.

The first half of an infant's first year is considered the **perlocutionary stage,** a phase in which communication is based primarily on caregivers' interpretation of infants' behaviors. It is assumed that infants lack conscious, goal-directed intentions in these earliest interactions. The **illocutionary stage,** in which intentions are signaled, emerges during the second half of the first year. By 8 or 9 months, infants begin to indicate identifiable intentions

The three dimensions of a speech act—perlocutionary, illocutionary, and locutionary—are discussed in Chapter 4. ▪

perlocutionary stage The stage of communication development from birth to approximately 6 months in which caregivers infer intentions on the part of infants.

illocutionary stage The stage in communication development beginning at approximately 6 months when the infant begins to signal intentions through gesture and vocalization.

locutionary stage The stage in communication development beginning when the first words are used to convey intentions.

with apparent awareness of achieving their goals through the caregiver's behavior. However, this is still accomplished primarily through gestures and vocalizations, leaving the **locutionary stage,** the use of words to express intentions, to emerge around the first birthday.

It should be recognized that the three stages are cumulative and overlapping, as illustrated in Figure 5–1. That is, the first stage continues as the second stage emerges and complements it. These first two stages, again, continue developing as the third stage evolves. Throughout the first year, the infant and caregiver both display behaviors that contribute to this evolution. Although the participants may be more or less conscious of their specific behaviors, researchers have noted their apparent significance in contributing to the development of communication.

Summary

- Infant communication has been characterized as passing through three cumulative stages that are analogous to the elements of a speech act.
- The perlocutionary period, during approximately the first 6 months, depends on the caregiver's interpretation of infant behaviors as signals.
- The illocutionary period occurs in the second half of the first year as infants develop behaviors to convey their intentions to caregivers.
- The final period of development, the locutionary period, arrives with the ability to produce words and phrases.

The Perlocutionary Stage of Communication

The first period, the perlocutionary stage, is essentially present from birth. The perlocutionary aspect of speech acts refers to the listener's interpretation of the speaker's message. Of course, infants do not truly represent "speakers" at the outset; after all, they are by definition "without speech."

It is also assumed that infants do not exhibit "intentions," as they are incapable of conceiving of cause-effect or means-end relationships. That is,

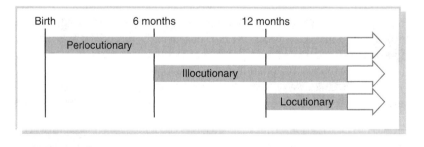

Figure 5–1. Development of pragmatic elements of speech acts.

infants would have no understanding of being able to achieve a specific result from their behavior. This leaves only the perlocutionary element of communication. Caregivers *infer* messages, imposing communicative significance on infants' nonverbal behaviors—cries, smiles, and vocal sounds. Communication at this point is a one-sided affair, based primarily on caregivers' willingness and ability to interpret their infant's behavior as signals. There are certainly moments when caregivers interpret signals that simply are not being sent. For example, caregivers might respond to gurgles and coos with *You like that, do you?* to fussing with *Oh my, you want me to fix that, don't you?* and to burps with *That feels better, doesn't it?*

It should be remembered that even for mature adult speakers, communication is a precarious enterprise. The effects our words have on a listener do not always reflect our intentions. Without the assistance of words from infants, caregivers' inferences are even more questionable. However, most caregivers make a gallant effort at discovering, even inventing, their infant's underlying message.

With some regrets, the following account does some violence to the fragile nature of the phenomenon it describes. The infant-caregiver dyad is so intricately and intimately intertwined that it should not be pried apart. However, to do so helps study the important elements more carefully. As the elements of this interaction become clear, it should be eventually possible to envision the infant and caregiver interacting in their natural state.

Infant Contributions to Communication

Infancy represents a period of communication that is nonverbal. At first glance, it may seem paradoxical to use "nonverbal" to describe "communication." However, we should be reminded that much of human communication is nonverbal. This includes extralinguistic aspects such as the paralinguistic and nonlinguistic cues.

Effective communicators use various cues (intonational contours, facial expressions, gestures, proxemics, etc.) that typically accompany and supplement their spoken words to make sense of the verbal or linguistic message. Infant behaviors generally include many of these aspects, although they occur unintentionally, often in reflexive response to the infant's physiological state (e.g., hunger).

Paralinguistic and nonlinguistic cues are discussed in Chapter 1. ▪

Even the earliest interactions between caregivers and their infants can be viewed as the foundation of social communication. Social because the behavior of one influences the behavior of the other. Communication because regardless of its source and form, there is a message transmitted by a sender to a receiver. Although this period precedes formal language, there still is communication between the infant and caregiver.

Infants become increasingly effective in engaging their partners in various interactions; caregivers continually adjust and expand the nature of their contributions to their infants' development. In the beginning, however, the two participants contribute to the interaction in ways that are quite

Recall that Chapter 2 noted preliminary evidence that the fetus is capable of hearing and responding to external sounds. Whether this constitutes communication is an interesting question to ponder. ▪

different. Caregivers may behave verbally with conscious intent, but the messages are less linguistic than social in nature. By talking in soothing or happy tones, caregivers intend to communicate emotionally, not verbally. On the other side, infants' behavior is neither intentional nor symbolic. Instead, it represents an outward manifestation of infants' inner sensations, whether that is hunger, pain, or pleasure.

Although inadvertent in nature, the first lessons learned through this partnership may be the most important foundation for all language learning. When infants act on a responsive environment, in some way they implicitly learn that those around them will respond in some way in turn.

Cry Behavior.   Infants' cries have inspired almost as much research on the part of scientists as they have aroused concern on the part of caregivers. Due to the heart-rending nature of infants' cries and their potential relationship to language, they have been the source of intrigue and inquiry for centuries.

To the inexperienced ear, all infants' cries might sound the same, just as some might think the cry of an individual infant is generally consistent. However, this is not the case. Some individual mothers can discriminate their infant's cry from those of other infants, suggesting that each cry possesses distinctive acoustic characteristics (Formby, 1967).

On another level, analysis of acoustic features such as intensity and pitch changes in the cries of normal and abnormal infants suggests that they may contain characteristics predictive of infants who are at risk for normal development (Zeskind & Lester, 1978). Finally, acoustic analysis has distinguished four types of infant cries: (a) a birth cry; (b) a hunger cry; (c) a pain cry; and (d) an angry cry (Lieberman, 1967; Wolff, 1969). However, in terms of communication, can caregivers differentiate among their infant's different cries?

According to Reich's (1986) discussion of this literature, the initial indications were negative. Early studies, using rudimentary procedures, indicated listeners could not perform much better than chance at discerning whether a given cry resulted from stimuli such as pain, startle, or hunger. Later, using more advanced procedures to control the amplitude and duration of each cry stimulus, researchers found this was still the case. One study (Petrovich-Bartell, Cowan, & Morse, 1982) has suggested mothers can interpret the degree of distress in their baby's cries, ranking them on a fuss-cry continuum.

But what about all the anecdotal evidence in which caregivers vow that they know the reasons for their baby's cry? The discrepancy may lie in the nature of the research (Reich, 1986). For purposes of control, experimental research generally presents isolated intervals of infant cries. Mothers are asked to respond to these brief samples. As natural occurrences, different cries may be preceded by distinctive periods of fussiness. Depending on their cause, different cries may vary in their intensity and duration, and the pauses between crying bursts may differ, too. Normally, all of this information is available to the caregiver as well as one other critical element—the situation itself. As in communication at any level, knowledge of the context (e.g., the caregiver's proximity, the infant's movements, intervals since the last feeding, changing, etc.) may assist caregivers' interpretations as much as any other cue (Haynes, 1994a).

Infants cry approximately a total of 2 hours out of each day in their first 7 weeks of life. Of course, this crying is episodic, not continuous (something for which we can all be thankful). Caregivers generally attend to their crying infants within 3 to 4 minutes after a cry episode begins and ignore very few occurrences (Reich, 1986). In short, in the first few months of life infants cry frequently and their caregivers react reliably. This contingency represents the perlocutionary effect that crying has on caregivers. Caregivers feel needed and infants are provided with prompt feeding, changing, and cuddling. But what other experiences are provided for infants in these episodes?

At the level of linguistics and speech, crying provides infants with early *stimulation* of laryngeal and oral functions. Later, with maturation, reflex inhibition allows voluntary cessation of crying, which may be a forerunner to voluntary control for speech breathing. In terms of social interaction, crying *functions* to prompt caregivers to provide basic needs (food, warmth, comfort), which requires their presence (cuddling, facial expressions), supplementing infants' attachment to their caregivers. Cognitively, to the extent that such social transactions reliably follow episodes of crying, the seeds of understanding *cause-effect* and *means-end* relationships are potentially planted. Ultimately, over these repeated episodes, infants are learning *natural contingencies*—that their behaviors have reliable social consequences.

 This information on infant cries and caregiver responses should not be overgeneralized to all cultures. Infants in some primitive societies cry very little because they are constantly with the mother. Infant cries in some cultures are not responded to as promptly because they are not viewed as communicative. And, even in Western mainstream societies there are differences based on family beliefs regarding "spoiling" the child.

Cause-effect and mean-end relationships are discussed in Chapter 3. ▪

Gaze Patterns. Eye contact for infants and newborns in particular is a fleeting and transitory event—by nature. This is because they spend so much of their first few months sleeping. Even when awake, their head control and visual focus are quite limited. As a result, even at the end of the third month they only scan their visual field approximately one third of their waking hours. Their initial limited visual acuity causes them to be primarily interested in objects that exhibit motion and geometric shapes with sharp contrasts. A convenient example of such a stimulus is the human face, with its moving mouth, blinking eyes, and surrounding hairline.

In the development of infant-caregiver interactions, eye gaze will play a central role. From an emotional standpoint, mothers have reported that once their infants were able to return their gaze, establishing mutual eye contact, they felt a much closer attachment to the baby (Klaus & Kennell, 1976). By the end of the second month, infants are able to maintain eye contact with their caregivers. However, this usually occurs when caregivers are currently gazing at their infants. Improving motor control permits infants to eventually combine head movements with eye movements for establishing

Visual acuity and tracking are also discussed in Chapter 2. ▪

Infants' recognition of facial features and infant-caregiver attachment are discussed in Chapter 3. ▪

or ending eye contact. These head positions are generally interpreted by caregivers as infants' signals of readiness to engage in eye contact.

Infants' ability to focus visually matures around 3 months and their visual behavior can more directly prompt interaction with the caregiver. Three basic patterns of infant visual behavior have been described: mutual gaze, gaze coupling, and deictic gaze.

Mutual gaze is intensified focus on the partner's eyes, what some might call "eye lock." The early occurrences often consist of prolonged eye contact. Later, eye contact evolves into an alternating, almost flirtatious pattern that has been referred to as *gaze coupling*. Gaze coupling is of interest in that it takes on the character of a conversation, with each partner alternately looking at the other, looking away, and looking back. *Deictic gaze* occurs when infants' eye gaze becomes fixated on some object, unintentionally "pointing" to it as an object of interest. The perlocutionary effect on caregivers is to interpret this as a signal, following their infants' "line of sight" to the object of apparent interest. Initially, infants are not *intending* to direct their caregivers' attention. Instead, infants merely react to an interesting visual stimulus and caregivers impose their interpretation that this is an invitation to interact. Research shows that caregivers pay close attention to their babies' eyes, reliably synchronizing their naming of an item during the brief time the infant is gazing at it (Collis & Schaffer, 1975).

It is interesting to note that we can actually "hear" a smile on the telephone. Smiling while talking affects the acoustic signal in characteristic ways that can be detected. ∎

Social Smiles.   In spite of its place in a beloved, classic movie, most would disagree with the verse, "a smile is *just* a smile." (For that matter, how could a kiss ever be *just* a kiss?) The smile has a peculiar place in human behavior and an even more puzzling history. Does it occur in our species out of a history of intimidation behavior—exposing our teeth to ward off aggressors and establish territorial domination? Or does it subtly convey submissiveness?

Locke (1993) summarized a hypothesis by Ohala (1980), which suggested the latter of these two possibilities. The acoustic result of smiling while talking is to raise the perceived pitch of the speaker's voice. In non-human primates, exhibiting high-pitched vocalizations with lips retracted (smiling) tends to evoke sympathetic responses from peers. Historically, aggressors may have been sympathetically moved to withdraw, increasing the survival chances for those who "smiled" at them. However the human smile came to exist, it is considered by many to be the "universal language" and it appears very early in our development.

reflexive smile   Infant smile behavior that is in apparent response to internal physiologic stimuli.

The first distinction that must be made is between infants' reflexive smiles and social smiles. **Reflexive smiles** are those that result from internal physiological stimuli. These occur in the first few weeks following birth primarily during sleep and are often associated with rapid eye movements that occur during dreaming (Wolff, 1966). Frequently, even awake infants smile for seemingly no apparent reason; many experienced caregivers have attributed some of these early smiles to "having a 'bubble' turned sideways in the tummy." Whatever the circumstances of each particular instance, it appears that such early smiles are simply a reflexive response to some internal stimulus.

In a matter of a few more weeks, auditory and visual acuity improves, and caregivers' voices and faces are more easily recognized. Infants then begin to exhibit *social smiles* that occur in response to another's social presence. In its appearance, the social smile does not differ from the reflexive smile. Instead, it differs in its apparent source. The social smile occurs in response to the human face and voice, especially those voices exhibiting greater inflection. Infants may see a familiar face, make eye contact, or simply hear a familiar voice, and smile in response.

Infants' first smiles are merely reflexive, not communicative. Neither are the earliest social smiles intentional or goal directed; they are more reactions than messages. Nonetheless, their appearance prompts caregivers to *invent* communication that is not really there. Imposing their interpretation on these early smiles, caregivers bubble over with praise and affection.

Later, infants' social smiles will become more meaningful as signs of recognition and attachment. Furthermore, the more reliably they occur in response to caregivers, the more they serve to reinforce and engage caregivers' continued interaction.

The human face and voice appear to be inherently intertwined. From the beginning, recognizable facial expressions are associated with certain distinctive vocalizations. Cries, laughter, squeals, and happy sounds are each associated with characteristic facial expressions. In this same way, social smiles, too, are typically associated with some form of pleasant infant vocalization.

Vocal Behavior.   In spite of the increased recognition that communication *at some level* does occur during the first year, the traditional vocal behaviors and their milestones have continued to serve as a measure of infant vocal development. Cooing, babbling, vocal play, jargon, and echolalia remain as reference points in infants' changing vocal repertoire. However, in the current view this repertoire is not simply a progression of isolated, one-sided behaviors. Although unintentional, these are important behaviors that evoke social interaction that evolves toward communication.

Again, it must be reemphasized that infants do not use early vocal behaviors to communicate with any intention. Early vocalizations are not goal directed, just as early crying, smiling, and gazing occur without any conscious intent. Nonetheless, infants' vocal behaviors do evoke their caregivers' attention. Cooing has a characteristic sound, often shaped by the smiles that accompany it. The perlocutionary effect on caregivers is to evoke attention, closeness, cuddling, and soft speech.

Impressively, it has been documented that infants' behavior frequently prompts vocal imitation within the infant-caregiver dyad (Locke, 1993). Given the occurrence of spontaneous infant vocalizations, caregivers then take the lead in the imitation game. In turn, infants frequently echo their caregivers' imitations, almost as though they were their own. Furthermore, as the nature of infants' vocal behavior evolves toward more "speech-like" sounds, caregivers' responses increasingly reflect these changes. In other words, caregivers modify their reactions to their infants' vocalizations. These modifications cause further changes in the infants' vocalizations.

Two mutually stimulating dynamics appear to be at work. First, infants' sound repertoires expand to include more speechlike sounds. Second, as these changes reflect infants' growing capabilities, so do caregivers' expectations of their infants' abilities expand. And, so continues this marvelous partnership!

Caregiver Contributions to Communication

In this partnership, caregivers unknowingly play a most important role by providing the perlocutionary element. In responding to infants' behaviors, caregivers *act as though* real communication is occurring. Realistically, given infants' initial capabilities, caregivers can only expect that communication will *eventually* occur with their child. However, that expectation is seemingly enough to prompt anticipation on the part of caregivers. The nature of caregivers' behavior suggests that communicating with their infant is a desire, so much so that they are willing to invent communication where it probably does not exist.

Perhaps in this way human communication development is a prime example of "self-fulfilling prophecy." Caregivers' behavior illustrates a premature expectation. This, in turn, may create a related expectation on the part of infants—that someone will respond in some way when they act on their environment. Caregivers' behavior makes their speech salient, identifies topics of interest, and establishes the natural cycles of expectation and fulfillment, and the participating and pausing found in mature conversations.

Baby Talk.   One of the most conspicuous ways in which the caregivers' behavior is made salient to infants is through their speech patterns. **Baby talk** (also *motherese* or **parentese**) refers to speech with several characteristic features directed at infants by adults and even older children. In using baby talk, caregivers make a number of modifications that appear to be instinctively related to the infant's current capabilities. Most adults would be at a loss to explain such behavior.

Over the years, researchers (Snow, 1977a; Stern, 1977) have documented what most have long recognized about baby talk from watching doting uncles, aunts, and grandparents. Baby talk features a number of distinctive modifications in the syntactic structure, semantic content, paralinguistic features, and nonlinguistic devices used by caregivers. Table 5–2 lists some of the key features of baby talk.

Structurally, in apparent recognition of infants' limited capacities, most caregiver *utterances are shorter in length,* exhibiting *simpler syntax and limited vocabulary.* Semantically, successive utterances in baby talk frequently relate to the same context. The words and phrases are often *redun-*

Some sources use *motherese* or *parentese* to refer to these early modifications in the caregiver's speech to infants. Others reserve these for speech directed to toddlers already exhibiting some language. ∎

baby talk Characteristic speech patterns, including shorter phrases and exaggerated intonation, used when talking to infants.

parentese (also **motherese** or **child directed speech**) Gender neutral term for the distinctive style of speech exhibited by caregivers with their toddlers.

Table 5–2. The features of caregivers' baby talk to infants.

Utterances are produced in closer proximity when infant is attending.

Utterances are produced at a higher pitch.

Utterances are produced with greater pitch fluctuations.

Utterances are produced at a slower rate.

Utterances are produced with more and longer pauses.

Utterances are simpler in construction.

Utterances are produced more fluently and clearly.

Utterances are based on a smaller, restricted set of words.

Words are frequently nouns for concrete objects.

Words generally refer to objects or events in the here-and-now.

dant and overlapping, labeling the same referent with related words and phrases. Another property of baby talk is the extent to which the context is tied to the "here-and-now." Caregivers implicitly recognize that infants have little awareness of the world beyond the immediate present so most utterances relate to objects and actions that are within their view.

With regard to paralinguistic features, caregivers exhibit several behaviors that apparently draw and maintain infants' interest. Caregivers' speech exhibits a *higher overall pitch,* a *broader range of intonation and stress,* and *longer pauses* between segments. These aspects give baby talk its characteristic "sing-song" quality. Finally, several nonlinguistic devices are used by caregivers to engage infants. These include using *more gestures, more varied facial expressions,* and consistently *positioning their face within the infant's field of view.*

Use of higher overall pitch and greater prosodic variations in baby talk have been documented across a number of languages (Ferguson, 1964; Fernald et al., 1989). Why do caregivers use such distinctive voices when talking to infants? Babies apparently prefer voices in higher pitch ranges. They are also more likely to attend to *novelty,* that is, changes in stimuli in their environment.

Episodes of baby talk typically occur as series of utterances surrounding a specific event. Early episodes occur following any of a number of insignificant behaviors such as a yawn, a sneeze, a burp, or a coo-like sigh. Later episodes will frequently center around the caregiver's manipulation of some object, thereby establishing it as the topic. As a result, most episodes are characterized by naming the object, perhaps with redundant labels repeated with various phrasing. However, the utterances are more than a simple string of successive statements. Caregivers instead weave them together

The development of joint attention, establishing a shared topic between caregivers and infants, is discussed later in this chapter. ■

with greetings and questions to impose a social framework in spite of their partners' communicative limitations. A typical episode might go as follows:

Hello sleepyhead! (caregiver approaches crib, pauses)

Not sleepy anymore? (brings face nearer, pauses)

Where's your bear? (raises open hands in gesture)

Here's baby's bear! (picks up, motions in baby's view)

Baby hug bear? Give big hug? Oh, nice hug! Nice bear!

Such an example illustrates object-centered naming, with repetitions and motions related to the topic. Unfortunately, it is not possible to illustrate the high-pitched, melodic character of caregivers' speech here. (Most of us have heard this sing-song speech and, embarrassingly, some of us have had our best baby talk caught on videotape!)

The overall effect in such episodes is to attract and hold infants' attention with eye-catching gestures and facial expressions, highlighted by sweeping vocal prosody. Then, while infants attend to a stable, available topic, caregivers present a series of overlapping comments related to it. Interestingly, each comment is followed by a brief pause that approximates the interval between turns taken in conversations between adults. Whether consciously or not, caregivers' pauses signal the expectation of a response from their infant.

Beyond embarrassment, what is in it for caregivers? It would appear that some desirable result comes from effecting these changes, even if caregivers are not conscious of making them. Perhaps engaging and continuing infants' attention, in the form of eye contact, social smiles, and vocalizations, reinforces caregivers for using baby talk.

On the other side, researchers have found that infants prefer the melodic character of motherese (Fernald, 1985). Furthermore, it may benefit infants' later language development. It has been found that caregivers' adjustments in length of utterance in speech to their infants is predictive of the infants' later language development (Murray, Johnson, & Peters, 1990).

Baby talk persists for some time and eventually evolves into a style characteristic of more mature verbal exchanges with older children (called motherese or parentese by some). The earliest episodes of baby talk are only suggestive of the conversations that these later exchanges will exhibit. However, there are other forms of interaction that, from the beginning, lay the foundation for later dialogue.

Joint Attention.   Speakers do not communicate in a vacuum and as a result their speech necessarily *refers* to something in the environment. For communication to occur, however, their listeners must also select and attend to the topic of speakers' utterances. In interacting with their infants, caregivers exhibit a variety of behaviors to establish joint or shared attention with their infants. In *joint reference,* the shared attention and caregivers' utterances are focused on an object. In contrast, in *joint action,* it is shared activity that provides the focus of attention and the topic of care-givers' utterances.

Joint reference involves speakers' identification of topics, objects, events, or relations about which they are talking. Such referencing helps the listener understand the speaker. Whether the referents for our speech are present, recalled from the past or anticipated in the future, located nearby or at a distance, mature speakers identify them for their listeners through vari-ous language behaviors. For example, a speaker might identify a remote ob-ject for discussion by saying something such as, *Remember on our vacation last summer how we admired that classic red Corvette in San Francisco? . . .* There is certainly communication value in being able to identify a topic to be shared (especially if one has an agenda related to the topic, as this spouse most likely does).

Although caregivers do not have a communication agenda beyond in-teracting socially and emotionally with their infants, their interaction gener-ally has some focus. Much of the early interaction occurs when caregivers must handle their infants more frequently. As caregivers verbalize in these face-to-face interactions the content is more social and emotional in nature, such as *Hello pretty baby! Momma loves you!* and so on.

Later, as infants' motor control matures and their ability to scan and focus improves, caregivers can direct their attention to objects of interest. Caregivers' speech will shift to naming and labeling objects, sometimes repeatedly and redundantly (as was described in discussing baby talk). Eventually, as infants' awareness of the surroundings expands, their care-givers begin to elaborate with increasingly descriptive comments.

Caregivers are aware of their young partners' limited abilities. Accord-ingly, they direct their infants' focus to items of interest in very natural ways as they talk to them. Caregivers might select items themselves for various reasons. Frequently, they single out items the infant has grasped or gazed at simply by chance, interpreting such behavior as expressions of interest in that item.

Several researchers have classified caregivers' techniques for achieving joint attention with their infants (Bruner, 1977; Collis & Schaffer, 1975). The various classifications include such techniques as indicating, marking, deixis, and naming. On some occasions, caregivers take advantage of their infants' current interests. When something catches infants' attention, care-givers exhibit **indicating,** in which they follow their infants' line of sight to the object of their curiosity. On other occasions, caregivers introduce the ob-jects of interest themselves. When caregivers select an object and strive to focus their infants' attention on it, they might use **marking,** in which they move or shake it conspicuously in their infants' field of view.

In utilizing **deixis,** caregivers use proximity as a way of channeling their infants' focus. Moving infants closer makes objects more prominent in their field of view. If the family cuckoo clock is to be the topic of discussion, mov-ing in closer will help focus an infant's attention on it (since it is probably not possible to shake it).

The caregiver's indicating behavior is the "flip side" of the infant's deictic gaze. ■

indicating Caregivers' use of their infants' line of sight to locate the object of their current interest.

marking Caregivers' means of attracting attention to an object by moving or shaking it in their infants' field of view.

deixis The ability of words and gaze patterns to "point to" objects being referenced.

naming   Caregivers' use of label to direct their infants' attention.

 Later, deixis will occur through verbal behaviors, such as using *this* versus *that* to indicate relative proximity. Development of this behavior is discussed in Chapter 7. ■

dialogue   A series of related verbal exchanges between at least two persons.

 The word *dialogue* derives from the Greek *dia,* for "between or through," and *logos,* for speech. Therefore, dialogue is speech between people. ■

Finally, with older infants beginning to recognize a few words, caregivers might use **naming** to prompt them to search for a familiar item or person before elaborating further. For example, once its name is associated with the characteristic sounds and actions, merely mentioning the word *cuckoo* will prompt the infant to look at it with anticipation.

Early referencing is, again, very much one sided throughout the perlocutionary period. Eventually, infants master their own devices for directing their caregivers' attention. In the meantime, caregivers are demonstrating to their infants that speech is intimately associated with the world that they are both experiencing and interacting with each day.

The other aspect of joint attention is joint action, shared participation in some activity that becomes the focus of caregiver-infant interactions. This occurs initially in the context of daily caregiving routines, bathing, feeding, dressing, and so forth. Later, joint action occurs in the context of games. In the earliest stages, infants are more passive partners. Most of us have put agreeable infants through the paces of "pat-a-cake" or "peek-a-boo" while they look on with idle curiosity. These early interactions are shared only because infants are usually compliant and captive partners. Infants soon begin to join in, throwing their arms up for "*So big!*" or squealing with excitement as our eyes reappear from behind our hands in *Peek-a-boo!* Eventually, infants signal their anticipation of these social games, clapping their hands together or covering their eyes to signal "let the games begin!"

Dialogues (Turn Taking).   The term **dialogue** technically refers to speech exchanged between at least two persons. Although infants are without speech, one of the most fundamental characteristics of dialogue has great significance for their development of communication. *Turn taking,* the alternation of responses and pauses between participants in an activity, is a basic element of dialogue. Without it, communication suffers severely since, at least in spoken language, each message has only a fleeting presence. Few of us can simultaneously speak and listen to someone else effectively. If one partner or the other fails to take turns, information is lost as their talking overlaps and collides (Lund & Duchan, 1993).

Similarly, if infants were incapable of pausing in their own behavior to attend to those around them, their opportunities to learn would be greatly diminished. Almost from the beginning, caregivers pattern their behavior so as to create predictable sequences of turn taking that seem to become second nature to the infant. Caregivers unknowingly accomplish this through several different natural interactions, including feeding sessions, game playing, and ultimately, through dialogues.

Although some mature speakers may struggle yet with turn taking (sometimes called "rudeness," if they fail frequently), this is not for a lack of developmental opportunity. Dialogues of a nonverbal sort occur with infants from the earliest

 Lund and Duchan (1993) remind us that later, in more formal contexts, turn taking is not always symmetrical. In formal settings, one might only get a turn when called on, as in a classroom setting. And, in a formal speech or sermon, the only turn is taken by one person.

moments. Researchers have found a primary biological basis for dialogue based on feeding behaviors of mothers and infants (Locke, 1993). Mothers quickly discover that their feeding babies suck in bursts followed by pauses. Most mothers attempt to adapt to this pattern by "jiggling" the baby or the nipple to restart the baby's sucking. The jiggle actually suppresses sucking, which usually resumes once the jiggling has stopped. Nonetheless, a distinct pattern of turn taking evolves and, significantly, in the context of a very impressionable and reinforcing interaction.

Another early form of interaction that is imposed on infants by caregivers is game playing. The earliest games are social in nature, based primarily on patterned interactions between caregivers and infants. Each game is patterned to contain a very consistent, predictable sequence of cues provided by caregivers. After setting the stage through a series of verbal and gestural cues, caregivers pause strategically for their infants' response.

Some typical games include *Gotcha, Pat-a-cake, So Big,* and the classic, *Peek-a-boo*! Each game presents a consistent sequence of gestural and verbal cues, making them very predictable for infants. This allows infants to eventually anticipate the course and outcome of each episode. Additionally, these may be incorporated into daily routines such as diapering, bathing, and dressing.

In the earliest sessions, caregivers must usually mold the response. For example, caregivers might have to initially guide infants' hands to cover their eyes and then lift them to play "peek-a-boo." Later, infants will anticipate the sequences in the game and contribute a motion or vocalization to signal its continuation. Eventually, infants may initiate the game by gesturing in distinctive ways (Ratner & Bruner, 1978; Sachs, 1985). Nonetheless, the overall structure of each series of turns is initially imposed by caregivers.

At the same time, caregivers also fine-tune their stimulation to maintain their infants' interest without causing overexcitement. Using baby talk, affecting looks of mock surprise, and changing facial orientation keeps infants' attention. When overstimulated, however, infants may strain to look away from their caregivers. Slowing the pace, softening the voice, reducing eye contact, and holding infants closer may calm the level of stimulation.

We should be careful not to assign too much significance to the games themselves. While they may be one interaction that facilitates language learning, they do not appear to be a necessary condition. There are groups in American society and other cultures in which such games are not an especially common activity between caregivers and infants (Sachs, 1985).

The length and sequence of games will vary between caregiver-infant pairs and also across different episodes. However, each session will characteristically involve predictable elements. Sessions begin with a *greeting* involving eye contact, smiles, and facial orientation. This is followed by *engagement,* or the game itself with its distinctive sequence of behaviors and pauses. Finally, there is a *pause* between game episodes. Infants suppress other behaviors during each pause in the game sequence and between game episodes in anticipation of their caregivers' next moves. This suppression of activity in alternation with caregivers' behavior is the essence of turn taking.

The value of suppressing one's own vocal behavior to experience another's seems to make an early impression on infants. It has been found that young infants will cease vocalizing to better hear a caregiver's voice. Furthermore, they will do so to a greater extent if they have demonstrated a preference for the voice of that caregiver over other caregivers (Barret-Goldfarb & Whitehurst, 1973). The extent to which this preferred voice has been associated with reinforcing activities (such as feeding, cuddling, etc.) may play a significant role in its appeal.

Vocal turn taking in infants appears to a notable extent around 3 to 4 months and steadily increases beyond that time (Locke, 1993). Three-month-old infants are twice as likely to vocalize again, if their caregivers vocalize in response, as opposed to gesturing or smiling. In addition, as infants grow older, caregivers are more likely to imitate speech sounds, as opposed to nonspeech sounds.

Clearly, a basic picture of a dialogue emerges out of these exchanges. So much so that such extended reciprocal vocalizations have been referred to as **protoconversations,** the first or earliest conversations, especially when other elements such as mutual gaze and social smiles are integrated into the interaction (Bateson, 1975). Although infants may not be transmitting a great amount of linguistic information in these earliest dialogues, they are taking turns sharing a great deal of unspoken social and emotional information for the time being.

> In this context, the prefix *proto-* refers to the earliest form of a behavior, just as the word *prototype* might refer to the first model of a new jet. ∎

protoconversations
Early interactions between caregivers and infants that include aspects such as turn taking.

Overview of the Perlocutionary Stage

During the perlocutionary period, infants and caregivers share a partnership based on innocence and trust. Infants' contributions seem to arise out of innocence, stemming from causes that are beyond their control. Infants present behaviors that are reflexive, physiological, or simply random events, with no conscious intention or goal, and no ulterior motives, if you will.

On the other side, caregivers trust that these cries, burps, gazes, and smiles are significant beyond their face value. Caregivers implicitly believe that their infants are attempting communication at some level. Caregivers even invent communication wherever interpretation allows. This trust is reflected in the baby talk that caregivers intone to their infants amid the feedings, games, and dialogues that precede any meaningful speech from their usually compliant partner. Furthermore, caregivers trust that true communication with this new and very precious person will soon be possible. In all likelihood, it is caregivers' expectations that unwittingly plant the first seeds of communication.

Summary

- Although communication requires partners, in the perlocutionary period, caregivers assume the lead role by interpreting their infants' behaviors.

- Infant behaviors that caregivers react to as signals for communication include various forms of crying, gazing, smiling, and vocal behaviors.

- Caregivers' behaviors reveal their expectation that their infant will communicate in some way.

- Caregivers use baby talk, which makes their speech more noticeable to their infant.

- Caregivers exhibit various means of establishing joint attention with their infants as they talk about them.

- The early interactions between infants and caregivers include many aspects of a dialogue and have been referred to as protoconversations.

The Illocutionary Stage of Communication

Throughout the first 6 months of life, during the perlocutionary stage, the responsibility for communication fell primarily on caregivers' shoulders. Infants were not yet capable of intending a specific goal or outcome and unknowingly relied on caregivers to infer or, just as often, invent them. As the next few months pass, this changes gradually, but significantly.

The illocutionary stage represents the emergence of intentionality on the part of infants. **Intentionality** means that infants' behavior is consciously directed toward influencing other persons to act on some object. For example, infants exhibit intentionality when they attempt to obtain a toy by directing their caregivers' attention to it. Between mature speakers, the most innocent utterances (*Do you have a watch?*) carry intentionality (the goal of finding out the time). However, infants are still making their way through the day without the advantage of words.

> **intentionality** Behavior that exhibits the conscious attempt to achieve some goal through influencing others' behavior.

During the second half of the infant's first year, the caregiver-infant dyad gradually moves into a somewhat more symmetrical partnership. This is due in part to infants' developing cognitive and motor abilities. Cognitively, infants have begun to understand the concept of cause-effect and means-end relationships; changes have causes and other people can be the agents of change. Not only do infants become cognitively more aware of their goals (desired objects, actions, and events), but the motor abilities for signaling these to caregivers are evolving every day. Ultimately, as infants' use of gestures and vocalizations becomes more effective throughout this period, this success provides even greater motivation to communicate more effectively. By 8 or 9 months, infants are capable of signaling desired objects or actions, even if still without true words.

The Foundations of Intentionality

At a most fundamental level, infants' understanding of cause-effect and means-end relationships is a basic requirement to developing intentionality. Beyond this, caregivers exhibit certain behaviors that set the stage for infants to begin indicating their intentions. These include establishing joint reference with infants and engaging them in joint action. Ultimately, infants mirror caregivers in acting to establish joint attention themselves.

Joint Reference and Joint Action.   Influencing another's behavior is not very useful unless they are also attending to some object of interest. It serves caregivers little purpose to describe or name an object if their infants are focused elsewhere on the myriad of other available stimuli. Similarly, before infants can eventually signal their intentions—obtain an object through their caregivers, cause caregivers to act on it, or engage them in a shared activity—infants must be able to direct their caregivers' attention. A prerequisite to developing intentionality will be infants' ability to establish mutual focus with their caregivers. This shared focus with caregivers may be object oriented or action oriented.

Caregiver behaviors for establishing joint attention are described earlier in this chapter. ▪

The foundations of joint reference, the shared focus of individuals on an identified object, is established by caregivers during the perlocutionary period. As caregivers achieved shared attention during the first 6 months, they demonstrated the tools infants need to eventually turn the tables as their capacities mature.

Infants' early visual abilities permitted tracking their caregivers' face, gaze, and reaching movements. By 7 months, infants can visually search for items that have disappeared, perhaps as caregivers manipulate them.

Auditorily, infants can respond discriminatively to utterances directed at them by 4 months and by 7 months they are beginning to recognize a few words. These are most likely the familiar names of significant objects or people frequently labeled by caregivers. The improving visual and auditory abilities certainly prepare infants for following their caregivers' referencing behaviors.

In terms of motor control, infants progress from grasping items placed in their hands at 2 months to coordinating the movements to focus on, reach for, and grasp items smoothly. Such skills were probably cultivated by caregivers' tendency to hold out objects of interest for infants to inspect or grasp.

The motor control for reaching may be a particularly significant development as it appears to guide infants toward the ability to direct their caregivers' attention with the ever so useful "pointer" finger. Early attempts at reaching for and grasping an object may evolve into simulated reaches that merely signal interest. Infants may extend an arm and hand without visibly straining to reach the item. This behavior is frequently accompanied by glancing at the object and their caregiver alternately, after which caregivers may respond verbally. Eventually, infants' pointer fingers are extended at the end of this reach, perhaps being generalized from previous experiences in touching and exploring other items of interest with their finger tip. Finally, infants combine this gesture with vocalization to emphasize the need for attention, thereby establishing joint reference.

Joint action also evolves during the second half of infants' first year, having been demonstrated by caregivers during the perlocutionary stage. In a manner similar to joint reference, the caregiver takes the lead initially. In the first 6 months, the early routines, games, and dialogues are initiated by caregivers. However, these activities are so structured and predictable (hence, the name *routine*) that infants are soon able to anticipate their beginning. At the appropriate times and in the appropriate settings infants may exhibit at least a partial response related to the interaction expected in that context. Whether this is truly conscious anticipation or just a response evoked through association is difficult to determine. Nonetheless, their behavior indicates recognition of a routinized series of behaviors that is intertwined with a given context.

Taking the interaction a step further, infants gradually learn their particular contributions at each step in the sequence. In contrast to the time when infants were simply compliant partners, maturation of cognitive and motor abilities permits them to take the lead in instigating the activity. The ability to recognize a familiar situation, initiate the routinized behaviors associated with it, and perform them sequentially in response to each cue is certainly suggestive of goal-oriented behavior.

Protodeclaratives and Protoimperatives.   The earliest infant communicative behaviors that signal intentionality occur near the end of the first year. Bates (1976) characterized these early communicative signals as protoimperatives and protodeclaratives. **Protoimperatives** are infant gestures that seem to signal that caregivers should retrieve an object that is of interest. In effect, protoimperatives are requests, commands, or demands for *action,* just as the term *imperative* would imply. A characteristic gesture may signal caregivers to retrieve a favorite teddy bear or pillow at nap time.

In contrast, **protodeclaratives** are more "conversational" in nature, just as the term *declarative* would suggest. These gestures seem to signal that infants' primary goal is to attain their caregivers' *attention*—objects are only a tool in doing so. With attentive caregivers, pointing at the simplest things—a button, an earring, or a watch—evokes their attention and perhaps a narrative about that object.

Over the first year, infants accumulate a wealth of experience playing give-and-take (or "please-thank you") games with objects. Eventually infants begin to anticipate these interactions, perhaps cued by the presence of some object. As the behaviors related to objects become more consistent and recognizable, infants' gestures may become recognizable as preverbal communicative signals.

protoimperatives Early infant vocal and gestural behaviors that suggest commanding or requesting action on the part of the infant.

protodeclaratives Early infant vocal and gestural behaviors that appear to note an object for the purpose of gaining the caregiver's attention.

The usual form of these signals is a reaching gesture. The form may be more or less sophisticated. It may include an actual pointing of the index finger or just an open or grasping hand directed toward the object. Infants may initially assume their caregivers' interest and later demand it more directly by looking back and forth between the object and their caregiver. Infants may eventually come to vocalize in unison with their characteristic gestures.

 A cautious reminder is in order here. As with any analysis of internal states, it is frequently difficult to confirm our impressions. Does the infant's apparent satisfaction with obtaining the object confirm that the gesture was a protoimperative? Or could it simply mean that the infant was not up to throwing a tantrum and simply acquiesced? Mind reading is not a perfect science, even with the best-trained observers.

This is a useful context to remind ourselves of the distinction between signals and symbols. Signals (or signs) usually involve some physical resemblance to what they stand for. An open-handed grasp at the end of an outstretched arm portrays its meaning pretty directly. ◼

Phonetically Consistent Forms (Vocables).   The gestures used as protoimperatives and protodeclaratives may suffice to achieve infants' desired goals. However, for gestures to serve effectively, the intended audience—caregivers—must be watching. In many cases, caregivers are not; they are busily attending to other matters while their infants play contentedly. Given a long history of successfully attaining caregivers' attention through vocal behavior, it seems only logical that infants would add this element in these situations.

Whining, crying, and grunting may provide the occasional prompt needed to gain caregivers' attention. However, as an apparent outgrowth of babbling, infants have been observed to produce a certain type of characteristic vocalization in such circumstances. Once researchers recognized these vocalizations as an identifiable step in the developmental process, they were very intrigued by them.

Just prior to the occurrence of the first word, the number of longer sentence-like strings diminishes and units with more word-like structure become more frequent. Infants appear to recognize the connection between producing sounds to convey meaning. These vocalizations sound very much the same from occurrence to occurrence. They supplement the gestures that typically accompany them and seem to signal the same intention each time.

These vocalizations have been variously called *protowords, prelexical forms, sensorimotor morphemes,* and *vocables* (Haynes, 1994d). The term **phonetically consistent forms (PCF),** provided by Dore, Franklin, Miller, and Ramer (1976), seems to be the most commonly used, perhaps because it is the most descriptive. Phonetically consistent forms have several common features. First, they appear to be "units," in that they have distinguishable utterance boundaries. Second, they can be recognized as reoccurring utterances. Third, they are reliably associated with certain situations or circumstances. And, finally, although they are not recognizable as attempts at true words, their phonetic composition is relatively constant. For example, an infant may produce "mabeebee" (/mabibi/) with a distinctive intonation and gesture every time more food is being requested.

phonetically consistent form (PCF)   Infant sound productions that are stable in form and seemingly refer to certain objects, but do not resemble conventional words for them.

Phonetically consistent forms do not appear to be attempts at real words. Their resemblance is rarely close enough to a real word that would be relevant. They do not appear to be attempts at more sophisticated babbling. Infants' PCFs are more phonetically stable and shorter than the jargon strings they produce otherwise. Instead, PCFs seem to be *quasi-symbolic* for infants. They signal that infants have begun to associate the connection between their vocal-verbal responses and the effects that follow in changing the behavior of those around them. Further, although PCFs are not symbols in the conventional sense of words, the caregiver frequently responds to them as though they are, reinforcing the infant's attempt to move ever closer to conventional communication.

The Communication of Intentions

Several researchers have recognized that a critical transition occurs in the evolution of communication toward the end of the first year. Intentional communication has evolved from infants' countless experiences in influencing the behavior of others through crying, gazing, vocalizing, and gesturing. Although still limited to relying primarily on gestures that are only amplified by their accompanying vocalizations, infants recognize the communication value of their behavior. Furthermore, as their motor and cognitive abilities mature, communicating their intentions will occur with increasing frequency.

Several different classifications of intentions have been published. Two commonly discussed classifications include Dore's Primitive Speech Acts and Halliday's Communicative Functions.

Dore's Primitive Speech Acts.   Dore (1974) outlined a classification of intentions conveyed by infants. *Primitive speech acts* (PSAs) represent categories of infant intentions expressed through characteristic patterns of gestures and vocalizations. Early vocalizations consist of distinctive intonational patterns; later PSAs may include a recognizable word. Primitive speech acts appear to be predecessors of the intentions expressed in adult speech acts, but are likely to be accomplished in a primitive manner, that is, without the use of conventional words.

> These intentions also apply and are more easily illustrated in the single-word stage. Therefore, tables illustrating these classifications are found in Chapter 6. ■

The early intentions communicated through PSAs come as no surprise when considering infants' perspectives and interests. Early PSAs may consist of *calling* or *greeting* the caregiver, *requesting action* from the caregiver, *protesting an action* proposed or initiated by the caregiver, or simply *repeating* or *practicing* a response. At this level of development, PSAs express only one intention per utterance. Although their form is primitive, the range of PSAs is similar to those that will be expressed during the second year of life when the child begins to use words and phrases.

Primitive speech acts begin first as highly discriminated behaviors, their occurrence being closely associated with particular contexts. With further experience, they begin to change subtly in form and occur in more varied situations. Later,

> The classifications provided by various theories correlate more or less well to PSAs or communicative functions. In the absence of words, there are no clearly related grammatical or semantic categories. On the other hand, because their function is defined by their contexts and consequences, these would correlate well with several of Skinner's verbal operants. Consider the parallels between PSAs and *mands,* *tacts,* and *echoics.*

with further cognitive development and the mastery of conventional language forms, the child's range of intentions will expand and the ability to express them more effectively will improve.

Halliday's Communicative Functions.   Halliday (1975) followed the development of communication in his son, Nigel, from approximately 9 to

communicative

functions Halliday's classification of intentions exhibited by infants and toddlers.

24 months. Among other purposes, Halliday attempted to classify the **communicative functions,** or pragmatic uses of gestures and vocalizations that appeared as Nigel developed language. Being essentially analogous to primitive speech acts, communicative functions at this stage of development also consisted of gestures and vocalizations. Of central interest was the role that these communicative functions played as catalysts in Nigel's language development.

At 9 months of age, Halliday identified the first two functions in Nigel's behavior. The first of these, *interactional,* was essentially a "me and you" function in which the infant's behavior was directed toward establishing interactions with others. Of course, several behaviors quite early in the infant's development—crying, cooing, smiling—have this effect, but the conscious intent of engaging someone else's attention is probably absent. The second function classified by Halliday at this age was the *personal* function. In these behaviors, Nigel was expressing a sense of himself and his personal feelings such as pleasure, frustration, disgust, and so forth.

A month and a half later, Halliday recognized two more communicative functions in Nigel's behavior, the *instrumental* and *regulatory* functions. The instrumental function essentially consisted of obtaining objects through the help of those around him, as in gesturing and vocalizing to obtain an unreachable juice bottle. Caregivers' behaviors in this case are simply an instrument to serve their infants' needs. In contrast, caregivers' behaviors are the central concern of the regulatory function. Infants in this case attempt to regulate their caregivers' behaviors to achieve a particular interaction, such as the classic when infants reach and grunt, wanting to be carried.

At 10½ months, Nigel had demonstrated four separate purposes or communicative functions served by his behavior, which was still nonverbal and nonconventional. By the time he was 18 months, a total of six communicative functions had emerged. These serve a variety of intentions and by that time may be associated with certain key words or phrases.

Overview of the Illocutionary Stage

Intentionality, infants' recognition that they can influence others to do things for them, is the catalyst for communication development in the illocutionary stage. Infants' use of gestures and vocalizations to convey their intentions is an important functional development for communication. However, there is perhaps a broader implication in recognizing the emergence of the illocutionary stage in infancy. That infants develop the ability to signal their intentions prelinguistically underscores that communication begins before conventional language.

The illocutionary period culminates in behaviors that appear to serve as a transition into conventional language. As they approach their first birthday, infants begin to produce utterances, phonetically consistent forms, that approach the nature of true words. Finally, several classifications of pragmatic functions describe the purposes intended by infants through their gestures, vocalizations, and eventually, their early words and phrases.

Emerging Literacy

Some years ago, it may have seemed premature to discuss "language development" in a chapter about infants. After all, for a number of years the prevailing view held that language did not begin until the first word appears. Similarly, it may seem odd to some to discuss "literacy" in a chapter about infants because reading and writing develop much later than even the first word. However, just as we now recognize that many of the foundational building blocks for language development are laid down during the first year, it appears that the seeds of literacy are sown much earlier than we once thought.

Planting the Seeds of Literacy

The seeds of literacy are sown during the first year in ways that many would not even suspect. After all, most of us have generally associated "learning to read" with the formal instruction that begins with elementary school. Yet, upon careful observation, it becomes apparent that some infant-caregiver interactions provide the basis for later development of some of the most basic literacy skills (Kamhi & Catts, 2005).

Earlier in this chapter, it was noted that in language development research a significant amount of attention has focused on the social interaction of infants and caregivers. This socialization is now viewed as providing one of the basic elements in infants' motivation to communicate. Infants and caregivers engage in a variety of social transactions throughout their daily routines of dressing, feeding, and game playing. These transactions become the essence of their communication together. With regard to literacy, many caregivers engage in a similar process that has been called *literacy socialization* (Van Kleeck & Schuele, 1987). Van Kleeck and Schuele described three areas of literacy socialization: (1) literacy artifacts; (2) literacy events; and (3) the knowledge gained from literacy experiences.

Literacy artifacts. **Literacy artifacts** are items associated with print and text, such as nursery rhymes, story characters, alphabet designs, company logos, t-shirts and sweatshirts with slogans, and the ubiquitous team ballcap. These items are everywhere in society as it is. In addition, caregivers in most middle- and upper-class homes draw on literacy artifacts for decorating children's rooms (Kamhi & Catts, 2005). Wall hangings, crib sheets, mobiles, and books surround infants with story characters, letters, names, and pictures. Infants may or may not appreciate the decorative flair, but at least in many homes they are exposed to literacy artifacts through such items.

literacy artifacts Items that commonly display stimuli associated with literacy, such as books, newspapers, nursery rhyme characters, t-shirts with slogan, logo adorned ball caps, and so forth.

literacy events
Interactions or behaviors related to literacy, including storytelling, book reading, letter writing, and so forth.

Literacy Events.   The **literacy event** that is of central importance to infants is joint book reading. This is an especially important example of the joint actions that are described earlier in this chapter. The caregiver uses a book as the focus of attention to engage the infant in various interactions. This may begin as early as 5 or 6 months, often at the time infants begin to sit up and focus their attention. In the earliest interactions, infants may only respond with curiosity and delight with the special attention that seems to surround these books. With improving motor control, books and alphabet blocks and such become objects for exploration and manipulation. Infants may spend time examining the movement of a book's covers and pages or the different images on each side of an alphabet block.

Literacy Knowledge.   Initially, the caregiver may simply display the book and label the objects, events, and characters illustrated in the pictures while pointing to each one. With time, caregivers will ask for actual evidence of comprehension, prompting their infants to point to or "find" the pictures that should be familiar from previous "readings." At this stage, the **literacy knowledge** gained by infants—the understanding that print exists in various forms, that it accompanies pictures, and that caregivers use both to engage their attention—is basic but important for future developments nonetheless.

literacy knowledge
Familiarity with the various aspects of literacy, including print awareness, book orientation, typeface styles, genres and styles.

Summary

- The illocutionary stage in communication development is the result of infants' emerging intentionality.

- Intentionality occurs as we recognize that our goals can be achieved by influencing others' behavior.

- Caregivers provide opportunities for infants to exhibit intentional behavior by establishing joint reference and joint actions.

- Infants' earliest intentions have been distinguished as protodeclaratives, gestures that merely direct caregivers' attention, and protoimperatives, those that direct caregivers' actions.

- Early intentions are expressed through gestures, vocalizations, and phonetically consistent forms, as the infant approximates the production of true words.

- The functions or purposes of behaviors used to achieve early intentions have been classified as primitive speech acts and communicative functions.

- The beginnings of literacy are introduced through literacy artifacts and literacy events, which begin to establish the foundations of literacy knowledge.

During the first year of life, infants' developing cognitive, perceptual, and motor capabilities are coupled together. Driven by the momentum of these converging developments, the infant's ability to communicate evolves from reflexive to intentional to conventional.

The newborn's auditory system exhibits some remarkable capabilities for speech perception. Beyond recognizing important voices, newborns (and some other mammals) evidence *categorical perception,* the ability to hear slightly different speech sounds as samples of the same phoneme category. Infants' emerging potential for speech has been marked by developmental milestones as they progress from reflexive cries through cooing, babbling, vocal play, and jargon toward their first word during the first year. Perhaps the most intriguing phase in this process is babbling, which appears to be related to eventual speech as described in the *continuity hypothesis.*

Research has revealed that infant-caregiver communication passes through two periods during the first year. The *perlocutionary period* occurs during the first 6 months and is characterized by the caregiver interpreting infant behaviors, such as cries, *social smiles, eye gaze,* and vocal behaviors, as though they are communicative. Infants attend to caregivers' speech, called *baby talk,* and caregivers also contribute to the foundations for eventual communication through establishing *joint attention* and *turn taking.*

During the infants' second 6 months, the *illocutionary period,* the infant begins to exhibit behaviors that are more goal oriented and exhibit increasing intentionality. These behaviors begin as gestures, called *protoimperatives* and *protodeclaratives.* Later, infant vocalizations called *phonetically consistent forms* approximate conventional forms of communication and their intentions can be categorized through classifications such as *primitive speech acts* or *communicative functions.*

In addition to the confluence of perceptual, motor, cognitive, and social developments, caregivers plant the seeds of literacy through the display of *literacy artifacts,* sharing *literacy events,* and developing *literacy knowledge* with their infants.

Chapter Summary

1. In reviewing infants' motor, social, and cognitive developments, how do these correlate to the evolution of communication during the first year?

2. Describe the two methods used to research infants' speech perception capabilities.

Review Questions

3. What are the infant behaviors and their expected ages that make up the developmental milestones of speech?

4. Characterize the position and manner of production for the most prevalent sounds in infants' babbling.

5. How do the *discontinuity* and *continuity hypotheses* relate to the classic "nature versus nurture" controversy?

6. Name the three types of designs used to research infant communication. What are their advantages and limitations?

7. List and compare the nature of infant behaviors exhibited in the perlocutionary and illocutionary periods.

Practice Questions

To the student: You are encouraged to use the following questions to prepare for multiple-choice examinations. This exercise is not intended to simply "provide the answers to questions." Instead, it is hoped that you will use the material to develop your ability to analyze questions and choices to identify correct answers based on a critical understanding of the distinctions among the answers. Use the answer key at the end of the book to prompt your analysis of each item and to confirm the correct answer. Remember that there is a difference between recognizing the correct answer and understanding why it is the correct one.

1. Which of the following terms is/are related to the observation that infants increasingly sound like those around them?
   a. discontinuity hypothesis
   b. continuity hypothesis
   c. phonetic drift
   d. a and c
   e. b and c

2. In Mowrer's Autism Theory it is suggested that infants' babbling sounds increasingly like their parents' language is explained by which of the following behavioral mechanisms?
   a. the LAD
   b. stimulus generalization
   c. self-reinforcement
   d. punishment
   e. negative reinforcement

3. Which of the following would *not* be considered "prelinguistic"?
   a. cooing
   b. first words
   c. babbling
   d. jargon
   e. vocal play

4. A caregiver who frequently says phrases such as "excuse you," "hello," and "I'm so sorry that you don't like that" to a 3-month-old infant is illustrating which stage of communication based on the speech acts theory?
   a. the perlocutionary stage
   b. the illocutionary stage
   c. the phonological stage
   d. the locutionary stage
   e. the politeness stage

5. Conversations are to "turn taking" as gaze patterns are to _____ .
   a. deictic gaze
   b. blinking
   c. gaze coupling
   d. mutual gaze
   e. sleeping

6. When caregivers attempt to establish joint reference with their infant and an object of interest by using "deixis," they would _____ .
   a. shake the object of interest in the infant's field of vision
   b. say the name of the object with exaggerated inflection
   c. bring the object closer or carry the infant closer to the object
   d. point to the item from across the room
   e. describe the color of the item

7. Which statement is *not* true regarding phonetically consistent forms (PCFs)?
   a. PCFs appear to be actual attempts at real words
   b. PCFs are used in consistent contexts
   c. PCFs sound consistently similar
   d. PCFs appear to be a transition between prelinguistic behaviors and the first word
   e. PCFs may be to "words" what jargon appears to be to "sentences"

8. When the infant begins to use relatively conventional gestures (e.g., pointing, reaching) and/or vocalizations to achieve some "goal" or result, this signals the beginning of _____ .
   a. the illocutionary stage of communication
   b. the perlocutionary stage of communication
   c. the locutionary stage of communication
   d. all of the above
   e. none of the above

9. Which of the following infant vocal behaviors would be the latest form to develop?
   a. cooing
   b. jargon
   c. vocal play
   d. marginal babbling
   e. reflexive cries

10. Which of the following terms is not related to game playing between infants and caregivers?
    a. greeting
    b. pause
    c. joint action
    d. engagement
    e. all of these are relevant

Suggested Readings

Crown, C. L., Feldstein, S., Jasnow, M. D., Beebe, B., & Jaffe, J. (2002). The cross-modal coordination of interpersonal timing: Six-week-old infants' gaze with adults' vocal behavior. *Journal of Psycholinguistic Research, 31,* 1–23.

Johnson, J. R., & Wong, M. Y. (2002). Cultural differences in beliefs and practices concerning talk to children. *Journal of Speech, Language, and Hearing Research, 45,* 916–926.

Locke, J. L. (1993). *The child's path to spoken language.* Cambridge: Harvard University Press.

Meadows, D., Elias, G., & Bain, J. (2000). Mothers' ability to identify infants' communicative acts consistently. *Journal of Child Language, 27,* 393–406.

Rollins, P. R. (2003). Caregivers' contingent comments to 9-month-old infants: Relationships with later language. *Applied Psycholinguistics, 24,* 221–234.

6

Early Language Development— Toddlers

Almost all of them had gathered in the twilight for the event. The sky had not yet darkened entirely even though the sun had now disappeared. A straight dark edge cut the world into two seemingly perfect halves. Above the black edge, an orange glow blurred into a velvety blue and finally became a sky of deep purple. At the sky's glowing margin, the horizon's line was dark, sharp, and level.

Slowly, more people silently gathered for the event. Although unspoken, all who were there and even those who were not knew it was expected soon. Four seasons had passed since the little one's arrival. All those who had arrived previously had waited the same number of seasons before their rite of passage. The time had now come for this little one. They waited silently in their vigil throughout the night, their excitement barely suppressed in an occasional murmur.

Suddenly, someone stepped out through the now sunlit opening. Those who brought this little one to their midst stepped out together, upright and proud. Unable to disguise their delight, they waited but a moment before exclaiming, "The logos! It has come!" Their delight was contagious. The crowd immediately cheered and hugged and slapped one another on the back! As they retreated into the morning haze, they were secure in knowing that all was right and well with this little one as well.

This chapter addresses the following questions:

- How does the locutionary period emerge?
- How do children expand their ability to express their intentions to those around them?

- What characteristics are present in the first real words?
- How do children's word mistakes reflect their understanding of the world?
- What hypotheses have been proposed to explain how children learn the meanings of words?
- How does the child make the transition from producing single words to multiword utterances?
- How do children express relationships in the word orders they produce?
- What behaviors do toddlers and caregivers exhibit in their interactions to facilitate language learning?

With *lingua* placed firmly in cheek, the previous scenario depicts the almost sacred aura that has traditionally surrounded the event of the first *logos*—the first word. Parents, grandparents, aunts, uncles, and neighbors find such excitement in its appearance. As the first birthday approaches, they listen intently, hanging on every syllable that their child produces hoping that this will be the one.

Parental pride seems to stimulate much of the excitement surrounding children's first words. However, beyond those parental feelings, the first word's appearance also has significant implications for children's development. It is recognizable evidence that true language behavior and improved communication with the child are imminent. Therefore, the first word's appearance around the end of the first year has traditionally served as a major milestone.

This chapter examines the developments that occur throughout the second year of life. As toddlers, many rapid changes will take place. Toddlers increasingly convey their needs through gestural, vocal, and eventually, verbal means. This emerging power to influence others' behavior serves as the catalyst for the first word to appear. It is rapidly followed by a few more, and then by what seems to be an avalanche of new words. Finally, this period culminates in toddlers struggling to put these words together to convey the relationships they perceive.

Development in Related Domains

To no one's surprise, children normally continue a rapid rate of development in the second year of life. Developments in motor capacities, cognitive understanding, and social skills accompany and even propel children's language development. The developments in these areas are all interrelated. Changes in one frequently serve as the foundation or even the catalyst for developments in the others. Additionally, the changes are generally continuous in nature, overlapping and blurring together.

The following summary lists various highlights that characterize developments in each area throughout the second year (Lane & Molyneaux, 1992; Nicolosi, Harryman, & Kresheck, 2003; Owens, 2005; Shulman, 1994).

Motor Developments

Toddlers will take significant strides (no pun intended) in coordinating their fine and gross motor control. Exploring their world is expanded during the second year as toddlers:

- Take their first steps around 12 months.
- Use common objects appropriately around 13 months.
- Use smooth reach, pick up small objects with the thumb, and develop finger opposition around 14 months.
- Build a simple tower of three to four blocks around 15 months.
- Scribble lines on paper around 16 months.
- Walk and run unassisted around 17 months.
- Walk up stairs unassisted, walk down stairs with assistance around 18 months.
- Catch and throw a ball crudely around 19 months.
- Scribble in circles around 20 months.
- Jump in place, lifting both feet off the floor around 21 months.
- Climb, squat, and kick a ball around 22 months.
- Put shoes on part way around 23 months.
- Turn book pages two or three at a time around 24 months.

Cognitive Developments

The process of relating experiences to abilities continues through the second year of life. In doing so, toddlers organize their understanding of the world in more efficient patterns. These developments become apparent during the second year as toddlers:

- Use common objects appropriately around 12 months.
- Imitate new movements not in the repertoire around 13 months.
- Search in a location where an object was last seen around 14 months.
- Follow simple directions accompanied by gestures around 15 months.
- Imitate absent models and small movements around 16 months.
- Give a mechanical toy to another for rewinding around 17 months.
- Enjoy picture books and begin to recognize familiar pictures around 18 months.

The reader might refer back to the developments in these domains in infancy described in Chapter 5. Such a review might provide a better sense of the continuity in development. ▪

As in Chapter 5, the developmental ages indicated are approximations. ▪

- Remember the usual location of objects around 19 months.
- Imitate adult use of an object around 20 months.
- Show interest in colors and shapes around 21 months.
- Actively experiment with objects around 22 months.
- Sit alone and look at books for short intervals around 23 months.
- Use the same toy in several different actions by 24 months.

Social Developments

Toddlers experience expanding social contexts in which a language is learned and used. These new experiences expand their social interactions as during the second year toddlers:

- Express needs and wants through vocalization and gesture around 12 months.
- Express preference for people around 13 months.
- Express many different emotions, give hugs on request around 14 months.
- Repeat actions for approving audience around 15 months.
- Exhibit resistance to changes in expected routines around 16 months.
- Search for the adult when left alone around 17 months.
- Begin to "test" caregivers' intentions around 18 months.
- Increase cooperative play with other children around 19 months.
- Develop attachment to various toys around 20 months.
- Play near, but not with, other children around 21 months.
- Hug when requested and spontaneously on occasion around 22 months.
- Engage in "soliloquies" about experiences around 23 months.
- Role play in a limited manner around 24 months.

Language Expectations

During this second year, toddlers build on the foundation that was laid down in the first year. Where responses were once primarily reflexive, the toddler has developed control over intentional behaviors. Gestures complement the intentions indicated through vocalizations. The word-like vocalizations at the end of the first year become true words at the start of this year. Toddlers' vocabularies build slowly at first and then explode by the end of the second year, at which time they have begun combining words into phrases. The following overview is intended to provide a picture of the overall developments expected during this period.

- Toddlers will produce their first true word—that is, an approximation that is recognizable as an attempt at an adult word and is used consistently and meaningfully.

- Toddlers will combine early words with gestures to accomplish an increasing variety of goals—requesting objects and actions, labeling objects and actions, imitating, and so forth.

- Topics will expand as toddlers' experiences and vocabularies grow, but dialogue is limited to a few brief turns during each "conversation" with caregivers.

- Toddlers' growing vocabularies will be composed of words that signal basic semantic categories and relationships that encode objects, persons, events, and their locations.

- Toddlers will begin to produce utterances that are initially trial-and-error attempts at combining words and gradually become reliable word orders that represent syntax.

- Toddlers will increasingly use the language they have learned to obtain more information about the world from those around them.

- Toddlers will become increasingly aware of the connection between various symbols they are consistently exposed to—signs, logos, and familiar words—and the way caregivers read them.

Development in Pragmatics

During the eventful first year, the flow of motor and cognitive developments carried the infant's social interaction along. Ironically, during the perlocutionary stage, caregivers' tendency to view their infants' reflexive and physiological responses as communicative may have provided the most compelling force drawing their infants into communication. During the illocutionary stage, as the end of the first year approached, infants have become not only communicative, but capable of communicating intentions, albeit without words. With their first word, infants enter the locutionary stage.

The Locutionary Stage

Recall that, according to Austin (1962), the locutionary element of a speech act refers to the words and propositions uttered by the speaker. Bates (1976) defined the beginning of the locutionary stage of communicative development in children by the emergence of conventional words. Along with the advent of words, toddlers enter a period of rapidly expanding challenges. Motor abilities continue to mature, bringing children's first steps. In fact, those early uncertain steps represent the source of their name change from *infant* (one without speech) to *toddler* (one who walks unsteadily).

Recall that Austin's three components of a speech act were introduced in the chapter on language models, Chapter 4. Bates's adaptation of these to communication development was introduced in Chapter 5. ∎

Standing and walking reveals a whole new world to toddlers. So many items slightly higher than caregivers' knees (coffee tables, bookshelves, etc.) now invite toddlers' interest and reach. When curiosity leads their eyes where their hands cannot reach, communicating intentions becomes an urgent need.

Accumulating experience with objects and people has expanded toddlers' understanding of the world. Cognitively, toddlers have begun to understand *cause-effect;* that is, that their behavior influences caregivers' actions. Furthermore, they have come to appreciate *means-end* relationships. Because caregivers reliably interpreted their infants' behaviors and responded to their needs, infants became increasingly responsive to their nurturing caregivers as means to an end. Finally, compounding caregivers' predicament is toddlers' increasing understanding of *object permanence;* all those interesting items and places are recalled, even when they are out of sight. These developments make toddlers become busy people and their caregivers' exhaustion serves as ample proof!

Pragmatic developments that accompany the onset of the locutionary stage occur in at least two areas. Toddlers refine the ability to communicate their intentions to caregivers, specifically, expressing them with words. Also, the nature of dialogues between toddlers and their caregivers evolves further as toddlers become verbal.

Expressing Intentions

When considering the illocutionary period, infants were characterized as *communicating* their intentions through gesture and vocalization. In contrast, toddlers can be characterized as *expressing* their intentions verbally. Toddlers enter the locutionary stage through appearance of their first words. Toddlers' communication then includes conventional language behaviors for expressing intentions to affect the behavior of those around them.

Dore's Primitive Speech Acts

The reader will recall that PSAs and communicative functions, described later, emerged in the illocutionary period and are introduced in Chapter 5. ■

A *primitive speech act* (PSA) is a distinctive vocalization or word, often accompanied by a gesture, to communicate intentions (Dore, 1974). Note that although gestures may be present throughout, the definition acknowledges the shift from infants' vocalizations to toddlers' first words. This illustrates the continuity of development; unlike books and their chapters, human development does not have clear breaks as it progresses.

With the emergence of intentionality, infants and then toddlers find they can attain various everyday needs through others who respond to their vocal and verbal behaviors. Just as with infants, toddlers express individual intentions with each PSA. Interestingly, this is still the case with the appearance of words, although a given word may be used to express different intentions in different situations.

Primitive speech acts have the appeal of describing in everyday terms the nature of the intentions they serve. Primitive speech acts include those that direct others' actions such as *requesting action* and *protesting*. Other PSAs are named for those that direct other's attention such as *labeling, requesting answers,* and *calling*. Some appear to serve social functions, as in *greeting*. Finally, others appear to be related to learning, as in *practicing* or *repeating*. Table 6–1 provides definitions and examples of the primitive speech acts and communicative functions described in the following section.

At the end of the first year, PSAs include gestures and vocalizations. During the second year, PSAs increasingly include words. ▪

Halliday's Communicative Functions

Halliday (1975) described *communicative functions* in toddlers as vocal, gestural, and verbal behaviors that serve their purposes in communication. They closely parallel PSAs in several ways. Like PSAs, the communicative functions in toddlers develop continuously out of those that occurred as infants. Although the particular functions expressed remain similar, the rate of expressing their intentions begins to increase, especially as more words appear. (This is no surprise to caregivers!).

Halliday, too, recognized similar purposes served by his son's utterances even after the first words appeared. It is not surprising that the goals or intentions conveyed in Halliday's communicative functions overlap with those conveyed in PSAs. Especially at such basic levels of functioning, children will tend to exhibit similar needs and interests. Halliday's different labels for these behaviors does not change their inherent nature.

Recall from Chapter 5 that Halliday's data came from observing his son Nigel. ▪

The six earliest communicative functions noted by Halliday occurred between 10 and 18 months. Three more functions appeared at approximately 24 months. Those that appeared to be used primarily to influence the behavior of others included the instrumental and regulatory functions. The *instrumental* function is demonstrated when toddlers attempt to satisfy their material needs (e.g., obtaining toys, objects, food). The *regulatory* function is exhibited in attempts to control caregivers' behaviors in ways that directly affect their toddlers (e.g., getting caregivers to play "horsie" or lift their toddler up).

The interactional and personal functions appeared to serve more social purposes. The *interactional* function might be apparent in toddlers' attempts to gain caregivers' attention (e.g., using greetings, calling to caregivers from their crib). The *personal* function would be illustrated in exhibitions of feelings or emotions about persons or events (e.g., rejecting a stranger's approach, expressing dislike for the lunch being served).

The *heuristic* function appeared to be intended toward directing the attention of others to obtain information about a shared reference. An example might include an object held out accompanied by *Wassit?* essentially asking *What is it?* The imaginative function appeared to provide a means of playing and perhaps learning through the child's own utterances. Narrating the same positioning of several favorite stuffed animals with *Sit!* may be part of discovering the generality of actions.

Table 6–1. Examples and definitions of Dore's Primitive Speech Acts and Halliday's Communicative Functions.

Examples of Behaviors	Primitive Speech Act	PSAs Defined	Communicative Function	Communicative Functions Defined
Shouts *Dada* from crib	Calling	Gaining another's attention	Interactional	Establishing interaction with others
Says *Dada* as he enters room	Greeting	Addressing persons when they appear	(Interactional)	Expressing personal feelings or attitudes
Asserts *No!* to unwanted food	Protesting	Expressing dislike or rejection of items or actions	Personal	Inquiring about or exploring environment
Points to dog and asks, *Doggy?*	Requesting answer	Asking for information with words, gestures, intonation	Heuristic	Attempting to control others' actions
Raises arms and says, *Up, up, up!*	Requesting action	Asking for others' actions	Regulatory	Attempting to obtain objects through others
Points and says, *Cookie, peez*	(Requesting action)		Instrumental	Demonstrating knowledge of world with others
Points, says *Here!* when asked "Where's your nose?"	Answering	Responding to others' questions	Informative	Using words to invent a play world
Touches nose and says *Nose!*	Labeling	Naming an object or event	(Informative)	
Says *Go!* while pushing toy car				
Echoes mother's exclamation of *Oh, no!*	Repeating	Reproducing an utterance in part or entirely	Imaginative	
Says *No, no, no!* while alone in crib	Practicing	Produces words or prosodic pattern with no apparent audience		

Note. Compiled from "Holophrases, Speech Acts, and Language Universals," by J. Dore, 1975, *Journal of Child Language;* and *Learning How to Mean: Explorations in the Development of Language,* by M. A. K. Halliday, 1975, New York: Arnold.

The purposes served by one-word utterances continued in two-word utterances as these developed during the second half of the second year. In addition, three new functions emerged around 24 months of age. The seventh communicative function, the *pragmatic* function, appeared to emerge out of a combination of the existing *instrumental, regulatory,* and *interactional* functions. The pragmatic function occurs in language used to act on the environment. In exhibiting the pragmatic function, toddlers might make requests to satisfy their needs and attempt to interact with and control others' behavior.

The eighth function, the *mathetic* function, is primarily involved in learning about one's environment. In exploring the environment through their language, toddlers question others, state their understanding, recall experiences of the recent past, or even guess future events.

The ninth communicative function noted by Halliday was the *informative* function, in which toddlers convey information about objects and events to their audience. This function may represent the essence of social verbal behavior. In these utterances, toddlers are being informative, but appear to be disinterested; that is, there is no specific motive such as obtaining objects or establishing interaction with others. The difference is that toddlers now use a *verbal* topic to engage a listener instead of resorting to obtaining objects or requesting actions.

Compare the nature of the *informative function* to Skinner's verbal operant tacting, described in Chapter 4. ∎

Toddlers' Intentions: A Caution

It has been thought that through their intonation, toddlers *might* signal their intentions, such as *labeling* (with a falling contour), *requesting* (with a rising contour), or *calling* (with an abrupt rise and fall). Although this possibility is intriguing, it should be noted that this ability has not been widely reported or verified (Bloom & Lahey, 1978).

In a related concern, some caution must be used in interpreting data regarding the relative occurrence of individual PSAs or communicative intentions. In conveying their intentions, toddlers may produce what appear to be meaningful prosodic patterns or accompanying gestures. In spite of any distinctive intonational patterns in toddlers' utterances, with only single words (or vocalizations) to interpret, caregivers must rely heavily on the situational context to determine their toddlers' intentions. For example, a cookie jar in the general direction of their toddlers' pointing finger may be the basis of caregivers' interpretations. In turn, while analyzing these interactions, researchers must rely on caregivers' interpretations, which may or may not actually reflect the toddler's intentions. When misinterpreted, toddlers might protest, but they frequently accommodate them as well.

It has been suggested that intonation might be an early form of Skinner's autoclitic behavior—a secondary aspect of verbal production that "comments" on relationships among the primary verbal behaviors (Segal, 1975).

▨ Summary

- The *locutionary stage* emerges with the first true words.
- Toddlers express **intentions** in the locutionary stage using vocalizations, gestures, and words.

intention   The effects speakers expect to follow their utterances.

- Most often, a single function is intended with each utterance.
- It appears that the earliest functions (obtaining objects, gaining attentions, etc.) are expressed by toddlers in most cultures.
- The same intentions are expressed in later two-word utterances.
- Interpreting intentions expressed by toddlers is subjective, as their reactions to caregiver responses may not reflect their true intention.

Developing Dialogue

As toddlers approach the task of conversing, several abilities have begun to develop, including gaining and directing attention, indicating understanding or lack of understanding. With toddlers' first words, conversations in the conventional sense can begin to take place (although many amused and bewildered caregivers have wondered what some conversations were actually about). During this second year, three areas develop further in toddlers' conversations: topic initiation, presupposition, and turn taking.

Topic Initiation

topic initiation
Introducing a topic in discourse.

Topic initiation is the act of establishing a subject for a conversation that a speaker is about to begin. In initiating conversations, mature speakers might utter any of various phrases to first obtain their partners' attention, such as *Oh, by the way* . . . or *You know what* . . . and so on. Next, they typically introduce subjects familiar to both participants, followed by related, but novel information about that subject. (Conversations that only revisit old information are less useful, even boring.) Finally, their partner acknowledges the information and perhaps expands on it.

Halliday (1967) referred to the distinction between familiar and novel information in conversations as the *given-new* distinction. That the topic is *given* means both participants should start out being familiar with it. In contrast, additional information about that topic provided by a speaker should be previously unknown or *new* to the listener.

As such, starting up a conversation might go as follows: *Remember the car salesman we talked to?* (given). *Well, he called me at work today and offered a better deal* (new). The listener may request a clarification (*Which salesman?*), acknowledge and extend the topic (*I thought he would. How much better?*), or indicate that the information is not new (*I know, Billy already mentioned that*).

Initially, toddlers bring to the task of conversing the abilities they developed as infants to establish a shared topic (joint reference) through gaze, gestures, and vocalization. These early forms of establishing reference restricted topics to those that are present. It has been suggested that early words are produced more as accompaniments to gestures than to carry information (Greenfield & Smith, 1976). Later, words increase not only toddlers' ability to establish joint reference more precisely, but also provide the *potential* to eventually introduce topics that are absent.

Although toddlers are by nature most likely to respond to stimuli that are present, novelty is already important in determining the next topic. Conversations with toddlers typically arise out of a stimulus that has just engaged their attention. A stimulus may have been present all along, but when it becomes salient or conspicuous to a toddler, it may prompt conversation, as when a toddler suddenly notices a favorite teddy bear, points and says, *"Teddy!"* The toddler's sudden awareness of its presence is all the novelty needed. Just as the same word may serve different intentions, different intentions may serve equally well to initiate topics of conversation. Whether the toddler's utterance of *"Teddy!"* turns out to be an instance of requesting or labeling, dialogue with interested caregivers frequently follows.

Presupposition

Presupposition refers to speakers' ability to judge how much their listeners might know about the subject being introduced and to adapt their utterances accordingly. Without context, the utterance *I had one exactly like it!* may be quite puzzling, perhaps prompting a listener to request more information (*What are you talking about?*). However, if uttered while both friends admire a classic car together, the immediate context provides all the information needed.

presupposition
Speakers' ability to adjust their message based on their listeners' abilities and knowledge of the topic.

Presupposition becomes more critical when the subject is not apparent to both partners. If the referent is absent, perceptive speakers sense the listener's needs and provide required background information. Less perceptive speakers may leave their listener confused and perhaps frustrated. With a greater variety of contexts remote in time or space, there is greater need for presupposition.

Fortunately, early conversations between toddlers and their caregivers are generally tied to the "here-and-now," usually centering around objects or actions that are central to their current interaction. As a result, conversations between caregivers and toddlers require less consideration of presupposition.

Younger toddlers without many words are frequently limited to establishing the topic by pointing to it, holding it out, or gesturing the desired action. With the first words, toddlers may still simultaneously gesture to direct caregivers' attention as the infant names an object. As the number of productive words increases, toddlers rely less on gestures to establish a topic. Instead, gestures may simply supplement the message intended by the toddler's words by demonstrating an associated action (Masur, 1983). For example, toddlers might cross their arms in a characteristic "cradle" while asking for their doll because they typically play with it in this manner.

As more words appear, and especially when toddlers begin to produce them without the presence of the primary stimulus, the burden of interpretation shifts. Most caregivers have experienced the frustration of not understanding the meaning of toddlers' utterances. Consequently, although caregivers may not be conscious of it, toddlers' ability to express additional information leads to more efficient and rewarding interactions.

Toddlers, too, suffer their own frustration when not understood. Gradually, as toddlers are able to convey more information about the context of their utterance, caregivers more quickly understand their intent. Early attempts may require toddlers to take their caregivers' hand and lead them to the relevant context. Later, with more words emerging, toddlers begin to more completely establish the contexts of their utterances verbally.

Turn Taking

Turn taking is a conversational skill in which speakers and listeners appropriately switch their roles. In adult conversations, polite partners wait for a signal that the other's turn is finished. Intonation, gestures, facial expression, and so on might provide the necessary signal that a speaker's turn has ended.

The number of turns taken on a given topic in a conversation can vary substantially. Each turn should contribute something new to extend the conversation. Several variables are at work, but a primary factor would be the amount of information partners have to share. Two individuals who are knowledgeable on a topic can converse for hours, each taking numerous turns.

Caregivers have provided children with cues for turn taking from the outset. Recall that while nursing, caregivers responded to their infants' pauses to prompt bursts of sucking. In talking to and playing with infants, caregivers consistently paused at strategic times, suggesting their expectation that their infants would fill their turn. Although caregivers eventually become less accommodating, they continue to generously provide their toddlers with appropriate and expectant pauses, anticipating and guiding their turn taking even in these early limited verbal exchanges.

The nature of turns taken by toddlers (e.g., evocative utterances) and caregivers (e.g., expansions) also contribute to the learning process. These aspects are discussed later in this chapter. ∎

For toddlers and caregivers, most conversations are abbreviated with few turns, primarily as the result of toddlers' limited experiences and information. For example, a toddler who requests objects with a reach and vocalization, might respond to the caregiver's inquiries (*What do you need?*) with a label (*Bear!*) to clarify the request. Upon receiving the object, the toddler might name it again in confirmation (*Bear!*) or announce some associated action (*Hug!*). In turn, the caregiver might echo and affirm the toddler's utterance or add a summary comment (*You like to hug your bear, don't you?*). As the toddler learns more words to label additional associated features (*Eyes!*), the length of such conversations can be extended (*Yes, your bear has big eyes*). However, even at the end of the second year, toddlers' turns will be few, conversations brief, and topics fleeting!

Summary

- In topic initiation, toddlers extend earlier behaviors used to establish joint reference by adding words.

- Novelty is an important characteristic that prompts toddlers to initiate a topic.

- Presupposition, understanding our listener's needs, is challenged as toddlers' boundaries and recall expand.

- As toddlers' recall of information and vocabularies expand, the number of conversational turns taken increases.

The First Words

Because this chapter is about toddlers, focus is on the transition from prelinguistic to linguistic behavior, which also signals the onset of the locutionary period. This transition is most clearly evidenced by the first word.

Many experts view the first word as the product of the pragmatic developments during infant communication. The first word is not merely the first step along the way to language. Instead, the first word is recognized as the natural outgrowth of communication established through the gestural and vocal precursors that evolved throughout the preceding year.

Infants' capacity to direct others' attention to objects of interest progressed through several abilities. Infants were first able to use head control and eye gaze to indicate an object of interest (visual reference). Later, reaching refined itself to include pointing and became an available means of directing attention (gestural reference).

In response to toddlers' reaching and pointing, caregivers frequently offered the objects of interest and labeled them. This perhaps provided the model for infants' next behavior, combining a gesture and a vocalization to obtain objects and attention (vocal reference).

Finally, the distinctive vocalizations that so often accompany gestures become conventional forms—the first words. Toddlers' attempts at using conventional words is of huge significance. There is strong evidence that they are responding to the connection between speech and the objects, events, and relations in their environment.

It is important to appreciate the distinctions among words, referents, and meanings before examining this important next step. It may be convenient to think that words have prescribed, assigned meanings. We have become accustomed to finding the meaning for a word in the dictionary. Dictionaries define words through other equivalent terms and concepts. However, a conceptual definition only represents that verbal community's commonly held associations for each word.

If the meaning of a word is based on our experiences, then we might reexamine Shakespeare's response to his own rhetorical question. He may have been only partially correct in writing "What is in a word? A rose by any other name is still as sweet." Those who have had considerable experience pruning or arranging roses, might add that, by any other name, they are just as thorny!

Meaning is not carried in the word. Neither does the referent contain the meaning. For each speaker, meaning, in its most fundamental sense, lies in the *relationship* between a word, the circumstances in which it has been experienced, and the effects it has had on listeners (Wood, 1986). As the young child accumulates experience with white coats, fever, illness, and hypodermic needles, the word *doctor* will be associated with meanings far removed from the dictionary definition.

Characteristics of First Words

With all the importance placed on toddlers' first words, researchers have examined their occurrence from various perspectives. Of interest has been the criteria that might be used to determine the typical or expected age of the first word. In addition, researchers have analyzed the phonetic characteristics of first words.

When Is It "The First Word"?

Traditionally, it is held that the first word occurs around the first birthday. However, we must emphasize *around* in this rule of thumb. The first word might appear as early as 8 months or as late as 16 months without necessarily signaling a serious concern.

Determining the average age of the first word proved to be a difficult process. Because researchers are unlikely to be present when the event occurs, they must rely on the recall of caregivers. Although understandably, anxious and proud caregivers may be unreliable observers. Caregivers often mistake early babbling as words, especially forms such as *mama* or *dada*. These may certainly be true words at some point, but probably not at 5 or 6 months of age.

To qualify as the *true* first word at least two criteria must be satisfied (Darley & Winitz, 1961). First, the utterance should occur with consistency in a given context in apparent response to an identifiable stimulus; that is, it should be produced consistently in the presence of the same person, object, or event. Whereas the infant's earlier productions of *mama* or *dada* were certainly exciting events, if they were isolated or random productions that did not necessarily occur in the caregiver's presence, they were not true words.

Second, the utterance must bear some phonetic resemblance to a conventional adult word; in other words, it should be a recognizable attempt at a real word that may be only an approximation.

What Do First Words Sound Like?

Although the actual first words attempted will vary from toddler to toddler, they appear to share certain phonetic characteristics (Ferguson & Farwell, 1975; Ingram, 1976). Most often the first word will consist of attempts at single words but might occasionally be approximations of common phrases (*allgone*) or social expressions (*bye-bye*).

Phonetically, the early attempts at producing words consist primarily of a subset of the sounds produced in the child's later babbling repertoire. For the most part, front consonants (/p, b, d, t, m, n/) are most common. These are combined in simplified syllable patterns, such as CV, VC, and CVCV. The CVCV utterances are typically reduplicated syllables in which the CV unit is repeated, such as *bye-bye, mama, dada.* (Finally, mom and dad can celebrate!) And, as toddlers successfully produce their earliest words using these syllable patterns (CV, VC, or CVCV), subsequent words added to their vocabulary tend to follow similar structure.

 It is interesting to note that cross-cultural studies have examined the phonetic nature of the equivalent terms for *mother* and *father* in other languages. It has been found that about 80% of the words for *mother* contain nasal-labial and dental sounds (as in mama and mother), whereas 80% of those for *father* contain nonnasal-labial and dental sounds. It has been suggested that infants' ability to produce nasal and labial sounds while nursing may explain the association of these sounds with the mother (Lane & Molyneaux, 1992).

Summary

- First words may evolve out of vocalizations that accompany gesturing or pointing to obtain objects.

- Transition utterances (vocables, PCFs, etc.) precede infants' first true words.

- First words generally appear around the first birthday.

- To qualify as true words, utterances must consistently refer to the same stimuli and be recognizable as attempts at conventional words.

- The phonetic composition of early words tends to be drawn from sounds in infants' later babbling.

The First Lexicon

The term *lexicon* (or *vocabulary*) can refer generally to the total words belonging to a particular language. It might also indicate the total words an individual knows. Determining the size of an individual adult's vocabulary certainly would be difficult as most adults probably know thousands of words. In addition, the task is even more elusive because it may appear that the individual does not know a word until it occurs in a certain context.

Please be reminded that lexicon and vocabulary are distinguished in Chapter 1. However, because toddlers use only single words without inflectional or derivational morphemes, either term would apply equally. ■

It would seem that the task of inventorying toddlers' smaller vocabularies might be easier. However, determining that an utterance actually qualifies as a word for a particular toddler is no less difficult.

What Is "Knowing" a Word?

Some difficulty in identifying the first words may stem from difficulty in determining what it means to "know" a word (Bloom & Lahey, 1978). Children's responses might give the impression that they know a word in the adult sense. For example, toddlers can echo a word, reproducing it acoustically, but they may do so without understanding the word or intending anything meaningful. Similarly, children might respond appropriately to words spoken in a certain context, giving the appearance of understanding them. For example, following bath time a caregiver might say, *Can you take your towel to the washer?* If the toddler does so, does that mean that the toddler understood each of the individual words? Or has the toddler simply learned from repeated experience where the caregiver puts the towel after bath time?

Beyond simply responding to and producing a word, Bloom and Lahey (1978) defined five levels at which children might "know" a word. The beginning level defined by Bloom and Lahey (1978) is knowing a word in its *referential sense.* In this level, a word simply refers to or stands for a particular object, event, or relationship. Initially, toddlers' production of *doggy refers* to the particular furry creature that lives at their house. Later, when toddlers produce *doggy* in response to similar creatures in the neighborhood, the word is known in the *extended sense.*

At another level, producing several words related by some meaningful context illustrates knowing words at a *relational level.* An example would be toddlers producing *dog* and *house,* or *dog* and *bark,* based on their pet's location or noisiness.

Eventually, in later developments, when the child responds to similarities among classes of stimuli, such as understanding that dogs are also *animals,* they demonstrate the *categorical level* of words. Finally, in achieving the *metalinguistic level,* children evaluate each word as a stimulus apart from its referent. This might be demonstrated when they note the number of syllables in a word or the fact that it rhymes with another word. Children who know that the word *caterpillar* is longer than the word *snake* are responding to them at the metalinguistic level.

Development through these levels is based on increasingly subtle relationships among stimuli and will develop only with appropriate experiences over several years. Closer to our present concerns, researchers have explored the meanings in toddlers' early lexicons.

Knowing words in categorical and metalinguistic ways develops more fully during the preschool and school-age years. These topics are discussed in Chapters 7 and 8. ■

How Fast Does the First Lexicon Grow?

An obvious fact is that toddlers' vocabularies normally grow. Traditionally, it has been suggested that following the first word at around 1 year of age, toddlers' expressive vocabularies will grow to approximately 50 words by 18 months of age. It is generally accepted that toddlers' receptive vocabulary (i.e., the number of words understood) grows faster than their expressive vocabulary (i.e., the number of words produced). The overall growth rate will vary across individual toddlers, and may even vary for a given toddler, with bursts and plateaus in learning new words within this time period.

The differences in rates of growth across toddlers may relate to various factors such as differences in experiences and exposure to language. Differences due to socioeconomic factors, caregiving styles, or health-related concerns (e.g., middle ear infections) have been historically assumed to play a role in a broad way. However, we must be cautious about attributing slower development in an individual toddler to any one of these factors.

An individual toddler's vocabulary may grow in spurts, then level off briefly, only to expand rapidly again. New words tend to be related to objects, events, and relationships that are already familiar. The toddler may be exposed to words incidentally as part of ongoing interactions with others or specific words may be singled out and directly taught by the toddler's partners. Furthermore, it has been noted that some words may emerge and subsequently disappear, at least temporarily, during this period. For example, a toddler's infatuation with airplanes might prompt learning related words (*fly, up, wing,* etc.). These words might all occur frequently for a period of time and then diminish as the toddler becomes intrigued with another toy.

Classes and Meanings of the First Words

Individual words can be analyzed according to several perspectives. As discussed previously, a word might be classified according to the pragmatic functions it might serve in different contexts. Analysis of toddlers' utterances according to the situations in which they occur also has led several researchers to distinguish several broad grammatical and semantic classifications among them.

Toddlers begin combining words when their vocabulary consists of approximately 50 words (Nelson, 1973b). As a result, researchers have been particularly interested in the proportions of different word classifications represented in the first 50 words.

Classes of First Words. Toddlers may utter "favorite" words more frequently and these can certainly be different among toddlers. Nonetheless researchers have found that, as a grammatical class, nouns appear to be the most prevalent words in toddlers' early lexicons. During this period of single-word utterances, nouns may constitute 50% or more of a toddler's vocabulary (Nelson, 1973b). Most instances are nouns for certain objects—persons, animals, toys, food items, and so on—that have frequently been involved in toddlers' interactions with others. Table 6–2 presents a classification of the first 50 words.

Table 6–2. Distribution of toddlers' first words in grammatical classes.

Grammatical Class	Description	Examples	Percentage
Nominal-Specific	Refer to specific, unique members of a category	*Mommy, Daddy, Nanna, Fido,* etc.	14
Nominal-General	Refer to items that represent general examples of a category	*spoon, cup, doggy, ball, book,* etc.	51
Action words	Refer to a requested, ongoing, or just completed action	*Go, Ride, Up, Play,* etc.	13
Modifiers	Describe the features or qualities of objects or events	*Big, Dirty, Yukky, Mine,* etc.	9
Personal-Social	Express feelings and indicate social relationships	*No!, Hi!, Bye-bye, Please,* etc.	8
Functional	Fulfill grammatical functions	*what, where, for,* etc.	4

Note. Adapted from "Structure and Strategy in Learning to Talk," by K. Nelson, 1973, *Monographs of the Society for Research in Child Development, 38.*

These early nouns are generally common nouns (*doggie*), in contrast to proper nouns (*Bowser*) or broad categorical names (*animal*). Although toddlers initially produce common nouns, these are typically based on narrow and isolated experiences. As a result it is reasonable to assume that toddlers are initially producing these nouns in response to the unique, individual item (the family pet) as opposed to an entire class (all canines).

Similarly, another smaller group of more specific proper nouns are generally present as well. These forms (e.g., *mama, dada, sissy, bubba*) continue to occur in response to specific persons for some time. Although the more common form is used, toddlers apparently produce them as proper names. In this sense, toddlers are indicating that their caregivers' *names* are *mama* and *dada,* as opposed to indicating that they have produced offspring.

 In reality, from the child's perspective it may be valid to view all the first words as "proper nouns," because they initially tend to occur in response to a particular item. Later, when those nouns that have the potential to generalize in response to numerous items do so, they become true common nouns.

The remaining words consist of several word classes of smaller proportions. Action words or verbs tend to name actions that are more general. That is, the actions named occur more frequently because they can relate to many different objects (*put, do, make*) in contrast to actions that are inherently related to specific objects (*eat, read, paint*). Other less frequent forms include modifiers that are related to the properties of objects (*hot, big, dirty*), personal-social words (*hi, bye-bye, no*) and functional words (*this, that*).

Researchers have speculated on the reasons that nouns would be prevalent in toddlers' early lexicons. Some have suggested that this is because early nouns refer to objects, which are more tangible and perceptually stable than actions. Objects can be experienced through several senses and they continue to exist, even if their location changes. In contrast, actions are intangible and transient; the opportunity to experience them generally occurs within the span of a moment. In addition, nouns name objects that are often the focus of toddlers' interactions; in most settings, numerous objects are present to experience, but most toddlers name items such as cups, spoons, and dogs, rather than walls, cabinets, dressers, and desks.

Other proposed explanations for the nouns' prominence point to their linguistic nature (Goldfield, 1993). Nouns tend to be the final, conspicuous word in sentences. In addition, nouns are perceptually more stable; that is, their forms are changed only minimally by perceptually subtle plural or possessive inflections (*-s, -z,* or *-ɪz*). However, these observations pertain mostly to English; other languages exhibit different word orders and apply a greater variety of morphological adaptations to nouns.

Finally, some have theorized that the prevalence of nouns might stem from their relative frequency. Although nouns occur less often in adult speech generally, they are more frequent when caregivers talk to their toddlers (Goldfield, 1993). The relative frequency of nouns and verbs in caregivers' speech to toddlers is influenced by the context. Nouns occur more often when toddlers are currently attending to an object; they occur less frequently in social interactions not involving objects. Also, nouns decrease in caregivers' speech as their toddlers' vocabularies approach the 50-word level (Goldfield, 1993). In contrast, verbs are most often modeled by caregivers prior to the impending action (Tomasello & Kruger, 1992).

Although caregivers may not consciously set out to teach specific words, they do make a number of significant modifications in how they talk to their children. The combination of caregivers' simplified, redundant speech to toddlers about perceptually stable objects that are functionally integrated into their interaction may account for the prominence of nouns in toddlers' first lexicons. Recent analyses of toddlers' attempts and caregivers' corrective feedback in language learning indicates far more "teaching" on the part of caregivers than had been acknowledged previously (Moerk, 1991).

 It must be noted that, although nouns are prevalent among the first words in most cultures, not all cultures exhibit these characteristics in their language or caregiver-child interactions.

Meanings of First Words. Researchers have distinguished several broad classifications related to the meanings of toddlers' early words. These broad categories are generally based on the extent to which words relate to objects themselves as opposed to the relationships between entities—objects, persons, and events.

Within the first 50 words Nelson (1973b) classified into grammatical categories, discussed previously, she also distinguished two broad classes of meaning in toddlers' first words. According to caregivers' reports, toddlers'

referential words   Early
words whose primary
purpose is to refer to
objects.

referential words   Early
words whose primary
purpose is to refer to
objects.

expressive words   Early
words whose apparent
purpose is to engage
others in social
exchanges.

Here again, toddlers'
maturing motor
abilities, developing
understanding, and
expanding social
interaction expose them to
a broadening array of
experiences. ■

Similar features or
functions may be
shared across objects.
However, some might say
that our similar responses
to them, due to stimulus
generalization, is what
defines them as a class. ■

substantive words
Classification of early
words that occur in
response to objects and
classes of objects.

As the child's
experiences and
understanding expand so
do the semantic relations
expressed. These
relationships will continue
to be expressed later, only
more precisely through
multiword utterances
described later in this
chapter and in subsequent
chapters. ■

meanings were broadly distinguished as either referential or expressive. **Referential words** were comprised of common nouns that primarily referred to objects; hence, the name of this class. In these instances, toddlers' words merely pointed out objects of interest with no further significance. The remaining words were classified as **expressive words** because of their personal-social significance. According to caregivers' descriptions, these words appeared to have more social significance, expressing more than just the name of an object.

Nelson also observed that the children themselves could be similarly classified according to their tendencies. Referential toddlers' nouns primarily indicated attention to an object. In contrast, expressive toddlers more frequently produced nouns as part of their social interactions.

Nelson's results must be qualified somewhat. The data collection relied solely on parental reports and children's actual productions were not observed. As a result, neither the frequency of individual words nor the reported significance of words used in a given context could be reliably verified (Bloom & Lahey, 1978). Perhaps words such as *Hi, Bye-bye,* and *Please* would appear in most interactions to be clearly expressive and social in nature. However, toddlers pointing to their chair, saying *Sit!,* could be naming the object by its function, requesting lunch, or simply making a bid for a conversational exchange. The nature of an utterance can only be inferred from analyzing the contexts and whether the effects satisfy the toddler in that instance.

Another distinction in the meanings of early words was noted by Bloom (1973). As was noted previously, toddlers' first words tend to occur in response to the original items experienced. At some point, however, toddlers confront new stimuli similar to originals in any of several ways— chairs shaped differently, cups in new colors, bigger or smaller dogs. When a word is prompted by new, similar items, toddlers' words are no longer tied to the original object. Instead toddlers are responding to the features and functions shared by other items, those aspects that define the substance of an object class.

In documenting her daughter's language development, Bloom (1973) took note of two broad word classes in her single-word vocabulary. Those vocabulary items referring to object classes were termed **substantive words** by Bloom. These words might include those produced for entities that are actually the only member of a class. For example, each toddler's *Mommy* is a unique, individual member of a class of one. (Most of us would agree that our mom is in a class by herself!) Children will eventually recognize that there are other mommies, but there will always be just one that they call *Mommy* (or *Mom,* or *Ma,* or . . .). Substantive words also name particular members of larger classes, such as a doggy, a blanket, a cup, or a toy. Again, these words start out naming original objects and soon generalize to other similar items. Eventually, experiencing a sufficient number of items that share features defines an object concept (Bloom, 1973).

The other broad class of words Bloom distinguished was **relational words.** These refer to several abstract relations objects might share with themselves or with other objects. **Reflexive relations** (Bloom, 1973; Brown, 1973) represent a major group of early words that indicate the state of objects—their own existence, nonexistence, disappearance, or recurrence. Also termed the basic operations of reference, they convey how the present circumstances "reflect" an object's status. For example, **existence** is expressed in words (e.g., *this, that,* or *wassat?*) that relate an object to itself, indicating that it exists. Toddlers might simply hold out a new toy and say *dis! (This)*, to acknowledge its existence. Table 6–3 presents these early reflexive relations.

Some words express **nonexistence,** that an object is not present where it was anticipated to be. Finding that Dad is not reading the morning paper in his favorite chair, the toddler might say *dada* in response to his unexpected absence. The reflexive relation **disappearance** indicates situations where an object that was present disappears, as when a child's ball unexpectedly rolls under the sofa. Uttering *Ball!* comments on its disappearance. The final reflexive relation, **recurrence,** indicates the reoccurrence of items or actions like a preceding one. Most toddlers express this relation at snack time. When the last cookie has been eaten, caregivers can expect to hear the proverbial *More!*

The remaining relational words express relationships that occur *among* objects. The first of these is **action relational words.** Beyond responding to objects of interest, increasingly active toddlers are also inclined to talk about actions associated with these objects. Hence, they announce *Throw!* as they send a ball across the room. In a related way, toddlers become more responsive to where things are—especially when they want them. This is expressed

relational words Words that refer to abstract relationships between objects.

reflexive relations Ways in which objects relate to themselves, including existence, nonexistence, disappearance, and recurrence.

existence Early reflexive relation in which a word denotes that an object is present.

nonexistence Early reflexive relation in which a word indicates an object is not present where it would be expected.

disappearance Early reflexive relation in which children's words indicates that an object has left their immediate experience.

recurrence An early reflexive relation in which a word indicates that an object or its duplicate has reappeared.

Table 6–3. Early reflexive relations expressed in one-word utterances.

Relation	Description	Typical examples
Existence	Child indicates awareness that an object exists.	Says *This, That,* or *Here,* while pointing to, touching, or holding out an object of interest.
Nonexistence	Child indicates that an object does not exist in a setting where it has come to be expected.	Says *Allgone* or *Bear* when placed in crib from which a favorite teddy bear is absent.
Disappearance	Child indicates that an object has been present is currently absent.	Says *Allgone* or *Ball* after watching a tossed ball roll under the sofa.
Recurrence	Child indicates either that an object that had disappeared has since reappeared or that another identical object has appeared.	Says *More, Again,* or *'Nuther* when a fallen cookie is retrieved or replaced with another cookie.

Note: Adapted from *Language Development and Language Disorders,* by L. Bloom and M. Lahey, 1978, New York: John Wiley & Sons.

action relational words
Early relational words that refer to actions associated with an object of interest.

location relational words
Early relational words that refer to the location of items of interest.

attribution relational words   Early relational words that refer to the attributes or characteristics of objects.

Brown (1973) referred to *existence* as *nomination*. ■

Chained associations also have been called *analogical overextensions.* ■

overextensions   Words that overgeneralize to items that do not represent the conventional referents for the word.

underextension   A word that is excessively discriminated in that it occurs only in response to a specific stimulus or context; compare **overextension.**

chained associations
Phenomenon in conceptual development in which a word occurs in successive contexts that are linked by one feature from the preceding situation.

through **location relational words** that occur in response to the locations of objects or the direction of their movement. Eyeing an interesting dish on a top shelf, toddlers might innocently say *Up!* while pointing to the object of their desire. The earliest expressions of locational relations often relate to locations of *dynamic* events (a ringing telephone) as opposed to *static* spatial locations (a pillow on the sofa) (Bloom & Lahey, 1978).

Finally, toddlers respond to individual features or attributes (size, shape, color, etc.) that distinguish one member of a class from other members. **Attribution relational words** occur, although infrequently in the early lexicon, to express individual characteristics such as *big, little, funny, hot,* and *dirty.* Toddlers might identify a pair of dad's shoes by noting a distinguishing attribute, *Dirty!* Those early attribution relations that are expressed may be more nominative than attributive. That is, for toddlers the attribute may initially name items rather than describing them. Instead of noting that a stubborn stain makes a bib *Yucky,* the toddler may initially adopt *Yucky* as the name of that bib.

Underextensions and Overextensions

A familiar experience for caregivers guiding toddlers through language is that the apparent meaning of toddlers' words extend beyond conventional boundaries. The "classics" include calling the neighbor's cat a *doggy,* calling a fork a *spoon,* or calling the mailman *daddy.* A toddler recently noticed my daughter's braces for the first time and asked his mother why that girl had "jewelry" on her teeth.

Less often, caregivers may note words with apparently restricted meanings produced only in limited contexts. Examples of this are fewer but include a child who said *car* only when looking out the apartment window at cars moving on the street below (Bloom, 1973).

Those instances in which toddlers' words extend beyond their conventional definitions are called **overextensions.** Conversely, occurrences of toddlers overrestricting words to particular contexts are called **underextensions.** These phenomena, overextensions and underextensions, have also been called *broad* and *narrow reference,* respectively (Bloom & Lahey, 1978).

Two primary patterns of overextensions have been identified. **Chained associations** occur when a word experienced in one setting is produced in subsequent settings based on similar features (Vygotsky, 1962). For example, having heard the word *milk* while holding a mug of milk, a toddler may later say *milk* in response to that mug filled only with pieces of cereal. Subsequently, when examining a toy with handles that resemble those on the mug, the toddler may respond to this connection, saying *milk.*

Chained associations appear to be more prevalent during the earlier stages of vocabulary development, when toddlers' experience in labeling objects is still limited. During this early period, word meanings may shift each time toddlers attempt a word. This might be influenced by their focus, the stimuli present, and their caregivers' feedback.

In contrast, **wholistic associations** occur when words are extended to items that share a greater number of similarities with the original referent. For example, the proverbial extension of *doggy* typically occurs based on a collection of similarities (fur, four legs, tail, etc.) shared with each mislabeled stimulus (cat, goat, fox, etc.). Wholistic associations become more common (than chained associations) as toddlers' word meanings and object concepts stabilize and approximate the adult model. The similarities that appear to prompt overextensions become more consistent with an overall concept or collection of features as additional experiences and caregiver feedback "fine-tune" and stabilize the toddler's concepts. For example, extending *doggy* to a goat becomes less likely than to a wolf.

Because overextensions are frequent (and often quite funny!) they have become the source of some curiosity. Caregivers understand that these occurrences are just "mistakes" with respect to the conventional adult word. On the other hand, researchers suggest that toddlers' mistakes are illuminating. Researchers have written extensively regarding what overextensions might reveal about how children form their early concepts.

Toddlers' overextensions might reveal the similarities or relationships that influence how they understand and organize objects and events. On the other hand, overextensions may simply represent toddlers' means for coping with a vocabulary that is still incomplete. When confronted with an unfamiliar object, toddlers may not have a word for it. However, engaging the attention of caregivers might be so compelling that toddlers attempt to respond with a word most likely to fit.

Such attempts are not unlike adult verbal behavior in similar conditions of uncertainty. When confronted with a truly unusual piece of furniture, for example, an adult speaker might qualify the strength of their response with phrases such as *I'm not positive, but I think it's kind of like . . . a chair.* The difference is that toddlers have not yet developed the verbal ability to express the uncertainty that underlies their responses in such circumstances. Based on conventional definitions, toddler's overextensions and underextensions might be considered mistakes. However, from the standpoint of learning they can be considered products of natural behavioral processes, stimulus generalization and stimulus discrimination (Winokur, 1976).

Stimulus generalization is the tendency for responses to occur in the presence of new stimuli or settings based on features or relationships similar to the original stimulus. Stimulus generalization accounts for many adult extensions of meaning. Most forms of figurative language (simile, metaphor, idioms, etc.) can be attributed to stimulus generalization. For example, referring to a leaked secret as "letting the cat out of the bag" is only useful if stimulus generalization makes the two circumstances analogous to the listener.

wholistic associations Extension of a word to items sharing a number of features with the original referent for that word.

Wholistic associations also have been called *categorical inclusions.* ■

Specific theories about concept development are discussed later in this chapter. ■

Stimulus generalization and discrimination are discussed in Chapter 4. ■

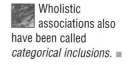

It has been suggested that humans (and primates in general) are good generalizers. This accounts for toddlers' rapid spread of language to new objects and settings. The greater relative frequency of overextensions (versus underextensions) seems to fit with this characterization.

In contrast, stimulus discrimination offsets stimulus generalization by establishing selective control between the features of a stimulus and the words that will be accepted in response. For example, children and adults know that an animal with four legs, fur, a tail, and so forth can only be called a dog if it barks; if it says "meow," we discriminate and call it a cat. Stimulus discrimination explains the nature of underextensions and why they are less common. When a word is experienced in a relatively constrained circumstance, that setting may become a unique context that influences the toddlers' production of that word. Anecdotal reports in the literature suggest that underextended (or highly discriminated) words are overcome through expanded experiences that prompt generalization of that word. Ultimately, when words generalize to objects (or events or relationships) that all exhibit relevant defining features, but do not occur in response to those that do not, they represent a concept.

Theories of Conceptual Behavior

At the core of vocabulary growth is the development of conceptual behavior. Toddlers, as their experiences accumulate, become increasingly responsive to similarities among stimuli. **Conceptual behavior** is the ability to respond selectively to a variety of specific examples representing a class of items related by some defining features. Concepts represented by their words allow toddlers (and adults) to more efficiently respond to our complex world. The process of concept formation as depicted in the evolution of toddlers' vocabulary has been the subject of several theories. Table 6–4 summarizes the main ideas associated with each theory.

conceptual behavior
Responding to a variety of items that are related by some feature defining them as a class.

Clark's Semantic Feature Hypothesis.   Clark (1973b) proposed a theory that emphasizes the role of perceptual features in defining classes of objects. Objects can be classified based on features such as shape, size, texture, color, and so forth. According to this theory, perceptual features most strongly in-

Table 6–4. Theories of conceptual behavior and word meanings.

Theory	Description	Example
Semantic Feature (Clark)	Concepts form around perceptual features: shape, size, color, etc.	Child calls the moon a "bowl" because it is round and white like his cereal bowl.
Functional Core (Nelson)	Concepts form based on the central use of an object.	Child calls a shovel a spoon because it digs dirt like he "digs" cereal.
Prototypical Complex (Bowerman)	Concepts form based on an early experience but shift with new experiences.	Child initially calls a book a "box" because of its shape, but later calls it a "door" because the cover opens and closes.

fluence the organization of children's vocabulary. As toddlers' concept of a word evolves through additional experiences and feedback, relevant features are added and irrelevant features are eliminated. This proceeds until toddlers derive a set of features that conform with those used by people around them.

Throughout this process, toddlers' overextensions hypothetically illustrate the features that most strongly influence their current concepts. When toddlers produce a word in response to fewer relevant features, the word will probably be overextended. Any four-legged feature will evoke *doggy*. Conversely, if a word occurs only in response to larger set of features, it will be underextended. That is, *doggy* may initially occur only for a furry, four-legged creature of a certain shape, size, and color living in a toddler's house.

According to Clark, the most salient feature for children is initially shape. This fits with the observation that many early overextensions appear to be based on shape. Accordingly, based on experience with a favorite red bowl, a toddler is more likely to extend the word *bowl* to a sink (no matter what color) than to a red building block.

Some have argued that certain overextensions are difficult to account for through the semantic feature theory. These include extensions involving imperfect exemplars (square bowls), quantitative or directional relationships (*allgone, up*), and functional similarities (Palermo, 1982).

Nelson's Functional Core Hypothesis. Nelson (1974) proposed an alternative theory. In analyzing toddlers' early lexicons, she noted many first words were in response to objects that toddlers acted on in their everyday interactions. From this perspective, Nelson hypothesized that toddlers' meanings for words are based on objects' movements or movements associated with using them. In other words, toddlers' core early meanings originate in the functions of objects.

This perspective has some inherent appeal. One way toddlers become familiar with new objects is to experiment with their associated actions. Infants first investigate objects orally, then through shaking them, and finally move them around in their field of view. As toddlers, new objects are often defined by discovering how they can be used. Even older children, when asked to define an object, such as a fork, will frequently begin with phrases such as *"it's something you eat with and . . ."*

There is no clear, overwhelming evidence that either the semantic feature theory or the functional-core hypothesis is exclusively correct. Each seems to apply in some instances, but neither is without limitations.

Bowerman's Prototypic Complex Hypothesis. Bowerman (1978) suggested that it is too narrow to think that children's overextensions rely exclusively on either perceptual features or functional similarities. Instead, Bowerman proposed that toddlers might first base their understanding of a word on early experiences with an associated object. These early experiences form an overall model—a prototype—that is representative of that category.

Although an early experience might provide the nucleus of a concept, the prototype will be refined over time. As toddlers' prototypes for a class evolve, their central concepts may alternate between emphasizing certain perceptual features or associated functions. It becomes a composite of the salient features and functions that accumulate with experience. The toddler's subsequent experiences with potential new members of that class are compared with this prototype to determine whether they belong and whether that word applies.

Like the other theories, this perspective has appeal for explaining certain observations. It permits the possibility that individual differences occur in how concepts evolve for each toddler. One toddler may focus on perceptual features. Another may attend more to movement and function. And both might vary in the complex of features or functions that define a concept at a given time.

Toddlers' Conceptual Behavior: Comments.   Some writers have characterized the cognitive process that might underlie vocabulary development as a process of hypothesis testing. In what he described as "the original word game," Brown (1958) asserted that children learn the meanings of words through a process of hypothesis testing. From this perspective, children's attempts at using words are a hypothesis or guess, subsequently confirmed or refuted by caregivers' responses. Other writers suggest further that toddlers refine word meanings by retaining or eliminating features based on their caregiver's feedback.

It should be cautioned that characterizing such phenomena in language development as "hypothesis testing" is based on inference. Toddlers' underlying mental processes cannot be directly confirmed, they cannot describe them, and we certainly cannot "read" their mind.

Interestingly, these characterizations appear to depict the same hypothesis testing a linguist might use to analyze an unfamiliar language. Linguists are fully capable of this process. However, Piaget asserted that hypothesis testing is an ability that does not develop until the child is capable of formal operational thought, which evolves after 11 years of age. Are toddlers in their second year somehow capable of this ability, even at a subconscious level? Does it contribute any more to our objective understanding to suppose that toddlers engage in hypothesis testing to select the features that define word meanings as the linguist might do?

"Linguistomorphizing" the child (i.e., attributing behaviors like those of a linguist) in this way is intriguing and perhaps insightful. However, it potentially misrepresents the actual process and risks delaying our objective understanding of it.

A more empirically based account of concept formation would be achieved by analyzing the responses classes that serve as evidence that children have "formed a concept." A concept is demonstrated when a class of responses is produced to similar stimuli under similar conditions with similar consequences. Documenting the relationships among the features and

In Chapter 4, it is pointed out that "meaning" refers to the relationship between stimuli and the utterances they influence. ■

functions of stimuli that influence toddlers' response classes might provide a more objective understanding of their development of word meanings.

Summary

- Words can be "known" at referential, extended, relational, categorical, or metalinguistic levels.

- Toddlers' vocabulary growth occurs at different rates, but generally approach 50 words by 18 months.

- The earliest words are predominately nouns, however, verbs increase as toddlers become more active.

- Toddlers' early words have been classified according to grammatical classes as well as their apparent meanings.

- Referential words occur in referring to things and expressive words express personal information.

- Substantive words also refer to objects, whereas relational words convey relationships among objects, persons, or events.

- Overextensions, in which a word is used for objects outside its conventional definition, are more frequent than underextensions.

- Stimulus generalization and discrimination are behavioral processes related to overextensions and underextensions.

- Theories of how children learn word meanings have suggested they focus on semantic features, or the functions of objects, or a prototype of the class based on both.

Combining Words, Meanings, and Functions

Through the first 18 months, children have normally passed a number of important communication milestones. From cooing and babbling, to signaling intentions through gestures and vocalizations, infants finally supplement gestures with their first words. Approximately halfway through their second year, toddlers will normally take the next big step.

This next milestone—combining words—is significant in several ways. Putting words together is evidence of toddlers' advancing motor coordination for producing longer, more phonologically complex syllable strings. Combining words reflects the cognitive ability that underlies perceiving and responding to relationships between objects or events. Behaviorally, it reflects toddlers' cumulative experience of past consequences resulting from communicating their ideas and intentions more effectively.

Linguistically, combining words represents the appearance of grammar, the next level of conventional language behavior. Of further significance is the recent finding that reaching this milestone generally requires some effort on the part of toddlers.

> Even though the individual words in the first lexicon can be fit into grammatical classes, most agree that single word utterances do not represent grammar. ∎

Transitional utterances are significant in that they illustrate the evolution of true two-word utterances and the beginning of grammar. ■

transitional utterances
Any of several utterance types that appear to represent a progression from single-word utterances to multiword utterances reflecting syntactic order.

dummy forms
Utterances consisting of a true word combined with an additional sound or syllable that give the appearance of approximating multiword utterances.

empty forms   Forms that are consistent but do not represent conventional words are combined with a true word and appear to approximate multiword utterances.

reduplication   An early approximation of a multiword utterance through repeating a conventional word within the same intonational contour.

pseudophrase   Early approximation of multiword utterances through production of conventional two-word phrases (e.g., *allgone, nomore*) in which the individual elements do not occur elsewhere independently.

Transition from Single Words

Although one-word utterances will continue to occur, toddlers normally begin to combine words into two-word utterances around 18 months of age. At one time, it was thought that in advancing to two-word utterances, toddlers immediately achieved correct word order or grammar. Characteristics defining true two-word utterances would include: (a) production of two true words; (b) no distinct pauses between the two words; and (c) a single intonational contour that envelops both words; as in the adult phrase *I know* ↓.

It now appears that a transition between single-word and two-word utterances occurs (Bloom & Lahey, 1978; Owens, 2005; Reich, 1986). During this transition toddlers may struggle through trial and error to produce more than one word. The forms of toddlers' various attempts at expanding their single-word utterances have been described as transitional phenomena (Dore et al., 1976; Owens, 2005; Reich, 1986).

Transitional Utterances

Toddlers' **transitional utterances** appear to be attempts at expanding the character of their utterances toward multiword syntactic utterances. Some expand only the phonological nature of utterances, whereas others appear as efforts to combine meaningful elements (Dore et al., 1976). There are several types of transitional utterances.

Dummy Forms.   **Dummy forms** are a transition phenomenon in which additional sounds or syllables are combined with a recognizable word. These additional sounds or syllables have no obvious referent and their phonological characteristics are variable. The toddler might precede words with one of several vowel sounds (e.g., *e baby, u cup*) or nonmeaningful syllables (e.g., *mu eat, wa ball*). The dummy forms expand what is otherwise a one-word utterance, but they add no new meaning.

Empty Forms.   Another transitional phenomenon is **empty forms.** These are still not recognizable as words, but they do evidence more consistent phonological structure. The same form is combined with different words as in *mama [didi], dada [didi]* (Bloom, 1973).

Reduplications.   Yet another way in which toddlers appear to expand the overall structure of an utterance is called **reduplication,** which consists of a repeated word. The two productions are distinguished by being uttered within the same intonational contour, as in *Car car* (Dore et al., 1976). They mimic the structure and rhythm of two-word utterances, but the additional word carries no additional meaning.

Pseudophrases.   Toddlers produce another transitional form called **pseudophrases,** which consist of utterances that appear to be conventional two-word phrases for mature speakers (e.g., *all gone, so big, no more*). On the surface, these appear to more clearly represent two-word utterances than the previous forms. However, on closer examination it seems that toddlers might initially learn them as single "big words." For example, a toddler might produce the individual elements *no* and *more* as isolated words at other times. However, if they are not yet combined with other words to make phrases, this suggests that they are just part of what is essentially a one-word utterance to the toddler.

Successive Single-Word Utterances. The most intriguing and significant transitional utterances are **successive single-word utterances.** These consist of productions of individual words in succession with a pause in between (Bloom, 1973). Beyond adding meaningless sounds or syllables to expand an utterance, these appear to be attempts at combining meanings in an additive way while only approximating grammar.

In these, toddlers produce two individual words in succession. Each is separated by a pause and produced with a separate falling intonational contour, as in *mommy↓* (pause) *sock↓*. Braine (1976) also observed such phenomena and called them **groping patterns.** Braine characterized these as "produced with evidence of uncertainty and effort, that is, haltingly, with repetitions or with hesitation" (p. 11).

On the surface, given the nature of their production, these utterances could be interpreted as isolated single words, each produced as though it is a separate statement with a separate referent. However, examining the context more closely may reveal that the stimuli toddlers responded to were actually related in some way.

Given the previous example (*Mommy - sock*), it might turn out that mommy was holding a sock at the time. In these occurrences, toddlers appear to perceive that the two items are in relation to each other and that this relationship could be conveyed by producing the two words together. However, they are not yet able to produce them as a single unit, achieving the grammar of a true two-word utterance. To do so would require producing the words without hesitation, enveloped under a single intonational contour, as in *Mommy sock↓*.

Trial and Error: A Comment. The most significant implication of these phenomena is the illustration of toddlers' efforts to gradually approximate the word orders (grammar) required to express relationships they perceive. This period of trial-and-error contrasts with earlier claims that toddlers' earliest two-word utterances immediately exhibit correct word order. It appears instead that consistent word orders might emerge more gradually as caregivers interpret (or misinterpret) their toddlers' attempts.

In all fairness to earlier researchers in language development we should recall that it was not until the 1970s that Bloom proposed the "method of rich interpretation," in which the linguistic and nonlinguistic contexts are considered in interpreting language transcripts. Prior to this, transcripts

successive single-word utterance Utterance composed of two words spoken separately, where both words are related to the same context; taken by some as evidence of successive approximation of grammar.

groping patterns Early attempts at true two-word utterances produced with effort and hesitation.

Groping patterns were noted to continue into multiword utterances, most often when new meanings were being expressed. ▪

generally recorded only the child's utterances with little of the context preserved. In that case, successive-single word utterances were probably noted as separate entries with no contextual evidence to link them.

▓ Summary

- At around 18 months of age, toddlers are expected to begin combining words into two-word phrases.

- Word combinations that express relationships are the first evidence of emerging grammar.

- It now appears as though toddlers might experiment and exhibit groping patterns for the word order that expresses their thought.

- Various types of transitional utterances appear to be evidence of the progression from single words to syntax.

Two-Word Combinations

The ability to order words appears to emerge gradually out of a period of trial and error. Toddlers' groping for word orders to express ideas and intentions continues. However, it has been found that by 24 months of age two-word combinations will be prevalent in toddlers' speech.

> Again, it is helpful to remember that the same utterance can be viewed under our three conceptual lenses—one each focused on grammar, semantics, and pragmatics—on our hypothetical "linguistic microscope" mentioned earlier.

The characterization of toddlers' multiword utterances has evolved over the decades. In the 1950s, children's language development was measured by productivity; that is, the number of utterances of various lengths produced at a given age was tabulated (Templin, 1957). During the 1960s, due primarily to Chomsky's influence, researchers began searching for children's underlying syntactic rules. In the 1970s, researchers attempted to identify the range of semantic relationships expressed in toddlers' utterances. Since the 1980s, the pragmatic functions apparently served by toddlers' utterances also have interested many researchers.

> ▓ Another measure used to characterize language maturity is *mean length of utterance* (MLU). Brown (1973) used MLU to characterize stages of development in his research. Brown's research is detailed in Chapter 8.▮

Traditional Syntactic Characterizations

Given that the prevailing theoretical environment in the 1960s was based on Chomsky's syntactic theory, researchers were understandably prone to viewing children's language from this perspective. The earliest characterizations analyzed toddler utterances by relating them to adult syntactic patterns.

telegraphic speech   A traditional concept of children's grammar that viewed their utterances as reduced forms of adult grammar.

Telegraphic Speech   One of the earliest terms applied to toddlers' multiword utterances was quite descriptive. Brown and Fraser (1963) coined the term **telegraphic speech,** noting the similarity of these early utterances to the nature of adult language used in telegrams where adults omit unnecessary words to save money. In traditional terms, telegram messages retain mostly *content* words (i.e., nouns, verbs, adjectives, etc.) while primarily omitting the *function* words (articles, conjunctions, etc).

Brown and Fraser (1963) noted that toddlers' utterances were primarily composed of content words, much like adult telegrams. Utterances such as *Daddy read* or *Mommy sit* were common.

The most significant limitation of telegraphic speech as a characterization of toddlers' multiword utterances is the implication for toddlers' underlying abilities. Taken literally, the analogy to adult behavior suggested that toddlers have the ability to generate complete grammatical utterances, but economize on their words due to limitations, perhaps in motor coordination or memory. Most researchers agree that, although telegraphic speech was a descriptive characterization, it was at best an oversimplification and at worst, misleading.

Pivot Grammar.   Another early characterization was provided by Braine (1963), who also observed that toddlers' early two-word utterances could be analyzed into two classes of words. However, in contrast to a pattern based on preferences for content words (as in telegraphic speech), Braine observed a pattern based on positional preferences. He called this pattern **pivot grammar,** in which *pivot words* from a smaller set occurred in certain positions and were combined with *open words* from a larger set. For example, the pivot word "that" might be combined with a number of open words to produce "That man," "That doggy," "That ball," and so on. Some pivot words occurred consistently in initial position, others only in final position. The remaining position was filled with open words consisting of the remaining words in the toddler's vocabulary.

A number of researchers quickly pointed out the shortcomings of pivot grammar. Among these were findings of children who failed to exhibit any utterances that fit pivot grammar. In addition, there were children whose utterances seemed to fit pivot grammar, but on closer examination a number of those utterances actually violated several of the position rules (Bowerman, 1973). Finally, Bloom (1973) argued forcefully that a pivot grammar ignored the influence of semantic roles that are expressed through word orders.

Linear Syntactic Relationships.   Toddlers' two-word utterances also have been described as representing **linear syntactic relationships** (Bloom & Lahey, 1978; Brown, 1973). In this characterization, it was noted that overall meanings are carried by simple, linear combinations of a function word (e.g., *more, allgone, there*) with a second word. Brown (1973) described the pattern as a formula, $f(x)$, where f represents a fixed value (the function word) and (x) represents any other word. The function word (e.g., *more*) is fixed, indicating that it carries the same meaning no matter which other words are combined with it (*more cookie, more milk,* etc.). These word orders are described as additive, indicating that no new meaning, beyond adding the individual meaning of each word, results from such combinations.

Content and function words are described as *lexical morphemes* and *grammatical morphemes,* respectively, in Chapter 1. ■

pivot grammar   A description of children's early grammar that described a limited number of words (pivots) occurring only in certain positions and a larger set of words (open) combined with them.

linear syntactic relationships   A description of children's early grammar that described the additive meanings of words combined in utterances.

Linear syntactic relationships are primarily useful in describing the nature of the earliest two-word utterances. It will be recalled that the earliest semantic relations expressed by toddlers' one-word utterances were described as reflexive, including existence, nonexistence, disappearance, and recurrence. Generally, the earliest two-word utterances reflect these same reflexive relationships with both the object and the relationship expressed.

Where toddlers once responded to the existence of objects with *this* or *that,* these terms are now combined with the name, as in *this kitty.* At the one-word level, requesting recurrence with *more* may have served to obtain additional cookies or another helping of strained peas. By expanding this to *more cookies,* the toddler can be more certain of obtaining the desired item.

Reflexive relations are the most frequently expressed meanings until the toddler approaches 2 years of age (Bloom & Lahey, 1978). As the toddler increasingly combines other meanings (especially action) in multiword utterances, the overall meaning is compounded beyond the individual words. As such, in many later word orders, the whole meaning is greater than the sum of its parts. At this point, linear syntactic patterns fall short in describing them.

Semantic-Syntactic Characterizations

Researchers eventually recognized that syntactic patterns failed to fully capture the essence of later two-word utterances. A study merely of structural aspects did not reveal the relationships perceived by toddlers when producing multiword utterances.

The *semantic revolution* is discussed in the context of the *semantic model* of language development in Chapter 4. ▪

The semantic revolution of the 1970s emphasized considering the overall context in which utterances occurred to fully understand them. In analyzing utterances like *Mommy sock,* Bloom (1973) recognized that a strictly syntactic approach revealed only a *Noun + Noun* structure. However, she pointed out that this utterance (as well as others like it) occurred in response to a variety of circumstances representing different relationships. If Mommy was holding her sock, she was a *possessor.* If Mommy was putting the sock on, she was the *agent,* and so on. Several different meanings arise from the same form depending on the context in which they occur. A number of researchers (Braine, 1976; Brown, 1973, among others) have made similar observations.

Semantic-Syntactic Rules.   Several other researchers (Bloom, Lightbown, & Hood, 1975; Bowerman, 1973; Brown, 1973) have examined the influence of underlying semantic relationships on toddlers' two-word utterances. As toddlers progress toward expressing themselves more completely, their word orders in responding to similar relationships in a variety of contexts become more consistent. This illustrates that they gradually learn the word orders that convey relationships they perceive as relevant.

semantic-syntactic rules Describes children's early grammar emphasizing that expressing meaning provides the motivation for attempting to learn correct forms.

These consistent word orders have been labeled with a variety of names. Bloom and Lahey (1978) called these word orders **semantic-syntactic rules,** emphasizing that meaning precedes and influences form. Because case grammar seemed particularly appropriate in describing the influence of semantic roles, such consistent word orders were called **case frames** by Brown (1973). Interestingly, although Skinner (1957) did not attempt to describe child language, his **autoclitic frames** are analogous to these conceptions and a fitting explanation of the learning principles underlying this verbal behavior (Moerk, 1992b; Segal, 1975; Winokur, 1976).

The meanings expressed by these word orders have been found to reflect toddlers' changing interests, abilities, and knowledge. It was noted previously that toddlers' one-word utterances expressing reflexive relations occur in response to objects of interest to them. Is it present, has it gone, or are there more? Early two-word utterances continue this reflexive focus on objects. However, at the end of the second year the meanings expressed by toddlers shift and expand to more frequently involve actions, locations, attributes, and possession (Bloom, 1973; Bloom, Lightbown, & Hood, 1975; Brown, 1973; Wells, 1985). Table 6–5 presents the prevalent semantic relations in two-word utterances found by Brown.

The meaning most frequently expressed by toddlers in two-word utterances increasingly shifts to *action*. Toddlers' word orders reflect their interest in who does what (*agent + action*), how actions affect objects (*action + object*), or who affects objects (*agent + object*). The actions expressed are typically more general in that they can occur across a wide range of objects— *put, make, get, go.* The generic nature of these actions means that there will be ample opportunity to talk about such experiences with many different objects. Other actions expressed are more specific, but also common to most toddlers' daily experiences—*read, color, eat, sit, walk.* The prominence of action related words should not be surprising, given the advances that have occurred in both fine and gross motor skills. Toddlers go places and do things—constantly!

case frames Brown's concept of the early consistent word orders used by children to express semantic relationships.

autoclitic frames Skinner's concept of certain orders in verbal responses that express relationships among stimuli.

It may be helpful to review both case grammar and the operant model. These are described in Chapter 4.

Table 6–5. Brown's prevalent semantic relations in two-word utterances.

Semantic Relations	Example
Agent + Action	*Daddy wash*
Action + Object	*Wash car*
Agent + Object	*Daddy car*
Demonstrative + Entity	*That soap*
Entity + Locative	*Soap car*
Action + Locative	*Put car*
Possessor + Possession	*Daddy key*
Attribute + Entity	*Pretty car*

Note. Adapted from *A First Language: The Early Stages,* by R. Brown, 1973, Cambridge, MA: Harvard University Press.

locative action relations
Spatial relationships or location of actions.

locative state relations
Spatial relationships between entities.

Cross-linguistic research suggests that the earliest semantic relations seem to be universal. That is, they occur in all languages. Although this is important to document, perhaps this observation could be expected since objects, events, locations, and so on occur in all cultures. We might ask whether these relations are universal to all languages or all environments in which languages occur. This presents one of those classic "chicken or egg" questions.

state relations   Several relationships regarding the status of objects such as location, possession, and attribution.

possession   The semantic case signaling that an entity is associated with, held, or owned by a possessor.

Toddlers' maturing motor ability and advancing cognitive ability combine to increase toddlers' awareness of the whereabouts of objects. This is exhibited through utterances expressing *locative relation.* Dynamic events involving objects changing locations are expressed earlier in utterances reflecting **locative action relation** (e.g., *Mommy go, Doggie down*). **Locative state relation** are expressed in two-word utterances (e.g., *Baby chair, Mommy bed*) that reflect objects in static spatial relation (Bloom, Lightbown, & Hood, 1975).

Other less frequent meanings expressed in early two-word utterances reflect **state relations,** which express the status of objects. **Possession** is expressed through juxtaposing two words representing the possessor ("owner") and the entity possessed, as in *Daddy chair.* However, toddlers' seem to be indicating only that an object is closely *associated* with the person involved in this relationship, as their understanding of possession is not fully developed (Bloom & Lahey, 1978). The association might be based on *proximity,* because that person always wears or locates near the object, or on *action* due to that person frequently using that item.

The other state relation expressed in two-word utterances is attribution, referring to the individual characteristics that distinguish between individual items of a class. Many words for attributes may have been so frequently associated with an item that they simply expand the name for those objects. For example, *Hot!* may have been associated with the stove so often (even though it is frequently not turned on) that it begins to serve as part of the stove's "full name"—*Stove hot!*

Combining Words: A Comment.   The accomplishment of producing two words integrated within a single intonational contour is a major motor accomplishment. However, perhaps even more significant is the accomplishment of expressing a relationship that transcends objects or events by juxtaposing two words in such utterances. As a single step, the ability to express perceived relationships through word orders may have the most far-reaching implications for language development.

Summary

- Accomplishing two-word combinations is a major indication of toddlers' cognitive, motor, and social development.
- Toddlers' two-word combinations become prevalent by 24 months of age.
- Toddlers' two-word utterances have been described by various syntactic formulations focusing on word order.

- Semantic models used to describe toddlers' two-word utterances have focused on the semantic roles expressed by the word orders.

- Word orders expressing relations among referents have been called case frames, semantic-syntactic rules, and autoclitic frames.

Tools for Language Development

The basic building blocks for language development evolved throughout the first 2 years of life. Several aspects of toddlers' verbal behaviors, however, continue to reflect a tentative connection between their experiences and the language skills they have not fully mastered. As a result, many toddler utterances signal their need for feedback. Caregivers, in turn, have proven to be capable of providing effective input and feedback.

Talking Together and Learning Language

Adult language that *surrounds* toddlers has been described as a stream of sounds, often interrupted, repeated, revised, or overlapping. The speech stream was deemed an inadequate sample of the language that toddlers are trying to decipher. Based on this characterization, the task of learning language seemed to be a formidable one. However, this is not the entire picture.

Researchers have shown that the language shared *between* toddlers and caregivers provides substantially different input. Researchers have discovered that toddlers are both resourceful and persistent in evoking information and feedback from their caregivers. In turn, caregivers also exhibit verbal behaviors that have a significant impact on toddlers' language learning. It has been estimated that in a typical 12-hour waking day, 2-year-olds produce from 10,000 to 20,000 words! And, their caregivers are conservatively estimated to respond with twice that many (Wagner, 1985). This represents a wealth of learning opportunities for caregivers and toddlers.

Toddlers' Tools for Learning Language

For toddlers, the complex, changing world is a challenge. It is for all of us! However, increasing mobility and limited experience frequently leads toddlers to unfamiliar contexts. To make matters worse, they are also confronted with trying to use and understand language—still a puzzle in itself!

Researchers have classified toddler verbal behaviors that prompt their caregivers to respond with feedback and information about language (Snyder-McLean & McLean, 1978). These toddler behaviors might reflect a range of certainty or response strength on the part of toddlers, indicating that, on occasion, they may be more or less certain of the connection between a stimulus and the words that apply.

evocative utterances
Assertions by toddlers that appear to anticipate affirmation or feedback from the caregiver.

Evocative Utterances.   **Evocative utterances** are those responses that occur when toddlers appear to make a statement with relative certainty, yet with the expectation of some feedback from the caregiver. In producing evocative utterances, toddlers produce a word in a declarative manner, with the falling, affirmative intonation of a statement. In these circumstances, the utterance may be more assertive because the history between a given word and an object is relatively established due to some experience with similar objects.

   If the word asserted by toddlers is correct, caregivers' responses will confirm it either directly (*That's right, it's a doggie!*) or indirectly (*I like cute doggies!*). If toddlers' words are inaccurate, the caregiver will provide some form of corrective feedback (*No, that's a kitty!*). In either case, in evocative utterances toddlers "take a shot" and benefit from the feedback it prompts.

hypothesis testing
Utterances by toddlers produced with rising intonation as an apparent request for confirmation or feedback from the caregiver.

Hypothesis Testing.   In **hypothesis testing,** toddlers attempt a word, but produce it with the rising intonation of a question. The questioning tone (*Doggie?*) more directly invites feedback to confirm or correct their utterance (which may take the form described for evocative utterances). Utterances reflecting hypothesis testing might reflect less certainty or response strength for the stimulus in question, perhaps due to relatively less experience with that stimulus.

   Here again, a caution should be noted. In spite of its name, whether this behavior actually represents the underlying mental process of hypothesis testing, a later developing cognitive ability, is not necessarily known. This behavior is labeled as such merely because it has the *appearance* of posing a "guess" with the expectation of caregiver feedback to confirm or refute it.

interrogative utterances
Toddler utterances that directly request information or labels.

Interrogative Utterances.   Occasionally, no response is available in a given context, perhaps due to very limited experience. In these instances, toddlers exhibit **interrogative utterances,** which generally take the form of a direct request for the appropriate word (e.g., *This?* or *Wassat?*). It appears that this behavior emerges nonverbally before the first words as infants use gestures and vocalizations to request information (Dore, 1974). After the first words appear, verbal requests for labels peaked later in the second year and then generally declined after the second birthday (Moerk, 1983). It has also been found that at 2 years of age vocabulary development correlates positively with this toddler behavior (Nelson, 1973a).

selective imitation
Children's partial imitations of adult utterances.

Selective Imitation.   The last behavior in this area is **selective imitation,** in which portions of caregivers' previous utterances are repeated within toddlers' next several utterances. Imitation has had a controversial history in the literature of language development. Its role in children's language learning has been strongly supported by some and vehemently denied by others. In examining this history, however, it appears that as the definition of imitation was modified, much of the controversy also dissipated.

Traditionally, some researchers held to a strict definition of imitation. For some (e.g., Ervin-Tripp, 1964), the utterance had to be reproduced immediately and in relatively unaltered form to qualify as imitative. Others (e.g., Bloom, Hood, & Lightbown, 1974), recognizing the overall limitations of toddlers and the nature of toddler-caregiver interactions, modified their criteria to accept partial repetitions that occurred within toddlers' next several utterances.

Selective imitation, the fact that toddlers do imitate, but not necessarily all that they hear, could represent either random occurrences or systematic behavior. Researchers studying selective imitation have found that it plays a sophisticated and predictable role in both vocabulary and grammatical development. Imitation is prevalent in the one-word stage, but the frequency of imitating caregivers varies with individual toddlers and eventually decreases beyond 2 years of age (Nelson, 1973b).

> The role of selective imitation in Piaget's sensorimotor learning is discussed in Chapter 3. ▪

For some time, most researchers have acknowledged the role of imitation in vocabulary development. It seems obvious that children must imitate a new word to merely gain control over its production. But do they actually imitate words they are learning? Ramer (1976) found that toddlers tend to imitate words they rarely produce spontaneously—those that are currently entering their vocabulary. In addition to focusing on new words, toddlers are more likely to imitate caregivers' utterances if a referent for the word is conspicuous. Apparently, imitation provides an additional opportunity to experience a word in the presence of the relevant object.

Similarly, others (Bloom et al., 1974; Moerk, 1977) have found that selective imitation is also grammatically progressive for toddlers. Toddlers selectively imitate grammatical structures they are currently mastering. They tend to not imitate structures they already successfully use, nor those they are not yet attempting to use.

In selective imitation, the response builds on one or several key words in the caregiver's preceding utterance (Bloom, Rocissano, & Hood, 1976). Frequently, these are at the ends of caregivers' utterances. For example, following the caregiver's statement, *It's time to play in your bath,* a toddler may simply echo *Bath!*

Toddlers' imitations become more sophisticated as their language abilities mature. In instances of selective imitation called *focus operations* the toddler focuses on several key words to repeat; for example, following the previous caregiver utterance, the toddler might repeat, *Play bath.* These are more common in younger toddlers. Older toddlers (and preschoolers) exhibiting *substitution operations* may selectively repeat one word from their caregivers' utterances and add another of their own as in, *Play bubbles!* Imitating words related to a current situation enhances toddlers' ability to produce those words when similar situations set the occasion again.

Caregiver Tools for Teaching Language

According to the early nativist theories that heavily influenced the prevailing view of language learning in the 1960s, this section on caregiver teaching tools would be unnecessary. It had been asserted that adult language was either too complex, inconsistent, or inadequate for children to learn language from them. Furthermore, it was claimed that adults did not modify their speech to children nor did they consciously attempt to teach them language.

These assertions prompted research on the nature of adult-to-child language (Lund & Duchan, 1993). Researchers determined that the nativist assertions had been premature. Caregivers do modify a variety of characteristics (phonology, vocabulary, and grammar) when talking to their children. They also exhibit a range of teaching behaviors that are finely tuned to the child's abilities and interests. Caregiver teaching tools appear to provide mechanisms for subtly reinforcing children's language attempts beyond the natural consequences of effective communication. Finally, caregivers unconsciously modify their use of these teaching tools as the child's language matures.

Input: Models and Child-Directed Speech. Caregivers' utterances serve many different practical purposes as they attempt to direct the course of events throughout each day. However, no matter their context or purpose, if caregiver utterances are audible to the toddler, they are a model. A **model** is any language behavior that is made available to the toddler. Caregivers provide models under a variety of circumstances and in a variety of ways. Every day caregivers talk about predictable objects and daily routines such as feeding, bathing, and dressing. Caregivers frequently narrate their own activities as toddlers look on.

In their speech to toddlers, caregivers exhibit a distinctive pattern that makes their models more conspicuous. This style of speech to toddlers has been called *motherese, parentese,* or **child-directed speech (CDS).** In CDS, caregivers' models are produced in a manner that makes them perceptually salient, contextually redundant, and linguistically simple (Lund & Duchan, 1993).

Caregiver models in CDS exhibit production characteristics that make the words and phrases more perceptually conspicuous to toddlers. In CDS, caregivers' speech displays an overall higher fundamental frequency, exaggerated stress, and sweeping intonation. In addition, more distinct pauses between utterances and a tendency to prolong the final syllable at the end of the utterance slows their overall rate. Finally, fewer errors and disfluencies contribute to greater fidelity and integrity in parentese.

Child directed speech is also perceptually salient by the fact that most caregiver (and toddler) utterances relate to the "here-and-now." By referring to objects in the immediate context, caregivers make the relationships expressed in the utterance more conspicuous. With their toddlers, caregivers frequently name the objects that are currently of interest to their toddlers. When toddlers' attention focuses incorrectly, caregivers will verbally and gesturally redirect their attention. This reliance on the "here-and-now" appears to be a continuation of the joint attention observed between infants and caregivers and plays a significant role throughout language development (Akhtar, Dunham, & Dunham, 1991; Tomasello, 1988).

model   Any behavior that is produced within the awareness of a child and presents an opportunity to be imitated.

Remember that the term *baby talk,* discussed in Chapter 5, refers to style changes that occur in speech to infants. ▪

Child-directed speech (CDS) (also **motherese** or **parentese**) Characteristic speech directed to toddlers and preschoolers by caregivers.

Motherese is the more traditional term. Parentese is gender neutral. However, CDS is the more inclusive term. This is appropriate as persons other than "parents" provide models to toddlers. ▪

Child-directed speech provides grammatically simplified models. This simplicity is reflected in caregivers' reduced utterance length when addressing their toddler. This adjustment occurs as infants begin to comprehend some words, around 6 to 8 months, and caregivers' utterance length remains depressed until about 24–27 months. This adjustment seems to positively influence eventual language development (Murray et al., 1990). It also appears that caregivers' utterances are adjusted based on their children's language development and on feedback (Snow, 1977b). In other cases, it seems to correlate more closely with the child's age.

A final way in which CDS provides input that is adapted to the needs of the toddler is through its lexical redundancy. Caregivers restrict their vocabulary to mostly concrete terms, but they also find ways to focus their language on the topic of interest. In doing so, they may repeat key words or substitute alternate forms as they produce successive utterances that paraphrase and overlap in meaning. For example, after noticing the toddler carrying a favorite stuffed kitten, the caregiver might say, "*You have your kitty. That's a cute baby cat!*" Overall, it turns out that through their parentese, caregivers provide models that are perceptually appealing, linguistically simple, and enriched with semantic information.

Continuity: Prompts and Turnabouts.   Beyond their models, caregivers also exhibit several behaviors that stimulate and maintain continuity in verbal exchanges with their toddlers (Kaye & Charney, 1981). Those that evoke toddler utterances have been called **prompts.**

Prompts take several forms which might reflect caregivers' assumptions about their toddlers' available responses. **Elicited imitations** take the form of prompts to imitate the word modeled by the caregiver, as in *Say, firetruck.* Presumably, in such instances, caregivers presuppose that their toddlers would not have an available response for the context. Under circumstances where it might be reasonable to expect that toddlers have an available response, caregivers might use a **fill-in** prompt. In using a fill-in, caregivers give toddlers a "fill in the blank" prompt, such as *This is a _____.*

It eventually becomes more reasonable to assume children have had sufficient experience to respond to different types of questions. **Confirmational yes/no questions** provide toddlers with more information as they attempt to respond. These take forms such as, *Do firemen drive firetrucks?* As such they require only simple comprehension and a *yes* or *no* response from toddlers. **Wh-constituent questions** require toddlers to recall associated information from their experience and formulate a specific response. For example, a caregiver might later ask, *What does a fireman drive?* Finally, toddlers who have demonstrated more advanced abilities might be prompted with a more challenging **open-ended question,** such as *What happens when there's a fire?* These obviously place a greater load on toddlers' abilities to recall and express information.

The nature of CDS helps toddlers attend to caregivers' models, and prompts stimulate toddlers to, in turn, reproduce the language modeled.

prompts   Caregiver utterances that stimulate responses from their children to continue their verbal exchange.

elicited imitation   Imitation by the child specifically prompted by the caregiver.

fill-in   A device used by caregivers to allow their child to complete a statement by supplying the correct word or label.

confirmational yes/no question   A caregiver prompt that requires a simple *yes* or *no* response.

wh-constituent question   A caregiver prompt used to evoke specific information in a child's response (e.g., *Where* questions to evoke locational information).

open-ended question   A caregiver prompt that allows for a variety of information to be included in the child's response.

turnabouts   Comments and replies used by caregivers to maintain the momentum in a conversation and shift the turn back to the child.

contingent queries   A conversational device used to prompt for specific information that maintains the conversational flow.

conversational repairs Devices used by individuals to clarify messages within a conversation.

Contingent caregiver responses have also been referred to as *consequating behaviors* (Owens, 2005). This suggests their role as a consequence that follows children's utterances in a contingent manner. ■

imitation   The relatively immediate reproduction of a significant portion of someone's preceding behavior.

expansions   Caregiver utterances that reproduce the child's utterance and include additional grammatical elements. Also, preschoolers' inclusion of additional elements in the noun phrase, which expands the length of their utterances.

Expanded imitations by caregivers have also been referred to as recasts (Farrar, 1992). ■

Caregivers also use **turnabouts,** a variety of various comments and questions that follow toddlers' utterances to maintain the interaction. In effect, the caregiver's turnabouts "put the conversational ball back in the child's court" to keep the interaction moving. Turnabouts often take the form of **contingent queries,** specific and nonspecific questions that request information (*Where did this happen?*), confirmation (*Do you mean horsie?*), or clarification (*Huh?*). Some differences between mothers' and fathers' breakdown-repair sequences with toddlers have been found, although this may be related to the caregivers' relative level of involvement in child-rearing activities (Tomasello, Conti-Ramsden, & Ewert, 1990).

When the purpose of contingent queries is to mend a breakdown in communication they serve as **conversational repairs.** Some have suggested that the negative feedback provided by contingent queries is insignificant (Morgan & Travis, 1989). However, at the least, these caregiver behaviors may provide feedback that indicates the child's utterance should be modified. The caregiver models that follow perhaps complete the tutorial (Moerk, 1994).

Contingency: Imitations, Expansions, and Extensions.   In responding to their toddlers, caregivers' utterances are more than conversational. Many caregivers' responses follow their toddlers' utterances contingently. Caregiver's responses are contingent when their timing and topic "hinge" on toddlers' preceding utterances; that is, they follow closely and address the topic introduced by toddlers. It is likely that such caregiver responses affect toddlers' language in several ways. These contingent caregiver responses include imitations, extensions, and expansions.

Caregivers frequently produce immediate **imitations** of their toddler's utterances, simply reproducing them in their original form. These caregiver imitations are, in turn, frequently repeated by toddlers. On at least one level, caregivers' imitations act to confirm that they heard their toddlers' utterance. However, it has also been found that a significant majority of caregiver imitations follow toddlers' well-formed utterances in contrast to those containing errors (Bohannon & Stanowicz, 1988). In other words, caregiver imitations seem to say to toddlers, "That was worth repeating!" And toddlers oblige, matching the utterance with the relevant context for a third time.

Another form of contingent caregiver responding takes toddlers' utterances one step further, grammatically speaking. In producing **expansions,** the caregiver reproduces the toddler's preceding utterance, but also includes several additional grammatical structures required to *expand* toward a mature form. For example, a caregiver might expand their toddler's exclamation, *Bird flying!* by following it with, *That's right, the bird is flying!*

In contrast to caregiver imitations of toddlers' correct utterances, the majority of expansions serve to correct toddler utterances containing errors (Farrar, 1992). Subsequently, most caregiver expansions are imitated in turn by the toddler, giving them immediate practice in producing the grammatically correct form.

Again, at a minimum, the immediacy of caregivers' expansions probably serves to acknowledge toddlers' utterances. However, the contingent nature of expansions goes beyond simple acknowledgment (which could be accomplished with a simple *Uh-huh*). The implication of altering the toddler's utterance to model the relevant grammatical structure is that a correction was needed. This apparently invites the toddler to imitate the corrected model (Moerk, 1994).

The third form of contingent utterance from caregivers is more conversational in nature. In producing an **extension,** the caregiver responds with additional semantic information related to the topic in the toddler's preceding utterance. For example, an extension to the previous toddler utterance (*Bird flying!*) might be *Birds have wings to fly.*

Again, extensions also acknowledge toddlers' utterances. However, they do so in a way that provides new semantic information which also appears to invite the toddler to *extend* the conversation on that topic. Interestingly, extensions, which reflect the semantic and pragmatic contingency of mature conversational utterances, become more common as children's language abilities mature (Lund & Duchan, 1993).

> **extension** Caregiver utterances that follow their child's preceding utterance and include additional related semantic information.

Learning and Teaching: Comments. It has become increasingly apparent that caregivers' behaviors impact toddlers' language learning in several ways. The distinctive production characteristics used by caregivers in CDS highlight language models for children. Caregivers use prompting and turnabouts to maintain verbal exchanges. Finally, the contingent utterances produced by caregivers in response to toddler utterances serve as teaching tools in several ways. Caregiver imitations acknowledge the toddler's correct language attempts. Expansions and extensions provide immediate feedback with grammatical and semantic information related to the toddler's utterance and topic (Moerk, 1992a).

The answer to one question central to explaining language learning might also have been illuminated by research in adult-to-child language. Researchers have wondered how caregivers' language teaching tools might serve as reinforcers for toddlers' language. Earlier attempts to identify the reinforcers that might be present in caregiver behaviors were focused too narrowly. It was thought that reinforcement might take the form of social praise (e.g., *Good!* or *That's right!*). Early research suggested that such specific praise usually depended on the semantic accuracy of the child's utterance. That is, even though the toddler might make a grammatical error, as in *It be's a horsie,* the caregiver will tend to confirm the "truth value" that the toddler named the correct animal (*That's right*).

It appears, however, that there are more subtle reinforcing consequences provided by other aspects of caregivers' contingent responses. First, the fact that caregivers respond contingently and acknowledge toddlers' utterances promptly reinforces their toddlers' attempts at language. Beyond this, however, the conditional nature of these contingent utterances may be significant.

In response to early attempts, it appears that correct utterances are imitated by caregivers while defective utterances are corrected grammatically through expansions. More mature utterances, less in need of grammatical correction, might be semantically extended by the caregiver more often.

The changes that occur in the nature of caregivers' input and children's responses are described further in Chapter 7. ■

Perhaps the theme that has been present throughout the child's life is also present in caregiver teaching tools used with toddlers. That is, that caregivers as sources of the most important primary reinforcers—nutrition, warmth, comfort, and affection—become the source of potent secondary reinforcers. Accordingly, their attention has become the most potent reinforcer from the beginning. In particular, caregivers' contingent responses go beyond simply acknowledging the toddler's utterance and modeling additional grammatical and semantic elements. They confirm that the caregiver is attending and invite the toddler to maintain that attention with their subsequent responses (Chapman, 1981).

Summary

- Toddlers and their caregivers experience many productive verbal exchanges daily.
- Toddler utterances frequently prompt certain caregiver responses that facilitate toddlers' learning of language.
- Although controversial, it is increasingly apparent that imitation plays a significant role in language learning.
- Caregivers' input, called child-directed speech, is well tuned to their toddlers' language abilities and challenges them to learn.
- Caregivers' contingent responses to their toddlers' language, including imitations, expansions, and extensions, provide various forms of feedback and reinforcement.

Emerging Literacy

By the time toddlers approach 2 years of age, their interactions reflect their ability to combine many basic elements of communication. They have expanded their vocabulary substantially and it has become more useful in their still short but developing narratives. Toddlers have a growing sense of the orderliness of language, responding appropriately to the contingent feedback provided by caregivers in their expansions and extensions. All this, in turn, contributes to their emergent literacy and appreciation of literacy events, in particular the joint reading of books.

Infants appreciated the physical presence of books that seemed to provide the joint attention for some enjoyable caregiver interactions. Infants explored the physical nature of books—the fact that they opened and closed, pages turned back and forth, and contained pictures. However, infants were passive in this exploration, generally left to the whims and schedules of their caregivers. Being more mobile, toddlers are likely to retrieve books independently to explore and page through the pictures themselves. They may point at pictures and call out labels that have been rehearsed with caregivers many times. They will recognize the presence or absence of print on a page and orient the book appropriately, front and back, with text left to right. Toddlers become increasingly aware of and are intrigued with the very nature of print. This evolving print awareness is viewed as a critical precursor to later reading proficiency (Gillon, 2004).

Caregivers are responsive to their toddlers' growth in vocabulary and comprehension. As a result, toward the end of the second year, caregivers will shift from selecting picture books that are restricted to simple labeling of pictures to story books that present storylines, albeit simple ones. This joint reading builds on the language abilities toddlers have developed and, in turn, expands their vocabulary and comprehension. Caregivers who are capable of gauging their toddlers' language levels can scaffold the text to provide an optimal learning experience. This involves using appropriate vocabulary and syntactic complexity as well as asking the right questions and providing targeted explanations (van Kleeck, 1995).

Chapter Summary

Around their first birthday, toddlers produce their first true word. This brings the toddler to the final pragmatic phase, the locutionary period, in which communication is accomplished verbally. Intentions, whether classified as *primitive speech acts* or *communicative functions,* continue to be expressed with gestures, but are now supplemented with words. Throughout the second year, toddlers learn to supplement gestures with words to initiate topics for discourse, or conversation, with their caregiver.

Toddlers' first words have characteristic phonetic structure and consist primarily of nouns. First words might be classified as referential or substantive (referring to objects), expressive (referring to personal feelings and interactions), or relational (referring to relationships between objects). Toddlers frequently exhibit *overextensions,* using a word for objects beyond the expected boundaries for that word. Conversely, *underextensions* occur when toddlers use a word for too few stimuli. Several theories describe toddlers' development of *conceptual behavior,* using words to appropriately name classes of objects.

By their 18th month, toddlers have learned approximately 50 words and are attempting to combine them in grammatical orders. These attempts, called *transitional utterances,* signify the toddler's recognition that ideas can be combined by putting words together. By the time of their second birthday, they are using frequent two-word utterances to express the relationships they have begun to recognize around them.

Toddlers exhibit verbal behaviors to elicit models and more information. They also make use of selective imitation to practice the language structures they are learning. However, toddlers are not simply left on their own to discover language. Caregivers fine-tune their speech, called *parentese,* to support their toddler's steps toward mature language. Caregivers also provide *prompts* and *turnabouts,* behaviors that keep the conversation going back and forth. With *expansions* and *extensions* they model syntactic and semantic aspects relevant to their toddler's utterances.

Finally, in most homes, toddlers become increasingly aware of the presence of print. They exhibit familiarity with the orientation of books—the fronts, the backs, and the right-to-left nature of the print. Toddlers begin to associate characters with stories, recall the storylines easily, anticipate story events, and may even begin to recognize whole words.

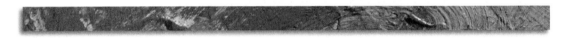

Review Questions

1. Consider how Dore's primitive speech acts and Halliday's communicative functions are similar. How do they relate to Skinner's verbal operants?

2. Contrast the similarities and differences between mature conversations and toddler-caregiver discourse.

3. What are five ways in which a toddler might eventually "know" a word?

4. Discuss how an utterance (e.g., "cup") by a toddler might be described from three different perspectives (or through three different "lenses").

5. How do Nelson's and Bloom's classifications for single-word utterances differ?

6. Which behavioral processes might explain the occurrence of overextensions and underextensions?

7. Describe how the theories of conceptual behavior describe what toddlers focus on as they learn the meanings of words.

8. How did the techniques used by linguists to interpret children's utterances change in the 1970s that would explain the recognition of transitional utterances?

9. Name at least three terms that have been proposed to describe the word orders seen in toddlers' early multiword utterances.

10. Discuss the significance of the term "contingency" when evaluating the role of caregiver responses (e.g., expansion, extensions) to toddlers' utterances?

To the student: You are encouraged to use the following questions to prepare for multiple-choice examinations. This exercise is not intended to simply "provide the answers to questions." Instead, it is hoped that you will use the material to develop your ability to analyze questions and choices to identify correct answers based on a critical understanding of the distinctions among the answers. Use the answer key at the end of the book to prompt your analysis of each item and to confirm the correct answer. Remember that there is a difference between recognizing the correct answer and understanding why it is the correct one.

Practice Questions

1. Clark's semantic feature hypothesis suggests that the early meanings of words for toddlers are probably based on _____ .
   a. the uses or actions associated with an item
   b. perceptual aspects as the shape, size, color of items
   c. their very first experiences of words and the immediate associations they make with the objects that were present
   d. genetically imprinted words that they know from birth
   e. none of these

2. The most frequent relational words in early language development according to Bloom and Lahey _____ .
   a. are called reflexive
   b. are words that relate an entity or event to itself
   c. encode meanings such as "existence," "nonexistence," "disappearance," and "recurrence"
   d. might take the form of "dis," "dat," "allgone," "more"
   e. all of these are true

3. How are the two words in true "successive single-word utterances" (SSWU) different from earlier "random" or true single words?
   a. each of the two words in SSWU is produced separately with equal stress, whereas earlier true single words are not
   b. each of the two words in SSWU is related to the same topic or context, whereas earlier true single words may not be
   c. the two words in SSWU evidence a pause between them, whereas earlier pairs of true single words would not
   d. each of the two words in SSWU would each evidence a separate intonational contour, whereas earlier true single words do not
   e. the two words would only be about football, other sports, and such, whereas earlier single words would be about food

4. Imitation appears to be useful to normal language learners for _____ .
   a. learning vocabulary or new words
   b. grammatical structures that they are not yet even trying to use

    c. grammatical structures that they are currently trying to master
    d. a and b
    e. a and c

5. Overextensions _____ .
    a. occur when children use a word in a manner in which the meaning is "broader" than the typical adult meaning
    b. usually occur with objects that look similar or are used in similar actions
    c. are more common than underextensions
    d. are evidence of stimulus generalization
    e. all of these are true

6. Classically, an adult who expands a child's utterance of "airplane flying" would most likely say which of these statements?
    a. "The airplane is trying to meet its scheduled connection in Denver."
    b. "If you'll wait, I'll put some ketchup on that hotdog."
    c. "That's right, the airplane is flying."
    d. "That's right."
    e. "That's not good grammar because you forgot your auxiliary verb."

7. In trying to learn first words, a toddler may hold out an item and say its name with rising intonation (e.g., cup?). The child's "strategy" in doing this has been called using _____ .
    a. hypothesis testing
    b. an interrogative utterance
    c. an evocative utterance
    d. imitation
    e. none of these

8. As children's utterances get longer, caregivers will most likely use certain "consequating behaviors" more frequently. Which of the following will become more common as children's utterances get longer?
    a. expansions
    b. imitations
    c. extensions
    d. a and b
    e. a and c

9. After hearing the caregiver say "Come on, it's time to play in the bath now," which of the following would a child produce using "focus operations"?
    a. "Come, mother, let us show frivolity in the bubbly bath."
    b. "No, eat cookies!"
    c. "Play bath."
    d. "Swing."
    e. "Don't like bubbles."

10. A child watches her Daddy using a rake to gather leaves in the yard and says, "Daddy leaves." This expresses _____ .
   a. agent + object
   b. entity + attribute
   c. entity + locative
   d. agent + possession
   e. agent + locative

Suggested Readings

Bauer, D. J., Goldfield, B. A., & Reznick, J. S. (2002). Alternative approaches to analyzing individual differences in the rate of early vocabulary development. *Applied Psycholinguistics, 23,* 313–335.

Goldfield, B. A. (2000). Nouns before verbs in comprehension and production: The view from pragmatics. *Journal of Child Language, 27,* 501–520.

McDonough, L. (2002). Basic-level nouns: First learned but misunderstood. *Journal of Child Language, 29,* 357–377.

Storkel, H. L. (2001). Learning of new words: Phonotactic probability in language development. *Journal of Speech, Language, and Hearing Research, 44,* 1321–1337.

CHAPTER 7

Pragmatic and Semantic Development in Preschoolers

Little Eddy Mology climbed up the stairs, paused in front of his dad's lap, and then climbed up. Although he was not yet 5 years old, he had been wondering for some time about something, and it was time to take care of it. He looked his now-curious dad in the eye and readied his big question. Placing his hand on his tummy, he said, "Daddy, why do we call it a 'buckle'?"

Mr. Mology paused and thought for a second—this is one of those funny questions. Parents either give too little or too much information. After settling on a strategy, he told little Eddy in a straightforward way, "Well, a long time ago, when French soldiers carried shields, there was a round part on the front or face of the shield. The Latin word for "cheek" was bucca, so this was called a boucle. Later, people used round pieces of metal to fasten their belts and they looked like the "cheek" on soldiers' shields. As a result, they were also called boucles. The English word for it became buckle."

Quite proud that he happened to know this tidbit of trivia, Mr. Mology looked into little Eddy's eyes. He was expecting to see a look of awe in response to his impressive store of knowledge. Instead, there was still bewilderment in Eddy's eyes. Lifting the hem of his T-shirt, Eddy exposed his bare tummy. He poked his finger in his belly button and announced with some amazement, "My 'buckle' came from a soldier's shield? Wait till I tell my friends!"

Before his dad could say another word, Eddy hopped down and excitedly ran out of the house. Somewhat humbled, Mr. Mology just shook his head and smiled. That day, Eddy Mology and his dad both learned a lesson about the history of word meanings.

This chapter addresses the following questions:

- How do the contexts and setting events for preschoolers' language expand through social interaction?

- How do the types of speech exhibited by preschoolers differ in levels of socialization?

- What degrees of social interaction are evident in preschoolers' different styles of play behavior?

- How do preschoolers' conversations and storytelling evolve as the contexts of their experiences expand?

- What skills evolve to make preschoolers' discourse or conversations more mature?

- What levels of narrative behavior are observed as children develop their storytelling abilities?

- How do preschoolers' vocabularies expand as they experience words for the objects, events, and relationships around them?

- In what ways can preschoolers' words be semantically related?

Although it is obvious that preschoolers' pragmatic, semantic, and grammatical abilities develop simultaneously, their development in grammar is dealt with separately in Chapter 8, to make the information more manageable. Nonetheless, the developments described in this Chapter and Chapter 8 are intimately intertwined. ■

The first 2 years of life present many challenges for children. During their infants' first 6 months, caregivers carried the burden of communication. Later, caregivers recognized intentional gestures as signaling specific needs. Soon, toddlers' first recognizable words gave caregivers some additional assistance. However, even with available context, those first words and their intentions were frequently difficult to interpret. Many times the guessing game was easy and the transactions remarkably natural. However, especially as toddlers' explorations and intentions expanded, one-word and even two-word utterances frequently failed to communicate enough, leaving both the toddler and the caregiver somewhat frustrated.

From 2 to 5 years of age, preschoolers' explore more, interact with a greater variety of people, and experience their world extensively. These intermingled developments are reflected in preschoolers' language. This chapter describes preschoolers' pragmatic and semantic development.

Development in Related Domains

As suggested previously, it may be helpful to review the highlights listed in the preceding chapters. ■

There is no adequate means of illustrating the relatedness of the many changes that drive children's development. Although we classify them separately, the child's domains are coupled together. As each develops, it stimulates changes in the others and the momentum of all these changes converge to propel the child's language development.

The following section lists highlights from each domain (Lane & Molyneaux, 1992; Nicolosi et al., 2003; Owens, 2005; Shulman, 1994). As with listings in previous chapters, these are certainly not intended to be exhaustive nor comprehensive. The items noted here characterize the changes occurring in each domain during this period.

Motor Development

Preschoolers' fine motor skills develop further and their overall strength and coordination in gross motor tasks continue to mature. These are reflected as preschoolers:

- Take simple objects apart and reassemble them around 24 months.
- Walk up and down stairs, but do not alternate feet, around 27 months.
- Start and stop running with ease around 30 months.
- Walk on tiptoes briefly around 33 months.
- Construct tower of seven to eight blocks around 36 months.
- Dress and undress themselves around 39 months.
- Imitate demonstrations of drawing vertical and horizontal strokes around 42 months.
- Copy cross and square around 45 months.
- Copy simple block letters around 4 years.
- Draw figures recognizable as a person with head, trunk, legs, and arms around 5 years.

Cognitive Development

Preschoolers increasingly exhibit curiosity and problem-solving skills. These traits are illustrated during this period as preschoolers:

- Follow simple verbal commands around 24 months.
- Point to and name familiar pictures around 27 months.
- Match familiar objects around 30 months.
- Identify simple actions in pictures around 33 months.
- Give "two" objects on request around 36 months.
- Match primary colors around 39 months.
- Give full name on request around 42 months.
- Enjoy "make believe" play around 45 months.
- Categorize objects around 4 years.
- Understand concept of today/yesterday/tomorrow and morning/afternoon/night around 5 years.

Social Development

Preschoolers' independence and personalities emerge throughout this period as they:

- Cooperate with adults in simple tasks around 24 months.
- Communicate desires and "order others around" around 27 months.
- Demand caregiver attention and throw tantrums when needs are not understood around 30 months.
- Show empathy for another's feelings around 33 months.
- Play independently in groups and select playmates around 36 months.
- Share toys for short periods around 39 months.
- Defend own possession with determination around 42 months.
- Play cooperatively and take turns around 45 months.
- Give up immediate gratification based on promise of a delayed privilege around 4 years.
- Show off and seek attention of others around 5 years.

Language Expectations (Pragmatic and Semantic)

During the preschool years, preschoolers' language learning accelerates across several dimensions. They communicate in an expanding array of settings and situations, but only gradually come to understand the nuances of doing so competently. Preschoolers will learn to manage the flow of conversations better and to consider their listeners' abilities and knowledge. They will become increasingly sophisticated storytellers. Preschoolers will begin the process of understanding the range of meanings represented by the array of words they are learning. The following overview is intended to provide an initial picture of the overall semantic and pragmatic developments during this period.

- Preschoolers will exhibit a range of communication modes in which they may talk to themselves as they play or even when alongside other children, as well as talking interactively with everyone in their presence.
- Preschoolers will continue to refine their conversational skills through more appropriate management of topics, turns, and background information.
- Preschoolers will become increasingly capable of telling stories that go beyond merely relating numerous isolated details to conveying themes and attitudes about events.
- Preschoolers will learn words in ways that reflect their rapidly expanding experiences and their understanding of those experiences.
- Preschoolers' utterances will increasingly include complete semantic elements—for example, the agent, action, and object complements of a sentence.
- Preschoolers will begin to recognize that stories read to them have beginning, middle, and ending elements that representing event sequences like those in their daily experiences.

Pragmatic Development

Preschoolers will evidence substantial growth in their use of language. The developments, however, will be as much qualitative as quantitative. As preschoolers' feet, hands, and eyes explore more of their surroundings, they certainly find more to talk about. And they talk more about it. However, the changes will reflect expansion, refinement, and elaboration of existing skills beyond the appearance of additional ones.

Where simpler utterances served basic uses, more complex utterances will serve similar purposes in a variety of situations. Where exchanging an utterance or two on a topic immediately at hand comprised a conversation with a toddler, additional turns and the ability to smoothly shift topics will extend the preschooler's conversational repertoire. Where toddlers' comments were tied to the "here-and-now," preschoolers' storytelling abilities will demonstrate that their recall and imagination reach beyond the present.

Preschoolers' Expanding Conversations

Between their second birthday and the momentous first day of school, preschoolers' conversations will mature in several ways. Conversations expand in their range of topics, reflecting the myriad of new experiences that their expanding social boundaries and motor abilities allow.

Growth is also evident in the increasingly sophisticated skills preschoolers develop for managing their conversations. Preschoolers' ability to guide the exchange of utterances and the flow of topics in their conversations improves. Finally, preschoolers become increasingly sensitive to their partners' needs for background information and clarification.

Expanding Contexts

Unlike toddlers, preschoolers develop more freedom of movement and therefore, soon become trailblazers in every sense of the word. They quickly discover that there is an entire world waiting to be explored! Conversations with preschoolers expand because their experiences and understanding expand with their motor and social development. The contexts that set the stage for preschoolers' language become more varied, often remote, and frequently less apparent to the listener.

Setting Events. A context or situation that sets the occasion for interaction is a *setting event* (Bijou & Baer, 1978). In the case of conversation, the interaction consists of a series of verbal responses to various stimuli occurring in the setting. Preschoolers' worlds set the stage for language with a rich supply of various stimuli every day!

New and varied stimuli—the lush forest of green grass, the soft colors in a sunlit bubble, the smell of fresh cotton candy, or the fantasy worlds of play—set the stage for language. Equally important are the predictable stimuli in daily routines, such as bathing, eating, dressing, and so forth. However varied or routine such experiences are, they play a central role in providing the setting events for preschoolers' conversations.

An overwhelming number, range, and diversity of setting events occur throughout each day. Also, each setting event is a myriad of stimuli. However, an analysis of each setting event shows the common threads that run through most of them.

There are four categories of stimuli that might contribute to a setting event: physical, chemical, organismic, and social stimuli (Bijou & Baer, 1978). It is impossible to list every stimulus that might fit into these categories, but some examples are provided in Table 7–1. *Physical stimuli* consist of objects and natural phenomena, including their movements. Such things as toys, eating utensils, furniture, buildings, waving trees, and falling rain all present opportunities to experience physical stimuli. *Chemical stimuli* consist of gases and solutions that we experience, such as the aroma of cooking food, perfumes, smoke, or the effects of soaps, lotions, shampoos, and so forth on our bodies. *Organismic stimuli* include the biological and physiological activities of our bodies. For example, we experience certain stimuli from internal processes such as breathing, eating, digesting, as well as from manipulation of objects and our own movements. Finally, *social stimuli* present themselves in the form of others' appearance, actions, interactions, and speech. Social stimuli may originate with people or even animals (i.e., pets).

For the most part, all of these classes of stimuli have been physically present and available to the child's senses from birth. However, only with

The eliciting function of unconditioned and conditioned stimuli in classical conditioning are contrasted with the discriminative and reinforcing functions of stimuli in operant conditioning in Chapter 3. ▪

Table 7–1. Setting event categories and examples of stimuli.

Physical	Chemical	Organismic	Social
Artifacts and natural entities:	Environmental gases and solutions:	Biological and physiological stimulation:	Others' presence, actions, or interactions:
Examples:	*Examples:*	*Examples:*	*Examples:*
Spoons, forks, bowls, cups, toys, books, mobiles, blankets, towels, chairs, houses, cars, lights, horns, trees, rocks, grass, clouds, wind, rain, lightning	Fragrances from fabric, wood, carpet, baking cookies, meat roasting, perfume, shampoo, flowers; Tactile sensations from soap, talcum powder, lotion, clay, food items	Hunger pangs; joint and muscle sensation from walking, climbing, reaching, eating; Pressure sensation from grasping objects, sitting on bottom, lying on back; goose-bumps, rashes	Appearance and speech or actions of mothers, fathers, caregivers, brothers, sisters, grandparents, pets, strangers, neighbors, babysitters, store clerks

experience do certain stimuli become significant or functional. A **functional stimulus** is one that influences an individual's behavior. Stimuli may function as reinforcing, discriminative, or eliciting events. Additionally, a stimulus might function in more than one way and even do so simultaneously. For example, a cookie received when a caregiver responds to a preschooler's request for a snack can serve as a reinforcer for the request and as a discriminative stimulus setting the stage to responding with a polite form, such as *Thank you!* As an eliciting stimulus, just the sight of the cookie may have also elicited salivation as well.

With their developing cognitive abilities, preschoolers' setting events may not be immediately present. Also, many of the seemingly different setting events preschoolers talk about may be related in some way that is not initially apparent. Most new settings present physical, chemical, organismic, or social stimuli similar to those experienced in other contexts. To preschoolers, something in the present setting might have a shape, color, smell, sound, or movement similar to that experienced previously. Therefore, it is not surprising that preschoolers generally find something to talk about even in seemingly unfamiliar settings. At the same time, what preschoolers say may be unique, and sometimes puzzling, because they are responding to unique combinations of elements in a new setting.

Private and Socialized Speech.   In addition to the expanding variety of contexts to talk about, preschoolers also talk in a variety of conversational modes. Reich (1986) described various modes or types of conversational styles in children, based in large part on the observations and writings of Piaget. Generally, the modes can be differentiated into private or socialized speech based on the degree of social communication intended.

Some preschooler "conversations" are not directed to another listener at all. When engaged in private speech preschoolers seemingly talk for their own satisfaction, although others may be present. They are apparently the only partner they need.

For example, **monologues** are instances of private speech in which children simply talk to themselves. Although these exhibit the least degree of social interaction, they qualify as conversations because preschoolers appear to respond in successive utterances that are related and even seem to expand on previous utterances. As an example, a child self-absorbed by a toy airplane simply might reflect, *I want to fly. Yeah, it'll be fun! I bet I see everything!*

Preschoolers' monologues might serve as self-guidance, as they talk to themselves while concentrating on a task. This is not unlike adults who "coach" themselves through a problem by talking aloud to themselves. While concentrating on a coloring book, a child verbalizes through some difficult decisions with, *Grass is green, mostly. But I'm gonna put in brown for the dirt. In between the grasses.*

In another type of monologue, **affect expressive monologues,** preschoolers might talk to themselves to express their feelings. Falling asleep

---

functional stimulus   A stimulus that is causally related to the occurrence of a behavior.

Recall that Skinner recognized this concept and referred to it as *multiple causation.* This is described in Chapter 4. ■

Piaget also referred to these types of private speech as *egocentric speech.* These noncommunicative utterances might be characterized as children talking to themselves aloud. ■

monologue   An instance of private speech in which children talk to themselves during play or to reflect on their emotional state.

affect expressive monologues   Instances in which preschoolers' talk to themselves as they reflect on their emotions.

at nap time, a child might quietly verbalize, wandering from thought to thought, *I love Mommy. Mommy hugs. I love Daddy. He laughs. I love Felix cuz he licks my nose. Don't like carrots!*

collective monologue   A phenomenon in which children playing in proximity of each other talk simultaneously but not necessarily to each other.

A **collective monologue** is a somewhat more socialized mode of conversation. These typically occur when several preschoolers are playing in each other's presence. Note how this differs from playing "with each other." Although the children take turns talking as though they are engaged in conversation, the content of each child's utterance is independent of those produced by the other children. As each child narrates his or her own play activity, there is simply a collection of monologues.

associated monologue A mode of play behavior in which children playing together contribute individual monologues related to the same topic.

Associated monologue is characterized by preschoolers' increased socialization in that each child in the situation contributes an individual monologue related to some central topic. The utterances all generally hinge on the same overall topic so that the preschoolers are at least talking about the same topic. However, each child's utterances are still not directly related to or contingent on any other child's preceding utterance. As a result, there is no apparent intention to convey information or to influence anyone else's behavior in the group.

socialized speech Speech that is addressed to others and acknowledges their needs and interests.

Eventually, preschoolers will exhibit more **socialized speech** in which they increasingly acknowledge their partners' utterances and begin to show a greater concern for the actual transmission of information. That is, they are more conscious of not being understood or failing to understand. This increasing responsiveness to their partner's language is reflected in the changing nature of preschoolers' responses. For example, from 21 to 36 months of age the proportion of contingent responses (those directly related to the current topic) increases significantly while noncontingent (unrelated) and imitative responses decrease proportionately (Bloom, Rocissano, & Hood, 1976).

Primitive speech acts, in the form of distinctive gestures, vocalizations, and eventually words, are introduced in Chapter 6. ■

The socialized speech of preschoolers will continue to serve the functions that emerged as primitive speech acts. Preschoolers continue to request action, request answers, call, greet, protest, and so forth. However, preschoolers develop increasingly sophisticated ways of managing these interactions verbally.

Symbolic play is an important aspect of the symbolic function described by Piaget and discussed in Chapter 3. ■

symbolic play   Play behavior in which one item is used to represent another.

Play Behavior.   Following the observations and writings of Piaget, the relationship between play and language has been studied by many researchers. (Fortunately, preschoolers cooperate by providing ample opportunities for their research!) Piaget and others have suggested that play behavior may provide a basic connection between cognition and language.

Symbolic play, in which the child allows one thing (e.g., a block) to represent another (a car), has been thought to be of particular importance. This appears to be closely related to children's development of the symbolic function in which words serve as symbols to stand for things. At more advanced stages of language, however, play behavior appears to provide other learning opportunities (Patterson & Westby, 1994). These opportunities include assimilating new information, developing abstract thought, and, of present interest, the uses of language through social interaction.

There appear to be three levels of play that can be differentiated on the basis of social interaction (Lane & Molyneaux, 1992). The first level involves the least amount of social interaction. This is called **solitary play,** in which the child plays independently, even if other children are present.

The second level of play, **parallel play,** consists of children playing near one another, perhaps using similar items in the same way, but not really playing with each other. Although there is a closer social connection in parallel play, it is not fully socialized in the sense of exchanging ideas or influencing each other's activity.

Finally, the third and most socialized level is **cooperative play,** in which children interact with each other in organizing and executing the structure of an activity. For example, in cooperative play children will negotiate who will play each role, the sequence of activities, and the story line, if indeed there is one. At this level, children's play is frequently based on pretending to be in social roles (mother, father, etc.) and real-life circumstances (going to work, making supper, etc.). Of course, just as often, the play may center on imaginary characters (Care Bears, Spider-Man, etc.) and fantasy tales of villains and heroes.

solitary play Play behavior in which a child plays independent of others, even those in close proximity.

parallel play Instances in which children engage in similar play activity in proximity to one another but do not actually interact.

cooperative play Play behavior in which children interact in organized goal-directed ways.

Play develops progressively and the levels overlap. Solitary play develops earlier with parallel play evolving as a transition toward cooperative play. However, children continue to exhibit solitary and parallel play throughout their preschool years. The progression of play behavior appears to reflect advances in social, cognitive, motor, and language skills. Conversely, it also provides a multitude of opportunities for these skills to develop further.

It is likely that playing is a universal behavior with children in all cultures. In some cultures, heavy chores are required of children. Yet children reportedly find ways to include play activities as they carry out their work. It has been suggested in some studies that the character of children's play in non-Western cultures is less abstract. However, others have cautioned that the bias of observers who are unfamiliar with a culture might cause them to miss the complexity in children's play behavior. More research is needed while applying culturally objective definitions and observational techniques (Patterson & Westby, 1994).

Dore's Conversational Acts

As toddlers, children's primary goals had been simply to obtain a desired object or engage their caregiver's attention. As preschoolers, they are not simply interested in obtaining the object or its label. They are curious about its uses, how to describe it, and perhaps the chance to use it. In addition, they are increasingly aware of the "give and take" in communication. The ability to "play the game" by verbally signaling the beginning, the direction, and the end of a conversation.

Dore (1978) developed a classification scheme for analyzing what he called **conversational acts** which serve various functions in discourse. These functions are evolved beyond those served by primitive speech acts (PSAs). Dore proposed that a conversational act is composed of grammatical form (the utterance), propositional content (its meaning), and an illocutionary function (the intended effect).

conversational acts Dore's classification of functions served by utterances within discourse.

Compare the nature of conversational acts and Skinner's verbal operants (e.g., mands, tacts), described in Chapter 4. ■

As can be seen in Table 7–2, the classes of conversational acts generally evolve out of the more primitive functions served in earlier communicative behaviors. This might be seen by comparing the underlying nature of the acts classified as PSAs and conversational acts. For example, the two most frequent PSAs, *requesting action* and *requesting answer,* are combined to become the most commonly occurring conversational act, *requests.*

The PSA *labeling,* which consisted of one-word responses, appears to evolve into the conversational acts of *descriptions* and *statements.* One-word responses to adult questions, classified as *answering* in PSAs, might evolve into more elaborate conversational acts called *responses to requests* and *acknowledgments.* The PSAs *calling* and *greeting* are elaborated into other forms that regulate the flow of interaction and conversations called organizational devices. The PSA classified as *protests* may evolve into more sophisticated forms, called *performatives,* that accomplish their purposes (e.g., protesting, complaining, or teasing) just by being uttered.

Table 7–2. Categories of Dore's Conversational Acts.

Conversational Act	Definition
Requests	Requesting information, actions, confirmation, clarification, permission, or acknowledgment from the listener.
Responses to requests	Responding to requests for information, confirmation, clarification, repetitions.
Descriptions	Providing information about events; labels and descriptions of objects, events, and persons.
Statements	Stating assertions, attitudes, feelings, beliefs, instructions, predications, inferences about other's feelings and explanations about causes.
Acknowledgments	Recognizing others' responses and requests, statements of approval/disapproval or agreement/disagreement.
Organization devices	Managing conversational beginnings, endings, and junctures, including addresses and polite forms.
Performatives	Producing utterances that perform their function by being uttered, such as teasing, joking, cautioning, and complaining.
Miscellaneous	Utterances that cannot be classified because they are unintelligible, incomplete, or unusual.

Note. Adapted from "Variation in Preschool Children's Conversational Performances," by J. Dore, 1978, in *Children's Language,* Vol. 1, pp. 397–444, by K. Nelson (Ed.), New York: Gardner Press.

Interestingly, two PSAs, *repeating* and *practicing,* do not have counterparts in conversational acts. This is fitting, however, as it appears that the frequency of imitation decreases as utterance length increases (Bloom et al., 1976). Certainly, these behaviors continue to occur, but are probably less functional in engaging the caregiver.

A number of useful schemes for classifying and analyzing children's discourse have been developed. These are presented in some detail elsewhere (Lund & Duchan, 1993; Retherford, 1993). Dore's conversational acts carry a descriptive quality that captures the character of children's utterances. However, several other conversational skills for discourse have been observed and described in the literature on children's language development. These are significant because they illustrate preschoolers' refinement of language use as their social skills mature.

Discourse Skills—the Conversation Game

Generally, *discourse* (or conversation) is thought of as a series of successive utterances shared by at least two persons. However, whether or not discourse results in true communication will rely on the extent to which each successive utterance is relevant and additive in adding information pertinent to the previous utterances. The accumulated utterances in a conversation should "stick together" and "add something new."

Cohesion refers to the relatedness of successive utterances in discourse. Researchers have described various behaviors that contribute to cohesion in discourse (Lund & Duchan, 1993). These include topic introduction, turn taking, presupposition, and topic maintenance.

cohesion The relatedness of successive utterances in discourse.

Topic Introduction.   Even as their language skills evolve, preschoolers' motor skills continue to serve them well in establishing topics of conversation. Preschoolers seek out, grasp, carry, and demonstrate those things that are topics of interest even more efficiently than they did as toddlers. However, as their verbal abilities develop, topics introduced into conversation by preschoolers are increasingly clarified with words and the accompanying gestures become less elaborate. Younger preschoolers may still rely heavily on physically bringing topics to their listener's attention (perhaps by gesturing with them or placing them on the listener's lap). However, in contrast to toddlers, preschoolers will more effectively label them or comment on them as they do so. Eventually, more verbally advanced, older preschoolers can rely solely on verbal comments to introduce a topic that is not in the present situation.

For younger preschoolers, conversations will frequently begin by addressing their listener to establish an audience. Even though they are nearby, caregivers frequently hear *Mommy?* or *Daddy?* at the outset of each exchange. If necessary, preschoolers will address their partner numerous times (*Mommy . . . Mommy . . . Mommy. . . .*) to be certain the person is attending. In contrast, when unable to "get the floor," older preschoolers learn to stop, wait for the next break, and then repeat their bid for an audience.

The conversations of younger preschoolers frequently center on familiar routines and objects. They may assert a topic by producing labels for objects, the objects' features, or their functions. Younger preschoolers converse to confirm action sequences or items involved in a familiar activity. These conversations generally follow a question-and-answer format. Interviews of caregivers on certain topics may be revisited frequently.

This familiarity with routine topics presents an interesting paradox. Normally, the purpose of a conversation between mature speakers is to share new information. Adults usually avoid telling each other things they already know or things that are apparent from the immediate situation. However, children frequently initiate topics with comments on information that is obvious (as in the "here-and-now") or with questions to which they already know the answers (Bloom & Lahey, 1978).

If these early conversations do not cover new information, what is their purpose? They may be produced merely for the sake of practice, with the caregiver's attention serving as feedback for new skills. Or, perhaps many of these conversations are intended to gain the parent's attention and interaction. The practice and feedback that result are just the natural and beneficial consequences of doing so.

The daily routines that provide the setting events for these conversations and play-by-play commentaries provide familiar contexts. These contexts provide a framework that supports and guides the conversations of younger preschoolers. As they become older, preschoolers may extend conversations by exploring likes and dislikes, ownership of objects, recall of recent events, and so forth. Additionally, older preschoolers begin to recognize and express emotions in themselves and others. Accordingly, conversational topics may begin to increasingly include inner states, attitudes, and feelings.

Turn Taking.   By definition, a conversation requires that two people take turns exchanging information on the current topic. Two obvious principles apply. First, if neither partner waits for a turn, their utterances will collide and little information will actually be shared. Perhaps surprisingly, this is rarely a problem between preschoolers and their caregivers. Even young preschoolers are sensitive to the need for taking turns in conversations and rarely interrupt their partner (Owens, 2005).

A second principle is that the more information each partner can share on a topic, the more conversational turns are possible. For most of us, the number of conversational turns would reflect that we have little knowledge to share on nuclear physics or paleontology, but most of us can contribute more on sports, politics, food, or movies.

Accordingly, preschoolers generally exhibit more turns per topic as their experience base and cognitive abilities expand. Expanded understanding of objects, events, and relationships combined with more words to express this information leads to an increasing number of turns (Bloom et al, 1976). One to two turns per topic would be typical in conversations with

The seemingly natural sense for turn taking in toddlers and preschoolers should not be surprising. Recall that Chapters 3 and 5 describe the turn taking that was occurring in the earliest days of infancy. These interactions in feeding sessions were even referred to as *protoconversations.* ∎

2- and 3-year-olds. However, on average, older preschoolers may produce as many as five turns per topic (Brinton & Fujiki, 1984).

In addition to the role of experience, the familiarity of topics and settings will influence the length of a conversation. For younger preschoolers, there may be more total turns in conversations centered on familiar routines, objects, or play sequences. The support of specific cues in familiar stimuli that are present will influence how much is available to be recalled and discussed. In contrast, new settings and experiences may only prompt standard requests for labels, roles, and relationships, as in *What that? What it do? Who's it is?*

Finally, another significant development that occurs is the preschooler's increased responsiveness to cues for turn taking. Beyond relying on conspicuous pauses, they become increasingly sophisticated at reading and using the more subtle cues for signaling turns, such as their partners' intonation, gaze, eye contact, and body language.

Presupposition. *Presupposition* is the ability of speakers to judge their listener's language abilities, experiences, and awareness of relevant information. Presupposition is actually demonstrated when speakers adjust their message for these considerations. This involves three types of perspective taking, or how individuals understand each situation (Geller, 1989). First, *linguistic perspective taking* involves our ability to adjust our language based on being able to gauge the language level of the listener. Second, *cognitive perspective taking* requires making judgments about the listener's level of understanding of the topic at hand. And, third, *perceptual perspective taking* involves the ability to infer what the listener is capable of perceiving (feeling, seeing, hearing, etc.) in the circumstances.

In introducing a topic, we generally make some assumptions regarding our listener's familiarity with the topic. As a result, mature speakers gauge how much information should be provided as they initiate a topic. As speakers, we can commit two different errors. First, by presupposing too little we may provide too much information. This might insult or bore our listeners. Second, presupposing too much and providing too little information may confuse or frustrate our listeners. Preschoolers usually commit the latter of these two errors.

Younger preschoolers are notorious for asserting information for which there is no apparent context. A young preschooler rushing in the door, blurting out something like, *She took mine. Now it's gone!* is not an uncommon experience for caregivers. Frequently, caregivers must follow with an in-depth "cross-examination" to determine exactly what crisis has occurred outside.

Beyond the age of 3, most preschoolers generally demonstrate improving presuppositional skills. There are several specific aspects that are indicative of maturing presuppositional skills. These include the emergence of anaphoric reference, deixis, grammatical ellipsis, and style shifting. As these emerge, they reflect not only preschoolers' growing linguistic abilities,

By the time we reach adulthood, some of us may average 11 utterances per topic. Aspects of adult language are discussed in Chapter 9. ■

The development of presupposition has also been related to decreasing egocentrism. Children are gradually becoming capable of "stepping into another's shoes" and seeing things from his or her perspective. ■

but also their social maturation and their cognitive ability to understand situations from someone else's perspective.

anaphoric reference
The linguistic effect in which pronouns replace nouns or noun phrases and refer to their occurrence earlier in the context.

The first of these aspects, **anaphoric reference,** is the role pronouns play in referring back to words that occurred just prior to them. In the sentence, *The boy ran and he fell down,* the pronoun *he* refers back to *The boy.* Pronouns rely on anaphoric reference for their meaning, because by themselves they have no established referent. Most words have specific referents that generally do not change. The word *toy* refers to an individual item or at least a single class of items defined by certain characteristics. However, pronouns such as *he, she, they,* and *it* are less direct or specific. They must refer to someone or something mentioned previously.

Pronoun development is discussed in more detail in Chapter 8. ■

When a child entering from the next room utters, *It broke!,* the referent for the word *it* is not immediately apparent. Unless the setting event that prompted this utterance is known, for most caregivers, determining what *it* means will be an urgent concern. In contrast, the child who presupposes what the caregiver may need to know about the context precedes this with, *Tommy took my toy.* Given the context for *It broke!* the word *It* makes anaphoric reference to the toy and aids the caregiver's comprehension.

A second related behavior that also reflects the developing ability to consider another person's perspective is *deixis,* in which words "point to" their referent according to the speaker's perspective. Words that are interpreted according to who spoke them are referred to as deictic words. For example, the meaning of each member of deictic word pairs such as *I/you, my/your, this/that, these/those,* and *here/there* can be interpreted differently depending on who said them. To illustrate, consider two people who are conversing while sitting in chairs across the room from each other. If one says, *I think this chair is more attractive than that chair,* the words *this* and *that* point to different chairs depending on which person expressed this opinion.

Preschoolers appear to go through several phases in learning that these words can have contrasting meanings (Clark & Sengul, 1978). Younger preschoolers may first use each member of a deictic pair interchangeably, using either *this* or *that* to call attention to an item regardless of whether they are pointing across the room or holding something out to the caregiver. Initially, preschoolers have learned from the caregiver's own use of these terms that they are used to direct attention. Subsequently, it is as though preschoolers know both terms (i.e., *this, that*) are related to the spatial distinction they are attempting to signal, but they are uncertain which term applies. In these earlier instances, preschoolers may rely heavily on accompanying gestures to signal the meaning of the deictic term. In the next phase, preschoolers may more frequently use one member of the pair correctly, but then overgeneralize it to incorrect instances. Finally, the terms are used discriminatively by preschoolers according to the setting event.

Generally, the pronoun contrasts (*I/you, my/your*) appear to be mastered earlier than the spatial contrasts (*this/that, these/those, here/there*). It has been speculated that this is because the pronoun contrasts are limited to more specific alternatives; that is, in most instances, the speaker and the listener in the situation are the only choices. By 30 months, most preschoolers use these pronoun deictic terms discriminatively (Owens, 2005).

In contrast, because they are based on proximity, the spatial contrasts are relative. For example, *here* essentially means "somewhere nearby" and, in contrast, *there* means "somewhere farther away." Depending on the context, then, *here* could mean "next to me" (as in, *Come, sit here*), "in this city" (as in, *We like our barbecue spicy here*) or "in this country" (as in, *I'm thankful we have freedom of speech here*). Of course, the corresponding contrasts for *there* are also relative. These relative contrasts are ambiguous, making the spatial contrasts more difficult to discriminate. Accordingly, it is perhaps not surprising that the age of mastery among these spatial deictic terms appears to vary from 4 to 7 years of age (Owens, 2005).

The third aspect of language behavior reflects preschoolers' developing awareness of their listener's knowledge of the context. **Grammatical ellipsis** is a device speakers use to eliminate information where it can be assumed that listeners are aware of it. Grammatical ellipsis may occur under either of two conditions. First, the information may have been provided in the linguistic context, having been just expressed by one of the partners. Second, the necessary information may be apparent in the nonlinguistic context, simply because it is available to both partners in the present circumstances.

grammatical ellipsis
Linguistic device in which speakers eliminate information apparent to listeners from the context.

In grammatical ellipsis, speakers assume that their listener's awareness of the linguistic or nonlinguistic context "fills in" the missing information in their utterance. For example, when a teenager asks in a panic, *Where's my homework?* a hurried parent can efficiently respond, *On the table.* Given the linguistic context of the teen's preceding question, the parent's utterance (*On the table*) is easily interpreted by the teenager as if it was preceded by *Your homework is.* Similarly, if a friend follows her neighbor to a window as she checks on her husband working in the backyard, the friend's question, *What's Bill doing?* can be answered simply, *Planting flowers.* Had the same question been posed over the telephone, more information, as in *Planting flowers in the backyard,* might have been necessary. Grammatical ellipsis is a complex process because it relies on understanding what information can and cannot be left out in a given situation with different listeners (Bloom & Lahey, 1978).

Grammatical ellipsis in preschoolers' language might also result in partial utterances. That is, one of the major constituent elements (subject-verb-complement) would be omitted, as in producing *Boy hit* (versus *Boy hit ball*). Preschoolers frequently produce such partial utterances that may be evidence of grammatical ellipsis. However, these would only qualify as elliptical if they are semantically related to the previous utterance. Prior to 3 years of age, this is generally not the case, indicating that younger preschoolers may not commonly use grammatical ellipsis. Older preschoolers, following the adult models around them, may attempt ellipsis. However, because of its complexity, it emerges only gradually after 3 years of age and may not be mastered until the school-age years (Bloom, Miller, & Hood, 1975).

style shifting
Modifications in style speakers make in response to social contexts or the status of their listeners.

Style shifting is also considered in Chapter 10 as an aspect of dialects and their variations. ■

Finally, the fourth aspect of developing language that demonstrates the preschooler's ability to infer information about the listener is **style shifting,** in which speakers modify how something is said based on the status of their listeners. The status of listeners might vary based on their age, familiarity, present role, and their assumed willingness to comply with a request. This would be illustrated by contrasting how we might ask someone at home to close a nearby window because we are chilly and how we might accomplish the same goal while interviewing in the office of a prospective employer.

Requests can be made in several ways. In the situation described previously, we might use a direct request (*Close the window*) with a more familiar listener. However, with a prospective employer, if we were chilly enough, we might soften this to a polite direct request (*I wonder if you would mind closing the window, please*). We might even attempt to convey our need through an indirect request, such as, *That wind sure feels like winter's on the way, doesn't it?* However, if we are hungry enough and intimidated by our prospective boss, we might say nothing, hoping that our goose bumps do the talking for us.

In preschoolers, style shifting first becomes apparent in the emergence of simple polite forms. Of course, the earliest polite form, *Please,* probably appears first under specific circumstances due to being prompted by the caregiver. It is possible that toddlers and younger preschoolers view this cued response as more of a practical device than a social nicety. However, its significance as a polite form may be more evident as *Please* appears more spontaneously in varied circumstances.

Later, with developing language abilities and a maturing sense of their listener's perspective, preschoolers as young as 3 years old begin to use modal auxiliaries (*Can you . . .? Would you . . .? Do you wanna . . ?*) to soften their polite direct requests. By the time they are 5, preschoolers have become quite sophisticated with indirect requests that take the form of justifications for the desired goal (*I played so hard, I need some ice cream to cool off*). Some have already learned that complimentary indirect requests are especially welcome to listeners, as in *Your cookies make the house smell so good!* (Flattery will get you somewhere sometimes!)

Topic Maintenance. To qualify as discourse, successive utterances should be related to the same topic. Speakers' ability to continue conversational topics by contributing comments related to their partners' last utterance is called **topic maintenance.** Topic maintenance is the conversational equivalent of returning the ball in bounds in tennis. As long as each partner's next utterance is related to the current topic (remains in bounds), that conversation (or point) continues. Similarly, the ability to contribute a greater number of conversational turns (or volleys) generally increases as the child's conversational skills improve.

topic maintenance The continuation of a topic in discourse through successive utterances related to that topic.

Topic maintenance has been measured in terms of contingency, the relatedness of an utterance to the preceding utterance (Lund & Duchan, 1993).

A contingent utterance depends on or "hinges on" the preceding utterance. Two types of contingency are possible, contextual contingency and linguistic contingency (Bloom & Lahey, 1978).

Utterances that share similar semantic information are *contextually contingent*. For example, in response to a caregiver's statement such as, *I think I'll bake some cookies,* the preschooler's supportive statement, *I find chocolate chips,* is semantically related. In contrast, utterances that overlap in topic and also share linguistic forms would be *linguistically contingent*. For example, following a caregiver's announcement, *It's time for bed,* a preschooler's response, *It story time,* is contextually and linguistically contingent.

The ability to maintain the topic through contextual and linguistic contingency probably improves with preschoolers' development in other areas. Preschoolers' additional experiences and expanding cognitive abilities permit responding with semantically related information through contextual contingency. Their expanding vocabulary and grammatical ability allow them to extend conversations by responding with forms that overlap with their partner's utterances through linguistic contingency.

Whereas toddlers generally could achieve only a turn or two in familiar circumstances, preschoolers are responsive to topics introduced by their partners. By 3½ years of age, a majority of preschoolers' utterances are on the topic established in their partner's previous utterance (Bloom et al., 1976). Furthermore, with additional experience, many 5-year-olds can maintain a topic for 10 or more turns (Garvey & Hogan, 1973) even though they are generally likely to change topics rapidly (Brinton & Fujiki, 1984).

An aspect of discourse related to topic maintenance is conversational repairs. *Conversational repairs* are behaviors that result in clarification of previous utterances and thus help maintain the flow of accurate information in a conversation. Conversational repairs can be initiated by either partner, depending on who is confused by an utterance.

The most common form of requesting a conversational repair is a contingent query. A *contingent query* is a request by the listener for additional information or clarification from the speaker. These might be nonverbal, in the form of facial expressions or body language. They might be neutral and nonspecific, as in *Huh?* or *What?* Or, they can be more specific, as in *What do you mean by "never"?*

In general, preschoolers do not frequently request conversational repairs from their adult partners. They may lack the skills to do so or be unwilling to indicate that the adult's message was flawed (Gallagher, 1981). On those occasions when they do signal the need for conversational repair, younger preschoolers' contingent queries may tend to take the form of quizzical or confused facial expressions. With experience, they become more likely to use the verbal forms of general contingent queries mentioned before. Only when they have advanced to a metalinguistic level, at which they can ask questions about specific words and phrases or relate specific words or phrases to information that is unclear, will they be able to specifically question their partner to clarify details.

Metalinguistic ability, discussed in Chapter 1, refers to the ability to evaluate a message objectively and determine whether it has been effective. ■

When their partner requests clarification, younger preschoolers are most likely to simply repeat what they just said, especially in response to nonspecific queries (Anselmi, Tomasello, & Acunzo, 1986). These repetitions will occasionally involve some minor revisions. Initially, younger preschoolers might make a phonetic modification in a word, changing *I hug bear* to *I hub bear,* seeming to respond simply to the sense that something in their previous utterance was not correct. Later, preschoolers may respond by omitting an element from their previous utterance, as in revising *I hug bear* to *Hug bear.* Finally, preschoolers begin to substitute increasingly elaborate forms to clarify, as in changing *I hug bear* to *Hug my red one.*

Eventually, some contingent queries from adult partners will be more selective in the information they request. For example, queries involving who, how, when, and where request details regarding the participants, methods, timing, and location of an event being discussed. The ability to provide more specific repairs that clarify the information requested by the form of the contingent query develops later during the school-age years. Again, being able to do so requires some metalinguistic ability to analyze the components of a message to determine where the confusion has occurred.

Summary

- Development in preschoolers' motor, cognitive, and social abilities provides much of the momentum that propels their language development.

- As preschoolers' understanding and recall of their experiences develop, the setting events or contexts for their conversations expand beyond the "here-and-now."

- Preschoolers' social and play behaviors place increasing demands on their developing language skills.

- Preschoolers develop discourse skills such as topic initiation and maintenance, turn taking, and presupposition to manage their conversations.

Preschoolers' Storytelling

A major theme in examining language development has focused on children's use of language to communicate their practical needs and wants. However, as children's social interactions evolve, language also serves beyond the practical acquisition of objects or actions.

Children's ability to gain the attention of those around them, whether as toddlers or preschoolers, is always a prerequisite for communicating their goals. However, on occasion preschoolers' primary goal may be to attain their caregiver's attention. The object they request is perhaps just a useful pretext for engaging the caregiver.

As children grow, explore, and accumulate experience, they simultaneously develop the ability to share their experiences through language. As a result, they develop an expanded means of engaging their caregivers' attention through narrative discourse or storytelling. Children find that not only do their stories gain the attention of the most important people around them, but their stories entertain them as well. In turn, caregivers' responses to such entertainment generally encourages more storytelling.

The Nature of Narrative Discourse

As the nature of discourse evolves, different styles are associated with different circumstances. These styles or types of discourse are called **genres** (Lund & Duchan, 1993). Some genres or types of discourse, such as conversations, discussions, arguments, and negotiations, require the participation of at least two people. However, some genres can be carried out by one person. Examples would include delivering lectures or sermons, giving descriptions, and telling jokes or stories (although an audience is helpful).

    Generally, at least five different discourse genres have been characterized by researchers. These include conversations, expositions, quizzes, descriptions, and narratives (Lund & Duchan, 1993). A property common to each of these is that they are all based on a schema. The *schema* is the underlying structure or organization of the interaction that the speaker and listener use to anticipate, understand, and organize the information being exchanged—their "mental set," if you will. For example, in delivering a lecture, the instructor assumes that the information is either not available or fully understood by the students. Conversely, the students should assume that the information is important, beyond serving as the source of test questions.

    Narratives have been defined as a minimum of two independent clauses produced in succession relating to a single event (Labov, 1972). Of course, this allows a range of possibilities that qualify as narratives, from the simplest of personal tales (*I was really tired last night. But, I slept great!*) to a monumental novel (e.g., Tolstoy's *War and Peace*). There are four major genres or types of narratives: recounts, eventcasts, accounts, and stories (Heath, 1986).

    Recounts report a past experience, usually in a chronological "blow-by-blow" manner. These are likely to occur in response to the proverbial question, "How did your day go?"

    An **eventcast** is a narrative that "sets the stage" by describing roles, relationships, and recent events that define a situation. In drama, it is the "stop-action framing" that sets the scene (*As Milicent enters, Marville is hanging up the phone after just hearing of Marlowe's demise*). In children's social role play, eventcasts define relationships and their qualities (*Remember, you have to talk like a mommy*).

    Accounts share experiences in a more detailed manner. These usually go beyond the chronological sequencing of events found in recounts, providing more of the individual's evaluation and interpretation of the events. Someone might spontaneously provide an account of how the last Thanksgiving dinner went, including who was and was not there, whether the gravy was too thick or the dressing too dry, and why relatives should never discuss politics!

genres Styles of classifications of discourse that occur in different circumstances.

narratives A series of utterances that relates an event or idea.

recounts A type of narrative that relates a series of events.

eventcast A type of narrative that relates the characters, roles, and relationships related to a situation.

account A type of narrative in which the speaker evaluates and interprets the significance of events.

Narratives, in contrast, are examples of **decontextualized language,** which refers to language about objects, people, and events that are not in the immediate context. There are two modes of thought that might be conveyed by decontextualized language. The *paradigmatic mode* represents academic, logical, and orderly thought. Examples of language reflecting paradigmatic thought include textbooks, classroom language, academic reports, and so on. In contrast, the *narrative mode* of thought emphasizes human interactions and goals. As such, the particular tone and style of the language reflects the personal perspective of the storyteller (Ely, 1997).

The fact that narratives are based on decontextualized language makes their development heavily dependent on the child's cognitive development. A narrative requires recall of settings, characters, and events apart from their immediate presence. The timing and sequence of events, and even the causal relationships among them must be understood by the storyteller.

Paradoxically, younger preschoolers, still struggling with these cognitive tasks, may get little help from their partners as they attempt their earliest stories. Because narratives are decontextualized language, caregivers will not necessarily know much about the context for the story. As a result, they are often unable to assist their preschoolers by prompting for relevant information. In spite of these early challenges for preschoolers and their audiences, the foundation for later, more complex narratives continues to develop throughout the preschool years.

Narrative Levels. The most basic forms of stories develop in preschoolers after 2 years of age and occur frequently by the time they are 3½ years of age. More often than not, preschoolers' earliest stories deal briefly and simply with some recent event that made a strong impression on them. These earliest stories have been called **protonarratives** (Miller & Sperry, 1988) or **prenarratives** (Westby, 1984). The primitive schema exhibited in these protonarratives have been analyzed into levels that progress toward mature narratives (Applebee, 1978; Westby, 1984).

The earliest protonarratives exhibit a characteristic organizational structure (or, more accurately, a lack of organizational structure). These protonarratives are termed **heaps,** suggesting that they are collections of seemingly unrelated elements. In a heap, there is no apparent relationship among the elements that are labeled and described in a series of simple declarative sentences. A heap story might sound like the following:

> There's a truck. The man has a red hat. This is smoke. I see a dog. That dog has spots. And here's a car and a bike.

Heaps generally emerge by approximately 30 months of age. It should be noted that, as with many areas of development, proceeding to the next level of organization does not mean that the previous levels cease to occur. In fact, some might note a striking resemblance between preschoolers' heap stories and many "stream of consciousness" novels (with apologies to James Joyce and Virginia Woolf).

decontextualized language Utterances that refer to objects, people, events, and relationships outside the immediate context.

protonarratives (or **prenarratives**) The earliest forms of children's stories.

heaps An early form of children's narrative in which unrelated elements are told in unorganized collections.

The relationships between story elements in these and later developing narratives are discussed in Chapter 8. ∎

sequences (or **chaining**) Early narratives that relate heaps of elements that are related to a central topic.

The next level of protonarratives emerges around 3 years of age and has been called **sequences** or **chaining.** In sequences, preschoolers produce a collection of story elements just as in heaps. In contrast to heaps, the elements in sequences do all relate to a central topic. In addition, the elements in sequences appear to be temporally related. However, they are not necessarily sequenced chronologically. Instead, each successive element (or each link in the chain) has some feature that overlaps with the preceding one. For example, a preschooler exhibiting a sequence (or chain) following a visit to the zoo might relate the experience as follows:

> The lion lives in a cave. The seal has a cave where he swims. And the monkey has trees in his cage. And the birds do, too. And, the hippo has a giant bathtub!

The elements in sequences appear to relate to a core topic according to attributes that are perceptually similar in some way. In the previous example, the elements are physically related to animal habitats. However, remember that the term "sequencing" may be a misnomer for such narratives. That is, these may only give the appearance of following a chronological order. The previous example may seem to approximate some order of animal exhibits. However, it does not necessarily mean that the preschooler attempted to recount any particular order in the story.

primitive narratives (or **centering**)   Narratives in which story elements are related in a conceptual way, but otherwise unorganized.

The next level, referred to as **primitive narratives** or **centering,** emerges around 4 years of age. Like sequences (or chains), primitive narratives generally have an identifiable theme that provides some overall organization. However, whereas the elements in sequence stories resemble each other in some perceptual way, the elements in primitive narratives are connected to the core topic in a conceptual manner. In primitive narratives, the elements center on connections between intrinsic qualities or feelings (e.g., goodness, anger, loneliness) and the events that apparently relate to them.

At this level, preschoolers begin to demonstrate the basic ability to infer information. For example, a person who is lonely will look a certain way and do certain things. A brief example of such a primitive narrative might go as follows:

> There were these lost children. They were alone and hungry in the forest. And they were scared. They cried and held their tummies and watched out for animals. And, their moms and dads were sad, too. They looked everywhere for the children. When the moms and dads found them, everyone laughed and hugged. And, they all went home to have supper.

Although preschoolers telling primitive narratives do see the relationship between circumstances and inner states, they do not yet fully understand cause-effect relationships. As a result, preschoolers may not be able to project the possible outcomes that could result from the characters' actions. The sequence of events in the previous example represents a story of sorts. Yet, there is no overall plot based on events that caused the story's circumstances or prompted a resolution (Westby, 1984).

Summary

- Verbal interactions such as discourse and narratives exhibit organizational structure called schema.

- Because narratives are examples of language produced apart from its original context they are referred to as decontextualized language.

- Preschoolers' narratives evolve from stories characterized as heaps to chaining to those that exhibit centering.

Semantic Development

The linguistic component of meaning in language is perhaps the least understood. Semantics, the study of meaning, takes into account individual meanings of words, or their *lexical meaning.* It also encompasses the relationships between words, their *semantic roles.*

Preschool children will evidence significant developments in both of these dimensions. Seemingly without effort, they will learn new words daily. Similarly, they will begin to combine words in ways that reliably indicate the relationships that they perceive among the objects and events around them.

> Semantics, the study of word meanings and word relations, is discussed as an aspect of language in Chapter 1 and as one theoretical basis for language learning in Chapter 4. ■

Word Meanings

How individual words gain their lexical meanings is not well understood by researchers. The histories of most word origins are quite long and meanings change slowly. In everyday use, we rarely concern ourselves with the history of a word. When we look up a word in a dictionary, the dictionary's copyright year is not normally of great concern to us. For the most part, the definitions in past dictionaries have been carried over to subsequent editions with little modification. The formal definitions for words might change depending on cultural influences, but this process is generally so slow that we are not aware of it.

As individuals, few of us are acutely aware of the subtle changes that might occur in individual word meanings. For even the most mature speaker, a given word may evolve to eventually carry several meanings based on that individual's experiences with that word. This transient, shifting nature of word meanings is especially evident in children's early vocabularies. Initially, the infant's first attempts at producing words may be more "vocal gestures" (sounds that accompany reaching and pointing) than true words carrying lexical meaning. Later, as a toddler, new words begin to occur apart from gestures, but their

The study of word histories, called *etymology,* can be fascinating. Many modern words have unexpected origins. For example, *Webster's Word Histories* (1991) explains that the word *gossip* comes from the Old English word *godsipp,* which meant godmother or godfather. Apparently, the word for someone close enough to you to provide spiritual guidance eventually referred to someone who also knows your deepest secrets—and shares them!

> The shifting meanings of toddlers' early words and the theories proposed to explain the underlying processes are discussed in Chapter 6. ■

meanings may still be unstable, shifting as the toddler focuses on different aspects of their referents.

Toddlers' first words appear to be responses that simply occur in close association with the gestures, items, or actions they have accompanied in the past. Some have characterized this early connection as words serving as *signs* for their referent. Later, those words occur in new situations with new people and, most important, in the absence of the items to which they refer. At that point, most agree that words "carry meaning" and have attained the status of a *symbol*.

Preschoolers' semantic development is closely coupled with developments in motor, social, and cognitive abilities. The interrelations among these domains should be apparent. As preschoolers' motor skills become more fully developed, they are better able to explore their environment and examine the things they find around them. At the same time, their maturing social skills and pragmatic language abilities typically allow them to at least temporarily obtain those things that interest them. Their growing language abilities allow them to comment on and inquire about the objects with their partners. And, ultimately, their expanding cognitive abilities permit them to more efficiently organize and store all the new-found information that results from such interactions.

The metalinguistic sense of language is discussed in Chapter 1. The developments that suggest evolving metalinguistic ability are described in Chapter 8. ■

Younger preschool children are not yet truly aware that words have lexical meanings, at least in the traditional sense of dictionary definitions. That is, they may not recognize that a word can exist apart from its meaning or that several words can share similar meanings. If a 3-year-old preschooler is asked to "say all the words that mean 'Yummy,' " the response would likely be to name a favorite snack or to simply say, "Yummy!"

Eventually, during the school-age years, children become more conscious of word meanings in the lexical sense. At a metalinguistic level, they recognize that different words share similar meanings and that the same word can carry several quite different meanings. For example, a fifth grader will typically know that the word *block* might refer to a section of land containing houses, or a unit of concrete used to build those houses, or the act of preventing someone from walking up to a house.

A helpful analogy would be to consider how much knowing a child's height tells us about that child's physical stature. Knowing how tall children are gives us only a general idea of their appearance. However, children who are all 48 inches tall, for example, can vary widely in their characteristics—body type, weight, hair color, and so forth. In the same way, two children who "know" the same number of words may use them in significantly different ways (e.g., different utterance lengths, sentence patterns, etc.) as they communicate.

Vocabulary Development

Vocabulary development is a commonly used measure of language development. Interestingly, most current researchers would question whether the ability to produce individual words (as in naming) is truly indicative of language (as in communicating ideas through sentences). However, perhaps the early interest in counting words makes some sense if we recall several traditional "rules of thumb." The first word occurs around 1 year of age and, by the time toddlers are

18 months, they will use approximately 50 words (Nelson, 1973b). Significantly, most toddlers begin combining words at this point. This relationship may have suggested the importance of learning words in relation to overall language development.

The growth of preschoolers' vocabularies is nothing short of striking. From 18 to 24 months, toddlers' expressive vocabularies expand from 50 to 200–300 words. By the end of the next year, 3-year-old preschoolers' vocabularies will triple to 900–1,000 words. By the time they head for kindergarten, usually at 5 years of age, their vocabularies will more than double to 2,100–2,200 words (Owens, 2005). Although rates will vary, children have been estimated to add new words to their expressive vocabulary at rates of two to five new words per day during the preschool years (Pease & Berko Gleason, 1985). It has also been estimated that preschoolers will learn 9 new words per day, accumulating a receptive vocabulary of as many as 14,000 words by 6 years of age (Carey, 1978).

As humans, we seem to be genetically well equipped with the motor, perceptual, and intellectual capacities required to rapidly learn complex behaviors such as language. Furthermore, perhaps our higher intelligence permits us to organize these abilities into learning sets. Actually, the entire picture may be completed by the social nature of caregivers' interaction with their children which may contribute to the development of children's capacity for "learning to learn" (Moerk, 1992a, p. 204).

Fast Mapping/Extended Mapping. We may never have a precise, objective understanding of the underlying processes that drive children's rapid vocabulary development. However, a hypothetical description of what may occur in the process of understanding new words has been suggested. It has been hypothesized that preschoolers' word learning involves two stages. The first stage is **fast mapping,** a hypothetical process in which children apparently associate a word and its referent after the initial exposure (Carey & Bartlett, 1978). Upon hearing a new word preschoolers may rapidly store some initial information—some temporary "first impressions" or associations—as to what the new word might mean.

In the second stage, **extended mapping,** this information will be gradually expanded and modified as additional experiences with that word clarifies its full meaning (Carey, 1978). This second stage might be a prolonged process, perhaps extending months or even years. And, of course, preschoolers might be simultaneously dealing with numerous words in this same way.

The research related to fast mapping in children is relatively recent and several methodological issues still need to be resolved. Nonetheless, researchers have suggested a number of factors that appear to influence how rapidly preschoolers map meaning onto a new word (Crais, 1992). These factors include each child's learning style, phonetic composition, syllable structure, situational factors, and linguistic context.

Children who exhibit a referential learning style (i.e., they tend to use words to name things) as opposed to a personal-social learning style (using

---

The difference between the sizes of expressive and receptive vocabularies also relates to the differences between the tasks of production and comprehension. This is considered in Chapter 8. ∎

fast mapping The hypothetical process in which children form initial associations when first exposed to a new word.

extended mapping The more prolonged process of modifying word meanings with additional experiences following their initial fast mapping.

words primarily for social interaction) are more likely to imitate new words. Phonetically, new words composed of phonemes already used by a child are more easily learned than words with phonemes absent from that child's phonetic inventory. In terms of syllable structure, words that consist of reduplicated syllables (e.g., /toto/) are generally learned more quickly than words consisting of nonreduplicated syllables (e.g., /fumo/).

The situational variables and linguistic context also appear to affect how quickly children learn new words as they occur (Crais, 1992). Object words are more quickly learned than action words. Of object words, those that refer to objects that are acted on in specific ways (e.g., only fry pans are used for frying) are learned more quickly. It has also been found that simultaneous pairing of the new word with its referent leads to more efficient learning for the child, as opposed to experiencing them separately. Research also suggests that children learn a new word more readily when it occurs in an unambiguous context, being the only new word with its referent more apparent (as opposed to being embedded among several new words and various referents).

In terms of linguistic context, the presence of related, familiar words (e.g., color words that are already known) makes it easier to learn new words for a new instance of that same property (e.g., a new color word). In other words, having learned *blue* and *red* means *yellow* might be learned more readily. This is an intriguing observation which Nelson (1993) described as an illustration of "the rich get richer" phenomenon. That is, knowing words facilitates learning new words (just as having money helps to make more money).

Lexical Learning Principles.   A number of researchers have speculated about the hypothetical principles that might guide children as they learn new words (Cairns, 1996). These principles describe children's patterns of responding to new words and may suggest how they have learned to interpret new words. The *principle of reference* states that children assume that words refer to the objects, events, and attributes around them. The *whole object principle* refers to the tendency for children to assume that a novel word applies to an entire object as a whole, not just parts of it.

The fact that children quickly generalize a new word to other similar objects is described by the *principle of extendibility.* In a related way, the *taxonomic principle* describes children's tendency to extend a new word to another similar object as opposed to an item merely associated with the original object. Finally, the *mutual exclusivity assumption* refers to the fact that children behave as though they assume that a new name applies to a category for which they do not yet know a name.

Creative Vocabulary.   Sometimes preschoolers produce some very interesting words that are not really words. These new words seem to fill the void somewhere between words that preschoolers have yet to experience and those they already know. Occasionally, a child is confronted with a situation in which the relevant word is simply not known or cannot be recalled, but some associated word might be. At these times, preschoolers have been observed to invent words out of these associations that seem to convey the meaning in an innovative way. These instances have been called *invented words* (Pease & Berko Gleason, 1985) and *idiomorphs* (Reich, 1986).

This phenomenon is not unique to childhood. Skinner's extended tacts, discussed in Chapter 4, explained the extension of a related word to an unfamiliar object or circumstance when a more specific label is not known. The difference is that a mature speaker would normally indicate or qualify it as an extension, as in, *It's kind of chairlike, isn't it.*

For example, children who cannot remember the word *stove* might call it a *cook-thing,* or a shovel might be called a *dig-spoon.* In a related way, children have been observed to use an object name in place of the verb for its action, as in *I knifed my sandwich in two.* (Actually, these improvisations are more useful than those by adults who apparently live in a world full of *whachamacallits* and *thingamajigs!*)

Development of Relational Terms

Preschoolers' vocabularies grow at remarkable rates as they learn to use and recognize various words, primarily for objects and actions that occur around them. We generally think of this growth as consisting of new nouns, verbs, and adjectives. However, also contributing to this growth is the development of several important groups of terms that describe relationships in more specific domains.

Preschoolers must master a number of terms that are critical to their basic understanding of day-to-day activities. Making choices, following instructions, understanding family roles, and doing things in the right order all rely on words that require some perception and experience to comprehend. Such terms are called *relational terms* because they express relationships in domains such as size, color, location, family roles, and temporal sequences. (James, 1990).

Relational terms cause some difficulty for preschoolers because, by definition, such terms do not always refer to properties that are all-or-none. In other words, as their name suggests, their properties are relative. The degree to which they are present in an object or circumstance is a matter of subjective judgment or determined by the relationships among the items in question. For example, it is unlikely that two avid gardeners will easily agree on whose roses are reddest. It is probably universal that children will disagree on whose daddy is the "biggest." The proverbial phrase, "Everything is relative" applies perfectly to these relational terms.

Dimensional Words.

Dimensional words refer to words that are adjective pairs used to indicate the various dimensions of objects. For example, dimensional word pairs include terms such as *big/little, high/low,* and *wide/narrow.* Each member of these word pairs refers to polar or opposite extremes of a dimension that exists along a continuum.

One member of each pair indicates the presence of that dimension or the positive end of that continuum. For example, *high* indicates the relative

dimensional words
Word pairs that refer to the physical dimensions of objects.

unmarked   Semantic aspect of words that refer to the presence of a dimension, including the positive end of that dimension (e.g., length); compare **marked.**

marked   Semantic aspect of words that refers to the negative end of a dimension or continuum (e.g., length); compare **unmarked.**

Quantifiers, such as *more* and *less,* or comparative and superlative forms, such as *-er* (e.g., high*er*) and *-est* (e.g., high*est*) express the degrees of a dimension. These are discussed in Chapter 8. ▪

presence of height, whereas *low* indicates its relative absence. The term for the positive end of the continuum (or the presence of that dimension) is said to be **unmarked.** The other member of the pair refers to the negative end and is referred to as **marked.** Furthermore, the unmarked member can generally refer to the entire continuum. For example, depending on the situation, either of the statements, *That shelf is 9 feet high* or *That shelf is only 2 feet high,* would be acceptable. In contrast, the marked member only refers to the negative end of the continuum, as in, *That shelf is extremely low.* However, we do not typically say *That shelf is only 2 feet low* (James, 1990).

Frequently, in the process of mastering dimensional pairs, preschoolers will tend to learn one member earlier. This is usually the positive unmarked member of the pair. Preschoolers are more likely to respond to (or use) the positive unmarked member as a signal that they recognize that the dimension is notably present or absent. Perhaps this is because the positive unmarked member reflects the presence of the dimension, which makes it more conspicuous; perhaps big items are perceptually more notable than little items. Additionally, because it can refer to the entire continuum, the positive unmarked member may tend to occur more frequently. In this early phase then, preschoolers may refer to both an ostrich and a canary as "big," simply because they are both remarkable in the extremes they represent along the size dimension.

It must be remembered that not only are these dimensions relative, but several pairs refer to dimensions that are restricted to specific circumstances. In addition, some are more perceptually subtle than others. The more general terms can be applied to a wider range of circumstances. For example, *big/ little* might be used to compare the relative sizes of items ranging from buttons to lakes. However, *deep/shallow* is limited to such things as lakes, rivers, ponds, canyons, and so forth. The perception of *deep/shallow* is also more subtle. Looking at the surface area of a lake or a puddle generally reveals whether it might be considered relatively *big* or *little* (or *large* or *small*), as lakes and puddles go. However, looking at the surface of a lake or a puddle does not necessarily tell us how *deep* or *shallow* either one might be.

Dimensions that are more commonly represented are experienced more frequently and, hence, tend to be mastered earlier. Conversely, those that relate to more specific circumstances tend to be experienced less frequently and are mastered later. Accordingly, the first pair to be mastered is *big/little* (or less commonly *large/small*), which is comprehended by about 3 years of age. The remaining pairs are generally mastered in the following order: *long/short* and *tall/short, high/low, wide/narrow,* and, finally, *deep/shallow* (James, 1990).

Color Words.   The ability to perceive colors is present at birth, even though overall visual acuity may not be. At least in Westernized cultures, infants are immersed in a sea of colors. Among their toys, clothing, mobiles, story books, and even eating utensils, they are exposed to a broad range of colors. Younger preschoolers are even able to sort and categorize items according to their color. In spite of all this experience, it is somewhat later in the preschool years before they begin to comprehend and express color names accurately.

In the process of mastering colors, younger preschoolers first demonstrate that they recognize color as a perceptible part of objects; that is, that it can be identified apart from the object. They demonstrate this understanding when they sort by color and by identifying items with color names, although they frequently use the incorrect name. Their preference for a red pillow might be erroneously asserted in a request such as, *Want blue pillow,* but it still indicates that they recognize the existence of color.

By about 4 or 5 years of age, preschoolers can name blue, green, yellow, and red. This, however, seems to represent only a basic connection between the concept of colors and their names. Naming subtle color differences with different names will be acquired later. Girls will tend to surpass boys in this process and, as always, there will be individual differences in the rate of mastery (Bornstein, 1985).

Spatial Words.   Spatial words indicate the location of a referent, typically in relation to some item. Spatial words can refer to relationships that are quite simple. For example, the spatial relation *in* is pretty obvious when a container is involved. On the other hand, some relationships are more complex. Whether something is *in front of* another item may depend on the speaker's point of view or whether the item has an identifiable front, as an automobile does, for example.

Children generally begin to comprehend spatial words before they use them expressively. However, they will continue to rely on the caregiver's gestures for additional cues for some time. In addition, it has been suggested that they may use the word order of the caregiver's utterance as a cue. Finally, the nature of the items involved in the situation may influence the younger child's interpretation. For example, depending upon whether one of the elements in the relationship is a container or provides a surface, the child may interpret an unfamiliar spatial word to mean "in" or "on."

By 4 years of age, most children have mastered the meanings of *in, inside, on,* and *under* (Clark, 1980). The term *next* is somewhat relative and, therefore, presents a little more difficulty; how close must one get to be "next to" something? However, because *next to* simply refers to adjacency without regard to orientation, it is somewhat simpler than *in front of* and *behind.* By the time preschoolers approach 5 years of age, they have generally mastered most spatial relations (Cox & Richardson, 1985).

Kinship Words.   Kinship words are the terms we use to indicate the various relationships among family members. Just as with dimensional and spatial words, how family members are named is also relative—pun intended! Depending on the overall family structure, a family member may have several kinship terms that apply. The appropriateness of each term depends on who is using it and in what context. For example, whether an adult male is called *son, dad, grandfather, brother,* or *husband* will depend on who is addressing him.

The complexity of kinship terms could prove to be quite confusing for young preschoolers, except that they naturally focus first on the relationships closest to them. Therefore, the first set of kinship words to develop are those that relate most directly to preschoolers—*mother, father, sister,* and *brother.*

The next kinship terms to develop—*son, daughter, grandfather, grandmother,* and *parent*—involve additional layers of relationships. For example, understanding *son* involves a vertical relationship linking two or three generations. For example, the word *son* implies a link between a parent and their male offspring. Similarly, *grandmother* involves three branches that link persons across three generations—from me to my mother's mother, for example.

In many cultures, including various regions of the United States, grandparents may go by informal names that have derived colloquially—within the family. Endearing forms like *mimi, meemaw, nanna, poppy, peepaw,* and *pawpaw* are sometimes carried across generations. Often these derive from the grandchild's unsuccessful attempts to say "grandmother" or "grandfather." Perhaps it is little wonder that younger preschoolers take longer to figure out these relationships, as the words mother or father are hardly recognizable in such terms. And, yet, who would ever wish to eliminate such colorful terms?

The lines of parentage associated with *grandmother* and *grandfather* may be first understood by younger preschoolers only at a superficial level—with a concept akin to, "my grandparents are people who are older and live where mommy used to live." Later, older preschoolers understand that this is "daddy's daddy" or "mommy's mommy." (At about 4 years of age, when answering telephone calls from their grandmother to their mom, my children loved to call their mother to the phone, saying, "Mommy, it's your mommy!")

Finally, the last terms to be mastered are those that indicate relationships involving a third, horizontal branching of the family tree. *Uncle, aunt, niece, nephew,* and *cousin* all refer to an additional link that shifts the relationship horizontally—that dad could have a brother, or mom a sister, and how their children are related to them can be somewhat elusive even to older preschoolers. In fact, it will not be until school age, at approximately 10 years of age, that most major kinship terms are understood.

temporal words Words that relate events in time.

Temporal Words.   The final group of relational terms, **temporal words,** refer to how events are related to each other in time. Time is perhaps the most abstract relationship any of us will contemplate. Einstein, who understood time's relativity, once said, "When you are courting a nice girl, an hour seems like a second. When you sit on a red-hot cinder, a second seems like an hour. That's relativity" (1949).

Children's ability to understand how events relate to each other in time develops slowly. Young preschoolers' limited cognitive abilities and experiences cause them to tend to live in the "here-and-now." They have yet to develop clear concepts for relating what has come before or what will happen later, after their present experience. Research suggests that children only begin to use temporal words for time relations that they have begun to understand (Cromer, 1981).

Temporal words address three basic time relationships between events. All events, no matter how brief, evidence *duration.* Events that follow other events illustrate *order* or *sequence.* And events that occur at the same point in time represent *simultaneity.* Table 7–3 presents these time relationships with examples.

Preschoolers tend to first master words used to indicate order, such as *after* and *before.* Generally, words indicating duration, such as *since* and *until,* are mastered later. And, finally, terms that indicate simultaneously occurring events, such as *while* and *at the same time,* are understood by the time the child reaches 5 years of age. This overall order has been viewed by some as fitting with children's cognitive development as described by Piaget.

Summary

- Preschoolers' vocabularies develop at remarkable rates, and can include 14,000 words that are understood at some level by the time they go to kindergarten.

- Fast mapping refers to the hypothetical process preschoolers use to initially associate new words.

- Extended mapping occurs as children refine word meanings through additional experiences.

- Preschoolers' vocabulary development exhibits patterns that suggest learning principles or "strategies" used as they encounter new words.

- Preschoolers demonstrate the ability to extend or generalize words in creative, but useful, ways as they accumulate their expressive vocabularies.

- Understanding relational terms for size, color, space, family, and time relies on cumulative experiences with them and occurs in predictable sequences based on the complexity of the relationship.

Table 7–3. Terms indicating time relationships.

Earliest forms—Order	After	*We played <u>after</u> we ate lunch.*
	Before	*We ate lunch <u>before</u> we played.*
Later forms—Duration	Since	*I have been waiting ever <u>since</u> you called.*
	Until	*Let's rest <u>until</u> it's time to go.*
Last forms—Simultaneity	While	*Daddy works <u>while</u> you're at school.*
	At the same time	*Mommy works <u>at the same time</u> as Daddy.*

Word Relations

The preceding section discussed children's development of word meanings—their individual lexical meanings. However, beyond the one-word stage, words rarely occur in isolation. More often than not, they occur together and relate to each other in any of several ways. One way in which words relate to each other is based on their semantic compatibility. As lexical items, certain words may or may not occur together because the semantic features of each word introduce *selection restrictions.* For example, mature speakers are unlikely to use the word *angry* in relation to the word *rock,* as inanimate objects are not capable of feeling emotions.

The concept of lexical *selection restrictions* is discussed in Chapter 1. ▪

Another way in which preschoolers learn to relate words to each other is through word orders. Word orders carry meanings above and beyond the words' individual meanings. The relationships between individual words in a sentence are called *semantic relations.* When the words *daddy* and *shoe* are produced together in a certain situation, their word order (*daddy shoe*) can convey *possession.*

The concept of semantic relations is discussed previously in Chapters 1 and 4. ▪

The semantic relations expressed in preschoolers' multiword utterances include those that were expressed as toddlers. (Refer to Table 6-5 in Chapter 6 to review the prevalent semantic relations expressed in toddlers' two-word utterances.) However, the number of relationships expressed in each utterance increases as utterance length increases—additional words generally convey additional relationships. Or, viewed in another way, the additional words reflect preschoolers' new understanding of other roles that can be played by the objects and people they talk about.

The semantic relations expressed by preschoolers gradually expand to include a broader range of relationships. However, longer utterances do not necessarily result from simply stringing together additional semantic relationships. Brown (1973) suggested that most early utterances are based on combining two or three basic semantic relations. Table 7–4 illustrates those basic combinations that occurred most frequently in Brown's research. Preschoolers' utterances appear to lengthen as they elaborate on one of the major terms in the basic relationship. For example, an early *agent + action*

Table 7–4. Prevalent semantic relations in early multiword utterances.

Construction	Example
Agent + Action + Object	*Mommy bake cake*
Agent + Action + Locative	*Mommy bake kitchen*
Agent + Object + Locative	*Mommy cake kitchen*
Agent + Action + Object + Locative	*Mommy bake cake kitchen*

Note. Adapted from *A First Language: The Early Stages* by R. Brown, 1973, Cambridge, MA: Harvard University Press.

utterance might take the form of *boy eat.* Later, this might be lengthened as preschoolers elaborate on the *agent* term with an *attributive* relation, as in *big boy eat.*

Basic relationships among an infinite variety of items and events can be conveyed by a limited number of word orders. However, beyond combining these basic relationships, preschoolers are soon compelled to express their ideas more clearly. As the variety of contexts and ideas preschoolers discuss expands, communicating clearly with their caregivers can become increasingly difficult at times. Soon after preschoolers begin combining words into basic relations, they elaborate or "fine-tune" the meaning with the production of grammatical morphemes (Brown, 1973).

Summary

- Beyond individual word meanings, preschoolers combine words to convey the semantic relations that they perceive between items and events.

- In their two- and three-word utterances, young preschoolers combine the basic semantic relations they expressed individually in one-word utterances as toddlers.

- As preschoolers understand more subtle ways that objects, persons, attributes, and events can be related, they combine words to specify these semantic relations.

Emerging Literacy

Preschoolers bring to literacy all the language abilities that blossom so rapidly between their second birthday and the first day of kindergarten. They have evolved to the point where they tell narratives that are more elaborate and carry on extended verbal exchanges in conversation, both in ways that parallel the increasingly complex stories that are read to them by caregivers. More importantly, they have actually reached the point where their metalinguistic ability allows them to analyze which element or information in the story needs clarification. Because they have developed the ability to ask questions more effectively, the process of "sense making" becomes a collaborative effort that builds their conceptual knowledge and reasoning (Kamhi & Catts, 2005).

Around 3 years of age, preschoolers may begin to develop *print awareness,* which may go beyond recognizing the correct orientation for print and its left-to-right flow. Some may begin to recognize individual letters and analyze text into letters, words, and sentences (Snow, Scarbrough, & Burns, 1999).

As preschoolers, many children may begin to attempt the task of reading, at least at a rudimentary level. This prereading stage has been called the *logographic stage* (Ehri, 1991) or the *prealphabetic phase* (Ehri and

McCormick, 1998). In this period, preschoolers establish associations between unanalyzed words or labels and some salient graphic aspects of a printed word and its context. They may recognize a word like "look" because they recall that it has two "eyes" in the middle, or recognize the word "Pepsi" when it appears on a bottle. The logographic stage is regarded as prereading because the preschooler is not actually utilizing any phonetic cues or sound-symbol relationships to analyze or read the word phonetically. In other words, preschoolers may "read" a logo (e.g., "Pepsi") based entirely on recognizing it as a whole symbol, or interpret it incorrectly when it is misplaced in another context, such as on a cereal box (Erhi & McCormick, 1998; Kamhi & Catts, 2005).

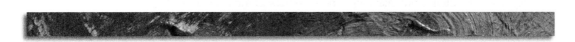

Chapter Summary

Following their second birthday, as preschoolers, children are exposed to an expanding variety of contexts. Their motor skills, cognitive understanding, and social interactions allow them to experience new collections of stimuli as *setting events* for language. As they increasingly exhibit *socialized speech* and *symbolic play* behavior, the need to negotiate verbal interactions more effectively expands. Pragmatically, as *discourse* skills and *narratives* develop, preschoolers become more effective and entertaining conversationalists.

Preschoolers' ability to explore and understand their world opens up to an avalanche of new words and meanings. Researchers have described preschoolers' attempts, including *fast mapping* and producing creative vocabulary, to make some initial sense of the rush of new information. Beyond the everyday words that become part of their vocabulary, preschoolers must deal with a number of *relational terms* that describe size, color, location, family, and time relationships.

Additional word relations develop and more are inserted into word orders that encode specific relationships among the elements. However, the typical length of utterances also increases because preschoolers encode additional information to elaborate on or specify an individual sentence element.

Finally, preschoolers have begun to exhibit a heightened awareness of the elements of literacy. They have begun to exhibit print awareness in recognizing certain letters. In addition, they may begin to analyze text into letters, words, and sentences. Some preschoolers begin to exhibit prereading behavior at the logographic stage. Although this involves more recognition than reading, the inclination to make an association between a symbol and a name at least signals an interest in learning to read.

1. Describe the types of stimuli that might contribute to a *setting event* for language.

2. What is the difference between a *stimulus* and a *functional stimulus?*

3. List three levels of *monologue* that precede *socialized speech.*

4. What are the cognitive and social contributions of play behavior toward language development?

5. Define *cohesion* and list three skills in discourse that contribute to it.

6. Describe the four major types of *narratives.*

7. Describe the four levels of narratives.

8. Describe preschoolers' vocabulary growth and the role of *fast mapping.*

9. Give four examples of the kind of information conveyed by *relational terms.*

10. What are two ways in which individual words can relate to each other semantically?

To the student: You are encouraged to use the following questions to prepare for multiple-choice examinations. This exercise is not intended to simply "provide the answers to questions." Instead, it is hoped that you will use the material to develop your ability to analyze questions and choices to identify correct answers based on a critical understanding of the distinctions among the answers. Use the answer key at the end of the book to prompt your analysis of each item and to confirm the correct answer. Remember that there is a difference between recognizing the correct answer and understanding why it is the correct one.

1. Which of the following statements regarding functional stimuli is true?
   a. stimuli present in setting events that we have not yet experienced would already be considered functional stimuli
   b. all the stimuli present in every setting event we have ever experienced would be considered functional stimuli
   c. those stimuli that become discriminative stimuli or reinforcing stimuli due to our experiences with them become the functional stimuli in later setting events

    d. setting events are made up of only our experiences, not functional stimuli

    e. all of these are true

2. Which of the following statements is/are true regarding children's learning of "dimensional words" such as big/little?

    a. they tend to learn the "unmarked" word earlier

    b. they tend to learn the word that refers to the *absence* of a dimension first

    c. they tend to learn words for dimensions that can be applied more broadly earlier than those that pertain to specific contexts

    d. a and c

    e. b and c

3. Which form of socialized speech is analogous to parallel play?

    a. monologue

    b. collective monologue

    c. affect expressive monologue

    d. primitive narrative

    e. associated monologue

4. Which of the following sets of relational words is *Not* in the general order that we would expect them to be learned?

    a. in, on, under, next to, in front, behind

    b. big, little, long, short, tall, wide, narrow, deep, shallow

    c. while, at the same time, since, until, before, after

    d. mother, father, sister, brother, grandfather, grandmother

    e. blue, green, red, yellow, mauve, chartreuse, taupe

5. A child who comments on the "yukky" smell coming from the pan of cooking spinach is responding to _____ .

    a. physical stimuli

    b. chemical stimuli

    c. organismic stimuli

    d. social stimuli

    e. metaphysical stimuli

6. The relationship between "fast mapping" and "extending mapping" might be expressed as _____ .

    a. fast mapping is the opposite of extended mapping

    b. extended mapping precedes fast mapping

    c. fast mapping follows extended mapping

    d. fast mapping is to extended mapping as the phrase "first impression" is to "getting to know you"

    e. a nonexistent relationship—they are not related

7. Which of the earliest forms of narratives are the first to involve temporal sequences?
   a. heaps
   b. chaining
   c. centering
   d. eventcasts
   e. none of these

8. Which of the following locational forms is the child most likely to accurately comprehend earlier?
   a. in, on
   b. right, left
   c. in front, behind
   d. above, below
   e. next to

9. Topic maintenance, turn taking, and presupposition are three important aspects in _____ .
   a. carrying on discourse
   b. vocabulary
   c. achieving cohesion
   d. a and b
   e. a and c

10. Decontextualized language refers to _____ .
   a. the basic utterances by toddlers trying to gain objects and attention
   b. the language exhibited by preschoolers who do not know how to maintain the topic
   c. the excessive use of pronouns
   d. language that is tied to objects, people, and events in the immediate situation
   e. language that is based on objects, people, and events that are in a remote context

Suggested Readings

Foy, J. G., & Mann, V. (2003). Home literacy environment and phonological awareness in preschool children: Differential effects for rhyme and phoneme awareness. *Applied Psycholinguistics, 24,* 59–88.

Ninio, A., & Snow, C. (1999). The development of pragmatics: Learning to use language appropriately. In W. Ritchie & T. Bhatia (Eds.), *Handbook of child language acquisition* (pp. 347–386). New York: Academic Press.

Winsler, A., Carlton, M. P., & Barry, M. J. (2000). Age-related changes in preschool children's systematic use of private speech in a natural setting. *Journal of Child Language, 27,* 665–687.

8

Developing Grammar in Preschoolers

EmmaLou did not know it, but her family had been quite concerned from the start. They were not obsessed with her development. There had been no complications or illnesses. They were simply concerned about whether she was developing like other children do. Like most other parents, they wanted to be reassured, but in very precise ways.

From the day she came home from the hospital, she was weighed almost daily. The numbers on her mother's tape measure were fading from being stretched along EmmaLou's length so frequently. It seemed silly, but while cuddling her weeks after her birth, her father would still silently count EmmaLou's fingers and toes just to be certain.

As the first year passed, even these anxious parents were satisfied with EmmaLou's development. Her weight and height had progressed as expected. As she happily dug her little fists into her first birthday cake, her father could even see that all 10 fingers had grown larger and stronger.

As the second year went on, however, her mother and father became anxious all over again. EmmaLou had begun talking. They were overjoyed at her first words, but now they worried, would her language develop properly? They could easily measure her weight in pounds, her height in inches, and count her fingers and toes for reassurance. But, what scale or ruler could measure her developing language? Should they gauge how loud she spoke each word, how many new words she spoke each day, or simply count them all?

Eventually, as EmmaLou began talking in two- and three-word sentences, her mother and father worried less. It became increasingly apparent that EmmaLou's language was developing just as it should. As her sentences lengthened, she added new meanings, new words and, most remarkably, as she added those seemingly insignificant "word endings," they understood her utterances with increasing frequency. Out of pride and in relief, her parents could only sigh, "That's EmmaLou!"

This chapter addresses the following questions:

- How have researchers defined and measured the language behaviors that have been studied?

- What factors appear to be most significant in influencing children's language development?

- How similar or different are children as they proceed in learning the structures of their language?

- How do different language structures develop as preschoolers learn to express themselves in basic and then more mature sentence forms?

- What differences are evident in preschoolers' abilities in comprehending and producing language?

- As preschoolers' language abilities mature, what changes occur in the verbal input and feedback they receive from caregivers?

Development in Related Domains

This chapter extends the discussion of the preschool child's language development to the learning of grammar. This chapter covers the same time period, basically 2 to 5 years of age, as is covered in Chapter 7. Therefore, the introduction and developments in the motor, cognitive, and social domains covered in Chapter 7 are relevant to this chapter also. The reader should review that information at the beginning of Chapter 7 as background for this chapter.

Language Expectations (Grammatical)

During their preschool years, children will learn how to fine-tune their utterances in ways that allow them to communicate increasingly complex and abstract ideas. They will learn to attach word endings that signal specific meanings—for example, verb tense, plurality, possession. Sentence structures become more complete and capable of expressing a full range of adult meanings. While preschoolers struggle with comprehending some complex sentence structures, even their misunderstandings are somehow logical. The following overview is intended to provide an initial picture of the overall *grammatical* developments expected during this period.

- Preschoolers will gradually master the use of word endings that inflect the meanings of their stem words.

- Preschoolers will learn to use most pronoun forms to replace many nouns while continuing to struggle with some.

- Preschoolers will eventually combine several ideas in one sentence through use of conjunctions or embedded phrases.

- Preschoolers will continue to struggle with comprehending sentences of greater complexity, applying strategies that lead to misinterpretations.

Grammatical Development

Soon after their first 50 words, at approximately 18 months of age, toddlers begin to combine words into two-word phrases. By the time most utterances are two words long, at about 2 years of age, the young preschooler begins to produce three-word utterances. Between 2 and 5 years of age, preschoolers will develop the ability to use grammatical morphemes, produce basic grammatical sentence types, and combine those into even more advanced grammatical constructions.

Mastering Grammatical Morphemes

Once preschoolers begin to combine two and three semantic relations, they begin to modulate or "fine-tune" their utterances through grammatical segments (Brown, 1973). In this fine-tuning, the preschooler produces grammatical morphemes—function words and word endings—that "modulate" the meaning of the more basic terms in their utterances. For example, in English, the present progressive verb inflection, *-ing,* signals that the action of the verb is ongoing. If the context is not available and only the stem verb is used, the listener may not understand if the action is ongoing, completed, or anticipated.

The emergence of these grammatical morphemes begins early in the preschool years. Their development represents a series of accomplishments that will occur throughout these years. Although other important aspects of language are also developing, as these grammatical morphemes gradually emerge, the preschooler's language takes on a more mature, adultlike texture.

Brown's *A First Language*

A landmark study in children's development of grammatical morphemes was conducted by Roger Brown (1973) and his colleagues at Harvard University. This work, described in his book, *A First Language: The Early Stages,* became the reference point for much of the subsequent research in child language. Brown's research is especially instructive for students of language development not only because it is well organized, but also because of its prominence in the literature concerning child language development.

The Research Design.   The research design was based on a longitudinal study of three preschool-age children called Adam, Eve, and Sarah—pseudonyms that protected their identities and signified their role in studying the *genesis* of language. These children were selected because they were especially intelligible and talkative; accordingly, they would provide full language samples that were easily understood and transcribed.

The data for the study consisted primarily of transcription of spontaneous conversations recorded in each child's home. With some variations, at least 2 hours of language were transcribed during each month. However, Eve moved away after 1 year; the remaining subjects, Adam and Sarah, were followed for another 4 years. Interestingly, it turned out that Eve was so advanced in her speech that the development evidenced in her 10 months of transcripts was equivalent to the development exhibited by Adam and Sarah in twice that time (Brown, 1973).

Some caution must be used in generalizing the results based on this research design. Can three (or, eventually, two) children provide a representative picture of the way in which all children develop language? Of course, this is precisely the trade-off these researchers knew they were making. Longitudinal research in language development provides detailed, intimate information about the continuous nature of development, but is so time intensive it requires a smaller number of subjects. Nonetheless, this is an important limitation that must be considered, especially if the few subjects chosen would happen to be verbally advanced. Other researchers have found similar results using cross-sectional studies including greater numbers of children (deVilliers & deVilliers, 1973).

Criteria for the Selected Morphemes.   The grammatical morphemes (to be discussed later) chosen for the study were selected for at least three practical reasons. The first criterion was that the grammatical morphemes had to be forms that have identifiable obligatory contexts. *Obligatory contexts* are linguistic or nonlinguistic aspects that require use of a certain form according to the rules of grammar. The linguistic context is provided by the child's or the listener's utterances. For example, a prompt to describe an *ongoing* action (*What's happening here?*) would require a response including a verb inflected for present progressive (*The boy is running*). The nonlinguistic context is also capable of obligating forms, such as the requirement for the plural inflection when eyeing the last two cookies in the cookie jar and saying, *May I have the last cookies?* (Saying *Please* also helps, but that is a pragmatic issue!)

It was fundamental to the research that the selected grammatical morphemes were obligatory, not optional. Some grammatical forms are optional—they appear only out of choice. For example, speakers may generally choose to substitute a pronoun (e.g., *he*) for a noun phrase (e.g., *The boy*). Including adjectives to describe objects is a speaker's option. If there is no obligation to produce a structure, its absence from an utterance

Moerk (1992a) performed a "microanalysis" of Brown's transcripts to examine the verbal interactions between Eve and her mother. ■

The dependence on linguistic and nonlinguistic aspects to determine obligatory context required use of the *method of rich interpretation,* described in Chapter 4. ■

is not necessarily right or wrong. Because the goal of the research was to examine mastery for each grammatical morpheme, it had to be possible to determine when the child used it correctly (i.e., it occurred when required) or incorrectly (i.e., it did not occur when required).

The second criterion was that the forms selected must exhibit a *high frequency of occurrence*. This was to ensure that the forms would provide a continuous picture of their development. If occurrences of a form were too rare, the opportunities to obtain an accurate picture of its development would be limited.

Finally, the third criterion related to the *speed of acquisition*. It was anticipated that it would be more instructive if the forms selected developed somewhat gradually. If, in contrast, a form made an isolated appearance in one sample and was then mastered before the next sample was obtained, there would be limited insight into the overall learning process. As we will see below, in applying these criteria, Brown's research focused on 14 grammatical morphemes.

Criteria for Mastery.   Brown anticipated that the data would represent a gradually changing performance curve. It was decided that mastery of a form was evidenced in the first of three samples in which it occurred at a level of 90% correct. This would represent a level of consistently correct production that subsequently showed stability. Although a level of 90% obviously meant errors were still occurring, it was decided that this criterion represented mastery.

Brown's Stages of Development.   Brown (1973) summarized the developments that seemed to characterize each level of development in five stages. The characteristics of each stage are outlined in Table 8–1.

According to Brown, the five stages represented an overview of the development in children's language. Stage I is characterized by individual words and semantic roles combined in linear simple sentences. In Stage II, what Brown called the modulations of meaning (specifically, the grammatical morphemes) emerge. Stage III is a period in which the major elements of simple sentences are rearranged into different sentence modalities, such as questions, imperatives, and negatives. In Stage IV, the preschooler begins to embed the elements of one sentence within another. Finally, in Stage V, utterances are coordinated, combining the content of two sentences into one.

Mean Length of Utterance (MLU).   Initially, it would not be surprising that stages of language development could be identified in detailed, longitudinal data such as Brown's. We might expect that chronological age would provide an obvious way of defining stages of development. For example, many of us might assume that most 2-year-olds are quite similar in their language development, as are most 3-year-olds, and so forth. However, as an indicator of children's language development, age level is not as precise as

Table 8––. Brown's stages of language development.

Stages	Characterized by	Features	Examples
Stage I MLU: 1.0–2.0 Age: 12–26 mos.	First words; semantic roles expressed in simple sentences.	Single word utterances. Combining semantic roles.	Naming significant objects, persons, and events in their daily experiences (*cup, spoon, Mommy, Daddy,* etc.). Agent + Action, Action + Object, Action + Location, Entity + Location, Entity + Attribute, Demonstrative + Attribute
Stage II MLU: 2.0–2.5 Age: 27–30 mos.	Modulation of meaning.	Emerging of grammatical morphemes.	Present progressive (*-ing*), prepositions (*in, on*), plural (*-s*), irregular past (e.g., *ran, ate*), possessive (*-s*), articles (*a, the*), regular past (*-ed*), third person regular, third person irregular, auxiliary and copula verbs (*is, are, was, were*).
Stage III MLU: 2.5–3.0 Age: 31–34 mos.	Development of sentence form.	Noun phrase elaboration and auxiliary development.	Noun phrases elaborated in subject and object positions (*Big boy running fast, Billy ate my cookie*). Auxiliary verbs allow more mature interrogatives and negatives.
Stage IV MLU: 3.0–3.75 Age: 35–40 mos.	Emergence of complex sentences.	Embedding sentence elements.	Object noun phrase complements (*I know you are my friend*); bedded wh-questions (*I know who is hiding*); relative clauses (*I helped boy who is nice*).
Stage V MLU: 3.75–4.50 Age: 41–46 mos.	Emergence of compound sentences.	Conjoining sentences.	Conjoining two simple sentences (*I have a book and you have a toy*).

Note. Adapted from *A First Language: The Early Stages,* by R. Brown, 1973, Cambridge, MA: Harvard University Press.

common sense might suggest. There can be wide variations in language development among children who are the same age.

Brown found instead that the typical length of a child's utterances was a far better indicator of grammatical development. As Brown explained, this appears to be so "because almost every new kind of knowledge increases length: the number of semantic roles expressed in a sentence, the addition of obligatory morphemes, . . . the addition of negative forms and auxiliaries, . . . and embedding and conjoining" all result in increased utterance length" (1973, pp. 53–54).

Specifically, Brown found that counting morphemes, as opposed to words, was the most sensitive measure of the important developments resulting in increased utterance length. This is because many of the grammatical morphemes are inflectional morphemes. Because these must be bound to words, they would not increase the word count for an utterance, but they would increase the morpheme count. For example, compare the word and morpheme counts for the following two utterances:

	Words	Morphemes
The two boy want two cookie.	6	6
The two boys wanted two cookies.	6	9

These two examples reflect a difference in their level of grammatical development that would not be apparent through counting words. On the other hand, changes in children's average utterance length in morphemes, their **mean length of utterance (MLU),** seem to index certain developments in their language behavior.

The 14 Grammatical Morphemes

The appearance and mastery of the 14 grammatical morphemes in relation to the stages of development became the central focus in Brown's (1973) research. Each of the morphemes appeared in Stage II. These morphemes generally convey meanings that could only be implied through the simple word orders exhibited in Stage I. They were then mastered at various stages as the subjects' language developed.

Brown ranked the overall order of mastery among the grammatical morphemes by his three subjects. Table 8–2 presents this ranking with examples of each morpheme. The nature of each grammatical morpheme is described here in their order of overall mastery.

Present Progressive Inflection. The first grammatical morpheme to be mastered, the present progressive verb inflection (-*ing*), indicates an action that is ongoing. In its mature form, it is usually coordinated with an auxiliary "to be" verb (*am, is, are, was, were*), which will be discussed later. In its early appearance, the inflection occurs without an auxiliary, as in *Boy running*. It was scored by Brown on the basis of the nonlinguistic context; that is, it had to refer to an ongoing activity. Significantly, the early appearance

It may be helpful to review the different types of morphemes described in Chapter 1. ■

mean length of utterance (MLU) Measure of language development based on average number of morphemes per utterance.

Actually, a broad correlation between MLU and chronological age has been found. For example, a child 3 years of age might be expected to exhibit an MLU of 3.0. However, this relationship does not hold beyond about 5 years of age. ■

Table 8–2. Order of acquisition in Brown's 14 grammatical morphemes.

Rank	Mastery Stage	Months	Morpheme	Example
1.	II	27–30	Present progressive inflection	*He eating.*
2.	II	27–30	Preposition *in*	*Juice in cup.*
3.	II	27–30	Preposition *on*	*Sleep on bed.*
4.	II	27–30	Regular plural inflection	*My toys.*
5.	II	27–30	Past irregular	*I ate cookie.*
6.	III	31–34	Possessive inflection	*Mommy's shoe.*
7.	III	31–34	Uncontractible copula	*Here it is! They were nice.*
8.	III–V	31–46	Articles	*A boy took the ball.*
9.	V	41–46	Regular past tense	*He walked fast.*
10.	V	41–46	Regular third person singular	*She bakes cakes.*
11.	V	41–46	Irregular third person singular	*He has some. She does, too.*
12.	V	41–46	Uncontractible auxiliary	*Is she reading? You were reading.*
13.	V	41–46	Contractible copula	*Tommy's tall! They are all tall?*
14.	V	41–46	Contractible auxiliary	*She's reading. They are reading.*

Note. Adapted from *A First Language: The Early Stages,* by R. Brown, 1973, Cambridge, MA: Harvard University Press.

and mastery of this form fits the observation, noted many times previously, that toddlers and younger preschoolers tend to live in the "here-and-now." Brown's preschoolers evidenced appropriate production of the present progressive inflection during Stage II.

Prepositions In *and* On.   The second and third grammatical morphemes mastered (they tied) were the earliest occurring prepositions, *in* and *on.* They actually make their first rare appearances in late Stage I. However, they are omitted more frequently than they are used. These particular prepositions exhibited learning curves that differed from the other grammatical morphemes in that, after some fluctuation, these forms more rapidly approach mastery. This ease of learning is perhaps because the semantic and grammatical judgments involved in their use are simpler.

These prepositions are semantically simpler because they are related to spatial locations that are determined directly. For the most part, to be *in* something, an item must simply be contained (as in *in a box, in a can,* etc.) and to be *on* something an item must be positioned on a horizontal surface (*on the shelf, on the desk,* etc.). Judging these topographical positions is less relational than *behind, beside,* and *in front of.* In addition, they are grammatically simpler because they only occur in one form, no matter what the context. These structures evidence mastery during Stage II (Brown, 1973).

Regular Plural Inflection. The fourth grammatical morpheme to be mastered is the regular plural inflection. In general, most items in the world occur in either a singular state (as one) or in a plural state (as more than one). In English, nouns are singular (unmarked) unless they are marked in some way for plurality. Nouns can be marked for plurality in either of two ways. The

 Inflectional morphemes assume various roles and forms in different languages (Reich, 1986). Arabic Egyptian uses different plurals to indicate a collection of a known number of items versus a group with an unknown number. Russian applies various word endings to nouns to mark their semantic role in the sentence. Finally, French-speaking children must figure out whether such things as tables, chairs, and trees are masculine or feminine to apply the correct gender suffix. Given modern fashion trends most of us have difficulty determining this with some people we see every day!

vast majority of English nouns are marked through a bound morpheme; that is, the regular plural inflection *-s,* as in *I found two coats.* A significantly smaller number of plurals are marked lexically, through words such as *men, women,* and *children.* Because the word varies in each instance, they are called irregular plurals.

An additional distinction that must be mastered in English is that mass nouns, such as *milk, sand,* and *hair,* do not accept plural inflections. We might ask for *more milk,* but we do not ask for *three more milks* (unless we are actually referring to cartons or glasses of milk).

In English, the regular plural inflection takes three different forms, /-s/ (e.g., *hats*), /-z/ (e.g., *cans*) and /-Iz/ (e.g., *busses*). Different phonological forms of the same structure are called allomorphs. The plural allomorphs all signal plurality, but differ based on whether the preceding sound is voiced, voiceless, or a sibilant.

Marking plurality evolves through several stages. Initially, the preschooler does not contrast singular versus plural and the listener must glean this information from the situation. Then, the plural inflection appears on a few nouns that occur frequently in the preschooler's language. Next, the form generalizes rapidly, even occurring on irregular forms that been previously correct. This overgeneralization (or overregularization) results in plural forms such as *mans, womans, childs.* Finally, the preschooler distinguishes between the regular and irregular forms. The regular plural inflection is mastered during Stage II, although the phonological distinctions among the allomorphs may not be mastered until much later.

Irregular Past Tense Verbs. Irregular past tense verbs were the fifth grammatical morpheme mastered in Brown's study. In English, like plurality, past events are also signaled in two ways. Verbs may be inflected with the regular past tense inflection *-ed* (discussed in greater detail later). Past tense may also be expressed lexically through words, such as *ate, sat,* and *ran.* Again, just as with irregular plurals, because each word is different, they are called irregular past tense verbs.

For younger preschoolers, there are a few irregular past tense forms that initially appear in correct form. These appear to be those that would be related to everyday activities, such as *sat, went, came, fell, ate.* These first instances may be learned simply as lexical items; they may not necessarily be understood to be past tense alternatives to the uninflected verb. As we will see later, when regular past tense inflections appear, they are overgeneralized to create incorrect forms, such as *goed, sitted,* and *runned.* Brown found the more common irregular past tense verb forms to be initially mastered in Stage II. However, after reverting to their incorrect, regularized forms, they are re-mastered by Stage V.

Possessive Inflection.   This inflectional morpheme, the sixth structure mastered in Brown's study, includes the same three phonologically based allomorphs as the regular plural inflection, /-s/ (e.g., *Pat's car*), /-z/ (e.g., *The man's coat*), and /-Iz/ (e.g., *The dish's design*). Possession is a multifaceted concept. Some items are inalienable possessions—most of us can safely assume that our nose will always be our nose. Other possessions are alienable. That is, their owners can change—our cars may not always belong to us, if we choose to trade or sell them (or park them on the wrong street). And, finally, some possessions are not even items. We "own" turns in a game (*It's Bill's turn*), parking spaces (*Mary's space is really close!*), or time in seats at events (*Save Tom's seat for us!*)—and we guard them jealously!

For the preschooler, "possession" is initially more a matter of association. The younger child does not truly understand ownership—daddy's coat is his only because he frequently wears it, not because he has a receipt for it somewhere. The relationship of possession is first marked by word order in Stage I, usually in the form of *Noun + Noun* (or *Possessor + Possessed*), as in *Daddy chair.* However, this requires the listener to have some knowledge of the context to interpret. With the emergence of the possessive inflection in Stage II, possession is more clearly signaled. In most cases, the earliest possessors will be those people in the children's environment and possessions will be those items which are most often involved in their interactions. The possessive inflection is mastered by Stage III. However, as with the plural inflection, the phonologically based allomorphs are not entirely mastered until later.

Aspects of the copula-auxiliary verbs can be confusing. Although the other copula and auxiliary verbs are mastered later, all of their features and distinctions are discussed at this point to allow the student to sort these out simultaneously. ∎

Uncontractible Copula.   The uncontractible copula was the seventh form mastered by Adam, Eve, and Sarah (Brown, 1973). In English, the copula occurs in the same forms—*am, is, are, was, were*—as the auxiliary "to be" verbs. Like the auxiliary, the different copula forms are used according to person, tense, and number. Their many similarities result in some confusion for those of us who struggle with the subtleties of grammar. Table 8–3 presents the similarities and distinctions between these two forms.

The most essential distinction to remember is that the copula serves as the main verb; it is not related to another verb. In contrast, the auxiliary is a helping verb, which means it is related to a main verb. The copula serves

Table 8–3. Features, roles, and examples of contractible and uncontractible copula and auxiliary.

Features of Copula/Auxiliary Verbs	Copula Verbs: Role and Examples	Auxiliary Verbs: Role and Examples
Copula and Auxiliary "to be" verbs (*am, is, are, was, were*) indicate: **Person:** First (*I am*), Second (*You are*), Third (She *is*) **Tense:** Present versus Past (e.g., I *am* vs. I *was*; You *are* vs. You *were*; He *is* vs. He *was*) **Number:** Singular versus Plural (e.g., He *is* vs. They *are*; She *was* vs. They *were*)	**Role:** Serve as the **main** verb (i.e., there is NO other verb) which "links" or "equates" the subject to a complement. For example, **Subject = Complement,** where the Complement can be a noun phrase, adjective, prepositional phrase, etc.	**Role:** Serve as the **helping** verb that supplements the main verb with information about person, tense, and number, as in **Subject + Helping + Main Verb.**
Contractible: It is permissible (i.e., optional) to use the contracted form.	**Examples:** *Mary is a girl. (or Mary's a girl.)* *He is tall. (or He's tall.)* *It is in here. (It's in here.)*	**Examples:** *They are walking. (or They're walking.)* *Pat is smiling. (or Pat's smiling.)* *It is burning. (It's burning.)*
Uncontractible: It is NOT permissible to use the contracted form due to sentence position or tense.	**Examples:** *Is he tall?* (Yes/No question) *Who's a girl? Mary is.* (Elliptical) *It was hot.* (Past tense)	**Examples:** *Are they walking?* (Yes/No question) *Who is smiling? Pat is.* (Elliptical) *It was burning.* (Past tense)

grammatically as a *linking verb* because it joins the subject to the predicate (usually a noun, adjective, or prepositional phrase) in a sentence. Semantically, it is called a *state* (or *equating*) *verb,* as it connects (or equates) the noun and some state. This might be conceptually thought of as *Subject = Predicate.* The copula occurs in expressing identity (*I am John*), membership in a class (*She is a nurse*), possession of an attribute (*He was very polite*), or a location (*We are in Disneyland!*).

A key feature of both copula and auxiliary verbs is their potential to occur in contracted forms. A central concept in this regard is *permissibility.* It is permissible to contract several forms of the copula, as in *I'm hot! She's cute! They're late!* In other instances, copulas cannot be contracted; either their form or the grammatical context makes them uncontractible. Uncontractible forms include the past tense forms *was* and *were;* contracting them would make them indistinguishable from their present tense counterparts. The normally contractible present tense forms cannot be contracted if they occur in certain grammatical contexts, such as a yes-no question (*Is he satisfied?*), or an elliptical response to a question (Where's my wallet? *Here it is*). In addition, the copula cannot be contracted simultaneously with a contracted negative; we do not say, *She'sn't the one.*

For Brown's preschoolers, the uncontractible copula appeared before the contractible copula and auxiliary forms. The early appearance of the copula might be due to its role in expressing the earlier appearing semantic relations (existence, locative, attribution). Additionally, the earlier mastery of uncontractible form might stem from the fact that it always occurs in its full form, making it stand out perceptually. As it turned out, two of Brown's three subjects mastered the uncontractible copula in Stage III. However, given their subtleties and complexities, it is possible that children will not fully master any of the copula or auxiliary verbs until Stage V or later.

Articles.   The eighth form to be mastered among the grammatical morphemes included the articles, *a* and *the.* Just as with the other forms, these also appear in Stage II, then require a substantial amount of experience to fully master. *The* and *a* are referred to grammatically as *definite* and *nondefinite.* Brown also used the terms *specific* and *nonspecific* to refer to the semantic aspects that differentiate their use.

In their mature use, the nonspecific article, *a,* is used to introduce an item by first referring to its entire class, as in *I saw a car run this stoplight today.* At this point, the entire class of cars—all makes and styles—is included in the reference (which would be of little help to a traffic officer). A subsequent reference might become more descriptive and include a specific article, as in *The car was blue and the driver's door was dented.* However, even with mature speakers, a number of factors complicate the use of articles, such as whether both speaker and listener have shared access to the supposedly new information. When you and your listener are both aware of a new student in class, the first mention of it will usually include the specific forms as in, *Do you know who <u>the</u> new student is?*

There are other articles (the indefinite forms *an, some, one*), but only *a* and *the* were tracked in Brown's study. By Brown's own admission, even this was difficult. Because it was not always possible to determine whether a reference to an item was the first one, it was difficult to determine which form was required. Because of this, Brown combined the data for both forms to establish mastery. Both forms appear in Stage II, but their mastery varied widely among the three subjects, from Stage III for Sarah, to Stage IV for Adam, to Stage V for Eve (the precocious one!).

Regular Past Tense Inflection.   The ninth grammatical morpheme mastered in the study was the regular past tense inflection. Of course, the term *regular* suggests that it always takes the same basic form, *-ed.* However, there are, again, three phonologically based allomorphs, /-d/ (lean<u>ed</u>), /-t/ (work<u>ed</u>), and /-Id/ (paint<u>ed</u>), which depend on whether the preceding consonant is voiced, voiceless, or a /t/ or /d/.

Although there are several quite subtle meanings that can be expressed through past tense, the primary meaning signaled by children's use is that of "earlierness" (Brown, 1973, p. 322). In this sense, past tense simply refers to an event that occurred prior to the time of the utterance. As was mentioned previously, the earliest past tense verbs were irregular forms referring to common daily activities—*ate, sat, ran,* and so forth. The earliest versions of regular past tense noted by Brown included a small set of verbs that referred to events of such short duration that they would almost always be completed by the time anyone mentioned them. These included, for example, *slipped, dropped, crashed.* Once the regular inflection appears, it generalizes to the irregular past tense words. Eventually, by Stage V all three of Brown's preschoolers had mastered most of the irregular and regular past tense forms.

Third Person Present Tense Singular.   The regular third person present tense singular verb inflection (3ppts), /-s/, and its irregular counterpart were ranked as the tenth and eleventh grammatical morphemes mastered. The regular 3ppts inflection includes three allomorphs, /-s/ (e.g., She hop<u>s</u>), /-z/ (e.g., He run<u>s</u>), and /-Iz/ (e.g., She wash<u>es</u>), which follow the same phonological patterns as the possessive and plural inflections. The irregular forms are limited to verbs such as *do/does* and *have/has.* These verb forms are required by English grammar when the subject of the sentence is in the third person. (Remember the person speaking is the "first person," the person spoken to is the "second person," and the person spoken of is the "third person.")

Ironically, the 3ppts is generally redundant in English. Most sentences in which it is required include the subject and the verb in its present tense and including it adds little information. This can be seen in comparing *He runs fast* and *He run fast;* although the latter sounds strange, it carries no less information. The 3ppts proves helpful in only a few specific instances involving nouns that do not change in their plural version. For example, in *The deer eat corn* versus *The deer eats corn,* the verb inflection clarifies whether one or more deer are feeding.

These forms also appear in Stage II and are generally mastered by Stage V. With all three of Brown's preschoolers, the regular inflection was mastered earlier than the irregular forms. A common observation, in fact, is that the regular inflection is overgeneralized as with several other regular versus irregular distinctions. As a result, preschoolers may be heard to produce such charming variations as, *He sure doos good, huh?*

Uncontractible Auxiliary.   The uncontractible auxiliary in the form of the "to be" verbs (*am, is, are, was, were*) was the 12th form to be mastered. The auxiliary is the helping verb in a sentence with another main verb, as in *He is painting a picture.* Its various aspects and characteristics were discussed previously in the context of its counterpart, the uncontractible copula. Recall that Table 8–3 also summarizes the relevant features of these forms.

The uncontractible auxiliary verb developed later than the uncontractible copula. Brown's preschoolers did not achieve mastery until well into or beyond Stage V. There may be a number of reasons for this. However, because using its various forms follows the same pattern as for the copula, it seems that it would be no more grammatically complex. On the other hand, the nature of their role may provide a possible explanation. In short, because auxiliaries only "help" the main verb, the information they convey about the action in the sentence is not as essential.

Contractible Copula and Auxiliary.   Most of the considerations related to the copula-auxiliary forms were discussed previously (see Table 8–3). The key distinction to be remembered about the contractible copula and auxiliary, the thirteenth and fourteenth morphemes mastered by Brown's subjects, is *contractibility.* In this sense, contractible simply means it would be *permissible* to contract a form. Whether the copula actually is contracted or not does not change its category. In both *Tommy is a nice guy* and *Tommy's a nice guy,* the copula is contractible.

The *is* form tends to be more prevalent resulting in some incorrect singular-plural distinctions. The *is* and *are* forms tend to emerge before *am.* Overall, Brown's preschoolers tended to fluctuate in their performance on the contractible copula (just as they did with the other copula-auxiliary forms) over a prolonged 2-year period. When these forms occur in their contracted versions, they are probably less perceptible to the preschooler.

The Nature of Mastery

Brown (1973) recognized that these 14 morphemes were not the only child language behaviors of interest. Nor were they necessarily the most important. (Who could choose?) Their usefulness would come from possibly illuminating the nature of the language learning process. As a result, much of his work went beyond tabulating and ranking these selected forms. His research also attempted to determine whether any of several factors might explain their development, with potential implications for language development in general.

Sequence and Rate of Mastery. Brown examined whether Adam, Eve, and Sarah differed in their sequence or rate in mastering the morphemes. It turned out that the sequences of mastery for the three children were quite similar, although not identical. In contrast, it became obvious that the rate at which the three children mastered the forms was quite dissimilar. Eve, in particular, was quite accelerated in her rate of mastery, whereas Sarah's rate was the slowest of the three, and Adam's fell between those of the two girls.

One subtle theme is woven throughout these results and much of Brown's discussion. That is, the extent of variability in the learning process that became apparent in at least three ways. First, the three children varied in their order of mastery, although less than they varied in their rate of mastery. Second, mastery of the morphemes themselves varied. Where some reached mastery in a fairly orderly manner (e.g., *in* and *on*), others stretched out over prolonged periods (e.g., copula-auxiliary). Finally, there was variability within certain morphemes. For example, significant fluctuations were evident in learning the copula-auxiliary forms and there were distinct differences in mastering the allomorphs related to several of the morphemes.

When the overall results are examined, a picture of *regularity* and *variation* emerges. The regularities or consistencies across children suggest that, at some level, there are similar dynamics at work. However, the variations should suggest that individual children learn language in different patterns and respond differently to various influences. The variations may also indicate that we have studied too few behaviors, too few children, or perhaps at the wrong level (Bloom & Lahey, 1978). Further, the possibility remains that the individual variations suggest that the sequences are not fixed and may be influenced by both linguistic and environmental contingencies. Some preliminary research has experimentally manipulated (reversed) the sequence of mastery for several of Brown's morphemes (Atherton & Hegde, 1996; Capelli, 1985; DeCesari, 1985).

Variables Related to Mastery. Brown examined three major variables to see if they related to the order of mastery in the 14 grammatical morphemes. The major variables included the semantic complexity, the grammatical complexity, and the frequency of occurrence in caregiver speech for each of the morphemes.

Semantic complexity was gauged by the number of discriminations required to use a morpheme correctly. For example, fewer discriminations are related to labeling the spatial relationship *on* (an item either is or is not) than are related to the use of *were* (more than one participant serving as agent in an action occurring in a previous time frame). **Grammatical complexity** of each morpheme was gauged by the number of transformations related to its correct use. And, of course, a simple tally of how frequently each form occurred in caregivers' speech samples measured the **frequency of occurrence** for each morpheme.

Recall from Chapter 4 that one of the goals of science is prediction. Like the weather, even variations in children's language development should be related to variables or patterns that can be identified. ■

semantic complexity
Measures the complexity of a linguistic structure by gauging the number of semantic relationships that must be discriminated to use it correctly.

grammatical complexity
The number of transformational rules related to the production or comprehension of a grammatical structure.

frequency of occurrence
The relative number of occurrences of a structure in a language sample.

Brown determined that the order of mastery correlated best with a rank order of combined semantic and grammatical complexity. Although semantic complexity seemed to be the more significant factor, Brown noted that it is not possible to entirely separate semantic factors from the grammatical considerations. Finally, according to Brown's analysis, the frequency of occurrence in caregivers' speech was not related to the order of mastery.

Learning Rules or Learning Contingencies?   An important implication of Brown's efforts was the potential for a better understanding of children's language development. Many researchers have speculated on how much children's language development relies on their ability to cognitively discover the rules of language in contrast to the role played by their interactions with others. Two questions that focus on this contrast are: Do children's language behaviors become consistent because they have discovered the rules of language? Or do children's repeated experiences as they learn to communicate result in increasingly consistent language behaviors, which can then be described by rules?

Brown (1973) and others (Bloom & Lahey, 1978; James, 1990; Pease & Berko Gleason, 1985; among others) interpreted his findings and similar data to suggest that preschoolers' grammatical development consists of "learning the rules of language." In arriving at this characterization, it was asserted that as preschoolers approach mastery of a morpheme, its correct production approaches the level of consistency that suggests preschoolers are "following a rule," even if they cannot state the rule. It is also suggested that preschoolers make "creative" errors as they apply newly learned rules to produce regular forms in place of irregulars, as in *sitted* for *sat.* Brown and others had also found little evidence of caregiver teaching behaviors, which would leave children to cognitively deduce the rules of language. Finally, it was reasoned that, if language development occurred through a simpler process, such as imitation, preschoolers would have mastered the morphemes in a sequence reflecting how often their caregivers had produced them.

Alternately, others (Hegde, 1980; McLaughlin & Cullinan, 1981; Moerk, 1992a; Segal, 1975; Skinner, 1974; among others) have pointed out that these assertions in a strictly cognitive characterization are not fully supported by the research that prompted them.

First, rule-governed behavior generally exhibits a rather smooth and relatively sudden acquisition (Brown, 1973). When we comprehend and apply a rule, our behavior conforms to it relatively rapidly. However, in achieving mastery, these morphemes did not follow an uninterrupted or rapid course. Instead, "there are unaccountable regressions and unexplained abrupt advances" (Brown, 1973, p. 388). From this per-

We should recall from Chapter 4 the principle of *scientific elegance.* To achieve elegance, an explanation should be as economical as possible. The inferences that children are learning rules adds little to our knowledge. Whether or not they might use some underlying cognitive process does not change what we can already observe in their language behavior. And since we cannot observe and they cannot describe it to us, any hypothetical mental process might end up being extraneous speculation.

spective, the gradual, almost painstaking way in which children's attempts slowly approach mastery appears to be the result of a prolonged accumulation of learning experiences. In fact, in a seldom quoted section, in which Brown (1973) described the variability in his subjects' language behavior, he suggested that

> the learning involved must be conceived as gradual change in a set of probabilities rather than as the sudden acquisition of quite general rules. If our conception is correct, it means that the learning of the . . . 14 grammatical morphemes is more like habit formation and operant conditioning than anyone has supposed. Skinner's definition of operant strength in terms of response probability is surprisingly apt. (p. 388)

Second, the "creativity" observed in children's early utterances would be better explained within the more comprehensive context of learning behavior. The fact that children are prone to *overgeneralize* certain inflections might be due to the lifelong human capacity for generalization, not necessarily to rule-learning that is restricted to this task during the preschool years. Some have asserted that the human ability to generalize is perhaps a defining difference between our ability to develop language in contrast to the more limited signal systems used by other species. Also, although imitation plays a role in learning new words and early attempts at learning new language structures, it is the accumulated learning from spontaneous attempts at communicating and their results that provide the driving force behind language learning.

Third, the search for caregiver teaching and reinforcement (e.g., Brown & Hanlon, 1970) appears to have been based on narrow definitions of these events. Researchers apparently looked for caregiver teaching of grammar in the form of explicit tutorials and for reinforcement following children's attempts only in explicit expressions of standard praise (e.g., *That's right! Good!*). Although these phrases occur, they are generally used to reinforce the semantic accuracy or "truth value" of children's utterances (*That's right, it's a doggy*).

Instead, it seems that reinforcement for grammatical development is also present in the complex and subtle interaction between children's attempts and the feedback they receive from caregivers. A reanalysis of Brown's (1973) original data by Moerk (1992a) revealed a striking contingency between Eve's attempts at language and her mother's responses. The mother's immediate expansions potentially reinforced Eve's attempts by signaling attention. The mother's expansions provided selective models for Eve, including an approximation toward the fully correct response. And, in many cases, the mother's expansions were reinforced with an action or object requested by Eve's utterance. In a survey of related research, Moerk (1994) found extensive evidence

 An illustration of natural consequences for advancing grammatical skills might be helpful. Picture a 2-year-old who happily enters the kitchen just as the caregiver decides they must go to the store. When the preschooler says, "I paint picture," the caregiver says, "No, we have to go!" Anyone familiar with 2-year-olds' trantrums can imagine the scene that follows. However, consider the difference had the child said, "I painted picture." Most caregivers would be wise enough to ask to see it, praise it, even bring it along. What a difference a syllable makes!

of this contingent relationship between children's attempts at grammatical structure and caregivers' corrective feedback.

Finally, when Moerk (1992a) reanalyzed Brown's frequency data, a stronger relationship than had been originally recognized became apparent. Brown had correlated the *overall* frequencies of caregiver usage with the order of mastery for the grammatical morphemes. In contrast, Moerk correlated the frequency of caregiver input in time periods *adjacent* to and preceding the emergence of the morphemes and found "impressively high correlations" (p. 49). Eve's mother appeared to mass her models of a structure just prior to its emergence in Eve's productive speech.

Children's language learning is more likely motivated by their social need to affect the behavior of others than it is by the need to "derive the rules" for grammar. From this standpoint, the development of grammatical behavior might be viewed as another form of complex human learning that is contingency shaped. This complex learning process may result from the countless, daily interactions between children, their utterances, and their caregivers' feedback. The natural consequences of these interactions in the form of relevant comments and appropriate actions by caregivers provide the reinforcement for communicating their ideas more clearly (or nonreinforcement in failing to do so).

Summary

- Preschoolers' grammatical development includes the emergence and mastery of grammatical morphemes.
- The development of various grammatical morphemes has been researched in longitudinal and cross-sectional studies.
- Preschoolers generally exhibit their first use of grammatical morphemes once they are producing multiword utterances.
- Mean length of utterance in morphemes (MLU) is a better overall measure of grammatical maturity of preschoolers' language than chronological age (CA) alone.
- Brown's subjects mastered the 14 grammatical morphemes in his study in approximately the same order, but at different rates.
- Brown found that a ranking semantic and grammatical complexity was closely related to the order in which his subjects mastered the grammatical morphemes.
- Some researchers describe children's language development as achieving "rule-governed behavior," whereas others believe that it is more accurately explained by the term "contingency shaped behavior."

Advances in Syntax

At the same time that preschoolers' utterances are expanding with additional grammatical morphemes, they are also being modified in other ways. By including additional elements and rearranging sentence elements, their ideas are expressed more completely and in new ways. These changes reflect preschoolers' advances in syntactic abilities.

Hierarchical Syntactic Relationships

The earliest multiword utterances (e.g., two-word utterances in Brown's Stage I) were characterized as expressing *linear semantic relations.* In these, the toddler seemed to produce word orders that expressed a simple additive relationship. Utterances such as *Mommy eat* seemed to reflect a relatively straightforward "one + one = two" proposition—this agent plus this action go together at this moment. Some utterances may even represent a "zero + one = one" expression. In producing *That car* while handing the item to a caregiver, the word "That" is somewhat superfluous, not adding any real information.

 Refer back to Chapter 1 to review discussion of hierarchical sentence structure. ∎

Once preschoolers are producing two-word utterances, at approximately 2 years of age, three- and even four-word utterances begin to appear. (See Table 7–4 for examples of common three-word utterances.) At this level, it is possible that the expanded sentence elements represent *hierarchical sentence structure.* That is, certain words may be more closely linked and may relate as a unit under the overall sentence organization. Two patterns in preschool language development that suggest the beginnings of hierarchical syntactic structure include recombinations and expansions (Brown, 1973).

It is worthwhile being reminded that children probably do not have a conscious goal of producing longer utterances. Longer utterances more likely result from their desire to be understood and have their needs met. Whether or not they are aware of it, their increasingly complex and remote ideas often require additional language structures to add clarity and make their utterances more effective.

Recombinations. **Recombinations** are the result of preschoolers combining utterances from levels that occurred previously, resulting in a single, longer utterance. For example, two common structures at the two-word level would be *agent + action* and *action + object,* as in *Mommy eat* and *Eat cookie.* In building up a longer utterance and expressing all the relevant relationships, the preschooler recombines these without repeating the common element to eliminate redundancy. An analogous formula might appear as follows:

recombinations The developmental process of combining two shorter language constructions into a longer construction.

$$\begin{array}{r} \text{Mommy + eat} \\ \text{eat + cookie} \\ \hline \text{Mommy + eat + cookie} \end{array}$$

Expansions. The other way in which utterances lengthen is from within. *Expansions* include additional information to elaborate on one of the terms in the utterance. These early expansions usually express attributive, possession, or recurrence information to elaborate on a noun in the more basic utterance. The following examples illustrate each of these:

Attributive:	Hold doll.	→	(Hold *new* doll.)
Possession:	Eat hotdog.	→	(Eat *Daddy* hotdog.)
Recurrence:	Want milk.	→	(Want *more* milk.)

The same patterns result in expansion to four-word utterances. However, preschoolers do not typically express any additional relations or semantic roles until sometime later with longer compound or complex sentence structures.

Basic Sentence Constituents

phrase   Groups of words that are structurally related but do not comprise a clause or sentence.

clause   A group of words that includes a subject and a predicate, but is not necessarily grammatically complete.

sentence   A group of words that includes a subject and a predicate and is structurally complete.

In syntax, individual words are combined or sequenced into larger, more meaningful units. **Phrases** are groups of words that are structurally or syntactically related, such as *Big boy.* A **clause,** however, is a group of words that includes a subject and a predicate, as in *Big boy eat.* This clause includes the basic constituents required for a sentence, but most would view it as grammatically incomplete. Finally, a **sentence** is a clause that is structurally complete, as in *The big boy is eating a cookie.*

Linguists point out that every sentence is composed of a *subject* and a *predicate.* This probably reflects the fact that the world we talk about is composed of people and objects involved in actions and or relationships. The sentence roles filled by people and objects are expressed through *nouns* or *noun phrases,* a group of words structured around a noun. These noun phrases serve as the subject, object, or complement of the sentence. The actions or relationships that are central to a sentence are expressed in *verbs* or *verb phrases,* again, referring to a group of words structured around a verb. See Table 8–4 for an illustration of the basic roles played by these sentence constituents in early sentence constructions.

Initially, in Stage I, in their early two-word utterances, preschoolers typically produce either a simple noun phrase (*a + Noun,* or *that + Noun*). Utterances with a verb include a noun as either the subject or object element (*Noun + Verb,* or *Verb + Noun*). (See Table 8–4.) During Stage II, preschoolers include the subject more consistently. By Stage III, their utterances may still frequently be grammatically incomplete clauses, but they will often contain all three major constituents of basic sentences—the subject, verb, and object/complement. Of course, as preschoolers learn to elaborate and express more ideas in a sentence, these basic constituents change to include a variety of other forms in grammatically complete sentences.

Noun Phrase Elements

Another term related to nouns is *nominals,* which refers to a word or phrase that acts like a noun. ■

The basic noun phrase contains at least a noun, called the head word. Frequently, a determiner of various forms precedes the noun, such as in *A car,* or *That boy.* Nouns can name common objects and their categories, specific people and places, and abstract concepts.

Table 8–4. Basic sentence constituents in early utterances.

Stages	Sentence Constituents	Examples
Stage I		
Word	Noun	*Doggy*
Noun phrase	Modifier + Noun	*A doggy* (or *That dog*)
Verb phrase	Verb + Noun	*Bite toy*
Clause	Noun + Verb	*Doggy bite*
Stage II		
Noun Phrase	Modifer + Noun	*A big doggy*
Clause	Noun + Verb + Modifier + Object	*Doggy biting my toy.*
Clause	Modifier + Noun + Verb + Modifier + Noun	*That doggy biting my toy.*
Stage III +		
Clause	Modifiers + Noun + Verb + Modifers + Noun	*That bad doggy biting my new toy.*
Sentence	Modifiers + Noun + Aux + Verb + Modifiers + Noun	*That bad doggy is biting my new toy.*

As was discussed previously, children's first words are mostly nouns used to label things. Eventually, these basic nouns are expanded and altered through various elements to communicate in more specific or flexible ways.

Noun Phrase Elaboration. To communicate more precisely, speakers elaborate on the nouns in an utterance with additional information. Speakers use a variety of forms to accomplish this, depending on the information they need to convey. In English, speakers precede nouns with forms called **determiners** (traditionally called *modifiers*), which qualify, specify, quantify, or rank the noun (Heidinger, 1984). Determiners include *prearticles, articles, demonstratives, possessives, ordinals, quantifiers, comparatives* or *superlatives,* and finally, *adjectives.* (Actually, nouns themselves can modify the nouns that follow them, as in *foot doctor* or *coffee shop.*) Table 8–5 presents examples of noun phrase elements.

> **determiners** Words, including articles, adjectives, and demonstratives, that modify the noun with which they are associated; traditionally called modifiers.

There may be characteristic patterns in which noun phrase elaboration emerges in children's language (Owens, 2005; Wells, 1985), although this is not well documented. In Stage I, toddlers modify nouns that might otherwise occur alone, usually with a nondefinite article (*a cookie*) or a demonstrative (*that cookie*). In Stage II, preschoolers begin to modify nouns occurring in the object phrase of longer utterances, even when subject phrases are also present (*Tommy ate big cookie*). By Stage III, modifiers appear in both the subject and object phrases, and by Stage V they may be using multiple modifiers (*My big blue car broke!*).

The earliest forms children include are the articles (*a, the*) and demonstratives (*this, that*). These are more generic in nature. Therefore, they can be used more widely and less discriminatively. However, this also makes

Table 8–5. Noun phrase elements and examples.

Prearticles	Articles	Demonstratives	Possessives	Ordinals	Quantifiers	Comparatives Superlatives	Adjectives	Nouns
just, only, even, all of, two of, some of, etc.	Definite: *the, each, every, either.* Nondefinite: *a, an, some, any,* etc.	*this, that, these, those*	*Mommy's, Daddy's, cat's, his, her, our, their,* etc.	*first, second, third, last, middle, next,* etc.	*one, two, three, many, several, few,* etc.	*more, fewer, better, most, fewest, best,* etc.	*green, round, heavy, rough, awful, cheap,* etc.	*cars, dog, ball, people, tree, night, love,* etc.

Rule for Determiners:

Det → (Prearticles) + Article / Demonstrative / Possessive + Ordinal / Quantifier / Comparative Superlative + Adjective + Noun

Examples:

Prearticles	Articles	Demonstratives	Possessives	Ordinals	Quantifiers	Comparatives Superlatives	Adjectives	Nouns
Only	the				three	biggest	green	balls . . .
	The			middle	two		tall	people . . .
		These		last	three		cheap	cars . . .
			Daddy's	first	three		big	bites . . .

them less communicative. Later, possessives (*my, Tommy's*), quantifiers (*all, some*), and adjectives (*big, blue, new*), which communicate more specific information, appear.

Pronouns. **Pronouns** (sometimes called *pronominals*) are a group of forms (e.g., *he, she, they*) that can replace nouns or entire noun phrases. The substitution process described by linguists is called **pronominalization.** In essence, through this process pronouns become equivalent to the words they replace. This results in **constituent equivalence.** In most cases, pronoun usage is based on *anaphoric reference*, in which the pronoun refers to a person or thing that has been mentioned previously. For example, speakers generally do not use the personal pronoun *he* until they have mentioned who it represents, as in *John ran away because <u>he</u> was scared.* (We would not typically say, *He ran away because John was scared*, unless *He* refers to someone else mentioned previously.) **Cataphoric reference** in which pronouns precede the noun they represent develops in later, more complex constructions, as in *When <u>he</u> was finished, <u>Dad</u> took a nap.*

Personal pronouns, perhaps the most complicated forms, are used to replace nouns referring to persons. As can be seen in Table 8–6, pronouns take various forms, depending on the context. Personal pronouns vary depending on the number, person, gender, and case.

Reflexive pronouns are forms that "reflect" back on the preceding subject of a sentence, as in *When I looked in the water, I saw myself.* Demonstrative pronouns include the demonstrative forms, *this, that, these,* and *those*, which replace nouns rather than modifying them. For example, if a certain book has already been mentioned, we might simply say, *<u>That</u> is mine,* as opposed to *<u>That book</u> is mine.* In the first sentence, *that* replaces *book,* whereas in the second *that* modifies *book.* Indefinite pronouns are compound words composed of *any, every, no,* and *some* combined with *one, thing, place,* or *body.* They are named *indefinite* for the fact that they do not have a specific referent, as in *Bring me something to drink.*

The English pronoun system is complex and confusing. Therefore, it is not surprising that pronouns develop slowly and variably in preschoolers. The variability in acquisition is such that only a general sequence can be identified. The earliest forms (*this, that, it*), which occur in Stage I, seem to simply signal existence. Most personal pronouns emerge after Stage II. Generally, subjective pronouns (*I, you, he, she, they*) tend to be mastered earlier. Next, objective pronouns (*me, him, her, them*) are mastered. The possessive pronouns (*his, her, theirs*) are acquired later. The exception to this is the first person forms (*my, mine*), which are acquired much earlier (to no caregiver's real surprise). The last pronouns to be mastered, the reflexive pronouns (*myself, himself, herself, themselves*), are acquired much later, after Stage V.

pronoun Words that can replace a noun or noun phrase through anaphoric or cataphoric reference; also called pronominals.

pronominalization The process of replacing a noun or noun phrase with a pronoun form (or pronominal).

constituent equivalence The status pronouns assume with regard to the nouns or noun phrases they replace.

cataphoric reference The linguistic effect in which pronouns replace nouns or noun phrases and refer to their occurrence later in the context.

Some linguists prefer the term *pronominal* because it suggests a form that can substitute for structures more substantial than a single noun, such as a noun phrase and even entire sentences. ■

Although pronouns are important grammatical morphemes, Brown did not include them in his study. Bascially this was because they do not meet the criterion for obligatory context. Pronouns may optionally replace a noun or entire noun phrase in a sentence. They might serve as the subject or object of the sentence or simply be used to indicate possession.

Table 8–6. English personal pronoun system.

Person	Subjective	Objective	Possessive
First	*I, we*	*me, us*	*mine, ours*
Second	*you*	*you*	*yours*
Third	*he, she, they, it*	*him, her, them, it*	*his, hers, its, theirs*

As preschoolers attempt to use pronouns some common substitutions occur. Most commonly, preschoolers substitute the objective for the subjective case (e.g., *me/I, him/he, her/she, them/they*). This results in almost stereotypical expressions, such as *Me want candy,* or *Her has new shoes.* With the exception of reflexive pronouns, most pronouns are mastered by approximately 5 years of age, although the sequence of mastery might be different for each preschooler.

Adjective and Noun Suffixes.   Finally, noun phrases might include several forms that result from adding suffixes to adjectives or verbs. Within the adjective class, preschoolers will develop the ability to express degrees of an attribute by adding inflectional suffixes to the relevant adjective—a building is *tall,* one is *taller* than another, and one is the *tallest* of them all. Using these suffixes is based on the cognitive ability to rank-order items along some dimension (e.g., length) or attribute (e.g., color). In addition, this ability plays an important role in many transactions that occur in preschoolers' daily social interactions. Although all persons are created equal, preschoolers know that all cookies are not!

Between 3 and 5 years of age, most preschoolers understand and begin to use the comparative and superlative inflectional suffixes, *-er* and *-est.* The **comparative** *-er* indicates a comparison between only two items, as in *This cookie is bigger than that cookie.* The **superlative** form signals that the comparison is among more than two items, as in *Of all the cookies, this one is the biggest.* The superlative form *-est* appears to emerge first, by 4 years of age, and the comparative *-er* is mastered by 5 years of age. The irregular versions (*better, best,* and *more, most*) go through a period in which overapplication of the suffix results in forms such as *bestest* and *more bigger.*

Another suffix applied to verbs derives nouns that can then become the head noun in a noun phrase. The **derivational noun suffix** *-er* changes a verb into a noun that names the person who engages in that action. For example, someone who *runs* is a *runner,* and someone who *paints* is a *painter.* In their early attempts at acknowledging the roles that people often play, younger preschoolers begin by attaching a *man* or (the less sexist) *-person* suffix, as in *storeman* or *cookperson.* Use of the derivational suffix *-er* appears to be mastered by around 5 years of age.

Recall from Chapter 1 that a defining difference between inflectional and derivational morphemes is whether they change the grammatical class of the stem word. ◼

comparative   Adjective form that expresses the relative degree of an attribute in comparing two items (e.g., *big* vs. *bigger*).

superlative   Adjective form that expresses relative degree of an attribute when comparing more than two items (e.g. *big* vs. *bigger* vs. *biggest*).

derivational noun suffix A type of derivational morpheme in the form of a suffix (-er) that derives a noun from a verb (e.g., the noun *runner* derives from the verb *run*).

Verb Phrase Elements

In every sentence there is a subject combined with a predicate. The predicate appears in the form of a verb phrase. Verb phrases can assume a variety of forms depending on the nature of the event or relationship they express. Verbs are classified according to the semantic relationships they convey and according to their syntactic restrictions.

Semantic and Syntactic Roles. Semantically, verbs assume the role of expressing different relationships. **Action verbs** refer to activity that can be seen, such as *eating, walking, painting*. We may be most conscious of these verbs because the actions or movements they refer to are visible, which distinguishes them from process and state verbs.

Semantically, **process verbs** refer to internal activity or to gradual changes in persons or things. Someone may be doing something where the "doing" cannot be seen, such as in *thinking, hearing,* or *seeing*. Similarly, people and things might change due to gradual processes that cannot be seen in any immediate sense, such as the aging process we all stubbornly go through or the process of oxidation ("rusting") that many items exhibit.

Finally, **state verbs** express a relatively static, or unchanging condition. State verbs generally link the subject of the sentence to some quality or condition, as in *That man is tall* or *That man is alone.* These have also been referred to as equative verbs because the verb essentially serves as an equals sign (i.e., *That man = tall*). The quality or condition is referred to as the *complement* of the verb because it *completes* the equation. State verbs that are lexical (described later) include such states as *wanting, remaining,* and *stayed.*

Syntactically, verbs can be classified according to the role they play in the sentence structure. From this standpoint, they might be classified as grammatical verbs and lexical verbs. **Grammatical verbs** include such structures as copula and auxiliary forms (e.g., *is, are, was, were*) that play a grammatical role in sequencing structures. **Lexical verbs** (e.g., *run, sit, write*) convey specific content in a sentence and are also classified according to what structures may follow them.

Transitive verbs are lexical verbs that are capable of carrying a direct object—something that is directly affected by the action of the verb. For example, the verb *hit* requires that something receive the force of the verb, as in *The boy hit the ball.* In addition to action verbs, transitive verbs might also carry a direct object that is experienced through a process verb, as in *The conductor heard the violins.*

As might be expected, **intransitive verbs** are lexical verbs that do not carry direct objects. Intransitive verbs include action verbs, although the action does not directly affect anything. For example, in *She is smiling*, there is nothing that is *directly* affected by the action. Although we might say *She is smiling at the baby*, she cannot *smile the baby*, and the baby is not physically impacted.

action verbs Words that refer to activity that is observable.

process verbs Words that refer to unobservable activity or gradual changes.

state verbs Words that link a subject to a stable or unchanging condition or attribute.

In contrast to lexical verbs, *grammatical verbs* are forms such as auxiliaries, copula, and modals. Rather than carry true meaning, they convey tense and number and also sequence the elements in a sentence. ■

grammatical verbs Verbs that play a grammatical role without conveying specific actions; compare **lexical verbs.**

lexical verbs Verbs that express a specific activity.

transitive verb Lexical verbs capable of carrying a grammatical object affected by the action of the verb; compare **intransitive verb.**

intransitive verb Lexical verbs that are incapable of carrying a grammatical object; compare **transitive verb.**

copula verb   A grammatical verb that serves to link or equate its subject to a noun phrase, adjective, or prepositional phrase.

auxiliary verb Grammatical verbs that serve as helping verbs by conveying number and tense.

modal auxiliary verbs Auxiliary verbs that express the speaker's attitude or mood regarding the main verb.

Copula and Auxiliary Verbs.   Copula and auxiliary verbs are grammatical verbs and were discussed previously in this chapter in the context of Brown's 14 grammatical morphemes. Briefly, when a "to be" verb (*am, is, are, was, were*) serves syntactically as the main verb in a sentence, it is a **copula verb.** Copula verbs are the syntactic equivalent of semantic state verbs. The copula acts as the grammatical link between the subject of the sentence and its complement, as in *The girl is (complement),* where the complement can be a noun phrase (*a Girl Scout*), pronoun (*it*), adjective (*happy*), prepositional phrase (*in her room*), or participle (*missing*).

In contrast, **auxiliary verbs** include the "to be" verbs and modals as helping verbs that accompany main verbs. The main verb usually carries the progressive inflection (*-ing*), as in *am sitting, is running, was eating.* The auxiliary verb supplements the main (lexical) verb with information about person, number, and tense.

Another quite varied group of auxiliary verbs is the modal auxiliaries. **Modal auxiliary verbs** are helping verbs that express the speaker's mood about the action indicated. These forms are semantically subtle and can be syntactically complex. The subtle shades of mood or attitude expressed by the modal auxiliaries below are familiar to us all:

Modal	*Mood expressed*
I *can* study.	Capability
I *could* study.	Possibility
I *should* study.	Obligation
I *will* study.	Promise
I *would* study.	Willingness
I *may* study.	Possibility
You *may* study here.	Permission
I *might* study.	Possibility
I *must* study.	Necessity

Finally, two other forms of auxiliary verbs play less common roles, but are nonetheless important. The first of these, the "do" auxiliary, normally appears for the sake of emphasis, as in *I really do like your hair that way.* However, it also plays an important syntactic role, being inserted when converting declarative statements into negatives (*I run every day* ⇒ *I do not run every day*) and interrogatives (*You run everyday* ⇒ *Do you run everyday?*). Of course, *do* can occur as a lexical verb, as in *I'll do the dishes tonight.* (Strangely, linguists have never explained why this form disappears in such utterances while children go through adolescence!) The second form, the "have" auxiliary, accompanies a main verb, as in *I have lost some money.* It, too, can serve as a lexical verb, as in *I have money.*

Development in Verb Phrases.   The previous information oversimplifies our complex English verb system. As preschoolers attempt to express their increasingly complex ideas, their task is especially difficult because of this complexity. Nonetheless, by approximately 5 years of age, they have mastered most of the forms in the English verb system (Wells, 1985).

During Stage I, when utterances are predominately one and two words, preschoolers produce primarily lexical verbs. These, of course, name the action that they are focusing on at the moment. The most common lexical verbs (e.g., *eat, put, make, get*) also tend to be transitive in nature, that is, they relate to an object affected by the action named (even though the object is not being expressed). Perhaps this prominence stems from these actions being more conspicuous in the effect they have on the concrete object involved.

In Stage II, the present progressive inflection, *-ing,* appears. Its early emergence may stem from two factors. First, the progressive inflection has perceptual salience—it is an entire additional syllable. Second, the progressive inflection is relevant to preschoolers' cognitive focus—it indicates the ongoing, "here-and-now" nature of the actions young preschoolers talk about with their listeners. The ever-present semi-auxiliaries (or catenatives) *hafta, gonna, wanna* also appear during Stage II. Preschoolers also begin to use what appear to be auxiliaries in the form of *can't* and *don't* during this period. With these forms, preschoolers appear to incorporate auxiliaries; however, the true auxiliaries *can* and *do* may not appear elsewhere in their language. This suggests that *can't* and *don't* are initially just "big words" used for negation.

In Stage III, the modal auxiliaries *can* and *will* and the "be" auxiliary verbs appear. However, the "be" auxiliaries require noun-verb agreement (*I-am/was, You-are/were, He-is/was, They-are/were*) and may not be completely mastered until after Stage V. During Stage III, preschoolers also begin to signal that they understand that not all events are in the "here-and-now"—events can be recalled from the past. They initially express this through the irregular forms for more common activities, such as *sat, ate,* and *ran.* However, once the past tense inflection *-ed* appears during this stage, it overgeneralizes to these previously correct forms, as in *sitted, eated,* and *runned.*

As preschoolers mature socially and cognitively, they become more aware of their emotions and attitudes. As might be expected, they express these more fully in their language in various ways. In Stage IV, modal auxiliaries such as *may, might,* and *must* emerge in verb system of preschoolers as they begin to express their attitudes when the need arises.

Finally, by Stage V, preschoolers will have mastered the distinction between regular tense inflections and irregular past tense forms. They will be able to use the third person present tense inflection and the contractible copula. Stage V is generally reached at about 5 years of age. If there is a "rule of thumb" that has emerged throughout the discussion of the many areas of children's language development, it would be that most of the grammatical aspects of language have been mastered by the time a child turns 5 years of age.

A number of grammatical aspects, primarily those that are less consistent or irregular in form, are mastered after Stage V. These include the various forms of the "to be" auxiliary, modal auxiliaries, and noun-verb agreement between the singular and plural subjects and their corresponding verb forms.

Basic Sentence Structure

From their earliest attempts at communication, children have announced their ideas, quizzed others on theirs, and expressed disagreement with those around them on various topics. By Stage III, preschoolers produce longer utterances and rearrange the words to produce more adult-like utterances that will increasingly serve their need to declare, question, and disagree.

Declaratives.   *Declarative sentences* assert some information, as in the utterance *That dog is cute.* Perhaps the toddler's first word, at 1 year of age, represents the first declarative. However, we must remember that interpreting intentions can be difficult even with careful observation of the context and the children's reactions to caregiver responses. Fortunately, one of the earliest speech behaviors to develop is intonational contour, which may serve as an additional clue. The earliest utterances with falling intonational contour and accompanied by gestures to direct attention (e.g., pointing as they say *Doggy*) may well be declaratives.

Of course, declaratives become longer and more complex as they communicate more information. This results from several factors. Maturing motor control permits improved coordination for physical production of longer syllable strings. Cognitively, preschoolers perceive new and more complex relationships among objects and events. Their expanding social interactions prompt the need to fine-tune the expression of these new ideas. In doing so, they incorporate additional grammatical morphemes, elaborate on nouns, and use more complex verb structure to express whether events are ongoing, completed, or yet to happen. And because this results in conveying their thoughts and interacting more effectively with others, these new behaviors become an integral part of their language behavior.

Interrogatives.   *Interrogative sentences* are forms that request confirmation, denial, or information, as in *Are you coming with us?* More commonly, these are called *questions.* There are three basic types of questions in English: yes-no questions, wh-questions, and tag questions. According to linguists, all questions are based on an underlying statement and the three types of questions differ in the hypothetical processes we use to form them out of this statement. Table 8–7 summarizes development of questions.

First, for both yes-no questions and wh-questions, the copula or auxiliary in the underlying sentence is *inverted* or moved to precede the subject. As can be seen in Table 8–7, when there is no copula/auxiliary, a "dummy" form (e.g., a *do* or *have*) is hypothetically inserted to be inverted. Second, in wh-questions, in addition to inverting the copula/auxiliary verb, a wh-word is substituted for the sentence constituent sought by the question, and

Recall from Chapter 5 that, even before the first word, infants' gestures and vocalizations have been interpreted as a form of assertion. Fittingly, these are called *protodeclaratives.* ◾

Recall from Chapter 4 that Chomsky described the deep structure of every sentence as a *simple active declarative.* It is the underlying statement in the hypothetical deep structure that we transform into a question. ◾

Table 8–7. Development of yes-no questions and wh-questions.

Period	Yes-No Question Formation	Examples	Wh-Question Formation	Examples
Early	Word + Rising intonation	*Milk?*		*What this?*
Stage I	NP + Rising intonation	*That kitty?*	What + NP?	*What Mommy doing?*
			What + NP (+doing)?	*Where Mommy go?*
			Where + NP (+go)?	
Stage II			What + NP + Verb?	*What Mommy make?*
			Where + NP + Copula?	*Where Mommy is?*
Late Stage II			Where + Copula + NP?	*Where is Mommy?*
Stage III	Aux + NP + Verb	*Do kitties swim?*	What + NP + Auxiliary + Verb?	*What Mommy is making?*
	Cop + NP + Complement	*Is Daddy happy?*	Where + NP + Auxiliary + Verb?	*Where Daddy can go?*
Final	Inverts all auxiliary and copula to form adult questions	*Can I go play?*	Preposes all wh-words and inverts all auxiliary and copula to form adult questions.	*How did he do that?*
		Are the boys here?		*When are they coming?*
		Does he like me?		*Why can't he help?*
				Who was at the party?

then *preposed* or moved to the front of the question. Finally, tag questions are a form of question in which a statement has a yes-no question tagged on at the end.

The nature of the three question forms differs in the kind of information they ask for and, therefore, the responses they require. The yes-no question asks for confirmation or denial of the information stated in the question. This form of question requires no more of the listener than a *yes* or *no* response; hence its name. For the speaker, the simplest forms of yes-no questions require only a rising intonation, as in *You're leaving now?*

The wh-question is sometimes referred to as the specific constituent question. Each wh-word (*who, what, where, why, when, which, how*) requests information that would be found in a specific sentence constituent. For example, if the information we needed were in the form of a statement, such as *Bill is washing the car in the driveway,* different wh-words could ask for different constituents from this hypothetical statement. (*Who is washing the car? Where is Bill washing the car? What is Bill doing to the car?* and so on.)

Tag questions also require only a *yes* or *no* response, as in *We're ready, aren't we?* However, they are more complicated than yes-no questions. Through tag questions, we are seeking to confirm that the relationship stated is true or untrue. If we want to affirm that something is true (i.e., we expect a positive response), we state it positively (*It is a nice day, . . .*), but the tag that follows includes a negative (*. . . isn't it?*). Of course, this is reversed if we are seeking to confirm a negative relationship (*This isn't easy, is it?*).

Developmentally, interrogatives (questions) have been evident from the first word and perhaps before. Facial expressions, gestures, and a characteristic rising intonational contour have been helpful in signaling curiosity even before the first recognizable word. Once the first word occurred, a word spoken with rising intonation provided the first truly verbal question. However, as we have seen, the adult forms of questions are quite complex. Mastery of the grammatical forms for questions is a prolonged process that has been described as occurring over three distinct periods (Klima & Bellugi, 1966).

In Chapter 5 it is pointed out that Skinner (1957) suggested that intonation might be the first form of autoclitic (or syntactically related) behavior. ■

Initially, a child's rising intonation applied to a nucleus word (*Ball?*) is all that is needed to evoke an answer (*That's right!*) from a responsive listener. Klima and Bellugi located the beginning of grammatical questions in Period I, when rising intonation is applied to basic nucleus statements, as in *That doggie?,* to produce yes-no questions. The three forms of wh-questions that emerge in Period I ask for information preschoolers talk about in their declarative utterances—information about labels, actions, and locations. Accordingly these take the form of *What + NP?* (*What this?*), *What + NP* (*+ doing*)? (*What Daddy doing?*) and *Where + NP?* (*Where sissy?*). These tend to be routine question forms; that is, they are familiar questions associated with everyday information.

Cognitively speaking, the other wh-words (*when, why,* and *how*) emerge later because they ask for relationships (time, causality, and manner) that are not yet understood by younger preschoolers (Lane & Molyneaux,

1992). In fact, Klima and Bellugi (1966) found that children did not consistently answer wh-questions like those they were using in Period I.

According to Klima and Bellugi (1966), no real growth in yes-no questions occurs in Period II. Development in wh-questions during Period II primarily consists of more frequently including both the subject and predicate. Additionally, preschoolers begin to comprehend most wh-question forms.

In Klima and Bellugi's (1966) Period III, the copula and auxiliary forms appear in most preschoolers' sentences. Accordingly, they also appear in preschoolers' questions in a limited way. Preschoolers begin to invert the copula and auxiliary verbs, especially the *do* forms, but only in yes-no questions. Although copula and auxiliaries are present, they are not yet inverted in wh-questions, resulting in forms such as, *What you are doing?*

Beyond Period III, preschoolers go on to correctly invert copula and auxiliary forms in wh-questions, insert dummy forms (e.g., *do* or *have*) where needed, and, basically, produce adultlike question forms. The final development, asking tag questions, occurs much later.

Negatives. *Negatives* are those forms that express nonexistence, disappearance, cessation, rejection, prohibition, and denial (Bloom & Lahey, 1978). For example, *I am <u>not</u> ready to go* illustrates one form of negation. Just as with interrogatives, negation clearly predates the first words. Although they may not be symbolic, infants' reactions, such as facial expressions, fussing, head turning, kicking, and arm waving, can speak loudly about rejecting unwanted attention, interruptions, strained peas and such!

The earliest form of verbal negation, *No!,* appears in the single-word stage (and never goes away!). Beyond this first step, the development of syntactic negation progresses through several periods (Bellugi, 1967). See Table 8–8 for examples of negation and their development. In Period I, toddlers' earliest multiword utterances express negation by placing negative forms (*no, not, allgone*) outside the nucleus statement, as in *not sleepy! no peas!* and *allgone cookie.*

Table 8–8. Development of negation.

Period	Negative Formation	Examples
Early	Neg (indicating nonexistence, rejection, or denial)	*No!, Allgone!, No-more!*
I	Neg + NP Neg + NP + Verb (presentence)	*No bath!* *No daddy play.*
II	NP + Neg + Verb (prepredicate) NP + can't/don't + Verb	*Daddy not sleep.* *I can't go.* *I don't like it.*
III	NP + can/do/does/did/will + not + Verb NP + isn't/aren't + Verb	*That boy will not play.* *She isn't helping me.*
Late	NP + wouldn't/couldn't/shouldn't + Verb	*She wouldn't believe it.*

The importance of observing the overall context and using the "method of rich interpretation" in determining the meaning of children's utterances is discussed in Chapter 4. ∎

It is sometimes difficult to determine if such forms truly represent syntactic negation (Bellugi, 1967; Bloom & Lahey, 1978). Some of these forms (e.g., *No Daddy read!*) may in fact represent two utterances. In producing these, preschoolers may reject caregivers' propositions (e.g., *Should someone read to you now?*) with an initial negative (*No*), and then state an alternative proposition in the immediately following sentence (*Daddy read!*). In this example, the preschooler's entire utterance sounds as though Dad should not read bedtime stories. In fact, a younger preschooler may simply fail to pause between the two sentence elements (*No / Daddy read*) when Dad is wanted as the reader that night.

Some have proposed that such *presentence negation,* when negative forms precede the full sentence, is not truly syntactic. In contrast, truly syntactic negation should only be credited when *prepredicate negation* occurs, in which negative forms precede the verb, for example, only when *Daddy no read,* is used to reject Dad's participation. Of course, taking note of the overall context would help clarify the meaning of such utterances.

In Period II, the negative forms begin to appear within the sentence, adjacent to the main verb, as in *I no take bath!* In this period, true auxiliaries have not yet appeared, but *can't* and *don't* have emerged. Younger preschoolers do not use these in their uncontracted forms (*can not, do not*) and appear to substitute them for *not* as though they are just big "negative words."

Finally, in Period III, the preschooler begins to use most of the copula and auxiliary verbs with *not* in both the contracted and uncontracted forms. At this point, they are able to express negation, with its various meanings, in more adultlike forms.

Imperatives and Passives.   *Imperative sentences* take the form of commands or requests with no expressed subject, such as *Pass the butter, Close the door,* or *Stop!* Each of these carries an implied subject, as in *(You) Pass the butter.* These appear to be present in children by the time they are 3 years old. However, this is difficult to confirm, as younger preschoolers frequently omit the subject of their sentences (Brown, 1973).

Passive sentences, in which the noun in the subject phrase is passive and acted on by the noun in the object phrase (e.g., *The <u>house</u> was painted by the <u>man</u>*) are difficult for younger preschoolers to comprehend. They are not produced correctly until the children are school age.

Complex and Compound Sentences

In basic sentences, words are strung together in certain ways that express the relationships among the elements they represent. Those relationships combine to convey an overall idea. Generally, with increased experience and understanding, preschoolers between ages 2 and 3 years begin to combine several ideas in longer utterances (Bloom & Lahey, 1978).

Two basic achievements accomplish this. Brown characterized Stage IV as the period in which preschoolers learn to embed additional information, creating complex sentences. And Stage V was described as the period in which conjoining ideas into compound sentences is mastered. See Table 8–9 for examples of both complex and compound sentence structures.

Complex Sentences. A **complex sentence** consists of an independent or main clause (a subject and a predicate that can "stand alone") with a dependent or subordinate clause embedded in it. As the name suggests, **subordinate clauses** are dependent or secondary clauses, meaning that their only purpose is to supplement or clarify the main clause. Embedding is the process that speakers hypothetically use to rearrange or order the segments into a complex sentence. Table 8–9 also presents examples of subordinate clauses embedded in the main clause to behave as though they are nouns, adverbs, or adjectives. Subordinate clauses acting as noun phrases include **object noun phrase complements** (clauses introduced by *that,* which follow certain verbs and act as nouns to complete the verb) and **infinitives** (phrases in the form of *to verb* that behave as nouns, adjectives, or adverbs). Subordinate clauses introduced by **subordinating conjunctions** (e.g., *when, where, if, until, before, after,* and *because*) act as adverbs to describe the time, location, cause, or condition related to the proposition in the main clause. Finally, subordinate clauses introduced by **relative pronouns,** such

complex sentence A sentence composed of a main clause with an embedded subordinate clause.

subordinate clause An embedded clause that supplements the main clause in a complex sentence.

object noun phrase complements Clauses introduced by *that* which serve as object phrases and complete a sentence (e.g., *I see that he is here*).

infinitive A phrase in the form of *to verb* that serves as a noun, adjective, or adverb (e.g., *To err* is human . . .).

Table 8–9. Examples of complex and compound sentence structure.

Sentence Structure	Sentence Elements	Examples
Complex		
Object NP complements	Main: I hope (X) Subordinate: (that) it's mine.	*I hope that it's mine.*
Wh-adverbial clauses	Main: I know (X) Subordinate: (what) you like.	*I know what you like.*
Infinitive phrase	Main: I want (X) Subordinate: to go home.	*I want to go home.*
Relative clause	Main: The girl was helpful Subordinate: The girl stopped.	*The girl who stopped was helpful.*
Compound		
Compound sentences	John walked. Mary skipped.	*John walked and Mary skipped.*
Compound subjects	John walked. Mary walked.	*John and Mary walked.*
Compound predicates	John walked. John sang.	*John walked and sang.*
Compound objects	John ate a sandwich. John ate a pickle.	*John ate a sandwich and pickle.*
Disjunction	John liked her. She didn't like him.	*John liked her, but she didn't like him.*
Alternation	We could eat pizza. We could eat Chinese.	*We could eat pizza or we could eat Chinese.*

subordinating conjunction A conjunction that introduces a clause that acts as an adverb to describe time, location, cause, or conditions related to the main clause.

relative pronoun Pronouns that introduce relative clauses, which act as adjectives for the noun they follow (e.g., *The boy who came thanked me*).

Be aware that some linguists use the term *complex sentence* to include any sentence with more than one clause. This use would include compound sentences also. ▪

The mental process of embedding hypothesized by linguists would be included in Skinner's autoclitic ordering, described in Chapter 4. ▪

compound sentence A sentence composed of two independent clauses joined by a conjunction.

coordinating conjunction A connecting word that links two structures into one sentence.

Some authors prefer the term *compound clauses,* because as described previously, clauses are a more basic unit of sentence structure. ▪

as *that, which,* and *who,* play the role of adjectives to follow and modify nouns (instead of substituting for nouns).

Developmentally, the earliest form of complex sentences to appear in preschoolers' language is based on *object noun phrase complements.* These have been observed in children between 18 months and 3 years, when MLU is between 3.0 and 4.0. These take the form of *I think (X),* where X is a clause introduced by *that,* as in *I think that I like candy* (Limber, 1973).

The second form of complex embedding observed at approximately the same time is the *wh-adverbial clause.* In these, the subordinate clause is introduced with a wh-word serving as a conjunction (e.g., who, what, when, where, which, how, why). These also take the general form of *I know (X),* in which *X* is the wh-subordinate clause. For example, *I know what I like to eat.*

The third form to appear as an embedded structure is the infinitive phrase. These take the form of *I like to play,* in which the *to verb* serves as an object of the verb. The infinitive phrase typically fulfills the notion of the "something" that completes the sense of the verb. These forms are observed during late Stage IV in 3-year-olds with MLUs between 3.0 and 4.0.

Finally, the relative clause is a later developing form in complex sentences, observed in Stage V and later, as the preschooler approaches 4 years of age with an MLU of 4.0 to 4.5. Earlier forms appear to modify abstract adverbial nouns (*This is the way that I walk*). Next, relative clauses are attached to "empty" nouns (*She's the one who I like*). And, later, relative clauses are attached to common nouns (*I talked to the boy who has red hair*).

Generally, the embedding of phrases occurs in developmentally expected ways. It is interesting that nouns tend to be the first words and, accordingly, the earliest embedding involves structures serving as noun phrases. Also, it should be noted that the general pattern in embedding these structures is to attach them to the ends of utterances to either serve as object phrases or to describe the noun in object phrases.

Compound Sentences. A **compound sentence** is one in which two basic sentence structures are linked together by a conjunction. A **coordinating conjunction** is a connecting word that links the two structures into one sentence. This connection can be between two clauses, two complete sentences, or it can combine multiple subjects, predicates, or objects. Conjunctions can convey a variety of relationships between the structures they connect. The ability to recognize these relationships appears to influence the order in which these forms appear. Table 8–9 presents the various forms of compound sentences.

Developmentally, toddlers probably expressed the notion of a compound sentence in Stage I as soon as they were able to simply string words together (Bloom, Lahey, Hood, Lifter, & Feiss, 1980). Such utterances as *ball block,* produced while emptying a toy box, suggest conjoining before the conjunctions are produced. Fittingly, *and* is the first conjunction to emerge in Stage II. Initially, *and* is used to express *additive* meanings, to express collections, such as *a ball and a block and a . . .* Next, *and* is used to express *temporal* relationships to order a series of events, as in *I fell down and got hurt and ran home.*

As it turns out, *and* is a versatile conjunction for preschoolers (and the rest of us). It is capable of conveying several different meanings, depending on the context. Later, *and* will also express *causal* relationships, as in *I ate too many cookies and I'm sick,* and to connect sentences with *adversative* meanings, as in *I don't want that and I do want this.* Of course, use of *and* to express these meanings does not emerge until preschoolers become cognitively aware of these subtle semantic relationships. Eventually, in Stage III and beyond, the adversative conjunction *but* and the alternative conjunction *or* appear. These express contradictory relationships, as in *I was thirsty, but the water was gone,* and alternative relationships, such as *I want popcorn or ice cream.*

 Children in other cultures have been found to develop use of conjunctions expressing these relationships in essentially the same order (Reich, 1986).

Summary

- Preschoolers' early multiword utterances are described as linear because the meanings are simply additive.

- Preschoolers' utterances become longer as they recombine shorter utterances and expand the structures used within existing utterances.

- Utterances take on hierarchical sentence structure when some words relate more closely as units or phrases.

- The basic units or constituents of sentences are words, phrases, and clauses with a subject and a predicate.

- Noun phrase elaboration is used to clarify or specify the referent of the noun through additional information conveyed by various structures.

- Verb phrases can take a variety of forms depending on the nature of the relationship they are communicating.

- Verb phrases can be described according to the semantic relationship they convey or the syntactic roles they indicate in a sentence.

- Preschoolers' development of the basic sentence types—declaratives, interrogatives, and negatives—has been described as going through characteristic periods.

- As a general "rule of thumb," most major language structures—grammatical morphemes, nouns, verbs, pronouns, sentence types—have been mastered by approximately 5 years of age.

Comprehension of Grammar

Comprehension, understanding the meaning of another's verbal behavior, has played a role in language development from birth. **Production,** the

comprehension Understanding or decoding the meaning of an utterance.

production The expression or encoding of an idea in an utterance.

The *interlocking verbal paradigm* described by Skinner similarly captures the nature of this reciprocal partnership between caregivers and toddlers as well as mature verbal interactions. See Chapter 4. ■

Myklebust's perceptual stages of sensation, perception, and imagery, are discussed in Chapter 3. ■

output of cries, gestures, words, or sentences, is of little communicative value if no one behaves according to our intentions. From birth, language learners and their caregivers develop a dynamic partnership based on comprehending behaviors produced by the other. Communication in this dyad, the reciprocal nature of producing and comprehending, has evolved from caregivers' interpretation of infant signals into more conventional conversations between caregivers and toddlers.

Comprehension versus Production

It is not entirely understood how comprehension and production relate to each other in early stages of language acquisition. Does one ability precede the other? It seems logical to assume that at least the basic steps in comprehension (sensation, perception, and perhaps imagery) must precede production; a child must have experienced a language form to eventually reproduce it. However, some have asserted that even beyond mere reception, comprehension consistently precedes production (Ingram, 1974). Others have maintained that this relationship might vary depending on the child's stage of language development (Bloom & Lahey, 1978).

On the one hand, toddlers have been found to comprehend as many as five words for every word they produce (Benedict, 1979). However, as toddlers, they do not have the experience base to fully comprehend them. Conversely, preschoolers frequently repeat nursery rhymes, familiar stories, and, to their parents' embarrassment, those more colorful words spoken in an emotional moment, without fully comprehending their meaning. It is not uncommon to hear proud caregivers report that their 3-year-old may not talk much, but their child understands "everything we say."

Does one ability differ from the other? It appears that the task requirements for comprehension are significantly different from those for production (Bloom & Lahey, 1978). In comprehension, the objects, actions, and relationships in caregivers' utterances are generally available for young children. Demonstrating comprehension might involve only a simple motor response of pointing to or retrieving an object named within an utterance. Everyday situations typically offer a number of cues that suggest the meanings of words. Familiar words and phrases spoken as part of daily routines are predictable and easily interpreted. Caregivers frequently include redundancies, restating and stressing segments to highlight key words or phrases. In addition, caregivers' eye gaze and gestures may signal which objects or actions are critical to interpreting their utterance.

In contrast, expression requires the preschooler to perceive the objects, actions, and relationships, formulate the appropriate words and phrases, generate, and then execute a motor pattern to produce the required series of sounds to produce the entire utterance. The difference in the task requirements relating to these processes could easily deceive us into believing that preschoolers are capable of comprehending much more than they are able to produce.

Comprehension Strategies

Even though context is generally available and caregivers instinctively adapt their language level, preschoolers are frequently challenged to understand the language directed at them. Researchers have studied preschoolers' development of comprehension of various language structures.

Changes in caregiver input and preschoolers' language are discussed later in this chapter. ■

Comprehension of Wh-Questions

A critical aspect of conversations between caregivers and preschoolers is the give-and-take of questions and answers. It is part of the tutorial nature of caregivers to pose numerous questions to their preschoolers. Perhaps it allows caregivers to assess their preschooler's level of understanding of the topic at hand. As long as preschoolers are capable or at least willing to provide an answer, caregiver questions certainly keep the exchange going.

Not surprisingly, research suggests that preschoolers first comprehend the wh-question forms that correspond to the questions they ask. And, as was noted previously, they ask questions about the kinds of information they understand and talk about—objects, locations, people, and actions. Accordingly, preschoolers comprehend *what* and *where* questions earlier, followed by *who* and *what-do* question forms. And, similarly, comprehension of questions involving *why, how,* and *when* must wait until preschoolers begin to understand causality, manner, and time relations sometime later. Until such time, preschoolers tend to answer wh-questions involving these concepts as though they were an earlier developing form. For example, in responding to *How do flowers grow?* a young preschooler is likely to answer, *In the garden.*

Comprehension of Active and Passive Sentences

The English language relies heavily on word order (syntax) to convey word relationships (semantic roles). The most basic and common sentence in English, the simple active declarative, presents a *noun-verb-noun* sequence, as in *Daddy hugged Mommy.* Semantically, this word order is interpreted as *agent-action-dative.* In other words, in the majority of sentences that confront preschoolers, the first noun is the instigator and the second noun is the recipient of the action. Should the nouns change places, so do their roles.

Passive sentences pose problems for preschoolers. The passive version of a sentence gives the appearance of this same *noun-verb-noun* sequence. However, even though the nouns change positions, their semantic roles remain the same. For example, the nouns in *Tom pushed Bill* (the active version) and *Bill was pushed by Tom* (the passive version) play the same roles despite their different orders.

Passive sentences are not consistently produced until the school-age years. This is discussed in Chapter 9. ■

reversibility The possibility that the subject and object phrase nouns could logically change places.

plausibility The notion that a relationship expressed in a sentence is a likelihood.

noun-verb-noun strategy Comprehension strategy that relies strictly on word order.

plausible event strategy Comprehension strategy that relies on determining the most probable state of affairs.

Two factors that influence the interpretation of active and passive sentences are reversibility and plausibility. **Reversibility** refers to the possibility that nouns in a sentence could be reversed (+Reversible); some relationships would make nouns irreversible (−Reversible). For sentences that are reversible, **plausibility** is the likelihood of the resulting relationship. A sentence is plausible (+Plausible), if the nouns might relate in that way; some resulting relationships are possible, but unlikely (−Plausible). The following examples illustrate these alternatives:

Active:

+Reversible/+Plausible	*Tom kissed Mary.*
+Reversible/−Plausible	*Tom kissed the kitty.*
−Reversible	*Tom kissed the trophy.*

Passive:

+Reversible/+Plausible	*Mary was kissed by Tom.*
+Reversible/−Plausible	*The kitty was kissed by Tom.*
−Reversible	*The trophy was kissed by Tom.*

Sentences that are reversible and plausible are the most difficult to comprehend; the other types are either unlikely or impossible. Younger preschoolers' experience leads them to initially rely on the **noun-verb-noun strategy** to comprehend such utterances. This would result in misinterpretation of many passive constructions. Preschoolers may also apply a **plausible event strategy,** determining which interpretation is most probable based on their experiences. Ultimately, preschoolers must rely on their experiences with language and the world to discriminate between the active and passive word orders, determine their meanings, and respond appropriately. Developmentally, children comprehend reversible active sentences by the time they enter Stage II. Passive sentences are not consistently interpreted until after Stage V, when the child is at least 5 years old (James, 1990).

The development of comprehension has been described as progressing from rigid to flexible interpretations. This pattern has been described in children's development of several languages, including Chinese, French, modern Hebrew, Hungarian, and Turkish (Owens, 2005).

An analogous concept is *bootstrapping,* in which the child uses current knowledge in one aspect of language to decipher information being presented in another area of language. ∎

Comprehension of Temporal Conjunctions

Statements that include temporal conjunctions also pose a special problem for preschoolers. Conjunctions like *before, after, until, while,* and *since* relate the timing of events by conveying sequence, duration, and simultaneity. These constructions are peculiar in that the conjunctions can occur in different sentence positions while conveying the same sequence. For example, *They left before Tom ate* conveys the same sequence of events as *After they left, Tom ate.* (I empathize with little ones—if it is possible to go "cross-eared," listening to these kinds of statements does it to me!)

In attempting to interpret these, most younger preschoolers apply the order of mention strategy. In doing so, they apparently attend strictly to the order in which events are mentioned in an utterance, which may or may not reflect their actual sequence. For example, using this strategy, preschoolers would likely interpret *Before they left, Tom ate* to be identical in meaning to the two versions in the previous paragraph. Interpreting utterances based on temporal conjunctions may still be a challenge for children well into their elementary years.

order of mention strategy
Comprehension strategy that assumes the first event mentioned occurred earlier than events in the remainder of the sentence.

Comprehension of Compound and Complex Sentences

Coordinating conjunctions create compound sentences (*Tom ran and Bill sat*). In addition, when combining utterances where a common element can be deleted (*Tom ate, Bill ate*), they result in compound subject phrases (*Tom and Bill ate*), object phrases (*Tom ate sandwiches and chips*), or verb phrases (*Tom sat and ate*). For mature speakers, compound constructions are economical and commonplace. However, for preschoolers they can be confusing.

There is some evidence that preschoolers may learn to interpret compound phrases earlier than compound sentences, perhaps at age 4. From this standpoint, a compound sentence like *The boy walked his dog and then he fed his kitty* would be more difficult than one with a compound predicate phrase such as, *The boy walked his dog and fed his kitty*. The difficulty with compound sentences could stem from their syntactic structure or simply from their greater length. However, the research is not yet clear in this regard (Lund & Duchan, 1993).

Complex sentences, with information embedded through various structures, also pose problems for preschoolers. Sentences with relative clauses, especially multiple embeddings, as in *The man that the dog that had fleas bit ate the hamburger,* can be quite difficult to interpret. (Who had fleas and who ate the hamburger?)

It appears that preschoolers may attempt different approaches to interpreting sentences with relative clauses. For example, they might use a **compounding strategy** in which they attend to the first noun phrase and apply the remaining verbs to it. In the previous example, a younger preschooler might tell us the man bit the dog, had fleas, and ate the hamburger! Generally, preschoolers appear to have the least difficulty with relative clauses that modify the object phrase, as in *The boy liked the car that had shiny wheels*.

compounding strategy
Comprehension strategy in which all actions in a sentence are attributed to the first noun mentioned in the sentence.

The interpretation of some complex sentences, such as those with infinitive clauses embedded in the predicate (e.g., *John told Mary to walk the dog*), may be confusing because their interpretation varies with the main verb. In most such cases, the subject of the verb in the infinitive clause is the noun closest to it—the **minimal distance principle.** In the example just given, Mary is to walk the dog. However, some verbs alter this interpretation,

minimal distance principle Comprehension strategy in which the noun closest to the verb is assumed to be the agent.

as in *John promised Mary to walk the dog;* in this case, John is to handle this chore. Young preschoolers might overgeneralize the minimal distance principle and misinterpret such sentences, thinking that Mary will be taking Bowser out.

Generally, the research in this area is inconsistent and incomplete (Lund & Duchan, 1993). In part, this probably is due to the ambiguous nature of comprehension. Researchers face difficult problems in this regard. What level of comprehension is required? What responses truly indicate comprehension? How should factors such as unintended cues and familiarity of context be controlled? Generally, we know a great deal more about production because researchers can more easily define the nature of the task—either a language structure has occurred correctly or it has not.

Summary

- In spite of its central importance to communication, the development of comprehension and its relationship to language production in children is not well understood.

- Most researchers agree that the nature of the two tasks—comprehension and production—are substantially different.

- Preschoolers apply various strategies in attempting to interpret more complex, unfamiliar language structures.

- Preschooler interpretations may be based on their experience with language (e.g., the noun-verb-noun and minimal distance principle) or with the world (e.g., reversibility and plausibility).

- Preschoolers' misinterpretations frequently result from overgeneralizing strategies that work with earlier developing sentence structures.

- Generally, comprehension of most sentence structure is achieved by around 5 years of age; more complex language structures (e.g., multiple embeddings, infinitive clauses) may not be easily interpreted until much later.

Language Taught and Language Learned

We can generally tell that a concept has attained a level of acceptance when it has been elevated to an acronym. In this case, the acronym for adult-to-child language, ACL, has appeared in the literature with increased frequency. ■

The title of this section has been borrowed from a book by Ernst Moerk (1992a). Moerk reanalyzed Brown's (1973) data, applying a culture learning and skill training model. In this conceptualization, caregivers are viewed as the "experts," children are the "novices," and language is one of several complex aspects of culture taught through this relationship. "The expert structures the training and monitors the novice's progress. The training is sequential, additive, and repetitive. . . ." (Moerk, 1992a, p. 3). Caregivers provide training experiences that are: (a) sequential in adapting to the child's abilities; (b) additive in building from simple to complex skills; and (c) repetitive in providing numerous opportunities to rehearse over a long period of time. In this partnership, caregivers' teaching is fine-tuned to their child's learning.

Changes in Caregiver Input

Adult-to-child language has been increasingly recognized as an important area of research. Caregiver behaviors such as modeling, questioning, imitating, expanding, and extending their preschoolers' utterances appear to be instrumental to early language development (Bates, Bretherton, & Snyder, 1988; Snow, 1977b). Through these behaviors, caregivers confirm their preschooler's language attempts, model corrections, and provide new information directly related to their immediate interest, when they might benefit most. The fine-tuning of adult-to-child language is evident in the gradual evolution of caregivers' responses to their preschoolers' language abilities and needs.

It has also been found that, although they may be unaware of it, adults adjust the degree to which they use these teaching tools as preschoolers mature. Caregivers' language changes most while the child is between 20 and 27 months of age. As caregivers continue to adapt, their subsequent adjustments are more in response to their preschooler's maturing language abilities than to simply their increasing age.

 It is important to recognize that the behaviors and, of course, the kind of adjustment seen in them are not universal. Not all cultures, or even socioeconomic classes in America, rely on the same kind of interaction between caregivers and children. Although the goal of the teaching behaviors generally described in the literature seems to be "get your child to talk," not all cultures value talkative children.

Caregiver Models

Some researchers have reported interesting differences in caregiver utterances, some of which occur when toddlers or younger preschoolers begin to evidence comprehension of language. Caregivers' mean length of utterance (MLU) may drop slightly at that point. Caregivers' rate of speech may be slower when addressing younger preschoolers. Typically, the number of grammatical errors is markedly reduced (although we all get tongue-tied sometimes). And, finally, caregiver models to younger preschoolers may be produced with distinctly longer pauses between them. These alterations become less remarkable as the child's language matures.

Caregiver models, imitations, expansions, extensions, and turnabouts are described in Chapter 6. ■

Imitations, Expansions, and Extensions

It has been generally found that, as preschoolers' MLU increases, caregivers are less likely to imitate their utterances or to provide expansions. Perhaps as preschoolers' well-formed utterances become more common, they are less remarkable. Similarly, because caregivers tend to expand preschooler utterances containing errors, as the preschoolers' language matures, expansions occur less often.

Finally, as preschoolers produce longer, more mature utterances, caregiver extensions increase in frequency. Because extensions contribute additional semantic information and, therefore, extend the interaction, this change is not unexpected as conversations between preschoolers and care-givers mature.

Turnabouts

Turnabouts, including prompts and contingent queries, are behaviors that maintain the momentum and integrity of a conversation. These behaviors also go through an evolution as preschoolers' language matures. With younger, less capable preschoolers, caregivers are more likely to use yes-no or tag question turnabouts to prompt for a clarification or the child's turn. Because the idea is to structure success, these are simpler for the preschooler to respond to correctly.

With older preschoolers, more specific wh-questions requesting infor-mation the caregiver is confident the child knows become more likely. Care-givers find that neutral requests (*Huh?, What?*) and open-ended requests (*Tell me how this happened*) for clarification are less successful with younger preschoolers, but will often elicit additional information with older ones (Kaye & Charney, 1981).

Summary

- Researchers are focusing with increased interest on the roles played by caregivers and preschoolers in teaching and learning language.

- Caregiver models become shorter, simpler, slower, and more precise when their child begins to evidence some comprehension of language.

- As their preschooler's language matures, caregivers respond with fewer imitations and expansions, but more extensions.

- The nature of caregiver turnabouts changes with their preschooler's ability to comprehend language and respond correctly.

Chapter Summary

Grammatical development begins with the appearance of two-word ut-terances, typically as toddlers. Researchers have investigated gram-matical structures that are reflective of the language learning process. Brown's research, focusing on 14 grammatical morphemes illustrates the emergence, gradual approximation, and mastery that characterizes much of language learning in preschoolers. Brown's stages, with boundaries defined by *mean length of utterance (MLU)*, depict the evolution of language that occurs from words and phrases in Stage I, through the fine-tuning intro-duced by grammatical morphemes in Stage II, to the development of major sentence types in Stage III, and the maturation found in *complex sentences* in Stage IV, and *compound sentences* in Stage V.

Research has suggested that, although preschoolers exhibit similar sequences of language learning, there is still a great deal of individual variation in both the sequences and rate of learning. Research with preschoolers suggests the role of *semantic relationships* and the related cognitive development in influencing which language forms are mastered earlier. It appears that overt *reinforcement* provided by caregivers plays a more significant role in vocabulary learning than in grammatical development. However, others continue to examine the nature of interactions between children and caregivers to identify the influence of reinforcement in the form of *natural consequences* in developing language. Whether children's language is simply the result of rule-learning or whether it is contingency-shaped by natural consequence continues to be an important question as researchers attempt to illuminate the nature of language development.

The nature of the respective contributions from *comprehension* and *production* to language learning have been studied. Researchers agree that the nature of the two tasks differ but their relationship is not clear. Several comprehension strategies used by preschoolers to interpret sentence structures that are complex or unfamiliar have been identified. Finally, changes in adult-to-child language have been found as preschoolers' language abilities mature.

1. Describe three criteria used by Brown to select the morphemes studied in his research.

2. Describe how Brown defined and characterized the five stages of preschool language development.

3. Why did Brown find MLU to be a more relevant measure of language development than chronological age?

4. How do the terms "rule-governed" and "contingency-shaped" relate to Brown's findings?

5. What are the basic elements of sentences?

6. What is the difference between linear and hierarchical sentence structure?

7. Distinguish between the semantic roles played by verbs and the syntactic roles they play in sentences.

8. How are copula and auxiliary verbs different?

Review Questions

9. According to linguists, what are the two underlying operations involved in forming questions? Which of these apply to yes-no questions? Which apply to wh-questions?

10. What are the differences between the tasks of comprehension and production?

11. What changes occur in caregiver input and feedback as their preschoolers' language abilities mature?

Practice Questions

To the student: You are encouraged to use the following questions to prepare for multiple-choice examinations. This exercise is not intended to simply "provide the answers to questions." Instead, it is hoped that you will use the material to develop your ability to analyze questions and choices to identify correct answers based on a critical understanding of the distinctions among the answers. Use the answer key at the end of the book to prompt your analysis of each item and to confirm the correct answer. Remember that there is a difference between recognizing the correct answer and understanding why it is the correct one.

1. When Brown analyzed the development of the 14 morphemes in his subjects, Adam, Eve, and Sara, he found that they exhibited _____ .
   a. similar rates of acquisition but different sequences
   b. similar rates and similar sequences of acquisition
   c. different rates of acquisition but similar sequences
   d. rates and sequences that were entirely different
   e. changes in their vocal pitch (fundamental frequency) at different ages

2. The difference between a clause and a sentence is that _____ .
   a. a clause does not have a subject and predicate, sentences do
   b. a clause is one word; a sentence always has two
   c. a clause includes a subject and a predicate; a sentence does, too; and it is grammatically complete
   d. a clause is simply two words that are structurally related; a sentence includes punctuation
   e. a clause is spoken quietly with hesitation; a sentence is asserted with confidence

3. According to Brown's research, the best index or indicator of expected development of the grammatical morphemes he studied is _____ .
   a. the child's height in centimeters
   b. the average number of morphemes in a child's utterances

c. the child's chronological age

d. the average number of syllables in a child's utterances

e. the child's birth date

4. In the utterance, "*Was* he at the house?" the underlined segment represents _____ .
   a. a possessive inflection
   b. a contractible copula
   c. a contractible auxiliary
   d. a regular third person, present-tense, singular inflection
   e. an uncontractible copula

5. Based on their cognitive development, the early wh-questions of young preschoolers would most likely request information regarding _____ .
   a. labels for objects and actions
   b. causality of events
   c. future time of events
   d. instruments used in actions
   e. ownership of objects

6. Bloom claimed that the earliest true form of grammatical (or "syntactic") negation was "prepredicate," not "presentence." An example of prepredicate grammatical negation would be _____ .
   a. "No baby sleep"
   b. "Me no sleep"
   c. "No cookie"
   d. "allgone cookie"
   e. all of these

7. Mastery of the pronominal (pronoun) system _____ .
   a. occurs in the same sequence and ages across all children
   b. usually starts with indefinite pronouns (e.g., "it," "that") or first person pronouns (I, me)
   c. has been found to be variable in sequence and age
   d. a and b
   e. b and c

8. Which of the following does *not* include a modal auxiliary?
   a. You should think about doing that soon.
   b. I might consider working on that tonight.
   c. She could be lost.
   d. I have been reading the same book.
   e. You can be certain about that.

9. Which of the following sentences would be considered "+reversible/+plausible"?
   a. The alligator bit the man.
   b. The cat licked the man.

    c. Bill was polishing the car.

    d. Tony was writing his paper.

    e. Mannfred was hugging Wilhamena.

10. In interpreting time relationships expressed in sentences, younger children might rely on an "order of mention" strategy. This means a younger child would interpret "Before he painted the house, Dad had some lunch" as something like _____ .

    a. Dad ate a sandwich and then got his paintbrushes

    b. the house was painted by the neighbors who made lunch for everyone

    c. Dad painted the house and then made a sandwich

    d. Dad held his sandwich in one hand and used his paintbrush with the other hand

    e. none of these would represent an "order of mention" interpretation

Suggested Readings

Brown, R. (1973). *A first language: The early stages.* Cambridge: Harvard University Press.

Fey, M. E., & Loeb, D. F. (2002). An evaluation of the facilitative effects of inverted yes-no questions on the acquisitions of auxiliary verbs. *Journal of Speech, Language, and Hearing Research, 45,* 160–174.

Moerk, E. L. (1992). *A first language: Taught and learned.* Baltimore: Paul H. Brookes.

Rispoli, M. (2003). Changes in the nature of sentence production during the period of grammatical development. *Journal of Speech, Language, and Hearing Research, 46,* 818–830.

Ryder, N., & Leinonen, E. (2003). Use of context in question answering by 3-, 4-, and 5-year-old children. *Journal of Psycholinguistic Research, 32,* 397–416.

CHAPTER 9

Language and Literacy during the School Years and Beyond

After moving to his new high school, Stuart had only been in classes with the same kids for a few weeks when they had already shortened his name to "Stu." It seemed he had been accepted. And, so far, he was well liked by his new teachers. Stu's grades were okay, but there were times when everyone wondered about him just a little.

He occasionally seemed a little strange. Sometimes he would tell a story, but it would meander through unrelated sequences. Although he seemed pleasant enough, in class he occasionally asked for help in a blunt manner that almost sounded impatient. And, sometimes Stu, in the most sincere way, would express himself awkwardly. Just the other day, he scolded a friend who had not finished her homework. He reprimanded her saying, "You buttered your bread, now you have to lay in it."

He did not seem to fit in entirely. Talking in the lounge one day, his teachers were all curious about his background. Was there anything that would explain his occasional odd behavior? Finally, someone got his folder. They came back looking dumbfounded! Stu's birth date indicated he was 3 years younger than the teachers had thought! But someone had marked the enrollment form to place him three grade levels higher than he should be!

When the principal called on his parents, she found they knew he was in the wrong grade. "We just figured you thought he was smarter than we thought," his mother said at first. Then, hanging her head, she confessed that Stu's records had been lost in the move and his father had to enroll him before the others made the move. She whispered in painful embarrassment, "Stu's dad can't read a stitch and he doesn't want Stu to know." The principal could only reply gently, "I understand. Don't worry. We'll take care of it. I'll find a way to explain the change to Stu." The next day, Stu was placed back in the proper grade where he fit in perfectly. And then, one evening the next month, Stu brought his father to the school building for his first adult literacy class. It turned out Stu Jr. was very proud that his father, Mr. Dent, had the courage to change his life, no matter how late in the game of life it was!

Of course, not all children are ready for kindergarten at 5 years of age. In spite of this individual variability, we will assume that the school-age years begin at 5. ■

This chapter addresses the following questions:

• What grammatical structures remain to be mastered during the school years?

• How does mastery of later developing grammatical structures reflect expansion in students' cognitive abilities and social interactions?

• How do receptive and expressive vocabulary change in size and organization during the school-age years?

• How are students' advances in abstract reasoning reflected in figurative language such as idioms and parables?

• How do developing metalinguistic abilities allow students to analyze and understand language in the classroom?

• How does classroom language differ from the language used in other interactions?

• How does the ability to read emerge in students and evolve during the school-age years?

• What kind of changes occur in language throughout adolescence and adulthood into our senior years?

This chapter addresses developments in language behavior during the school years and the school-of-life that follows throughout adulthood. In the earlier sections of this chapter, the term "student" is used. As a parent, I recognize that being students is only one dimension of who children are during these years—they are first and foremost sons and daughters. However, the term "student" conveys the significant changes that are occurring in them. They are venturing into important new relationships, settings, and activities that affect them beyond their home life. Even at home, much of the interaction focuses on their lives as students.

By the time preschoolers come of age and caregivers prepare to send them off to school, they have already developed skills in a number of areas. It has been traditionally held that about 90% of grammar has been learned by the time children are 5 years old. By the time they enter their kindergarten classroom the basic language tools are normally in place. Through their lan-

The impressive development of language during the preschool years has been interpreted by some to support the notion of a "critical period" for language learning. Much of the support for this concept comes from information regarding language learning following brain injury and second language learning. Younger individuals seem to recover their language learning abilities following brain injury. Learning a second language appears to be easier for children prior to adolescence.

guage behavior they gain others' attention and get help, share tidbits of interest, and tell tall tales. They have the tools to ask whether they understand the world correctly or to ask for specific details they need to know.

In spite of the now famous adage by Robert Fulghum (1986) that "all I really need to know I learned in kindergarten," there are many changes yet to come. Students' bodies, coordination, emotions, social interactions, and even their thought patterns change. Although a major share of language is already mastered, there are still developments left to occur. A handful of grammatical structures are yet to be consistently understood or produced by young students. Subtle but significant changes will occur in their semantic and pragmatic abilities throughout their years as students and adults.

Development in Related Domains

As time goes on, it becomes more difficult to clearly number the individual developments. Major changes may be less specific, result from several converging developments, and stretch over a broader period. For example, the motor changes in the school years are spread across numerous areas (e.g., athletics, fine arts, technical skills) and build on earlier developments. This is in contrast to the more clearly defined early developmental milestones—crawling, walking, running—that we looked for in the infant and toddler.

Nonetheless, it is possible to outline some major changes related to the motor, cognitive, and social domains. The following summary lists various highlights that characterize developments in each area throughout this span of years (Lane & Molyneaux, 1992; Nicolosi, Harryman, & Kresheck, 2003; Owens, 2005; Shulman, 1994).

Motor Development

Motor developments are refined as previous developments are applied to more specific skills. This is illustrated as maturing individuals:

- Exhibit improved coordination and balance for climbing, bike riding, and beginning sports activities by around 6 years.

- Exhibit physical growth in limbs, hands, and feet, and maturation in nervous, respiratory, and circulatory systems that approach adult levels by around 10 years.

- Exhibit physical changes associated with onset of puberty by around 12 years.

- Exhibit increased vocal fold size resulting in a drop of one octave in pitch of male voices with less change in females beginning around 14 years.

- Develop increased muscle mass, facial hair, greater height in males, and breasts and broader hips in females by 16 years of age.

- Exhibit characteristic physical and physiological changes that accompany the aging process as young adults, mature adults, and seniors.

Cognitive Development

Cognitive development occurs in refining and applying accumulated understanding to specific academic and vocational skills. These changes are illustrated as individuals:

- Develop longer attention span and more easily focus on problem solving by around 6 years.
- Develop clearer concept of classification, similarities and differences, cause-effect relationships by around 10 years.
- Develop independent abstract reasoning, problem solving, and anticipation of reversible consequences by around 14 years.
- Exhibit ability to envision hypothetical outcomes, apply deductive reasoning, and examine own thought styles by around 16 years.
- Focus learning on career-related information and terminology as adults attempt to develop and advance in chosen careers.

Social Development

Expanding roles in more diverse social contexts require increasing independence. This is evident as individuals:

- Develop abilities to express own feelings and empathy for others' feelings by around 6 years.
- Develop stronger sense of peer group through structured games, sports, and hobbies by around 10 years.
- Develop interests that differentiate between sexes, but begin to engage in social activity centered around the opposite sex by around 14 years.
- Develop personal responsibility and ability to complete tasks without adult supervision by around 16 years.
- Shift obligations as adults manage responsibilities for careers, marriage, family, and civic responsibilities.

Language Expectations

Extensive language and literacy expectations across grade levels are summarized in Appendix B. ■

As children become students, they experience language from a new perspective—an academic perspective. Vocabularies are reorganized in hierarchical classifications seemingly imposed by academics. As students, they become more conscious of language as something that can be analyzed, manipulated, and used for entertainment and persuasion. Classroom language and textbooks pose a new challenge for students. As literacy skills develop, younger students who initially "learned to read" become mature readers who "read to learn." Vocabularies grow and specialize, especially in relation to career developments. In the elderly, a number of changes occur that are related to the aging process. The following overview is intended to provide an initial picture of the overall developments expected during this period.

- Students will make final gains in the structures of language as they master irregular forms, complex sentence structures, reflexive pronouns, and the distinction between mass nouns and count nouns.

- Students' greatest area of development will be growth in vocabulary, greater awareness of the features of language, and literacy.

- Students will intuitively begin to organize their vocabulary according to hierarchical categories—classifying words according to superordinate and subordinate categories.

- Students will begin to become increasingly conscious of the metalinguistic aspects of language—syllabification, rhyming, multiple meanings, ambiguity, and so on.

- Students will consistently improve in decoding the special meanings carried by "teacher language" and "textbook language."

- Students, as adults, become lifelong learners, understanding the role of language in social and vocational settings and using their literacy skills in their career development.

Grammar: The Final Pieces of the Puzzle

Beyond 5 years of age, preschoolers become students. Perhaps one of the most exciting parts of this big step is those school supplies! Caregivers and their young students carefully purchase all the items on the supply list provided by the school. The smell of new pencils, brightly colored pencil boxes, perfectly shaped new crayons with their labels still in place—all the right tools, all brand new, make that first day seem special! What many caregivers overlook in these moments is the fact that for the previous 5 years they and their children have been perfecting the most important tool for learning—language! During their school years, growing cognitive abilities and increased social interactions will cause students to gain more experience with later developing grammatical structures.

Advances in Grammar

The aspects of grammar to be mastered during the school years are not categorically separate from the achievements of the preschool years. They are extensions of the same "slow, gradual continuum of change and modification" (Wallach, 1984, p. 82). There is not a categorical difference in the basic grammatical skills being learned just because children have become students. There is instead a continual evolution of more complex and more elaborate forms of language behavior.

There does appear to be a qualitative change in students' approach to learning language that comes with their advanced understanding and experience. As preschoolers, children tended to apply literal translations to language. In contrast, school-age children begin to integrate more information from their experiences into their overall understanding and use of language. Students gradually use language with more insight into what their words might mean to others and, similarly, they comprehend much of others' language by "reading between the lines" (Wallach, 1984, p. 83).

The grammatical developments that take place over the school years involve a variety of language structures. Growing students will achieve more consistent comprehension and production of wh-questions, compound and complex sentences, passive sentences, and various morphological features related to nouns and verbs.

Two qualifications should be noted. First, much of the data regarding mastery of these grammatical forms are based on comprehension studies. Second, paradoxically, this reliance on comprehension data probably stems from the fact that many of these structures are produced before they are fully understood; a carefully structured comprehension task may be the best way to determine if school-age children know what they are saying when they use these structures.

Wh-Questions

Questions appeared as early as the infant's gestures and vocalizations could request labels from caregivers. Asking questions, in the verbal sense, emerged in toddlers and evolved during the preschool years in a fairly predictable sequence. The earlier wh-questions generally reflected the information that preschoolers were aware of and curious about.

As described in the previous chapter, the wh-word in questions essentially serves as a pronoun for the sentence constituent it requests. Generally, the earliest wh-questions request information about objects (*what?*), actions (*what-do?*), agents (*who?*) and their locations (*where?*). The remaining wh-forms emerge as older preschoolers and younger students begin to understand time (*when?*), causality (*why?*), and instrumental (*how?*) relationships.

Anyone who has raised children will recall the unrelenting *Why?* questions of the preschool years. However, these probably expressed the communicative equivalence of "talk to me some more." It is unlikely that these were inquiries about causality, as preschool children were probably incapable of understanding the subtleties of why dogs howl at sirens, why kittens purr, why toast turns brown, or why rainbows follow a storm.

Older preschoolers actually express relationships involving time, causality, and instruments prior to asking about them. Their later appearance in questions could stem both from semantic and grammatical considerations. Not only do these later forms ask for information about more subtle semantic relationships, but they also represent sentence constituents that are more elaborate than those represented by earlier developing wh-words. Given a sentence such as *Billy ate some pizza with a fork at home after the game,* the sentence elements requested by the who or what in a wh-question (*Who ate pizza? What did Billy eat?*) can be as simple as a noun. However, *how?* and *when?* questions will generally require an entire adverbial phrase (*with a fork, after the game*). A w*hy?* question typically requires an entire clause (*Because he was hungry*), which is frequently based on inferred information. These later wh-question forms will probably be used consistently by most 8-year-olds (Wallach, 1984).

Complex and Compound Sentences

Young students improve in understanding and producing complex sentences with subordinate and relative clauses and compound sentences. Interestingly, these forms play an especially important role in the verbal reasoning abilities that evolve during these same years.

> The grammatical aspects of complex and compound sentences are discussed in Chapter 8. ∎

Complex Sentences. Complex sentences are produced when a main clause has a subordinate clause or relative clauses embedded within it. The earliest subordinate clauses usually indicate causal relationships introduced by *because. Because* appears late in preschoolers' language, although it is not until the early school years that younger students begin to use it appropriately. Initially, it appears to play the role of a coordinating conjunction, simply connecting two main clauses. Preschoolers and younger students may use *because* the same way they use *and;* that is, to simply signal some order of events, as in *I got sick because* (= and) *I woke up.* In these early instances, the actual order of events and their relationships may not be entirely clear.

Later, as students begin to understand causal relationships more clearly, *because* begins to assume its role as a subordinating conjunction. However, younger students may still have difficulty producing *because* in word orders that express the causal relationship clearly. The causally related events may be reversed as in, *I got sick because I went to the doctor's.* (Although that can happen, it is not the usual order of events.)

Eventually, students' early productions of *because* statements become more frequently correct, even though they still do not consistently comprehend those they hear. This may be related to the tendency for students' early *because* statements to convey meanings that occur simultaneously and are closely associated, as in *He's laughing because the show is funny* (James, 1990).

Experience and cognition play significant roles in the eventual mastery of *because*. The earliest versions of *because* sentences to be understood are those in which interpretation is assisted by logical probability. For example, there is only one logical interpretation of *The water leaked out because there was a hole.* However, those that express a reversible relationship, as in *The boy ran because the dog barked* (or *The dog barked because the boy ran*), may not be consistently comprehended until 8 years of age. Based on earlier experiences of interpreting such word orders in the context of present or probable relationships, students are eventually able to independently interpret the grammar of such complex sentences (Wallach, 1984).

Interpretation of conditional *if* sentences progress similarly. In these, one proposition is dependent on fulfillment of a stated condition. Those that express logically related conditions (e.g., *If the sun shines, I feel warm*) are understood earlier than those that are reversible (e.g., *If you win, I will leave* and *If I leave, you will win* are both possible). Here again, most students will be able to understand even the more complex version by the time they are 8 years old (Wallach, 1984).

As adolescents, students may engage in higher level abstract or hypothetical reasoning. This goes beyond understanding conditional relationships based on experience. The ability to think flexibly and consider several possible outcomes of a condition, as in *If this, . . . then that,* statements probably evolves beyond 12 years of age.

Finally, two other later developing subordinating conjunctions express contrasts between a condition and a proposition. The conjunction *although* juxtaposes a condition against a contrasting proposition, as in *We kept walking, although we were tired.* The conjunction *unless* expresses a negative conditional relationship, as in *Unless we find the tickets, we can't go.* By 11 years of age, students should understand the conjunctions *if* and *although.* However, they may be 15 years old before they fully comprehend and use *unless* correctly.

The ability to interpret and produce embedded clauses also improves throughout the school years as well. Preschoolers demonstrate the ability to produce complex sentence structures with an embedded clause. These included noun phrase complements, embedded wh-questions, infinitives, and relative clauses to replace or describe noun phrases. During the school years, students learn to interpret and produce these elements in more flexible ways. The primary advances relate to their changing positions and potentially related changes in their roles. For example, relative clauses might be center-embedded to modify nouns in the subject phrase, as in *The boy <u>who has red shoes</u> took my candy.* Similarly, when *that*-clause complements are positioned at the beginning of a sentence, as in *That the boy cried was sad,* they serve as subjects instead of objects.

Preschoolers and younger students come to rely on the prevalent *noun-verb-noun* order in English sentences to interpret constructions. However, center-embedded relative clauses interfere with this sequence, apparently making it more difficult to interpret sentences containing them. By junior high school, most students are able to consistently interpret sentences with relative clauses in either object or subject phrase positions.

Compound Sentences.   Compound sentences are created when two clauses (e.g., *He ran, She walked*) are connected through the use of coordinating conjunctions (e.g., *He ran <u>and</u> she walked*). Because both independent clauses could stand as independent clauses, neither is made subordinate to the other. Compound subjects, predicates, and objects are further results of combining sentences where the elements are shared.

The earliest and most prevalent conjunction, *and,* connects propositions that are concurrent or consecutive. Another early conjunction, *but,* expresses propositions that are adversative; that is, they are contradictory or unexpected. Finally, as preschoolers become capable of considering several possibilities, *or* emerges as a conjunction expressing alternation.

The later developing conjunctions are more complex (Wallach, 1984). Paired conjunctions involve coordinating two elements to express alternatives, as in *both-and, either-or,* and *neither-nor.* Some tend to appear only in formal speech or writing to relate propositions logically. Conjunctive adverbs are used when one proposition is the result of (*therefore, consequently*) or in contradiction to (*however, nevertheless*) the other. The level of abstract verbal reasoning at which these occur is probably not reached until well into the adolescent years, which coincides with the development of logical thought in the formal operations stage described by Piaget (Ginsburg & Opper, 1969).

Passive Sentences

At the end of the preschool years, children produce truncated or shortened passive sentences. These are based on verb participles, verbs ending with *-ed* or *-en* serve as adjectives, and usually omit the agent. For example, *It was broken* would imply that there was an agent, but the agent is omitted. The underlying relationship actually may have been *It was broken (by me);* passive sentences have an interesting effect of shifting focus away from the agent.

Preschoolers' difficulty in comprehending passive sentences is discussed in Chapter 8. ■

At 5 years of age, preschoolers do produce a number of full passive sentences (including both the agent and object). These early types tend to be reversible passives. However, due to their reversibility, it may be that on closer examination many of these still exhibit incorrect word order and we simply cannot be certain sometimes. Younger students also tend to cue on specific words as opposed to sentence structure to detect passives. For example, they may focus on *by* to determine that a sentence is passive (*John was kissed by Mary*), but fail to detect passive sentences with *to* (*The money was taken to the bank*) (Shorr & Dale, 1981). The fact that at 5 years of age, preschoolers still inconsistently interpret passives makes it a strong possibility that their word orders do not always accurately reflect production of passives.

The notion of reversibility is discussed in Chapter 8 in regard to comprehension of active and passive sentences. ■

Beyond the age of 5, students gradually learn to interpret passives correctly. A number of interesting differences have emerged in the research regarding their production, however. Although both reversible and nonreversible passives occurred in the preschool and school-age subjects in at least one study (Horgan, 1978), no one subject produced both types. Agentive nonreversible passives, which include an agent that could not be the object of the action (e.g., *The car was dented by <u>the boy</u>*) are more frequent for students under 11 years of age. Instrumental nonreversible passives, which include the instrument used in the action (e.g., *The car was dented by* <u>*the*</u> <u>*ball*</u>), are reportedly more frequent for students between 11 and 13 years of age. However, this is based on limited data because passives occur so infrequently until adolescence.

Grammatical Odds and Ends

Preschool language left a number of grammatical odds and ends undone. These are aspects of grammar that are confusing either in their structure or the contexts that control them. In other words, either the response patterns or the stimuli that call for them are inconsistent.

Count and Mass Nouns.   Generally, most items can occur singularly or in some quantity. The nature of the items and the forms used to describe their quantities can be confusing for young students. This confusion is sorted out gradually throughout the school years (Gordon, 1988).

Some items occur in quantities that can be distinguished as individual, countable units (e.g., spoons, rocks, trees). The nouns that label such items are called **count nouns.** Other items (e.g., milk, hair, sand) occur in quantities that are perceived as indivisible. These are labeled **mass nouns.** (Expressing quantities of these items in units that can be counted—cartons of milk, strands of hair, grains of sand—only means that the units are count nouns.)

Beyond perceiving the distinction between such quantities, using count nouns and mass nouns correctly requires knowing which ones take plural inflections and which quantifiers go with each. Count nouns accept the plural inflection, whereas mass nouns do not. We can have *rocks,* but we do not have *sands.* Mass nouns accept quantifying modifiers such as *much* and *little.* Count nouns are modified by *many* and *few.* Someone can find *many rocks,* but they cannot find *many sands.* Once younger students have mastered regular plural forms used with count nouns, they begin to modify them with *many.* It may take until adolescence to become consistently accurate in using *much* with mass nouns. In the meantime, like so many of us, young students find that *lots of* (or, more likely, *lotsa*) is adaptable to either type of noun.

count noun   Nouns that represent items that can be counted as individual units (e.g., pennies, forks); compare **mass noun.**

mass noun   Nouns that express items perceived as integral wholes that cannot be divided (e.g., milk and sand); compare **count noun.**

Reflexive Pronouns.   The English pronoun system is complex and confusing. It is not uncommon for young students to still confuse subjective (*he, she, they*) and objective (*him, her, them*) pronouns. The typical error is to substitute objective for subjective pronouns, as in *Him is my friend.* For the most part, students have mastered the subjective, objective, and possessive pronouns early in their school-age years. The final accomplishment, mastering reflexive pronouns (e.g., *myself, yourself, himself, herself, themselves*) may not come until the later elementary grades for some students.

The complexity that underlies learning the pronoun system is discussed in Chapter 8. ■

Irregular Past Tense and Plurals.   It will be recalled that expressing past tense and plurality in English can involve both regular and irregular forms. Regular forms, of course, consist of inflections that are consistent, at least within the phonological constraints that specify their allomorphs (i.e., /-t/, /-d/, /-ɪd/, and /-s/, /-z/, /-ɪz/). Irregular past tense verbs and irregular plural nouns are forms that each vary from their base form in ways that do not follow any regular pattern (e.g., *run-ran, eat-ate, child-children, man-men*). In both, it has been found that common irregular forms appear early in toddlers and young preschoolers, only to vanish when regular inflection forms are learned.

One of the difficulties for English-speaking children is the inconsistencies in the language. Not that English has a monopoly on inconsistency, but faced with all the irregular forms, it must sometimes seem to children learning English that the only real "rule" is that there are no consistent rules.

Linguistically, this phenomenon has been called overregularization; behaviorally, it is called overgeneralization. The irregular forms are then relearned in a rote, case-by-case manner. The most common forms are generally remastered by the early school years. Those that are less familiar and present more variations (e.g., *lie-lay-lain, swim-swam-swum*) may still pose a challenge to adolescents and adults. Some of us still are not clear about whether we *lie down* or *lay down* for a nap!

Summary

- During their school-age years, students master the remaining aspects of grammar.
- Much of what is known about the later developments in grammar is based on comprehension studies.
- Students become increasingly capable of using their experience to infer the meanings of utterances.
- Students expand their repertoire of wh-questions to ask for information regarding instrumental, adverbial, and causal relationships.
- By the time students are adolescents, they are capable of using complex structures that express causal, conditional, and relative relationships.
- As adolescents, students begin to use higher level conjunctions in their verbal reasoning.
- Although preschoolers appear to understand some **passive constructions,** they do not use passives correctly until they become older students.
- Students will become capable of modifying **mass** and **count nouns,** and using reflexive pronouns and irregular past tense and irregular plural forms.

Semantics: Growth and Changes

The majority of grammar develops in the preschool years, generally leaving higher level and irregular forms to be mastered during the school years.

Conversely, although children accumulate significant vocabulary as preschoolers, they have only laid the groundwork for the impressive semantic development that occurs as students. During their school years, students' maturing physical stature, developing cognitive abilities, and broadening social interactions will significantly expand their experience base. With each new setting, challenge, and role, students are exposed to new words and, just as important, new meanings for old words.

Vocabulary grows rapidly throughout the school years. However, the changing nature of students' word meanings during this time is just as significant. As students accumulate experience with new situations and words, they perceive the many ways in which various stimuli, contexts, and words are interrelated. As they recognize these interconnections, they use their existing vocabulary more flexibly and they more efficiently add new words to it. As students, they will learn more words, learn more about words, and learn how to learn words.

Growth of Vocabulary

Researchers have estimated vocabulary development at various points throughout the school-age years. First graders are capable of understanding approximately 20,000 words. By the time they have reached sixth grade, students reportedly understand about 50,000 words. And, by high school, although the rate of growth slows to a more steady pace, students are eventually capable of understanding around 80,000 words.

Vocabulary growth is not a simple accumulation of new words stacked like index cards in the dusty corners of our long-term memory. For toddlers, each new word probably reflects a new tool—another means to obtain objects and attention. For preschoolers, words begin to accumulate the semantic features that correspond to their growing perception of the attributes, actions, locations, and agents associated with them. As students continue to learn new words, they also recognize additional features associated with each word, and they discover additional meanings for each word.

Toddlers' and preschoolers' overextensions, discussed in Chapter 6, diminish as they recognize additional features for discriminating the adult meaning of a word. ■

horizontal vocabulary development The process of adding associated features that expand the meaning of a word; compare **vertical vocabulary development.**

Vertical and Horizontal Development

The growth of vocabulary has been conceptualized as occurring in two directions—horizontally and vertically (McNeill, 1970). **Horizontal vocabulary development** is characterized as the process of associating additional features with a word. The additional features fill out the meaning of the word—expanding its horizons, if you will—to eventually approximate its more adultlike meaning. Initially, a word may have a narrow meaning. It is quite likely that in its earliest occurrences *mama* may have only one referent with specific features. Eventually, the meaning is broadened horizontally to include other children's mothers, dogs that have puppies, and even necessity (which happens to be the "mama" of invention).

In **vertical vocabulary development,** the separate, multiple meanings of words are learned. The earliest meaning of the word *block* was probably based on the toy item. However, eventually, a child is told that his "blocks are blocking the doorway" and to "never cross the street or leave the block." For preschoolers, additional meanings may have coexisted, each understood in its own context, but not necessarily associated with the other meanings. During the school-age years, however, not only will other meanings be added (e.g., dad may "block out" a section of yard to become a garden, he may select a "block" of text to edit on his computer), but older students will begin to recognize the conceptual relationships among them.

vertical vocabulary development The process of associating additional meanings and contexts with a word; compare **horizontal vocabulary development.**

Word Definitions

How children define words has been a source of some curiosity for researchers. The nature of their definitions has been thought to reflect how they organize their information about the world. Several shifts in children's approach to defining words have been described as they move from the preschool to school-age years and beyond.

Defining words is probably an infrequent task for toddlers and preschoolers. The most likely reason to do so might have been in response to a confused caregiver's plea for clarification, *What is an "abbo?"* If one was present, the "definition" probably consisted of a pointing gesture and the utterance, *This!* Later, when truly attempting to give a verbal definition, toddlers and younger preschoolers were likely to provide a functional definition, indicating only the action associated with it, as in *You eat it.*

As younger students, definitions change in two related ways. They are said to become less concrete and functional, and instead become more abstract and conceptual (Pease & Berko Gleason, 1985). From another perspective, this shift might be characterized as growing beyond definitions based on personal experience to definitions based on socially shared information. Young students come to rely less on their private, episodic recall to define a word and more on their accumulated understanding of the conventional, semantically related information that others associate with it.

By the time students have progressed through the sixth grade, they can provide a relatively formal, conventional definition. Being conventionalized, these might follow a formula of sorts, typically starting with the item's category (e.g., *A [noun] is a [category] . . .*) and matching this with its functions and features to distinguish it from other items (*. . . that [functions] and has a [feature] and [feature]*). Translated, this might go something like *A car is a vehicle that carries people and has a motor and a trunk.*

Changing Organization of Vocabulary

One of the telling behaviors in students' maturing semantic domain is their ability to relate words to each other with increasing flexibility. Words become

As students progress toward an abstract level of understanding words, they illustrate the perceptual levels of *conceptualization* and *abstraction,* described in Chapter 3. ■

associated through contexts that overlap in a physical or conceptual way. When these connections are perceived and expressed in students' language, it signals that they are able to understand and respond to their world at an abstract level.

Changes in the organization of vocabulary have been characterized in several ways. These shifts appear to occur at different age levels; yet, there are no clear-cut age boundaries at which one ceases and the next emerges. Additionally, although these conceptualizations are not integrated under any overall theoretical framework, they may provide an interesting illustration of the changing levels of stimulus features children perceive as they continually learn more about the words that become their vocabulary.

Thematic-Taxonomic Shift

thematic organization
Associating words based on their relationship to a theme or context.

An early change in children's word associations has been described as a shift from thematic to taxonomic organization of responses (Locke, 1993). **Thematic organization** is based on associations that relate words to some integrated context in which they are experienced as a whole. For example, when asked to think of words that "go with" wagon, children exhibiting thematic associations might respond with *the sidewalk, my dollies, our playhouse,* and *dirt.* The experiences associated with playing with their wagon has provided the theme that pulls these words together into a cohesive collection. When asked to sort a pile of toys—such things as toy cars and trucks, toy furniture and household items, people and animal figures—into groups that "go together," children making thematic associations would tend to assemble groupings based on themes or stories. They might make a typical "family" as they perceive it, complete with the usual furnishings, pets, and two cars.

taxonomic organization
Associating words based on hierarchical categories.

In contrast, **taxonomic organization** is based on associations or classifications in which items share features that define them as a class. For example, taxonomic responses to the word wagon as presented in the task described previously, would probably include such items as *my trike, daddy's car, a truck,* and *a bus.* Items associated from a taxonomic perspective will tend to share similar features or functions, which classify them as a group. Children exhibiting taxonomic organization would sort that same pile of toys into separate groups of people, animals, furnishings, and vehicles.

Children's tendency to generalize, even to the extreme seen in overextensions, may set the stage for the eventual taxonomic organization of vocabulary. As children successfully generalize a word to new, but similar stimuli, in some way, it may demonstrate that several objects can share the same label. In this sense, the word is freed up from the specific features of the individual objects they know and becomes a much more flexible and useful response. For example, when children learn that all dogs are not the same color or size as their own, the word dog can be used with other dogs, and even some other critters (at least, until the defining features for dogs are more completely discriminated).

Through interacting with their caregivers, children gradually learn to discriminate among the essential semantic features for the myriad of items they name. As they do so, the classifications in their taxonomic organization are shaped by their caregivers' input as they evolve beyond simple, unidimensional classifications into hierarchical categories. The student's categories are continually refined. More specific subgroups called **subordinate categories** are associated under the broader, more conceptual groups, called **superordinate categories.** This process probably extends throughout the school years and beyond.

As children attend to the various features of an item and attempt to produce a label for it, caregivers may initially assist them by providing the name for the most typical members of that entire category. For example, in supplying the name for a large bird floating lazily in the sky, the caregiver is more likely to initially call it a *bird,* regardless of its specific name. In doing so, caregivers are providing the label for the mid-level superordinate category for the item. A higher level, more superordinate label, such as *animal,* is apparently so broad that perhaps caregivers sense that their children will not be able to recognize any commonly shared characteristics. To illustrate, bears, hawks, penguins, and pigs are all animals. Nonetheless, their most conspicuous features do not associate them in a way that might be obvious to younger children.

Depending on their estimation of children's vocabulary level, caregivers might go on to mention that the previously described bird is a *hawk.* Also, in another situation, if the exemplar is so unusual that its closeness-of-fit to the superordinate category is not apparent, caregivers may opt to use only its specific label. For example, caregivers might be satisfied to call a penguin a penguin, and not get into an involved analytical discussion.

The age of this shift from thematic to taxonomic organization of words is not clear. It may begin as early as the onset of overextensions, as toddlers begin to rapidly generalize words to a variety of stimuli. On the other hand, thematic associations may not cease to occur entirely. Given their imaginations and fondness for stories, many children may be still be inclined to associate words thematically as they approach school age. However, soon thereafter and increasingly throughout their school years, children will organize words taxonomically, according to superordinate and subordinate classifications.

Syntagmatic-Paradigmatic Shift

Preschoolers go through a period of rapid grammatical development, mastering a number of morphological and syntactic structures within the few years prior to entering school. Perhaps this is related to another shift noted by researchers, the **syntagmatic-paradigmatic shift.** Prior to reaching school age, it has been observed that word associations in older preschoolers have a syntactic basis. This is called a syntagmatic association. For example, when prompted to think of a word that goes with *car,* preschoolers tend to respond with words that follow a syntactic pattern, such as *drive.*

subordinate category
Subgroup of objects defined by a greater number of specific features than those defining the overall or superordinate category.

superordinate category
The highest conceptual level in a hierarchical classification of meanings, which includes all of the subgroups or subordinate categories in a given class.

syntagmatic-paradigmatic shift A transition in which word associations shift from a syntactic to semantic basis.

Shortly after entering school, the nature of students' word associations changes. Instead of a syntactic connection between words, their associations become semantically based. By associating members within the same semantic class, students exhibit paradigmatic association. In the previous instance, school-age children operating with paradigmatic associations are more likely to respond with *truck* or *bus.* This shift appears to proceed most rapidly in the first few grades, but does continue into adulthood. The basis of this shift and its timing is not fully understood. It may be an extension of the thematic-taxonomic shift that emerged early in the preschool years. On the other hand, it may be a reflection of increased emphasis on the analytical, categorical reasoning style that is integral to the language and curriculum in the classroom.

Semantic Networks

Preschoolers' *fast mapping* of new word meanings is discussed in Chapter 7. ■

As preschoolers, the initial learning of a new word—the process of storing the first associations for it—was called *fast mapping.* However, it is also noted that, beyond their initial associations, children continue to add information and refine the total meaning of the word in a prolonged, continuous process. For many words, new experiences and associations will modify our meanings for them throughout our lives.

A significant part of a word's meaning is derived from the information we relate to it. The related functions, contexts, stimuli, agents, and so forth gradually fill out the student's meaning of a word. Maybe just as important, all of this related information interconnects a host of other words with the original word of interest. In a semantic sense, a web of words and concepts develops around the original word. This web collects even more words to supplement and resonate the total meaning of the word.

semantic network The pattern of associated words and concepts that evolve out of experiencing a word.

This web of related words and concepts interconnecting individual words in a variety of ways has been called a **semantic network** (Pease & Berko Gleason, 1985). Semantic networks appear to evolve later as students become increasingly aware of the relatedness among certain words. These relationships may be thematically based, as in being aware of all the words that relate to the concept of a fire truck—firefighter, axes, hoses, sirens, and so forth. In turn, associations may become organized according to conceptual categories—events, objects, people. Ultimately, other associations that are superordinate-subordinate in nature may evolve—*firefighter* represents a career, *red* is a color, *axes* and *hoses* are tools, *siren* signals an emergency, and so on. Figure 9–1 illustrates this semantic network.

These interconnections may also contribute to two other related abilities that illustrate the vocabulary organization during the school years, divergent semantic production and convergent semantic production (Guilford & Hoepfner, 1971). As students' vocabularies grow, the patterns of association among words become increasingly familiar. This enhances the ability to produce related words or recognize a specific word related to other words.

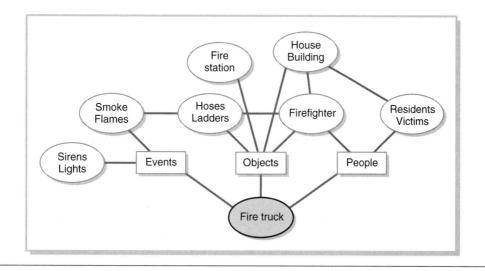

Figure 9–1. Illustration of a hypothetical semantic network for "fire truck." Bidirectional arrows indicate convergent and divergent semantic meaning. Dashed lines indicate likely associations between conceptual categories—events, objects, and people.

Divergent semantic production is demonstrated when a word prompts expression of a variety of related words, information, and concepts. As a result, students become capable of expressing ideas with greater flexibility by using a variety of related words. For instance, in the previous example, the network of words associated with *fire truck* provides a variety of relevant information and topics to use in discussing such emergencies.

Conversely, **convergent semantic production** is evidenced when the production of a specific word is prompted by other words that semantically point to it. That is, students are capable of inferring a meaning that has been expressed indirectly through associated words and concepts. In the example above, having overheard only scattered references to sirens, smoke, hoses, and so forth, students applying convergent semantic abilities would be able to guess that the conversation had something to do with a fire emergency. The ability to recognize semantic clues that lead to such inferences is a skill that is fundamental to the verbal reasoning abilities so critical to academic success.

divergent semantic production   The ability to produce a diverse collection of words based on their association with a topic.

convergent semantic production   The ability to identify a topic based on inferences from associated words.

Summary

- Beyond the preschool years, vocabulary represents a major area of development throughout the school-age years.

- Vocabulary expansion results from new experiences stemming from maturing physical abilities, cognitive understanding, and social interactions, which are all coupled together.

- During the school years, students become increasingly aware that word meanings are flexible in that they may apply to different contexts, carry altogether different meanings in other contexts, or share similar meanings with other words.

- Students' word definitions gradually become more conventional and formal as they adopt definitions that are less specific to their own experiences.

- The way in which students organize word meanings shifts from associations based on personal experiences, to associations based on syntactic patterns, to associating words based on features that define superordinate and subordinate classes.

- The interconnections that associate a variety of words across classes and contexts enhances students' abilities to use words flexibly and analytically.

Metalinguistics—Rising Above Language

Metalinguistics is introduced in Chapter 1. ■

Frequently, mature speakers think about language apart from simply communicating. When we analyze and evaluate language as something separate from our own behavior, it becomes an object of sorts. We might notice that certain words have the same number of syllables or even rhyme. We like the "sound" of certain words together. Or we intentionally choose to use certain words either to impress our listeners or avoid angering them. **Metalinguistic ability** refers to a speaker's ability to make a conscious evaluation of language behavior.

metalinguistic ability
Speakers' ability to consciously evaluate their language behavior.

Metalinguistic Abilities

Metalinguistic abilities are evident when our awareness shifts from the meanings of our utterances to the utterances themselves. Children do not evidence clear metalinguistic abilities (i.e., they cannot talk about language itself) until they are 6 and 7 years old. However, several subtle precursors to metalinguistic abilities appear prior to reaching school age. As toddlers and preschoolers, younger children self-correct words, recognize special or brand names (e.g., McDonald's, Dairy Queen), substitute or make up words to be "silly," refuse to attempt "hard" words, and adjust their language level for older and younger listeners. However, as school-age children, they will develop the ability to think about language, analyze it, and make conscious decisions about its status. See Table 9–1 for examples of metalinguistic abilities present during the developmental stages as individuals grow from toddlers into adults (Wallach & Miller, 1988).

As complex as human intelligence and language are, there are a myriad of ways in which metalinguistic abilities might be exhibited. Four major domains in which metalinguistic abilities become increasingly apparent in

Table 9–1. Selected developmental metalinguistic abilities.

Approximate Age Group	Metalinguistic Abilities
Toddler	Asks for labels when confronting unfamiliar objects.
	Revises utterances to repair communication.
	Requests that caregivers read text (versus only talk about pictures in books).
	Repeats words and sounds for practice.
	Associates graphic figures or trademarks with favorite cartoon characters, foods, drinks, restaurants, etc.
Preschooler	Adjusts speaking style for different listeners.
	Isolates individual words from spoken sentences.
	Produces different sounds in familiar words to create "funny" words.
	Judges others' utterances as grammatically correct or incorrect.
	Responds to words as inseparable from the items they name.
	Affects speech styles for different characters in play.
Elementary student	Appreciates humor in jokes involving lexical ambiguity.
	Judges appropriateness of different forms for different situations and listeners.
	Understands flexible or multiple word meanings.
	Segments words into syllables and syllables into phonemes.
	Understands more transparent idiomatic expressions.
Adolescent and Adult	Analyzes sentences at various levels.
	Understands various forms of figurative language, including idioms, metaphors, similes, proverbs, and so forth.
	Creates humor through lexical ambiguity.
	Judges sentences' correctness and explains the source of their incorrectness.

Note. Adapted from *Language Intervention and Academic Success,* by G. P. Wallach and Miller, 1988, Boston: College-Hill Press; and "Metalinguistic Skills: Cutting Across Spoken and Written Problem-Solving Abilities," by A. van Kleeck. In *Language Learning Disabilities in School-age Children,* pp. 128–153, by G. P. Wallach and K. G. Butler (Eds.), 1984. Baltimore: Williams and Wilkins.

students are segmentation abilities, word awareness, word order awareness, and ambiguity.

Segmentation of Linguistic Units

A fundamental step to developing metalinguistic abilities is metalinguistic awareness; that is, the awareness of language as an arbitrary system of sounds and symbols (van Kleeck, 1984). The first step toward this awareness might be **segmentation,** in which speakers analyze the stream of language into linguistic units.

The prefix *meta-* includes the sense of transcending, going beyond, or rising above. ∎

segmentation The ability to analyze the stream of speech into units such as phonemes, syllables, and words.

Printed text may give us the false sense that our speech is produced as segmented words. You might be aware that ancient documents were written in unsegmented "strings" of letter symbols. In the 1400s, Gutenberg's printing press introduced the convenience of preformed blocks for letters and words to mass produce texts. As a result, we are now accustomed to seeing spaces between printed words, even though they are not there in our speech.

Consider the experience of trying to understand a foreign language. It not only appears to be an uninterrupted stream of sounds, it is! Although our own language is also an uninterrupted stream, through our extensive experience with it, we have learned to discriminate the segments that represent "individual" words.

The younger child must go through the process of discriminating which series of sounds are relevant to a given situation. For example, toddlers hear frequent phrases such as, *Let's wash your bowl, Keep the cereal in your bowl, Put the bowl down, Take the bowl off your head!* The toddler eventually discriminates the one thing that is always present. It must be what that series of sounds (*bowl*) in the caregiver's utterances stands for.

As toddlers and preschoolers, children initially view words as an integral and inseparable part of their referents (van Kleeck, 1984). For example, although younger children might agree that a cat could be called a dog, they will assume that doing so would mean that cats can bark. Eventually, children separate the word from its referent, understanding that the word is merely a conventional, but arbitrary, name.

Once children are aware that words are arbitrary, it means that they can play with, analyze, examine, and substitute for them, without doing any harm to their inherent role as symbols for communicating. As such, students begin to notice rhyming words and homonyms (*If I'm at the beach, I can see the sea!*), find a word within a word (*Hey, hamburgers don't have ham in them!*), note that some words are longer or shorter, or use different words because they are "favorite" or "funny" words.

Word segmentation, the ability to analyze words into individual syllables and phonemes, develops later than sentence segmentation skills. For example, a younger child who has not developed word segmentation skills is likely to choose *snake* over *caterpillar* as the longest word. Younger children have not metalinguistically separated the word from its referent and fail to analyze words into syllables. Students may begin segmenting words by substituting initial or final sounds to make rhyming words. It appears that segmenting words into syllables and phonemes might be especially important in learning to read; however, reading may conversely enhance the ability to segment phonemes. Also, children who have progressed to associating letter symbols with specific sounds or phonemes tend to be advanced in their reading and writing skills (Westby, 1994a).

Word Awareness

word awareness The conscious awareness that words are objects with phonetic structure and can have multiple meanings.

Another metalinguistic ability that develops in the early school years is **word awareness,** the understanding that words can have multiple meanings and a referent can have multiple names. For preschoolers, words have specific, inflexible meanings closely tied to objects' physical features or their personal experience with them. For example, *sharp* will be narrowly understood from an experiential standpoint; only knives and scissors can be sharp.

Young students' awareness of word flexibility may be first evidenced by recognizing familiar words in unfamiliar contexts and asking what they mean in those situations. With additional experience, young students accept word meanings that become more flexible and abstract. Young students might say a person has a *sharp sense of humor,* although they may not be able to clearly explain the relationship. By the time they are in junior high, most students will give a sound explanation of the logic behind such expressions (Westby, 1994a).

In a similar way, after a widened exposure to the language of their community, students recognize that other people have different names for things. Families differ in what they call a *cup, mug,* or *glass.* (At our house, anything that does not have a handle tends to be a *glass,* regardless of its composition.) If you show up for *dinner* at some households, you may have missed the noon meal they invited you to share and find them scraping together enough *supper* to serve you that evening.

Academically, this increased awareness of words probably enhances comprehension of new information due to increased semantic flexibility. Recognizing that a word is not in its usual context may prompt a student to examine the context and consider the different meanings that might be associated with it in this new circumstance.

Word Order Awareness

Judging the acceptability of speakers' utterances is another way in which children's metalinguistic abilities are revealed. Researchers have presented children with sentences that exhibit incorrect word order or word pairs that violate lexical restrictions (e.g., "hungry rock," "married bachelor"). In their responses, children might reveal whether they can evaluate the form apart from the message (van Kleeck, 1984).

Preschoolers tend to judge a "good" or "bad" sentence based simply on their personal experience and understanding of its "truthfulness." The preschooler might reject *Daddy washed his car* as "wrong" on the basis that "Daddy has a truck." On the other hand, they may accept *Baby the wash* because based on their experience that is something you do with babies. Younger school-age children, however, will begin to react to the form of an utterance, apart from its relevance to their personal experiences. Initially, they may be able to only identify incorrect sentences as "bad" or "silly," without being able to tell why. But, eventually, they will be able to correct them and even explain the difference.

Ambiguity: Figurative and Funny Language

Different words can have essentially the same meaning and the same word can have different meanings. Different sentences can mean the same thing

ambiguity The observation that a sentence has more than one interpretation.

and the same sentence can convey different meanings. This illustrates the concept of **ambiguity,** in which two or more interpretations are possible for the same utterance. For example, the statement *They are baking potatoes* might describe the activity of some cooks or might refer to the best use for a certain type of potato.

The potential for confusion stemming from ambiguity would seem to pose problems for mature speakers as well as for young language learners. Linguists (e.g., Chomsky, 1957) have suggested that the underlying deep structures of ambiguous sentences assist listeners as they interpret such sentences. However, others (e.g., Fillmore, 1968; Skinner, 1957) contend that it is the context that helps the listener decide which interpretation (or deep structure) applies. Without a context for reference, the listener would be left in an endless state of indecision. Based on their experience with ambiguous utterances and the relevant situations, speakers eventually learn to consider the possible contexts that might support an ambiguous utterance as they attempt to understand them.

Some ambiguous utterances, such as the "baking potatoes" example just given, are meant to be interpreted in either of two ways, both literal. Other ambiguous utterances can be interpreted at two levels, literal or figurative. A literal interpretation presumes that the utterance means just what it says. Most utterances are intended to communicate directly through literal interpretation; that is, they mean just what they say. My wife's statement, *I'd appreciate it if you'd take the garbage out,* usually means just that.

figurative language Language that conveys meaning through analogy based on stimulus generalization rather than through literal interpretation of the words and phrases.

simile Figurative language that directly states an analogous relationship (e.g., *He's as clumsy as an ox!*).

metaphor Figurative language that implies an analogous relationship (e.g., *He's an ox!*); compare **simile.**

idiom Figurative language that express ideas through analogy (e.g., *Don't let the cat out of the bag*).

proverbs Figurative language that expresses truths or gives advice through analogy (e.g., *Look before you leap!*).

The verbal operant that explains *figurative language* is called an *extended tact,* and is described in Chapter 4. ■

Figurative language consists of utterances that convey meaning by suggesting a connection between two contexts that share features or relationships. Stimulus generalization is the behavioral process that makes figurative language possible for speakers and useful for listeners. Most settings or contexts are complex clusters of stimuli. Two different clusters may share similar features, parts, or relationships (Skinner, 1957; Winokur, 1976). Figure 9–2 illustrates a stimulus cluster in figurative language. In using figurative language, speakers mention one cluster to indirectly suggest the features or relationships shared by the context we are actually describing. Although this results in ambiguity, experienced listeners disregard the literal translation and generalize the significance of the figurative one. Figurative language results in some of our most colorful verbal behaviors, such as **similes,** which directly state an analogous relationship (e.g., *She is as light as a feather*); **metaphors,** which imply analogous relationships (e.g., *He's a bull in a china shop*); **idioms,** short analogous expressions (*Don't let the cat out of the bag*); and **proverbs,** analogous statements that express truths or advice (e.g., *Don't put all your eggs in one basket*).

Generally, the learning of figurative language is a prolonged process that involves substantial experience and the ability to generalize through analogy (Nippold & Rudzinksi, 1993). Younger preschoolers may learn a particular idiom by rote when exposed to it frequently. After challenging my own children's balance of imagination and logic, I would frequently prompt them with, "Am I pulling your leg?" They were quite young when they came to understand that idiom, whereas several others continued to puzzle them.

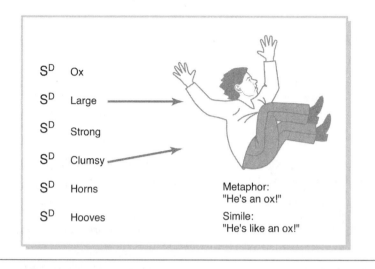

Figure 9–2. Illustration of the role of stimulus clusters in figurative language. (S^D = Discriminative stimulus.)

Even with experience, some figurative expressions are more or less concrete than others as a result of their **metaphoric transparency,** the degree of similarity between the literal referent and the figurative relationship. For example, the literal level of an idiom such as *Don't let the cat out of the bag* shares a stronger concrete resemblance (and greater metaphoric transparency) with its figurative interpretation, and would therefore be easier than an idiom such as *He kicked the bucket* (Gibbs, 1987). Familiarity from experience and transparency based on concreteness have been shown to make figurative language easier to understand (Nippold & Haq, 1996).

To demonstrate mastery of figurative expressions, children must be able to use, understand, and even explain a variety of them. Metaphors and similes appear to occur more often in preschoolers than in school-age children. However, it may be that the earlier occurrences represent true figurative language less often than thought, and are more often cases of "stretching" a limited vocabulary (as in extended tacts, if the pun can be excused). By school age, students' vocabularies have improved enough that conventional words are used more, and, although fewer, the metaphors and similes are perhaps used more consciously. Understanding of idioms and proverbs develops later, in older students and adolescence (Nippold & Erkine, 1988; Nippold & Martin, 1989). Even into adulthood, some of us fail to comprehend the wisdom in proverbs.

A strange and wonderful part of human anatomy is our funny bone! Ambiguity also creates utterances with multiple meanings that may be humorous, especially if one of the meanings is unexpected. Although some humor is strictly situational, most higher level humor is based on ambiguity in language. Puns, riddles, and jokes are metalinguistic behaviors in which we respond to double meanings as being funny.

metaphoric transparency   The extent of similarity between a figurative expression and its literal referent.

Some do not consider situational humor and slapstick humor to be "higher level" humor. But try to convince a die-hard Marx Brothers or Three Stooges fan of that! Or that they should care! ■

Table 9–2. Levels of ambiguity in humor.

Level	Basis of Ambiguity	Example
Phonological	Two words differ by a single phonetic contrast resulting in different meanings.	A house painter economized in painting his pastor's house by watering down the paint. When it rained and the paint washed off, his pastor told him to *repaint and thin no more.*
Lexical	Two words sound alike (regardless of their spellings) but have different meanings.	What did the beach say to the wave? *Sea ya' later!*
Surface-structure	A word or phrase carries different meanings, often figurative versus literal, depending on the context of the sentence.	1st lady: *Whenever I'm down in the dumps, I just get myself a new dress.* 2nd lady: *I wondered where you found this one.*
Deep-structure	A word or phrase results in two underlying meanings or relationships for the sentence.	Mom: *Should we take the kids to the zoo today?* Dad: *Heck, if the zoo can handle them, they can come and get them.*

Note. Adapted from "Communication Refinement in School Age and Adolescence," by C. E. Westby. In *Communication Development: Foundations, Processes, and Clinical Applications,* pp. 341–383, by W. O. Haynes and B. B. Shulman (Eds.), 1994, Englewood Cliffs, NJ: Prentice-Hall.

There are four levels of ambiguity that lead to humor in language. See Table 9–2 for examples of linguistic ambiguity in humor. Phonological ambiguity, in which the meaning is changed in an unexpected way by altering a key sound in the utterance, develops earliest, around 7 years of age. Next, lexical ambiguity develops, which depends on the double meaning of a key word. Ambiguity in surface structure and deep structure, in which the interpretation is focused on the wrong phrase or the wrong underlying meaning, is the last to develop, around 11 or 12 years of age (Westby, 1994a).

Summary

- Metalinguistic awareness occurs when speakers shift their attention from the meanings of their utterances to the form of the utterances themselves.
- Toddlers and preschoolers evidence the beginnings of metalinguistic abilities when they make up words, self-correct words, and adjust the level of their language.
- Segmentation refers to analyzing the speech stream into words or words into sounds and syllables.
- As students develop word awareness, they restrict word meanings less and accept more flexible word meanings which lays the foundation for abstract thinking.

- Students become capable of evaluating sentences that are grammatically acceptable and, eventually, become capable of explaining inadequacies that need correcting.

- Younger students first become capable of understanding metaphors, similes, and idioms in context and only as adolescents can they understand and explain the underlying analogies of proverbs.

- Humor as a form of ambiguity is only gradually understood as children progress toward adolescence.

Pragmatics: Conversations, Anecdotes, and Classrooms

The basic functions of language have been in place since the child's first words (and perhaps before). They evolved and differentiated during the preschool years. However, the basic functions will not be further distinguished during the school years. Instead, how the basic functions are served through language in the contexts of conversations, storytelling, and the classroom will be refined.

School-Age Refinements

The school-age years bring many changes and challenges to communicating as students mature physically, cognitively, and socially. Conversations with people outside their family will refine their ability to communicate more explicitly. With a growing variety of experiences, they will be presented with more opportunities to refine their storytelling. In addition, they will experience the classroom—perhaps the single most influential setting outside their home. Students are compelled to develop greater sophistication as they verbally negotiate complex social transactions, relate experiences to familiar and unfamiliar audiences, and learn from their interactions within the classroom setting.

Conversational Discourse

As a student, conversational discourse becomes increasingly fluid and sophisticated. Students apply their experience with an improved understanding of others. They become more perceptive in making assumptions about their listeners. The ability to specify topics with greater clarity is improved. As their audiences become more varied, so does the range of styles they are able to exhibit with them. Should the conversation break down in some way, students become increasingly capable of making the repairs.

Presuppositional skills, the ability to adjust the message to the needs of the listener, begins to develop rapidly in the preschool years. As preschoolers begin to initiate conversations about topics that are less constrained to

Perspective taking, as an aspect of *presupposition,* is introduced in Chapter 7. ■

the "here-and-now," it becomes increasingly important for them to understand who their partners are and what they do and do not know.

As preschoolers, children begin to adjust the level of their language and they become more capable of perceptually "stepping into their listener's shoes." These two abilities are called linguistic and perceptual perspective taking, respectively. A third aspect of presupposition that develops significantly in school-age children is cognitive perspective taking, which is the ability to infer others' feelings, thought processes, and intentions. Not only do students become more sensitive to their listener's language level and point of view, but they perceive more subtle clues that suggest their personality and educational traits. This permits even more sophisticated judgment regarding their level of language and overall understanding of the topic (Geller, 1989).

An area of improvement that reflects this growing sense of audience is *style shifting.* School-age children become increasingly adept at judging social and role status. Younger students, one would hope, learn to address adults other than their own caregiver in a different, more formal tone. Polite forms (*Please, Thank you,* etc.) may become even more likely with these individuals than they are with caregivers. More often, students' requests become softened with modal auxiliaries (*May I, Would you, Could you,* etc.). Finally, they become masters at using indirect requests, which only hint at the goal or object of desire. Teenagers quickly learn that a phrase such as *Your car is sooo cool!* translates into "I'm low on gas, so can we use your car?"

Improvement in presuppositional skills is also evident in students' improving use of deictic terms, such as demonstratives, to specify referents for their listeners. As preschoolers, children began to use the demonstratives *this* and *that;* however, they were used in ways that made them almost interchangeable. Using the full set of demonstratives competently requires judgment of several aspects, including singularity-plurality (*this-these, that-those*) and the relative dimension of proximity (*this-that, these-those*). In addition, it must be understood that proximity is based on the speaker's perspective (Webb & Abrahmson, 1976)

Other later developing pairs of terms that are also based on semantically subtle relationships include *here-there, ask-tell, bring-take,* and *loan-borrow.* These, too, involve proximal and directional judgments that must be understood from the standpoint of the speaker. These terms may still confuse older students but should be understood by most adolescents.

The final areas of improvement in conversational discourse to be addressed here are the abilities to maintain and repair conversations. Preschoolers are limited in the number of conversational turns taken on a given topic. In part, this probably relates to their limited experience and information on most topics. Generally, the number of subsequent turns that maintain a given topic will increase with age, and especially so from throughout adolescence into adulthood (Brinton & Fujiki, 1984). One means for maintaining the connection between subsequent comments in conversation is through the use of adverbial conjunctions to signal logical connections between sentences. Younger students may rely on simpler notions of connection expressed by *then* and *so*. By the time they reach sixth grade, students will expand their repertoire to include such sophisticated forms as *otherwise, therefore,* and *however* (Scott, 1988). Adolescents and young adults continue to have difficulty correctly using more advanced forms (e.g., *similarly, consequently, nevertheless*) of adverbial conjuncts (Nippold, Schwarz, & Undlin, 1992).

In a related way, the number of topic shifts within a conversational episode decreases. This perhaps results from the expanded experience base and information that older individuals have to draw on for a given topic. In other words, it becomes easier to maintain a topic longer and still contribute fresh comments. Similarly, this may also reflect the social maturity of older individuals wishing to acknowledge their partner's interest in a current topic. Additionally, topic shading, which occurs as individuals become more sophisticated about shifting topics, may account for the perception of fewer topics as individuals mature. In **topic shading,** a subsequent utterance maintains one aspect of the previous utterance but shifts to a related topic. A series of such shadings will cause the topic to drift without either partner realizing they have changed topics.

Finally, older students begin to repair conversations in ways that are more deliberate and effective. As preschoolers, repetition was a typical response to the listener's request for clarification. As younger students, they generally repair a breakdown with relevant information, and are likely to add supplemental information to clarify their statements. Successive repetitions in which additional elements are included to supplement the previous information are called **stacked repair sequences.** Finally, by the time they are 10 years old, students will be generally capable of providing definitions, descriptions, or background context to assist their listener (Brinton, Fujiki, Loeb, & Winkler, 1986).

Storytelling and Narratives

Preschoolers' storytelling evolves from prenarratives, to heaps, to chains, to primitive narratives. Preschoolers become capable of longer stories and even began relating the increasing number of elements in their stories. However, few preschooler stories introduce true cause-effect relationships, and fewer yet contain any sense of a plot, which is necessary for the final three narrative levels to be discussed later: unfocused chains, focused chains, and true narratives (Westby, 1984).

In the school-age years, several developments set the stage for progressing to true narratives. School-age children develop a better understanding of cause-effect relationships. In a related way, they develop the ability to use adverbial conjunctions to connect elements that are causally related. Also, students become increasingly aware of inferred information and, conversely, how to imply information through indirect cues.

topic shading   Subtle shifts in the conversational topic through addressing an isolated aspect of a previous utterance.

stacked repair sequences Successive attempts to clarify an utterance in which additional elements are included in each subsequent attempt.

Early narrative development during the preschool years is discussed in Chapter 7. ■

Connecting elements through adverbial conjunctions is discussed earlier in this chapter under Conversational Discourse. ■

plot   The central theme that provides the focus for story elements.

setting   The characters, location, and circumstances for a narrative.

episode   A part of a narrative that relates a series of events as part of the overall plot.

unfocused chains   Narratives based on elements linked together logically, but in an unorganized manner.

focused chains   Narratives that organize a sequence of events around a character but omit reasons for the character's actions.

complete narrative   Story that includes all of the required elements of mature narratives.

complex narrative   Mature narratives that include subplots that are related to each other and an overall plot.

Perhaps the essential defining characteristic of true narratives is the presence of a **plot.** A plot is the central organizing theme for the story—romance, victory, vindication, and so forth. Organized under the plot are the two main elements, the story setting and the story episodes. The **setting** includes the story's characters, location, time, and circumstances. **Episodes** are composed of seven elements: (a) the *initiating event;* (b) the main character's *internal response* or feelings about it; (c) the main character's *plan* of action; (d) the main character's *attempt* at executing the plan; (e) the *consequence* of the plan; (f) the *resolution* as portrayed through the main character's reaction to the consequence; and (f) the *ending* or moral principle of the story.

As young as 5 years of age, students begin to include episodes with cause-effect relationships in their narratives. The earliest of these, **unfocused chains,** consist of individual elements linked together through logical or cause-effect relationships, perhaps expressed by adverbial conjuncts (e.g., *because*). However, in unfocused chains, even though the events and elements relate to each other, they are not well organized (or focused) under an overall plot.

By approximately 9 years of age, the sequences of events expressed in students' narratives become more centrally focused on a character. These are called **focused chains,** which may consist of a central character and a true sequence of events, but omit characters' internal plans or intentions. As a result, they take on the superficial appearance of a mature narrative, but do still fall short because characters and events are not related in a dynamic plot.

In contrast, the next level of narratives, **complete narratives,** includes dynamic and reciprocal relationships among events, character's attributes, and achievement of the goal. The characters achieve their goal because the events change or reveal their inner attributes. Finally, adolescents achieve **complex narratives,** which are based on multiple embedded episodes or subplots. These develop as older students learn to consider and intertwine multiple relationships and consequences in their plots (Westby, 1984).

Classroom Language

As students, children must deal with language in an entirely different context. Prior to entering kindergarten, language was primarily a naturally occurring behavior in preschoolers' everyday activities with familiar people and settings. Preschoolers certainly learned through the language exchanged in their interactions. Although their focus was on learning about their world and social transactions, they certainly learned about language as well.

As students, from kindergarten on, language will be the most critical learning tool. And, yet, the nature of the language game changes signif-

 American classrooms continue to consider the issues that arise from our cultural diversity. Our composition is rapidly approaching a point when one third of the population will be composed of minority populations. Classroom language and textbooks must account for a wide range of cultural and linguistic differences. Our diversity truly is our strength, if we allow ourselves to be challenged to learn from it.

icantly once students find their seats. Two kinds of language occur in the classroom, teacher language and textbook language. Both have teaching and learning as their primary purposes, but classroom language is quite different from "everyday" language.

Teacher Language. Research has described the differences between "everyday language" and teacher language. Although we can describe the characteristics of teacher language, we do not necessarily know which features contribute most effectively to learning (Nelson, 1984; Wallach & Miller, 1988).

The language of teachers will vary across individual instructors; realizing this and adjusting to it are two of the annual challenges faced by students each school year. However, a number of broad characteristics of teacher language and how it differs from everyday language have been documented. These include differences in contextual support, rate and proximity of presentation, levels of presupposition, and the opportunity to request clarification (Lane & Molyneaux, 1992; Nelson, 1984; Wallach & Miller, 1988).

The utterances shared in everyday communication and those that occur in the classroom differ significantly in the extent of available contextual support. In everyday language, as preschoolers and at home during their school years, children have been afforded the luxury of communicating with familiar partners in daily routines with a supportive setting and a known context. The utterances in everyday language are highly *contextualized,* meaning they are supported by referents or stimuli in the situation. In contrast, the utterances that occur in teacher language in the classroom are highly *decontextualized,* that is, presented apart from the context or situation to which it relates. Teacher language is addressed to a group. The referents for teacher utterances may not be immediately apparent to all students, especially in a classroom filled with bulletin boards, blackboards, different textbooks, and so forth. In later grades, teachers introduce posters, transparencies, slides, and other visual aids that may be difficult to relate to their comments. Even the high-tech classroom with individual computers risks the possibility that students may unknowingly arrive at a screen that is not relevant to the discussion.

A significant difference that weighs heavily on students, especially the younger ones, is the diminished *presupposition* between teachers and their students. In everyday language, family members have an intimate, ongoing understanding of a child's language abilities and world knowledge. Teachers are left to make broad assumptions about the abilities and experiences of their students. The smaller the classroom and the more attentive teachers are to individual differences, the more this can be offset, but it is the rare teacher who knows each student's experiences and language abilities better than the family.

Another set of variables that distinguishes everyday and teacher language is *speaking rate* and *proximity.* Researchers have found increased speaking rate in teacher language through the grade levels. In addition, teachers in lower grade levels are more likely to maintain proximity and face-to-face contact while talking to younger students. As grade levels increase, students may find more teachers are not only less conscious of their proximity to students, but are also more prone to "lecture to the blackboard."

Teacher language has also been found to differ in *complexity* and *style*. It is not surprising that syntactic complexity of teacher language increases with grade levels. However, the language of instruction also tends to use more imperatives and interrogatives (to direct attention and question for comprehension) in contrast to a predominance of declaratives in everyday language. Generally, most would describe everyday language as exhibiting an informal and social style; in contrast, teacher language has been described as having a more formal, **expository style,** in which relatively structured information is presented in a logical and tutorial manner.

The final difference to be noted here is the logical result of all of the previous characteristics. Given the nature of the classroom situation—the rate of presentation, the formal interaction, the lack of proximity, and so forth—the typical student will find it challenging, if not intimidating, to request clarification when a communication breakdown has occurred.

Textbook Language.   In addition to teacher language, students are also challenged with another form of classroom language, textbook language. It might be assumed that spending so much of our lives as students, we would come to know the characteristics of textbook language. However, textbook language is not something that all students are necessarily conscious of, which may hinder their comprehension and recall of printed information.

Texts are organized to present their content in predictable styles and patterns depending on their purposes (Westby, 1994a). The books students are confronted with in the earliest grades are more narrative in nature, generally consisting of "readers" and "storybooks." Early books are intended to expose younger students to written language about familiar or entertaining topics. By second grade, books begin to take on more of the distinctive style of "textbooks" to convey academic information. This organization, called **text grammar,** presents information in an expository style similar to teacher language. However, being written language, expository text tends to be even more structured and formal. There will tend to be distinct sections that serve as introductions, discussions, and reviews.

The specific expository style varies depending on the information that is being conveyed, and there are a number of key phrases and words that characteristically signal which type of expository pattern follows (Westby, 1994a). For example, **descriptive patterns,** which simply describe something, might be signaled by phrases such as *is something that, refers to,* or *is similar to.* **Collection patterns,** in which the text will list related items, are marked by phrases such as, *for instance, including,* and (guess what) *such as.* Information presented in **sequence patterns,** which relate a series of events or steps, might be introduced with *first, next,* or *subsequently.* **Comparison patterns,** contrasting items as similar or different, might be signaled by *similarly, although, in contrast,* or *conversely.* The reasons for an

---

expository style The structured and formal style of tutorial language in classrooms and textbooks.

Literacy and the process of learning to read and write is discussed later. ■

text grammar Characteristic styles associated with language found in textbooks.

descriptive patterns Syntactic devices found in text grammar that signal a topic is being described.

collection patterns Syntactic devices associated with text grammar that indicate a listing of items.

sequence pattern Syntactic devices associated with text grammar that signal the description of a sequence of events or steps.

comparison patterns Syntactic devices associated with text grammar signaling that similarities or differences are being noted.

event are conveyed in a **cause-effect pattern,** which might be prefaced with words such as *because, consequently,* and *therefore.*

By fourth grade, students are somewhat aware of text grammars. As this ability improves it might help students anticipate the kind of information that will follow, which in turn may facilitate their comprehension and recall of it. Although the research is not consistent, generally it appears that some types of text patterns are more difficult to comprehend and recall than others. For example, descriptive and collection patterns may be more difficult to recall than comparison and sequential patterns. Fittingly, cause-effect patterns tend to be recognized much later in adolescence, perhaps not until high school (Westby, 1994a).

cause-effect pattern
Syntactic devices in text grammar that signal a cause-effect relationship is being proposed.

Summary

- Language assumes an entirely new importance and nature when children become students.

- School years bring new settings, audiences, roles, and experiences that provide the motivation for further refinement of language skills.

- Conversational skills mature as students improve their ability to perceive others' abilities and knowledge and their ability to shift topics in subtle ways.

- Narratives become more mature as students create more complex plots with cause-effect relationships and dynamic characters.

- Students are challenged to adapt to teacher language and textbook language, both of which are qualitatively different from the everyday language they experience outside school.

Language for Literacy

Literacy is the ability to communicate through visual symbols. Although the visual symbol system involved might vary across settings and cultures, most of us think of **graphemes,** the letters or letter combinations of the alphabet for phonemes as the primary symbols for visual communication. It is important to stress that literacy involves more than just "reading" and "writing." Calling out the sounds of letters to say words or making letters to form words on paper do not represent mature literacy; the intended meanings must be fully comprehended or expressed within an overall context to truly demonstrate literacy.

Literacy may be to present and future generations what tools and agriculture were to our prehistoric ancestors. It is almost impossible to imagine survival in today's "information explosion" without the ability to read and write—to readily access and transmit verbal information. From reading a want-ad to writing a check, from navigating interstate systems to navigating the information super-highway, it would seem to be an overwhelming task

literacy The ability to communicate through written language.

graphemes Letters or letter combinations that represent the phonemes of a language.

The verbal operant called *textuals,* discussed briefly in Chapter 4, was how Skinner analyzed the behavioral processes of reading and writing. ∎

to survive without literacy. There is nothing so sadly moving as the image of grown adults who are actually frightened of the bewildering sea of words that swirl around them. Their needless shame and loss of potential is a private tragedy. The deplorably low literacy rates world wide represent a great collective tragedy.

Traditionally, reading and writing as forms of literate language have been separated. This has occurred in ways related to distinctions in research methodology, instructional methods and materials, and even separate professional organizations. However, some view them as much more analogous than these distinctions might suggest (Fitzgerald & Shanahan, 2000).

It has been proposed that both reading and writing processes are based on analogous mental processes and share forms of knowledge that are superordinate. The four types of knowledge have been described as metaknowledge, domain knowledge, knowledge about universal text attributes, and procedural knowledge (Fitzgerald & Shanahan, 2000). Table 9–3 presents these types of knowledge shared by writers and readers. *Metaknowledge* is pragmatically based understanding that reading and writing have purposes that allow writers and readers to interact in a unique manner while exchanging information. *Domain knowledge* is readers' understanding words based on their "world knowledge." It may be based on prior experiences or even knowledge constructed from interacting with the text itself. The knowledge that readers and writers demonstrate regarding graphemes, phonemes, morphology, and syntax is the *knowledge of universal text attributes*. Finally, *procedural knowledge and skill to negotiate reading and writing* is the understanding of the processes involved in reading and writing that allow intentional strategies such as predicting information or finding analogies for comprehension.

Emerging Literacy

Literacy opens doors to a whole new world. Readers can travel anywhere and see anything through the words in a book. However, the process of unlocking those doors is not an easy one. Two observations must be appreciated as we consider the development of literacy. First, although oral language obviously lays the foundation for literacy, the processes of reading and writing differ from talking in several ways. Because they are based on language, reading and writing are also complex symbolic behaviors involving higher level perceptual, cognitive, and linguistic abilities. However, there are notable differences between language in interaction and language in print that may not be immediately obvious to us.

Second, unlike developing oral language, developing literacy appears to be a more formal and explicit process. For most children, literacy does not emerge as effortlessly as oral language appears to do. Although the underlying process is not fully understood, at a minimum it will involve different perceptual and cognitive abilities to discriminate individual letters, associate their sounds, synthesize them into words, and eventually comprehend the meaning that transcends all those "little black marks."

Table 9–3. Categories of knowledge shared by readers and writers.

- **Metaknowledge (*Pragmatics*)**
  Knowing about functions and purposes of reading and writing
  Knowing that readers and writers interact
  Monitoring one's own meaning making (metacomprehension) and word identification or production strategies
  Monitoring one's own knowledge.
- **Domain knowledge about substance and content (prior knowledge, content knowledge gained while reading and writing)**
  Semantics
    Vocabulary meaning
    Meaning created through context of connected text
- **Knowledge of universal text attributes**
  Graphophonics—Letter and word identification and generation
    Phonological awareness
    Grapheme awareness (letter shapes, knowledge of typographical representations such as punctuation and capitalization)
    Morphology (word structure and orthographic patterns)
  Syntax
    Syntax of sentences
    Punctuation
  Text format
    Syntax of larger chunks of text (e.g., story grammars and expository text structures)
    Text organization (e.g., sequence of text, graphics)
- **Procedural knowledge and skill to negotiate reading and writing**
  Knowing how to access, use, and generate knowledge in any of the previous areas
  Instantiating smooth integration of various processes

Note. Adapted from "Reading and Writing Relations and their Development," by J. Fitzgerald and T. Shanahan, 2000, *Educational Psychologist, 35*(1), pp. 39–50.

To a great extent, there seems to be an assumption on the part of many caregivers that literacy must be developed through the formal instruction received in school. Nonetheless, it appears that many students arrive at school having had certain experiences that give them an advantage in learning this process.

Literate Language Differences

Although oral language is the basis for written language, it does not follow that written language is oral language on paper. Written language as a process allows for a different style and level of integration (Westby, 1994a). In written language, more concise vocabulary is typical and the syntax is generally more complex. The writing process itself normally permits the selection of more specific words and the construction of sentences that make explicit, but complex, connections among ideas. The connected statements within written language are more centrally focused on a topic. This focus results in a more predictable organization of most written language, especially as more advanced levels are achieved. The result of this process is called **literate language.**

literate language The style of formal written language that is structured and organized in distinctive ways.

To achieve this specificity and complexity, written or literate language relies on certain structures. Because written language is generally decontextualized (perhaps with the exception of picture books), literate language cannot rely on the deictic role of pronouns and demonstratives. Shared context in conversation allows listeners to track the shifting referents for *this, that, he, him, her,* and *them.* Literate language, however, must name the referent or person more frequently to help the reader track the story. In addition, sequences and connections in most conversations are indicated with simpler conjunctions (*and, then,* and *but*). Literate language relies more heavily on subordinating and adverbial conjunctions (*because, although, whereas, however*) to express the relationship between sentences.

Deictic roles of pronouns and demonstratives are discussed in Chapters 7 and 8. ■

Another difference that may cause some confusion along the way is punctuation. Speakers signal utterance boundaries with intonational contours. They use pauses and prosody to emphasize or de-emphasize words and phrases. However, in printed form, language is now embedded with periods, commas, semicolons, colons, quotation marks, apostrophes, and so on. Students must decipher the significance of these as they master reading.

Oral Language Skills—Predecessors to Literacy

Although they are not identical, it appears that many of the skills developed while mastering oral language provide some basis for emerging literacy. There are perhaps three major developments that relate most strongly to eventual success in reading.

The foundations to literacy laid down with infants, toddlers, and preschoolers were discussed in Chapters 5, 6, and 7. ■

The first major related development is comprehensive mastery of oral language. In this context, comprehensive refers to the integration of world knowledge and linguistic abilities. Throughout the years preceding school, children have been simultaneously collecting experiences and learning the language that accompanies the objects, people, events, and relationships experienced. Ultimately, because storytelling reflects the extent of integration and organization achieved in their oral language, a strong indicator for reading success is children's development of oral narrative abilities (Norris & Brunig, 1988).

A second related indicator predictive of successful reading is development of metalinguistic abilities. Preschool children who enter school with a metalinguistic awareness of sounds, words, word order, and meanings are more likely to successfully learn to read. These abilities are fundamental to the cueing systems used by successful readers and will be discussed later.

Appendix B presents detailed academic expectations for language and literacy grades K–12. ■

A third and final factor that is perhaps the strongest indicator of potential for reading success is the extent of exposure to literacy prior to school. Although this is not a feature of children's developing language, homes in which adults read, read to preschoolers, and have books tend to be homes that produce students who become strong readers. Although these experiences do not directly teach reading, they may make the preschooler more conscious of the parallel nature of oral language and written language and more likely associate reading with close, meaningful interactions. Years later, my children (who are now adults) and I still share a favorite line (*"Do you like my party hat? I do. I do like your party hat!"*) from a favorite childhood bedtime story, *Go Dog Go!*

Development of Reading

Reading has been characterized according to several models. Two contrasting models have been dubbed the top-down and bottom-up models. The **bottom-up model** describes reading as the process of translating graphemes into phonemes, phonemes into words, words into sentences, and sentences into ideas. The bottom-up model probably represents the more conventional view of reading and would correlate with the traditional phonics approach to teaching reading, which emphasizes decoding sound-symbol associations as the fundamental level.

A **top-down model** of reading is based on the concept of hypothesis testing to derive meaning. As individuals read, they form guesses about the print and the meanings that are upcoming. As they read further, subsequent words confirm or conflict with their hypotheses. Readers continue integrating information until the entire meaning of the text has been derived. In this view, the ability to decode individual symbols in a text is secondary to extracting its meaning. The top-down model is associated with the whole language approach to teaching reading.

These models represent extreme theoretical positions. In reality, most researchers and teachers probably agree that some aspects of both models apply in an interactive process (May, 1990). Obviously, the process of reading must begin with some decoding of symbols just to identify a word or topic. However, as readers anticipate subsequent words, they also question their decoding of earlier words in light of the overall fit with other cues.

There are four cueing systems that readers learn to use in reading interactively (May, 1990). These are: (a) *graphophonic cues,* hints provided by the letters and associated sounds in the text; (b) *syntactic cues,* hints carried by the order of words; (c) *semantic cues,* clues provided by the meaning and relationship of surrounding words; and (d) *background cues,* inferences provided by associations, memories, and expectations based on related experiences. All of these contribute to the reader's *schema* or overall mental set for what the text is going to tell them.

A number of authorities have outlined and described various stages that children pass through as they become proficient readers (Chall, 1983; Ehri & McCormick, 1998). Chall's classic six stages of reading development are

bottom-up model The model that proposes reading proceeds from interpreting phonemes to words to phrases to sentences, and so forth.

top-down model The model that proposes reading progresses from confirming ideas about overall content as additional written material is decoded.

It is unfortunate that these models and their approaches to teaching reading too often become "political footballs." Groups with political agendas treat one or the other approach as the only available choice. In all likelihood, the most effective teachers find a middle ground and encourage learners to use both strategies in their reading.

presented in Table 9–4. The earliest phase, prereading (also called the logographic phase), begins when children are still young preschoolers. This phase consists of simply recognizing a limited number of highly familiar words or phrases (e.g., commercial logos) as an unanalyzed whole. It is also known as the *pre-alphabetic phase* because children are not responding to sound-symbol (or letter) associations.

print awareness   The recognition of print and its distinctive patterns (left-to-right flow, character orientation, etc.) as meaningful symbols related to reading and writing.

In the years prior to and including kindergarten, the prereading stage, most children are consistently exposed to print and develop **print awareness.** That is, they recognize the presence of individual letters as figures and shapes of significance, but without any corresponding sounds. This recognition occurs in expected places (e.g., books) and in other settings as well (e.g., commercial logos, store signs, road signs). A preschooler or kindergartener may recognize a number of "whole words" (e.g., Coke), each as one integral symbol as opposed to a series of letter-sound associations.

Table 9–4. Stages of reading development.

Stage	Age Range	Description
Prereading	1–6 yrs. Preschool to kindergarten	Exposure leads to recognition of printed material (books with print versus pictures), trademark logos (e.g., McDonald's, Coca Cola). Experience leads to recognition of own name in print and attempts at printing own name. Exposure to caregiver reading models results in left-to-right scanning of printed material.
Stage I	6–7 yrs. Grades 1 to 2	Instruction leads to recognition of symbol sound associations, the ability to sound out single words, and reading of simple stories composed of simple words.
Stage II	7–8 yrs. Grades 2 to 3	Instruction results in more automatic decoding, improved fluency in reading simple materials. Continued application of sound-symbol skills leads to more conscious attack strategies in reading unfamiliar words. Continued exposure to results in expanding base of sight words.
Stage III	9–14 yrs. Grades 4 to 9	Application of established reading skills leads to improved comprehension of larger, more complex segments of text. Exposure to varied materials and information leads to reading for entertainment and learning.
Stage IV	15–17 yrs. Grades 10 to 12	Established reading skills serve the conscious pursuit of specific information, differing perspectives, and new knowledge.
Stage V	Adult years	Broader knowledge base and individual beliefs lead to efficiently reading for inquiry, critical analysis, integrating information into new ideas.

Note. Adapted from *Stages of Reading Development,* by J. S. Chall, 1983. New York: McGraw-Hill.

In Stages I and II, spanning first through third grade, students perhaps rely more heavily on the bottom-up process, because learning to read is a goal in itself. (This may also be the case because so many curriculums are based on this model.) This period would correlate to what many refer to as the *alphabetic stage* in which children begin to process sound-symbol associations to read individual words (Kamhi & Catts, 2005). Some have broken this period down into several phases: partial-alphabetic, full-alphabetic, and consolidated-alphabetic (Ehri & McCormick, 1998). During this period, **phonological awareness** develops, in which the young student develops sound-symbol associations, the ability to segment words and sentences, and skills that allow them blending and analyzing sound-symbol combinations. As has been suggested, these abilities may not develop naturally on their own; hence the need for academic instruction—teachers and schools!

In the middle period, Stages III and IV, students in Grades 4 through 12 may rely increasingly on a blend of the bottom-up and top-down models, using both to read interactively. Because reading should be more established by this time, it is less of a goal in itself. Further, because academic demands continue to expand the need, reading for the sake of learning increasingly becomes the motivation.

Finally, at Stage V and beyond, skilled readers are capable of reading rapidly and automatically, efficiently scanning and comprehending larger chunks of material. Skilled readers integrate information and analyze it in light of their own knowledge and beliefs. They predict upcoming segments (words, phrases, and sentences) and hypothesize about broad underlying meanings with improving skill. The later period includes an *orthographic* stage, in which children begin to recognize words based on analyzing them visually in terms of familiar letter patterns or sequences (Kamhi & Catts, 2005). Chall (1983) also described the final phase as the *automatic phase,* in which the student develops highly skilled automaticity and speed in identifying even unfamiliar words. The reader is allowed to become "unglued" from the words and is freed up to concentrate on the ideas conveyed by the text. It is at this level that readers truly pass beyond the "learning to read" and can participate in "reading to learn" and, ultimately, in "reading for pleasure" (Kamhi & Catts, 2005).

Research indicates that a number of specific linguistic abilities, such as phoneme segmentation, short-term verbal memory, and word finding are associated with good readers (Lane & Molyneaux, 1992). Figure 9–3 indicates a number of component skills that are considered fundamental to proficient reading. However, one of the key characteristics appears to be that proficient readers see reading as communication—they sense that there is a message in the text and they search for it. In contrast, poor readers tend to have significant difficulty with decoding graphophonic cues, getting tangled up in the sound patterns indicated by letters. They also tend to be deficient in the abilities related to other cueing systems that help carry the message as well (May, 1990).

phonological awareness
An aspect of metalinguistic abilities in which the child becomes conscious of the sounds of language in words, as evidenced by skills such as syllabification, segmentation, rhyming, alliteration, and blending.

These component reading skills are interrelated and do not develop independently of one another; rather, skills must develop in the context of a curriculum that applies effective reading strategies to become an effective reader.

Print Awareness—is the ability to understand how print works, which includes knowing that the print on the page represents the words that can be read aloud.

Phonological/Phonemic Awareness—is the understanding that words and syllables can be broken down into smaller units or phonemes. This is an oral prerequisite to phonics and one of the best predictors of later reading success.

Phonics/Decoding—requires developing strategies to apply sound-symbol relationships in the identification of unfamiliar words.

Vocabulary—is the store of word knowledge that is essential to understanding and comprehension, which comes chiefly from his or her vocabulary base.

Reading Fluency—develops as decoding skills develop to the point where the child becomes "unglued" from the print and frees a student's attention to comprehend the text and achieve speed and accuracy.

Comprehension/Critical Literacy—is the ability to understand the meaning or point of the text; it is the essence of reading. Comprehension in reading serves a variety of purposes, including locating information, becoming informed, being entertained or persuaded, and so on.

Figure 9–3 Component reading skills. These component reading skills are interrelated and do not develop independently of one another; rather, skills must develop in the context of curriculum that applies effective reading strategies to become an effective reader.

Note. Adapted from *Priority Academic Student Skills (PASS),* by the Oklahoma State Department of Education, July 2002, Author.

Development of Writing

Children go through characteristic stages as they learn to write. Caregivers who have raised children through adolescence might accurately describe the progression of writing as follows. Toddlers make marks just to mark (anywhere!). Preschoolers make marks and shapes to make "letters" (and they will tell you exactly what it all says). Young students "make" letters to write. Older students write letters to write. And, adolescents and adults write to communicate.

These stages have also been more formally described by researchers (Gentry & Gillet, 1993). Table 9–5 presents the stages of spelling development. In the first stage, *precommunicative spelling* (called "featural spelling" by May, 1990), children from 3–5 years of age explore the features of spelling through scribbling. Of course, no one but that child can read the scribble, so it does not communicate any ideas without that child's interpretation. In the next stage, *semiphonetic spelling,* children of 5 and 6 years of age show recognition that symbols represent sounds, although entire words may be represented by one or two key sounding letters. For example, in writing "I love you, Mommy," semiphonetically, a child might use "I LV U MME." When children around 6 and 7 years of age begin to symbolize all

Table 9–5. Developmental stages of spelling.

Stages and Their Approximate Ages	Characteristics Exhibited in Spelling
Precommunicative 3 to 5 years	Scribbles with no systematic sound-symbol relationship.
	Scribble emulates the general shapes of written language, as in lines of scribble representing lines of text or paragraphs.
	Lines of scribble may flow from left to right, top to bottom, or occur randomly on the page.
Semiphonetic 5 to 6 years	Exhibits awareness of relationship of letters to sounds.
	Lacks understanding that words are written as distinct units.
	Ideas are written in strings of letters (not words), apparently reflecting the stream of speech.
	Spellings are economical, relying on single letters for syllables or sounds; e.g., TDA for *today*, M for *me*, U for *you*.
Phonetic 6 to 7 years	Spellings begin to represent most or all of the perceptible sounds in words; e.g., YU R MI FRND TUDA for *You are my friend today*.
	Words are not directly recognizable, but are decipherable by considering basic sound-symbol associations.
Transitional 7 to 8 years	Applies most basic conventions for spelling easier, more familiar words.
	Reverses or transposes letter sequences in words confronted less frequently (e.g., GAOTS for *goats*, or SLIED for *slide*).
Conventional 8 years and older	Knows conventional spelling for a large number of familiar words.
	Considers possible alternatives when spelling unfamiliar words.
	Judges spellings for unfamiliar words as correct or incorrect based on appearance and knowledge of both conventions and exceptions in spelling.

Note. Adapted from *Teaching Kids to Spell,* by J. R. Gentry and J. W. Gillet, 1993. Portsmouth, NH: Heinemann.

of the sounds, even though not in the conventional way, they are exhibiting *phonetic spelling.* Transitional spellers, at around 7 and 8 years, begin to use most of the conventions of spelling, but continue to occasionally reverse or transpose letter sequences (e.g., RIED for ride, HORES for horse). Finally, when the rules for mature spelling are applied consistently, the individual is using *conventional spelling* (May, 1990).

Beyond spelling, others have analyzed the writing styles and organizational schemes exhibited as written language develops (Ely, 1997). Expressive writing is writing that expresses personal thoughts, ideas, feelings, and memories. This is generally easier for younger writers because it generally flows much the same as it would if we were speaking the same thoughts. As was discussed above, narrative writing is organized as a story, with a plot and characters. Because even the earliest levels can be structured to follow chronological organization, this style of writing is not as difficult as the final level. Expository writing requires concise organization, a logical

executive function The ability to review, evaluate, proofread, and edit one's own writing.

structuring of the points to be made, and precise vocabulary to express them. This style of writing will be fostered in the late elementary grades, but may not be mastered until high school or college, by which time the student should also be developing **executive function,** the ability to proofread, evaluate, and revise one's own writing.

The development of writing has been described in various ways. The connection between oral and written language is universally noted. Paradoxically, the two language systems—oral and written—are actually viewed as starting out as separate systems. As writing evolves, the two language systems eventually converge on one another and then, in its ultimate form, writing is consciously understood as a somewhat separate and integrated system with rules of its own (Silliman, Jimerson, & Wilkinson, 2000).

The earliest period is the *preparation* or *emergent writing phase* and generally occurs between 4 and 6 years of age. During the period, children's writing can be characterized as "draw-write," in which children draw to express ideas and begin to write words (or at least attempt at words) to supplement the drawings. In this process, the children's print awareness, which developed through watching caregivers read stories to them, is inverted to produce print that supports the stories they create through pictures.

The gradual shift from emergent writing to the *convergent phase* in the early elementary grades reflects children's injection of discourse and grammatical styles used in their oral interactions. In this phase, features of oral language converge with written language to give writing a "write like talk" quality. Although their writing abilities are not fully developed, children at this stage believe they are capable of writing, even in different styles.

In the later elementary years, during the *differentiation phase,* children begin to distinguish between talking and writing. Although they viewed them as closely related forms of communicating ideas, children begin to differentiate the syntactic styles, motivations, and tones associated with writing versus talking. They begin to recognize that, depending on the audience, they can fashion language to express internal states, entertain, or persuade (Silliman, Jimerson, & Wilkinson, 2000).

Ultimately, some writers proceed to the highest level, the *integration phase,* in which writing is consciously understood as a tool that can be used in many ways with many audiences. Fully mature writers at this stage develop a "voice" that engages readers and draws them into complex relationships with the words and relationships that comprise the text.

The process of writing can be broken down into basic steps, shown in Figure 9–4. In addition, the process of formulating or composing written material requires addressing a number of components that vary depending on the context and the task: mode, tone, form, purpose, and audience. *Mode* refers to style or genre of the writing and includes narrative, descriptive, argumentative, and expository writing. *Tone* is the "voice" of the writer and may vary from personal and quite intimate to business-like and quite formal. *Form* is the "shape" of the written work and includes essays, poetry, letters, and research papers. *Audience* is the intended consumer of the written work, which might

Prewriting—This process helps the writer get ready to write through gathering ideas and organizing them. During this stage, the topic is generated and purpose, audience, and form are clarified.

Drafting—This stage involves putting ideas down on paper with a focus on content, and begins with notes or ideas generated during prewriting.

Revising—This stage involves the refining of content, not mechanics. Revision ("to see again") begins during the prewriting activity and continues through the final draft.

Editing—This stage is the point at which the writing is made suitable for publication.

Publishing—Publication (or simply printing) provides an opportunity for the writer's product to be shared with and/or evaluated by the intended audience or reader in general.

Figure 9–4. Basic steps in the writing process.

Note. Adapted from *Priority Academic Student Skills (PASS),* by the Oklahoma State Department of Education, July 2002, Author.

consist of peers, colleagues, teachers, relatives, or others. The reason for writing is the *purpose,* which indicates the writer's intention. The writer's goal may be to discover and express personal feelings, to conduct everyday business, to communicate information, or to describe, entertain, and persuade.

A concept that is thought to be critical to successful writing is *executive function.* This refers to the mental capacities necessary to control our overall output, including how we initiate, sustain, regulate, and monitor behaviors. For the writing process, it is thought that the capacity of working memory, which allows organizing, linking, and monitoring the ideas expressed in writing, is crucial. This may influence every level of writing from spelling and punctuation to the conceptual arrangement of information for the purpose intended (Hooper, Swartz, Wakely, de Kruif, & Montgomery, 2002).

Summary

* Literacy is an important survival skill for school and life.
* Literacy develops more formally in the school years, but has its foundations in the oral language that develops before.
* Although literate language is based on oral language, there are significant differences in style, including vocabulary level, grammatical complexity, and organizational structure.
* Children's development of oral language skills, especially metalinguistic and narrative abilities, is a strong predictor of reading success.
* Development of writing occurs in characteristic stages and writing styles evolve as individuals grow older and the demands for scholarly writing increase.

Language Changes Across the Life Span

Aging is a continuous, lifelong process. Aging begins from the moment of conception. Adulthood (and some would claim life) begins after high school. There are characteristic changes that occur over the decades that follow (Atchley, 1987). Table 9–6 presents the changes associated with the stages of adulthood.

Language also changes in a continuous, lifelong process. The foundations are laid in the first 5 years and the language we will use as adults is nearly complete by adolescence. Still, language continues to change in subtle ways, reflecting the role of changes that occur throughout our adult lives. As senior adults, normal aging brings subtle changes in the physical state of the structures we use for communication.

Language in Adulthood

In our adult years, there are few significant grammatical developments, other than further refinement of complex constructions, especially in written language. Instead, changes in semantic and pragmatic aspects primarily

Table 9–6. Stages of adulthood and associated changes.

Age Range	Life Stage	Educational Changes	Occupational Changes	Family Changes
Age 18 to 30	Young adult	Complete high school, then vocational or professional education	Temporary jobs to support education and experimenting with jobs	Transition from dependent to adult status; marriage for some.
30 to 45	Adult	Specialized training to promote present career or change careers	Job commitment and advancement	Marriage and developing family; relating to own parents adult to adult.
45 to 60	Middle age	Less formal training	Job plateau	Adjustment to "empty nest"; return to spouse-spouse relationship; increased care of dependent parents.
60 to 75	Later Mature		Retirement	Possible widowhood.
75 years	Old age		Retirement	Dependence on children for support and possibly care.

Note. Adapted from *Aging: Continuity and Change* (2nd ed.), by R. C. Atchley, 1987. Belmont, CA: Wadsworth.

reflect the cognitive and social influences in adulthood—developing careers and maturing roles.

Semantics: Vocabulary Growth

It has been estimated that the typical college graduate has a vocabulary of approximately 22,000 words. By age 65, the typical individual will have a vocabulary of 45,000 words (Lane & Molyneaux, 1992). Adult vocabulary growth comes primarily from new bodies of information, expertise, and technical terms associated with training for and even changing careers—something we will reportedly do five or more times during our adult life.

The vocabulary growth of adulthood, however, is more than the accumulation of specialized, technical words associated with a chosen career. The independence and mobility that comes with adulthood expands opportunities to accumulate additional experiences and world knowledge. As a result, adult vocabularies also continue to grow both horizontally and vertically. Vertical growth is evident in the additional meanings that are compounded as adults continue to experience known words in new contexts. Horizontal growth is apparent in the accumulation and refinement of associated information and concepts for words in their vocabulary.

For example, even as educated adults, the levels of meaning (vertical growth) and a new range of associations (horizontal growth) are experienced for a word such as *accident* after becoming parents. From the thought of a wet bed, to a carpet stain, to the prospect of a tragic auto accident, parents experience the varied meanings of *accident* with a wide range of associated emotions.

Pragmatics: Registers and Genderlect

Although much of our personality was formed in childhood, as adults we are still establishing how we will talk to friends, spouses, children, strangers, work associates, and so forth. As adults, we develop different styles of communication, called **registers,** to talk to people in different circumstances (Lane & Molyneaux, 1992). Perhaps the most universally recognized register would be called the politeness register. Although this is instilled in childhood, it is refined as adults attempt to conform to social expectations, especially in formal events such as parties, receptions, and so forth.

As adults, we assume membership, formally and informally, in many different groups—religious, civic, professional, athletic, and so forth. The different styles that are associated with each group may include more or less structured agendas and specialized vocabulary or phrases, such as the *rituals* and *jargon* of various religious, professional, fraternal, and recreational groups. In contrast, when people are especially close, their conversations might assume an intimacy register, which exhibits casual language forms and may not exhibit an agenda other than reminiscing, planning, or simply passing time. The intimacy register may also include affectionate "pet

registers Speaking styles that are characteristic of certain roles of social contexts.

Registers are a variation of *alternations,* discussed in Chapter 1. They also reflect the influence of *audience* as a controlling variable, described by Skinner and discussed in Chapter 4. ■

names" shared only between those two persons—those names no one else even wants to hear!

Another kind of register that may become more noticeable as we mature and assume more clearly defined adult identities is **genderlect,** the styles of communication that seem to characterize the two sexes (Tannen, 1990). Although it would be inappropriate to stereotype either males or females, on the whole, there are characteristic differences in the way they communicate (Tannen, 1990).

genderlect The communication styles that appear to be characteristic of each gender.

Traditionally, women tend to be less direct or confrontational than men. Although typically unaware of their behavior, men tend to use more intimidating behaviors such as interrupting others, making direct eye contact, and displaying body language that suggests dominance. Where men seem to be more topic focused, women seem to focus more on people and are more receptive to their nonverbal cues. On the other hand, with changing roles and opportunities in the workplace for women, these differences may be increasingly blurred. Today, more than ever, females in more countries see increased opportunities to assume professional positions, leadership roles, and administrative responsibilities. Conversely, men see that the ambition to succeed "in a man's world" is just one option; many males are assuming the roles of raising children and providing domestic support for their wives as they pursue professional careers. Over time, these shifts could alter the nature of genderlect. In the 1960s, Bob Dylan wrote that "the times, they are a-changing," and they still are!

Aging and Communication

Perhaps the most important (and reassuring) theme to emphasize as we consider this information is that aging does not have to mean "growing old." Many individuals continue to function at high levels of both physical and mental activity well into their senior years.

On the other hand, there are certain immutable truths about spending 7, 8, or 9 decades facing the challenges of living. Structures do begin to change, whether due to disease, genetics, extreme living conditions, or just the wear-and-tear of normal living. As aging occurs for most of us, changes that are considered normal will affect our hearing mechanism, speech mechanism, and our language skills to some degree.

Changes in Hearing

Perhaps the most consistent change affecting communication in the elderly, at least in most Westernized cultures, is hearing loss. Approximately one out of two individuals over the age of 50 will suffer from some degree of hearing loss. This affects men more than women, although it evens out as aging progresses. Most cases of hearing loss in the elderly are **sensorineural,** meaning that it is caused by the deterioration of the nerve endings for hearing. Although hearing loss in the elderly is called **presbycusis,**

sensorineural Hearing loss due to damaged nerve endings.

presbycusis Hearing loss associated with aging.

which means "old hearing," the deterioration is not simply a matter of getting older. Noise exposure, certain diseases, and even genetic patterns can influence at what age an individual begins to lose hearing acuity.

Sensorineural loss typically affects sensitivity for the higher frequency sounds, which affects the ability to discriminate between certain consonants. As a result, these elderly individuals have difficulty with speech discrimination, especially in listening situations with competing background sounds (e.g., equipment, television, other voices). Sadly, not as many of the elderly who could benefit from the amplification of hearing aids actually seek professional help. As a result, they may frequently misunderstand others, get frustrated, and withdraw further from social interaction.

> A number of studies have found that, although hearing loss has been assumed to be a fact of old age, it is not necessarily so. In a number of simpler cultures, individuals well into their senior years have been found to have essentially normal hearing. It would appear that hearing loss is a fact of life—as we know it. It is more than likely the price many of us pay for the excess noise and stress of our "advanced" culture.

Changes in Speech

The structures for speech also exhibit some change during the later years. The most significant physical changes in the speech mechanism occur in the larynx. The laryngeal cartilages become more rigid with ossification and the vocal folds may atrophy and become less elastic. As a result of these and other changes, individuals who are elderly exhibit voices that are higher in pitch (due to the decreased vocal fold mass) and more breathy (due to the weaker seal between the folds when adducted). Older speakers may also exhibit shorter phrasing when aging vocal folds are combined with reduced lung capacity (due to weakening respiratory muscles). These changes appear to result in a characteristic quality; a number of studies have shown that individuals can judge the approximate age of a speaker from their voice (Lane & Molyneaux, 1992).

The other aspects of speech—articulation, fluency, and resonance—are less affected by aging. In the absence of specific disease or injury, the articulators continue to function adequately with normal aging. The elderly also maintain their previous level of fluency. That is, if they did not stutter previously, the elderly rarely begin to do so in their senior years. However, there are often an increased number of disruptions in the flow of speech that have been described as **uncertainty behaviors** or **verbal fragmentations** (Shadden, 1997). These consist of increased interjections (*um, well, er*) and revisions (*Then he . . . Then Bob said*). These behaviors, however, appear to be more closely related to word-finding and formulation difficulties than to stuttering, which typically begins in early childhood.

uncertainty behaviors (or **verbal fragmentations**) Excessive interjections and filler sometimes noted in utterances of aging individuals.

Changes in Language

Even the otherwise healthy brain shows some changes as a result of aging. The brain generally loses density, with the atrophy resulting in wider sulci ("valleys") and narrower gyri ("ridges"). There is a loss of functioning neurons, especially with smaller, association neurons that are most likely involved in discriminating and associating information.

In spite of these microscopic changes in the brain, language abilities in the elderly are generally durable. Of the three language domains—syntax, semantics, and pragmatics—syntax has been found to be generally more well preserved. Research with regard to utterance length and complexity has been variable. Some studies actually indicate an increase in length and complexity, although most have suggested reduced complexity. Nonetheless, there are no notable increases in syntactic or morphological errors (Shadden, 1997).

Basic semantic abilities in comprehending and defining words are also relatively unchanged. Interestingly, it appears that elderly persons may shift their word association pattern from semantically based *paradigmatic associations* (i.e., associating words based on their meanings—*cup* and *glass*) to syntactically based *syntagmatic associations* (i.e., associating words in terms of word order—*cup* and *spill*).

The most likely change to occur with aging is a decline in word-finding skills. This may be reflected in the verbal fragments and uncertainty behaviors mentioned earlier. It also appears that seniors may use less precise naming strategies, relying on fewer and broader categories in organizing their vocabulary. In those moments when a specific word is not promptly recalled, as when intending to say, *"My wife is shopping for a parka,"* they may substitute a superordinate term, in saying, *"My wife is shopping for a coat"* (Shadden, 1997).

In spite of these subtle changes in semantic organization, in the normal aging process pragmatic behaviors appear to remain relatively intact. Some studies have found some elderly to be better conversationalists than younger speakers. They can be more sensitive about turn taking, more adept at maintaining topics, and even more sophisticated at shifting topics based on their partner's previous turn (i.e., topic shading). In terms of their narrative abilities, seniors have also been found to be masters at weaving tales, bringing together their historical perspectives and personal experiences (Shadden, 1997). Although there are certainly wide individual differences among the elderly, these characteristics are not entirely surprising to anyone who has taken time to appreciate the seniors around them.

> The syntagmatic to paradigmatic shift that occurs in the school years is discussed in Chapter 8. ■

Summary

- Changes in vocabulary beyond the school years reflect growth due to education and changing social roles.

- Adults develop specific styles called registers when speaking in certain circumstances.

- There appear to be characteristic gender differences between the communication styles of men and women.

- The aging process results in identifiable changes in the hearing, speech, and language of the elderly.

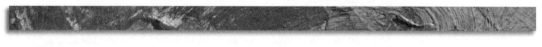

A s students, language expands from being a tool for interaction to becoming a tool for learning. There is a reciprocal relationship between learning and language that becomes evident at this stage. Most of the remaining grammatical development represents complex language that will be founded on experience with and understanding of *abstract relationships.* Conversely, these language behaviors probably enhance the verbal reasoning that facilitates understanding these abstract relationships.

    Vocabulary growth during the school years and beyond represents a major area of language change. New experiences and roles prompt *horizontal development,* which fills out and refines the semantic features associated with a word, and *vertical development,* in which new meanings of words are added to existing ones. School-age children develop *conventional word definitions.* They shift from *thematic* and *syntagmatic associations* as preschoolers, to *taxonomic* and *paradigmatic associations* as students, when they begin to associate word meanings in increasingly flexible ways.

    During the early school years, children exhibit the *metalinguistic abilities* that allow them to focus on language itself, rising above the messages it conveys. The flexibility in understanding that results allows students to consider *ambiguous meanings* in *figurative language* and language for humor. In adjusting to the classroom, students' pragmatic strategies expand to comprehend classroom language and textbook language. The foundations established in oral language are soon extended to *literate language* as students learn to read and produce written language.

    Language continues to change, even throughout our adult and senior years. Adults develop distinctive communication styles or *registers* that accommodate their changing roles. Finally, aging brings physical changes that affect the structures for human communication.

Chapter Summary

Review Questions

1. What is the apparent connection between later developing grammatical structures and advanced understanding of abstract semantic relationships?

2. What shifts occur as school-age children become more aware of the additional features and multiple meanings that might be associated with words?

3. In how many ways does metalinguistic awareness change students' view of language behaviors?

4. How are interactive language and classroom language different?

5. What are the stages of development for reading and writing?

6. What general changes in language behaviors are expected throughout our adult and senior years?

Practice Questions

To the student: You are encouraged to use the following questions to prepare for multiple-choice examinations. This exercise is not intended to simply "provide the answers to questions." Instead, it is hoped that you will use the material to develop your ability to analyze questions and choices to identify correct answers based on a critical understanding of the distinctions among the answers. Use the answer key at the end of the book to prompt your analysis of each item and to confirm the correct answer. Remember that there is a difference between recognizing the correct answer and understanding why it is the correct one.

1. Which of the following is *least* related to "figurative language"?
   a. idioms
   b. metaphoric transparency
   c. metalinguistics
   d. embedding
   e. humor

2. As the shift from a syntagmatic style of word association to a paradigmatic style of word associations occurs, children would tend to make associations as follows. They would _____ .
   a. shift from "car – drive" to "car – truck"
   b. shift from "car – drive" to "car – ride"
   c. shift from "car – blue" to "car – red"
   d. shift from "car – car" to "truck – truck"
   e. none of these represent what would occur

3. Figurative language abilities would include the ability to _____ .
   a. interpret idioms, metaphors and proverbs
   b. use language creatively
   c. correctly inflect nouns and verbs
   d. a and b
   e. a and c

4. Which of the following concepts or components is/are related to the development of humor?
   a. ambiguity
   b. metalinguistics

    c. phonological and lexical
    d. surface structure and deep structure
    e. all of these

5. Which of the following structures is/are most likely to be mastered after 6 years of age?
    a. present progressive inflection
    b. personal pronouns
    c. reflexive pronouns
    d. the "be" verbs "is" and "are"
    e. prepositions "in" and "on"

6. Which of the following best illustrates the vertical development of vocabulary during the school years?
    a. a student learns that a "frame" has corners, hangers, wire, and is sometimes fit with matting around the picture it holds
    b. a student comes to understand that the word "frame" has one syllable and rhymes with "tame"
    c. a student understands that "frame" can refer to something that holds a picture, might be the supporting structure for a building, and could also mean that someone has been wrongfully convicted of a crime
    d. a student learns the rule about "silent e" and spells the word "frame" correctly
    e. all of these are correct examples

7. Which of the following statements *does not* correctly describe the relationship illustrated by a child's statement that "tables are furniture"?
    a. it relates a subordinate category to its associated superordinate category
    b. children always learn the word "furniture" before the word "table"
    c. the use of these words suggests a shift from thematic to taxonomic organization of vocabulary
    d. this phrase reflects a later developing stage in children's vocabulary organization
    e. this is a categorical statement that would be more likely as a child progresses through the school years

8. Text grammar used in academic textbooks might include words such as *similarly, although,* or *conversely,* which signal the expository pattern called _____ .
    a. descriptive patterns
    b. comparison patterns
    c. collection patterns
    d. cause-effect patterns
    e. sequence patterns

9. The differences in how adults speak to their spouses, friends, and
   employment supervisor ("the boss") has been called _____ .
   a. jargon
   b. genderlect
   c. dialect
   d. register
   e. illocutions

10. Generally, the most likely change to be noted in the language of elderly
    persons who are otherwise healthy is in their _____ .
    a. grammatical ability
    b. comprehension ability
    c. word-finding ability
    d. abstract-reasoning ability
    e. sense of humor

Suggested Readings

Catts, H. W., & Kamhi, A. G. (Eds.). (2005), *Language and reading disabilities* (2nd ed.). Boston: Allyn & Bacon.

Ehri, L. C. (2000). Learning to read and learning to spell: Two sides of a coin. *Topics in Language Disorders, 20*(3), 19–36.

Ely, R. (1997). Language and literacy in the school years. In J. B. Gleason (Ed.), *The development of language* (4th ed., pp. 398–439). Boston: Allyn & Bacon.

Fitzgerald, J., & Shanahan, T. (2000). Reading and writing relations and their development. *Educational Psychologist, 35*(1), 39–50.

Hayes, P. A., Norris, J., & Flaitz, J. R. (1998). A comparison of the oral narrative abilities of under-achieving and high-achieving adolescents: A preliminary investigation. *Language, Speech, and Hearing Services in Schools, 29,* 159–171.

Nippold, M. A., & Haq, F. S. (2003). Mental imagery and idiom comprehension: A comparison of school-age children and adults. *Journal of Speech, Language, and Hearing Research, 46,* 788–799.

Scott, C. M. (1999). Learning to write. In H. W. Catts & A. G. Kamhi (Eds.), *Language and reading disabilities* (pp. 224–258). Boston: Allyn & Bacon.

CHAPTER 10

Language Differences: Diversity and Disorders

Carlos focused closely on the ribbon of paint that marked the side of the road. He hugged his car tightly to the road's edge so he could see the white ribbon as it stretched ahead into the dense fog. He had driven this stretch many times, through fog much worse than this. However, his confident, steady gaze was betrayed by his knuckles, which were hard and white as he tightly gripped the steering wheel.

Around a wide, easy bend in the road, he could make out lights ahead. Some poured out their light softly on the ground below them. Others flashed in a slow, pulsing rhythm. An accident, perhaps, but this felt different. He had no choice but to stop.

In a moment, someone appeared at his window. The dark figure was tall, so tall that he could not see a face above the door frame. Yet, he knew to get out. Without speaking, the figure led him toward the lights. Again, he knew to follow.

This couldn't be an accident; he sensed no alarm. Instead, it all seemed so planned, so expected. As he passed around the circle of lights, he realized they were not headlights. Their radiance was simply not light at all. Just beyond their liquid glow, was a shadow sloping up into darkness—a black ramp extending into the blacker night sky. Again, he followed without really knowing why.

Somehow, someone was communicating to him. He was not even convinced that it was the dark figure moving silently ahead of him. But, how did he know what was being asked of him? How would he express himself when the time came to transmit his own thoughts?

Suddenly, an icy cold penetrated between his shoulders! He shuddered, drew back, and looked around bleary eyed. His wife said, "Sorry, my hands are so cold. You were having that dream again, weren't you? Carlos Aygan, what will I do with you?!"

This chapter addresses the following questions:

- How are human languages simultaneously similar and different?
- What variations are found within a primary language?
- What are the effects of learning two or more languages?
- What variations occur within the same major language?
- How are individual differences apparent in children's language learning?
- What causes children to vary from the expected or normal learning of language?
- What characteristics are found in children who exhibit disordered language development?
- What procedures are available for treating children with disordered language development?
- Which professionals can contribute to the treatment of children with language disorders?

language universals
Those features that are considered to be part of every human language.

language variations
Structural or phonological differences in individuals' or subgroups' production of a major language.

The various aspects of language that appear to be universal are introduced in Chapter 1. The concept of formal linguistic universals is discussed in Chapter 4. ■

We can only speculate, with a measure of childlike awe, on how universal the basic elements of language might be. The opening vignette for this chapter—with respectful apologies to the fond memory of scientist Carl Sagan—was a tongue-in-cheek exercise in imagining how the most universal of all languages might be experienced.

Human language behavior presents two paradoxical dimensions. At one level, all human languages exhibit fundamental similarities; so much so that some of those similarities are considered **language universals**. In contrast, human language also exhibits differences, within the same language and across languages. In other words, human languages exhibit **language variations** (Parker & Riley, 2004).

That all human languages exhibit basic similarities should not be surprising. Language does not exist apart from human behavior. Human behavior arises from our basic makeup and experience as humans, factors that are universal to the human condition. As humans, we all share the same basic genetic foundations. The essential anatomical and neurological makeup of humans as a species has evolved, regardless of race, culture, religion, and so forth. In learning to communicate, humans share the same structures for experiencing and responding to their world.

In addition, the physical world all humans experience and respond to presents universal similarities. All cultures have evolved around people, objects, and events that are related through the same universal dimensions of mass, energy, time, and space. From this standpoint then, we would expect that all human languages would share certain features. For example, one of the proposed universals of human language is that all human languages make use of nouns and verbs (Parker & Riley, 2004). Because all humans have experienced objects and events as verbal behavior developed, is it surprising that they would produce words that symbolize them (i.e., nouns and verbs)?

In spite of the underlying similarities, each human language is also different in several ways.

Each is composed of varying subsets of all the possible speech sounds. These are combined in different ways to compose words unique to each language. Also, words are sequenced and marked for meaning in ways that vary from one language to another. In short, human languages each exhibit variations that reflect their unique historical and cultural evolution. This chapter is devoted to describing the variations that occur across languages and within a given language.

These features that vary across languages are related to those described by Hockett and presented in Chapter 1. ∎

Diversity in language behavior reflects the diversity present in the human experience. As a result, variations are expected. We expect broad differences in languages that have evolved in different cultures; when the contrasts are so significant that people from two cultures do not understand each other's utterances, they each speak a **primary language.** Some variations within a primary language reflect subtle differences found within the same culture; when people exhibit these variations, but still understand each other, they exhibit *dialects.*

primary language The major language spoken and understood by a population.

Individuals within a verbal community might use words or styles that are unique to them; if they are still understood by those around them, the idiosyncrasies might be called an **idiolect.** Many children will vary substantially in how they learn language; when we determine that the differences are extreme enough to interfere with communication, it might be concluded that a child exhibits a **language disorder.**

idiolect Language variations unique to an individual speaker.

language disorder Language behaviors that exhibit slower than expected development or variations in development that significantly interfere with an individual's communication abilities.

Language Diversity

Diversity in language occurs across different domains and to different degrees. The variations in language might occur in any of the major domains; there may be phonological, syntactic, semantic, or pragmatic differences. The degree of these differences may be so significant that they define a separate primary language, or just degrees of variation that result in variations of the same language.

Separate primary languages exhibit significant variations that prevent or extremely limit communication between their speakers. For example, Chinese and English each exhibit so many contrasts that neither one can be readily understood by native speakers of the other. Within a given language, there may be subtle differences that evolve out of regional or social influences that result only in variations of the primary language. Regional influences on the sound of English are heard in speakers from Georgia, Oklahoma, Minnesota, and New York, but they still generally understand each other. Finally, speakers within a language community might exhibit some unique variations that set them apart, although they remain speakers of the primary language.

Cross-Linguistic Differences—Languages of the World

Throughout history, the world's populations, boundaries, and cultures have shifted in response to forces such as famine, religion, and war. Even today, with precise maps to define national boundaries, boundaries are not visible to the naked eye. They were even more blurred as our ancestors wandered the earth. As people moved and intermingled, so did their languages. Given the long, convoluted history of humankind, it is not surprising that the family tree of language has many diverse branches.

There are over 6,000 different languages spoken in the world. A number of these—Chinese, English, Spanish—are major languages spoken by large numbers of people in various regions of the world. Others have only a few thousand speakers in isolated areas. All these languages exhibit some characteristics that are shared and many that are unique (Allen, 1996).

language families
Groups of languages that share historical roots.

Most languages are hybrid languages with historical ties to several others. These interconnections form groups of related languages in **language families.** For example, the Indo-European family includes various languages belonging to the Germanic (including English), Romance, Balto-Slavic, Celtic, and Indo-Iranian groups. Some languages appear to have no historical ties to any other languages. For example, Japanese, Korean, and Vietnamese are *each* a unique language, unrelated to any other! (This would probably surprise most speakers of English.)

As might be expected, the most obvious area of difference between languages is vocabulary. Words for the same things are different in different languages. Even words for the same thing in different languages might have slightly different meanings, based on the cultural experience of that object. For example, in English there is only one word for "snow." However, Eskimos have a number of separate words for snow—falling snow, wet snow, icy snow, blowing snow, drifting snow, and so on.

 Another area of cultural contrast and potential conflict is gestural language. Although the smile continues as a universal sign of friendship, when traveling in foreign countries, Americans must be sensitive to the possibility that their hosts assign different meanings to seemingly innocent gestures. For example, two commonplace gestures for Americans, the "okay" and "thumbs up," are extremely rude gestures in Germany and Nigeria, respectively (Axtell, 1991).

There are words in some languages that simply do not have a counterpart in another language. The respective words for "house" probably carry drastically different connotations for speakers of English and Hausa (a Chadic language of West Africa). The Russian phrase *Ja govorila* can be interpreted as "I said" in English. However, the verb in this phrase (*govorila*) carries much more information than its English counterpart. That is, it also conveys that the speaker is female, has spoken more than once, and is not finished speaking. It is easy to see why translation is a very sensitive part of world diplomacy.

The sound systems for languages also vary. For example, in English the sound /ng/ can only end a syllable; it cannot start a syllable. However, in several African languages it can start a syllable. Similarly, many words in English start with the cluster /sp/. Ironically, this combination never begins a word in Spanish.

Another contrast exists between English and languages that are tonal, such as Chinese. In English, intonation changes the meaning of the overall utterance; we might inflect a statement to make it a question, as in *I'm late* ↑.

In contrast, changes in intonation change the meaning of a set of phonemes in Chinese; for example, *chyan* can mean "thousand," "money," "shallow," or "owe" depending on whether it is produced with a level, rising, dipping, or falling tone.

Finally, both inflecting and combining words differ significantly across languages. In contrast to English, Japanese has no plural inflection. The French would say that they see *a sky blue,* instead of *a blue sky.* Turkish uses what are called postpositions, meaning they would say that they are *house your in,* as opposed to the English preposition, *in your house.* Japanese relies on markers or tags such as *wa* and *o* to indicate the subject and object in a sentence, in contrast to English, which relies primarily on word order.

In spite of boundaries, imaginary or real, another aspect of diversity in human languages is that some people speak more than one. For example, many Canadians speak both French and English. In the United States, in many areas of the country there are groups that regularly speak Spanish, Chinese, or Vietnamese in addition to English. As this becomes more commonplace, it will be important to consider the effect it has on children who must deal with more than one language at home, in their neighborhood, and in school.

Bilingualism

Bilingualism is the ability to speak two languages fluently. (*Multilingualism,* of course, would suggest that a speaker is fluent in more than two languages.) As mentioned previously, speaking more than one language is common in several countries—Canada, Switzerland, Belgium, for example.

bilingualism The ability to speak two languages.

Historically, English has been the predominant language in the United States. However, due to the immigration that has contributed so significantly to the United States, ours is also the quintessential multicultural society. Our cultural roots now include European, African, Asian, and Hispanic immigrants. As a result, many children are born into circumstances where they will eventually learn at least two different languages—whatever language is native to their family's cultural roots and English.

 The British playwright, Israel Zangwill (1864–1926) introduced the term "melting pot" to describe the growing multicultural society in America. However, more contemporary views avoid the notion that cultures must melt together and be lost in one homogenous society. Instead, most see America as a tapestry that derives its strength and beauty from its many different cultural strands.

There are several perspectives to consider when evaluating the effect of bilingualism. The initial concern is the implications of bilingualism for children's language development. In addition, there are concerns about its effect on children's educational and societal adjustments.

Developmental Patterns

Children who learn two or more languages may do so because of family circumstances or as a result of school experiences (Erickson, 1985). Given the increase in the number of children raised in culturally diverse homes, an increasing number of children will become bilingual. The process of acquiring more than one language can occur in either of two ways: simultaneous or successive acquisition.

simultaneous acquisition
Learning two languages at the same time.

Simultaneous Acquisition.   **Simultaneous acquisition** refers to the learning of two languages at the same time prior to 3 years of age. Simultaneous acquisition tends to be associated with situations in which more than one major language is spoken as part of the child's natural communicative interactions. This may occur exclusively in the home (as with two caregivers who each speak a different primary language) or may be divided between the home and other child care settings. Most research indicates that children in such circumstances learn both languages with equal facility. The rates and sequences of development tend to be similar in both languages, regardless of how different the languages may be.

There are apparently three stages that children pass through as they learn two languages simultaneously (Volterra & Taeschner, 1978). Initially, younger children's vocabularies are a mixture of individual, nonoverlapping words from both languages. That is, if a vocabulary item is learned from one language, it prevails over the corresponding word in the other language. At this early stage, the words are used without regard to the situation or audience.

Later, children begin to "sort out" the words belonging to each language. Although they may not yet be conscious of two separate languages, they tend to use words from each more discriminately, in the situations where they originally experienced them. In contrast to this lexical sorting, children during this period may apply similar grammatical rules to both sets of words. They also progress from simpler toward more complex sentence structure, just as they would if only one language were being learned.

Finally, the child sorts out both the vocabulary and the grammatical systems for the two languages. Initially, the preschool child may simplify the task of maintaining the separate languages by restricting them to particular audiences. However, children are frequently bilingual by their early school years, appropriately switching from one language to another automatically.

successive acquisition
Learning a second language following establishment of a first language.

From the standpoint of "semantics," it would follow that only *successive acquisition* can really result in "second language acquisition." ■

Successive Acquisition.   **Successive acquisition** describes learning a primary native language first, usually prior to 3 years of age, and then learning a second language at a later time. This may result when a child grows up in a home where the only language spoken is one other than English. Ultimately, upon entering a preschool or school situation, the child is subsequently exposed to English.

It is widely agreed that success in learning the second language will depend on the nature of the individual's experience with it. Younger children will learn a second language more readily when they are motivated to use it frequently in natural contexts for true communication. Younger children more readily acquire second languages, especially with more natural pronunciation, than do teenagers and adults who attempt to learn a language later in life as an academic subject (Oyama, 1976).

Some have suggested that this difference in children's and adults' abilities to learn a second language illustrates a "critical period" for language learning. There have been isolated findings of some neurological differences in contributions of the two hemispheres in learning a second language. However, the interference of responses learned in a primary language and increased metalinguistic awareness of language might cause differences in the way language is processed in later language learning. In addition, the sheer number of adults who have successfully learned multiple languages should cause some skepticism about the reality of a "critical period."

In second language learning, it appears that many of the same broad principles from first language learning apply (Lane & Molyneaux, 1992). Understanding generally precedes expression, comprehension initially relies heavily on cues in the "here-and-now," sentence construction proceeds from simple to complex, and interactive language precedes decontextualized (academic or expository) language.

Decontextualized language is discussed in Chapter 9. ■

There may also be three general stages in successive acquisition of a second language (Grosjean, 1982). The earliest stage appears to be based on the social functions of language. Children first learn to interact, rather than inform. In the next stage, children seem to press themselves to communicate in the new language. All of the available words and phrases may be drawn on, although incorrectly at times, to be certain that ideas are somehow conveyed. Finally, the child is able to communicate while also attending to the details of correctness.

Interference and Code Switching. Traditionally, there has been concern about the overall impact of bilingual language development. Some have feared that **interference,** features or rules that conflict between different languages, will disrupt the overall language development of a child who is becoming bilingual. This appears to not be the case. Generally, it appears instead that long-range positive effects might be observed, including enhanced awareness of language, greater flexibility in using language, and, certainly, a better understanding of cultural diversity.

interference The observation that features or rules of one language conflict with learning another language.

One phenomenon that can be distressing as children are becoming bilingual is code switching. **Code switching** occurs when a bilingual speaker unknowingly inserts elements of one language into the other. Children's code switching tends to be primarily semantic in nature, inserting words (typically nouns) from one language into sentences being produced into the other. This is especially likely when the word is being switched between sentences that are similar in structure.

Code switching is related to alternation and style shifting, introduced in previous chapters. ■

Code switching is not indicative of a language deficit nor is it restricted to children. Adult bilingual speakers also code switch, but they tend to substitute entire phrases and sentences from a pragmatic standpoint. That is, depending on the formality of the situation, they may insert conversational devices (*By the way, . . .*), stylistic devices (*. . . , if you will*), or informal

code switching A phenomenon in bilingualism in which speakers unknowingly include elements of one language in the other.

expressions (*Oh, my gosh . . .*) that are fitting, but may only be available from the other language (Haynes & Shulman, 1994).

Educational and Societal Effects

standard language
The primary language expected by most speakers in formal contexts.

Most cultures have a **standard language.** That is, there is often a version of the primary language that is expected in most formal situations, such as in schools, businesses, newspaper, radio, banks, and so forth. In the United States, use of Standard American English (SAE) is generally expected in these settings and interactions. In some countries the standard language is established formally through legislation or by decree. Although making English the "official" language in the United States has been attempted from time to time, SAE is the standard only by historical consensus.

The overall composition of the United States population is expected to shift over the next few decades such that there is a greater balance of cultural groups. Many of the children in these groups may develop a language other than English as their first language. Even for those children who are not exposed to an alternative language at home, there is a growing likelihood that their educational experience will include significant exposure to a second language at some point.

In contrast to this, because our historical, legal, financial, scientific, and educational foundations are documented in Standard American English, it is very likely that English will continue to be our standard language. Therefore, the effect of bilingualism on children's educational experience, and their adjustment into adult roles, must be considered.

The concern then becomes one of allowing speakers of non-English languages to achieve their academic, social, and vocational potential, without sacrificing their cultural identity and values. To do this, it is important to do more than just recognize the existence of other cultures. Their cultural contributions to our society as a whole need to be acknowledged at all levels of education.

Bilingual education continues to be controversial, not so much from the standpoint of *whether-or-not-to,* but from the standpoint of *how!* Some stress the importance of presenting academic information in students' first or native language, while they learn English as a second language. Others assert that the more quickly non-English-speaking students are immersed in the English language, the sooner they will learn it and be assimilated into the mainstream culture.

The first position has the practical drawback that teachers who can instruct academic subjects using languages other than English are difficult to find. On the other hand, the second approach may give students the sense of "sink or swim." Also, because it implies that the primary concern is to quickly absorb them into the mainstream culture, it may diminish their own cultural identity. To this point, there has not been extensive research done to compare the relative effectiveness of specific approaches in bilingual education.

Dialects

Another level of diversity in languages occurs *within* primary languages. In a community of speakers, each speaker probably exhibits some minor and unique variations from the primary language (i.e., an idiolect). However, in all likelihood there are groups of speakers who also vary similarly in their production of the primary language in some way. If their variations are consistent and recognizable, but they are still understood by other speakers in the primary language, their collective variation of the language is a *dialect.*

The collective variations that become recognizable as dialects might result from several different influences. Some dialects might consist of variations associated with geographical areas. Other dialects evolve within groups who have become socially homogenous, either through their common socioeconomic status or through their shared ethnicity.

Regional Dialects

When a group of people has existed and interacted over an extended period of time within a geographical region, certain distinctive variations in speaking patterns evolve. The variations might be exhibited in phonological, semantic, or syntactic variations. Ultimately, these differences may become recognizable and closely identified with that geographical region.

Speakers might pronounce words that are common to the primary language differently. Certain vocabulary items or phrases might be peculiar to that region. In addition, certain word sequences or "aberrations of the grammar" might be a recognizable characteristic of a certain region.

The United States is said to have initially developed three major dialect areas running as horizontal bands from east to west. These consisted of a Northern, a Midland, and a Southern dialectal band. These regional groups apparently resulted from the migration patterns in the early years of our country. The Atlantic coastal areas were settled first. Then, as people sought out new land to settle, it was more fruitful to move inland or

Of course, the United States does not have a monopoly on dialects. The Chinese language has approximately 300 individual variations.

westward, as the areas to the north and south were already occupied. This resulted in a relatively homogenous community of speakers spanning each of these geographic tiers (Parker & Riley, 2004).

At this point, the United States is thought to have at least 10 distinct regional dialects; these are illustrated in Figure 10–1. The regions on the East coast (i.e., Eastern New England, Upper North, Lower North, Upper South, Lower South) are more compact and represent a greater range of distinctive patterns. Consider the differences one might hear from speakers ranging from Maine to New York to Georgia. These differences would probably be more noticeable than the range we would hear with speakers from Seattle to San Francisco to San Diego. It is likely that as populations moved west of the Mississippi, they intermingled more extensively, especially as modern transportation became increasingly available.

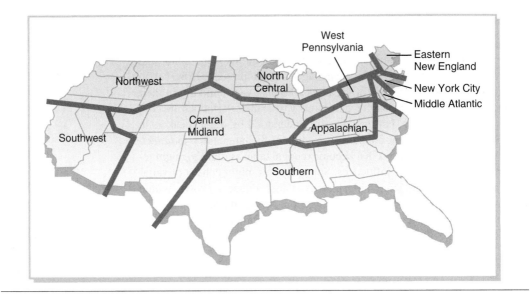

Figure 10–1. Dialectal regions of the United States.

The regional differences we might hear in traveling around the United States are a symphony of diversity, with each region exhibiting a characteristic personality through its speaking patterns. Some phonological examples include the New Yorker's linking /r/, in which an /r/ is inserted to link a word ending with a vowel when it is followed by a word beginning with a vowel, as in *The island of Cubar is near Floridar's Atlantic coast.* Many Southern dialects neutralize vowels that precede a nasal consonant. As a result, pairs that would otherwise contrast, such as *pen-pin, been-bin, ten-tin, him-hem,* and so forth, would all sound alike.

In addition, each regional dialect will also exhibit certain lexical differences. Commonly recognized differences include the use of "soda" in the Eastern New England area in contrast to "pop" in the Central Midland states, where both refer to carbonated beverages. Again, in the Central Midland states, most people sit on a "couch" and bring their groceries home in a "bag." In the south, people sit on the "sofa" and use a "sack" for their groceries.

Finally, there are distinctive phrases and syntactic patterns that characterize certain regions. For example, speakers in the South usually take the time to mention themselves as the indirect object of a sentence, as in *I'm gonna get me a drink of water.* In colder northern climates, this is assumed unless otherwise stated; compare *I'm gonna get a drink of water* and *I'm gonna get you a drink of water.*

These examples do not begin to capture the variety of regional expressions, from the bizarre to the quaint, that decorate our diverse language. One very subtle, but meaningful, variation came from my wife's aging grandmother, who, even when ailing, would always say when we had to end our visit by saying *I'm so proud that you came!* At first it seems to be a very odd expression, until you listen again, with your heart.

Social Dialects

Within a society, some groups and their dialects are defined by barriers that are not necessarily geographical. Some groups are defined instead by boundaries formed by socioeconomic status, ethnicity, and even by the influence of a surrounding language on a group's primary language. Dialects associated with socioeconomic status are perhaps less well defined in societies that are more open with broad-based educational systems, such as the United States. In contrast, the dialects spoken within the more rigid Hindu caste system of India carry clearer signals to suggest a speaker's social status. On the other hand, the more conscious societies are of ethnic origins, perhaps the more likely they are to focus on the dialectal variations associated with ethnic groups.

Regardless of the level of openness, probably no society is free of "linguistic chauvinism." This is the mistaken belief that your own version of a language is inherently the best, the most correct, or most pure version (Warren-Leubecker & Bohannon, 1985). As a natural result of this attitude, some dialects acquire a negative stigma. This attitude has led to what has been called the "deficiency model." This model assumed that dialects resulted from deficient learning of the primary language and were, therefore, a mark of socially inferior persons.

 We should be aware of distinguishing carefully between race, culture, and ethnicity. Racial groups are defined by a set of biologically determined physical features. Cultural groups are defined broadly by the sum of their living patterns. Specific cultural patterns common to members within a society define ethnic groups.

Our understanding of dialects has expanded significantly over the past 30 years. Since the 1960s, sociolinguists have thoroughly analyzed the structure and organization of dialects. What has become apparent is that all dialects are systematic, consistent subvariations of their primary language. They represent variations in the primary language that have evolved as different conventions for a specific verbal community. In other words, a "difference model" recognizes that dialects simply represent differences, not deficiencies, in using the primary language.

The terms used by sociolinguists to designate the social status of a dialect can be confusing. A **standard dialect** is the most broadly accepted version of the primary language and is said to draw no negative social attention to its speakers. In the United States, this would be Standard American English (SAE). The term **nonstandard dialect,** then, refers to those dialects other than the standard dialect, which may result in negative social attention. However, this is a social judgment, not a linguistic one; note that the term is <u>not</u> *sub*standard dialect. Designating a dialect as nonstandard does not mean that it is linguistically deficient. Nonetheless, the sad reality of linguistic chauvinism is such that speakers of nonstandard dialects might be viewed as not meeting the standard (Parker & Riley, 2004).

standard dialect The generally accepted version of the primary language used in a group.

nonstandard dialect Variations of the major language spoken by the overall population.

Within the United States, there are three major social dialects, Black English, Hispanic English, and Asian English. These dialects appear to be originally based on ethnicity in that the native languages of these groups were influenced by the surrounding English language. However, it is likely that geographic and socioeconomic factors have played roles in their evolution as well. In addition, each of these variations shows evidence of influence from primary languages other than English. Characteristic features of each of these dialects are presented in Tables 10–1, 10–2, and 10–3.

Black English.   The dialect spoken by many, but not all, African Americans has become known as Black English (BE). The term *Black English* is a misnomer to some extent, because it is not used by all African Americans and actually occurs in many non-African American, lower working-class speakers. And different versions of Black English have evolved within various regions of the United States.

There is some controversy about its origins. Some authorities have held that BE was simply a defective version of the dialect spoken by poor whites in the South. Others have suggested that it shows traces of *Creole,* a language of the Caribbean that evolved out of languages that were mixed through the trade and colonization that populated that region (Parker & Riley, 2004). Some of its features have been traced back to *Pidgin,* a reduced and simplified version of English that Europeans and Africans first used to communicate (Terrell & Terrell, 1993).

Technically speaking, BE is a nonstandard dialect of Standard American English (SAE). However, this does not suggest that it is linguistically deficient or inferior. The patterns of BE are consistent, not erratic. BE exhibits patterns that are as logical and complex as any primary language. In fact, the differences between BE and SAE are relatively minimal, as they share most vocabulary and overall grammatical systems. Some prominent contrasts noted by researchers between BE and SAE are summarized in Table 10–1 (Taylor, 1986).

The common phonological variations in BE have, in fact, a linguistic basis. For example, the substitution of /d/ for /th/ (e.g., *dis* for *this*), probably reflects an expected linguistic principle based on the fact that stops (such as /d/) are more natural and more prevalent in human languages overall.

Many of the grammatical variations in BE reduce the redundancy of SAE. Possessive inflections are eliminated where word order otherwise indicates possession (e.g., *Find daddy hat* versus *Find daddy's hat*). Similarly, third person present tense inflections, a redundancy in SAE, are similarly streamlined (e.g., *He run every day*). On the other hand, redundancy is introduced in double negatives, such as *I haven't eat nothing today.* This rule, in which indefinites are negated through the verb, is not unique to BE. There is a similar rule in Russian. Also, BE introduces additional complexity through its use of the auxiliary *be* to express aspect. In this distinction the auxiliary *be* is used to indicate an ongoing state in contrast to a temporary state. For example, someone who normally drives to work and is currently

Table 10–1. Some contrasts between Standard American English and Black English.

Features in Standard American English	Variations in Black English
Medial and final consonants /b, g, d, k, t, θ/: released, unaspirated, or unreleased depending on phonetic context (e.g., tab, table, bag, baggage, bad, batter, lick, locker, pit, putter, bath, bathtub).	Weakened, unreleased, or unaspirated as in *ba'er* for batter, *be'* for bed, *baf* for bath.
Final consonant clusters: released, unaspirated, or unreleased depending on phonetic context (e.g., best, desk).	Reduced, as in *las'* for last.
Possessive /-'s/: Obligatory, regardless of context (e.g., *Find Billy's book, please*).	Optional when word position signals possession, as in *Find Billy book, please.*
Plural /-s/: Obligatory regardless of context (e.g., *I found two dimes*).	Optional when quantifier provides context, as in *I found two dime.*
Pronouns: Used separately in anaphoric reference to noun (e.g., *Daddy called. He's happy you're here*).	Pronoun follows noun immediately, as in Daddy called. *Daddy he happy you're here.*
Contractible copula (is - 's): Copula obligatory, but contractible with context: (e.g., *She is tall vs. She's tall*).	Optional when contractible, as in *She tall.*
Regular past tense /-ed/: Obligatory with context (e.g., *He talked to me last night*).	Optional or reduced as part of consonant cluster, as in *He talk to me last night.*
Regular third person present tense /-s/: Obligatory with context (e.g., *He always works too hard*).	Optional, as in *He always work too hard.*
Irregular third person present tense (do/does, have/has): Obligatory with context (e.g., *He does my taxes every year*).	Optional, as in *He do my taxes every year.*
Future tense (am going to, gonna, will be): Commonly occurring forms used optionally (e.g., *I'm going to go home later, I'm gonna go home later,* or *I will be going home later*).	Common usage of be going to, gonna, or omission of *will* when followed by *be,* as in *I be going to go home later, I gonna go home later,* or *I be going home later.*
Negation: Marked once in each sentence; *ain't* regarded as nonstandard (e.g., *Nobody came to see me,* and *I'm not upset*).	Triple negatives occur as in, *Nobody didn't never come to see me. I ain't upset.*

Note. Adapted from *Nature of Communication Disorders in Culturally and Linguistically Diverse Populations,* by O. Taylor (Ed.), 1986, San Diego, CA: College-Hill Press.

doing so would be described in BE with *He be driving to work.* In contrast, someone who only drives on occasion would be described in BE with *He driving to work* (Warren-Leubecker & Bohannon, 1985).

Generally, the developmental trends in BE have been described in three stages. The younger child first learns the basic phonology, vocabulary, and grammar from caregivers. Next, during the school years, from 5 to 15 years, BE speakers assimilate more of the dialectal variations from their peers. Finally, as they approach young adulthood and become more aware of social situations, BE speakers begin to use more features from the standard dialect

Table 10–2. Some contrasts between Hispanic English and Standard American English.

Features in Standard American English	Variations in Hispanic English
Final Consonants: released, unaspirated, or unreleased depending on phonetic context.	Numerous final consonants (e.g., /p, m, w, b, g, k, f, d/) omitted, weakened, or distorted.
Consonant clusters: released, unaspirated, or unreleased depending on phonetic context.	Frequently preceded by schwa vowel, as in *astep* for step, or *aschool* for school.
Possessive /-'s/: Obligatory, regardless of context (e.g., *Find Billy's book, please*).	Postnoun modifiers mark possession, as in, *Find the book of Billy's, please.*
Plural /-s/: Obligatory regardless of context (e.g., *I found two dimes*).	Optional, as in *I found two dime.*
Pronouns: Used separately in anaphoric reference to noun (e.g., *Daddy called. He's happy you're here*).	Optional if subject occurs in preceding context, as in *Daddy called. Happy you're here.*
Regular past tense /-ed/: Obligatory with context (e.g., *He talked to me last night*).	Optional with context, as in *He talk to me last night.*
Regular third person present tense /-s/: Obligatory with context (e.g., *He always works too hard*).	Optional with context, as in *He always work too hard.*
Future tense (am going to, gonna, will be): Commonly occurring forms used optionally (e.g., *I'm going to go home later, I'm gonna go home later,* or *I will be going home later*).	Frequent use of *go + to,* as in *I'm go to go home later.*
Negation: Marked once in each sentence; *ain't* regarded as nonstandard (e.g., *Nobody came to see me,* and *I'm not upset*).	*No* is inserted before the verb, as in *I'm no upset.*
Interrogative: Marked with rising intonation and noun-copula/auxiliary inversion (e.g., *Is Bill coming?*).	Marked with rising intonation without noun-copula/auxiliary inversion, as in *Bill is coming?*

Note. Adapted from *Nature of Communication Disorders in Culturally and Linguistically Diverse Populations,* by O. Taylor (Ed.), 1986, San Diego, CA: College-Hill Press.

(Warren-Leubecker & Bohannon, 1985). In this regard, it is important to note that not all African American children will be exposed to or speak BE. Additionally, it is very possible that with increased integration, the variations of BE will become less distinct.

Hispanic English.   The Hispanic population is the largest ethnic group in the United States. Individuals with Spanish heritage are considered members of the Hispanic ethnic group. As a result, the Hispanic population is quite varied, as is the extent of their integration with surrounding groups. In the United States, individuals who are Hispanic may have their cultural origins in Cuba, Puerto Rico, or Mexico. Some Hispanic communities, such as those in New York City and Miami, are more locally concentrated. In con-

Table 10–3. Some contrasts between Asian English and Standard American English.

Features in Standard American English	Variations in Asian English
Final Consonants: released, unaspirated, or unreleased depending on phonetic context.	Numerous final consonants (e.g., /p, s, z, t, θ/) omitted.
Possessive /-'s/: Obligatory, regardless of context (e.g., *Find Billy's book, please*).	Omitted, as in, *Find Billy book, please.*
Plural /-s/: Obligatory regardless of context (e.g., *I found two dimes*).	Omitted, as in *I found two dime.*
Regular past tense /-ed/: Obligatory with context (e.g., *He sat with me last night*).	Sometimes omitted, as in *He sit with me last night;* or, sometimes overgeneralized, as in *He sitted with me last night.*
Perfective aspect (have + verb + -en/-ed: Obligatory with context (e.g., *I have taken the check*).	Omitted, as in *I have take the check.*
Copula (am, is, are, was, were): Forms obligatory based on person, number, and tense (e.g., *I am eating, I was eating, You are eating, You were eating,* etc.).	Omitted, as in *I eating;* or, used without regard for person, number, or tense, as in *I is eating.*
Adjective inflections (comparative -er): Optional forms depending on context (e.g., *My picture is prettier/more pretty than yours*).	Incorrect forms, especially with irregulars, as in *My picture is gooder than yours;* or, double marked, as in *My picture is more prettier than yours.*

Note. Adapted from "Cross-cultural and Linguistic Considerations in Working with Asian Populations," by L. Cheng, 1987, *Asha, 29*(6), pp. 33–38.

trast, other individuals of Hispanic origin are widely dispersed and integrated throughout southwestern regions of the United States.

Although their Spanish heritage may define them as Hispanic, individuals may vary widely in the extent to which the Spanish language has influenced their English. Hispanic individuals may differ in the form of Spanish in their background; there are differences between Caribbean and Mexican Spanish. There are differences in the amount of Spanish used by Hispanic individuals based on their individual family characteristics. Nonetheless, there are general characteristics that have evolved out of the interference between English and Spanish that we will distinguish generally as Hispanic English (HE) (Taylor, 1986). Table 10–2 presents some prominent characteristics that contrast HE and SAE.

There are phonological differences, such as a number of sounds in English that do not occur in Spanish, including several fricatives, (/θ/, /th/, /z/,/zh/, /sh/) and vowels (/ɪ/, /æ/, /ʌ/). The two sound systems, especially in regard to differences in vowels, can be a source of significant interference between the dialects.

Hispanic English, like BE, also eliminates many of the grammatical features that are redundant in SAE. For example, possessive inflections are replaced by postnoun modifiers, as in *This is the dog of my <u>brother</u>*. Plural noun inflections are optional in HE (e.g., *The two boy are going home now*), as are verb inflections for past tense (e.g., *He walk me home last night*) and third person present tense (e.g., *Each day, she write in her book*).

Asian English.   Asian languages came to the United States from diverse origins—China, Taiwan, Japan, the Indian subcontinent, the Philippine Islands, Korea, Cambodia, Laos, and Vietnam. To underscore this diversity, recall that it was noted previously that the Chinese language actually represents a large collection of dialects. In contrast, Japanese, Korean, and Vietnamese are unrelated to any other language. Further, some languages of the Indian subcontinent belong to the Indo-European family of languages.

From this standpoint, it would seem difficult to characterize any pattern as representative of a true Asian English (AE) dialect. Nonetheless, some common features have been observed where Asian communities and their languages have been influenced by Standard American English (Cheng, 1987). Table 10–3 presents some features that contrast AE with SAE.

Style Shifting.   Style shifting is a phenomenon that has been observed in dialectal behavior. *Style shifting* occurs when a speaker alternates between using the devices and styles of two dialects. It appears to be closely related to the notion of alternation described by sociolinguists, in which speakers use alternative forms and styles depending on the context, including the listener. It is also analogous to code switching, in which bilingual speakers switch between the linguistic codes of two or more languages.

These phenomena are not necessarily restricted to bilingual or bidialectal speakers. Most of us alter the forms and styles we use in response to different speaking contexts. Competent speakers respond differentially to different settings and audiences. Varying settings, such as classrooms, playgrounds, or home, and audiences, including teachers, peers, or parents, provide young speakers the opportunity to learn how to best communicate in each circumstance. The critical concern in facilitating this ability is to preserve the integrity and validity of the child's home dialect, while providing alternative models of the standard dialect in real opportunities for communication.

Summary

- Human languages have evolved with fundamental similarities called language universals.
- As human cultures have evolved and diversified, so have their languages, which resulted in language variations.
- Groups of languages that have descended from similar historical and cultural roots are called language families.
- In many societies, learning more than one language, whether through simultaneous acquisition or successive acquisition, is common.

- Within a community of speakers, there will be subgroups who develop variations of the primary language, called dialects.

- Most bilingual speakers learn to code shift between the languages they use; speakers of dialects may learn to style shift between the dialect of their community and the standard dialect.

Language Disorders

When groups of individuals collectively use a variant of the primary language, they are speaking a dialect. When individuals use unique words, phrasing, and devices within that language, it is considered an idiolect as long as the message is understood by those around them. These variations in mature speakers, whether they constitute a dialect or an idiolect, may occasion times when communication is difficult and some clarification is needed, but the repairs are generally made effectively and naturally.

Children also exhibit variations in how they develop language. This has been stressed at various points throughout this book. Children's individual development will vary based on biological foundations, motor capacities, cognitive abilities, and social opportunities to learn from their interactions.

This textbook has focused on the learning that generally is expected when all of these factors contribute appropriately to children's development of language. However, not all children benefit to the same extent from one or several of these factors and, as a result, their language development might vary substantially from the children around them.

When a child's inability to communicate—gain attention, express ideas, obtain needs, and so forth—compromises his or her interactions with caregivers and others, it represents a language disorder. Ultimately, a child whose language is disordered is also at risk for development in those other domains—motor, cognitive, and social—that are coupled to language.

Adult language disorders generally result from neurological injury and disease. Due to the complexity of the related information, this text focuses only on children's language disorders. ∎

Individual Variations in Language Development

Prior to the 1970s, the goal of language researchers was to describe normal development as a common path followed by all children. The focus of early theories was the universals of language and finding commonalties in children that would illuminate these universals. In contrast, variations in children's language development were often treated as aberrations or artifacts; differences were often ignored or excluded so that the similarities among children could be used to describe "the norm." However, in spite of this orientation, researchers continued to find ample evidence of individual variability in the midst of the collective similarity (Haynes, 1994c).

Variations have been noted in age of first word production (Darley & Winitz, 1961), phonological development (Ferguson & Farwell, 1975), the first lexicon (Nelson, 1973b), early word combinations (Bloom, Lightbown, & Hood, 1975), and even the rate of acquisition of later structures (Brown, 1973).

Children's Language Disorders

As strange as it sounds, then, variability is the norm. The challenge for professionals interested in language becomes one of determining how much variability is indeed expected and, therefore, "normal." Conversely, children exhibit a *language disorder* when their language varies from their peers to the degree that it significantly impairs social and academic communication.

Aspects of Children's Language Disorders

Professionals want to research various aspects of children's language disorders. Describing the characteristics of language disorders based on their origins may result in useful classifications. Understanding this information would assist in assessing children who are at risk for disordered language development. This is especially important because researchers and clinicians have learned that early intervention is the most efficient way of maximizing a child's overall potential.

Characteristics of Language Disorders.   Children who exhibit language disorders will present a variety of difficulties in learning language. These difficulties may be evidenced in quantitative differences, in which they learn less language in a longer period than their peers. Alternately, some children may talk as much as their peers, but, qualitatively, their language is not as effective in communicating.

There may be significant delays in developing functional oral communication. Children with language disorders may present vocabulary development that is limited to fewer words than expected for their age. They may have difficulty expressing relationships and ideas through grammatical word orders. Even with the expected level of vocabulary and the development of grammar, some children with language disorders struggle with the subtle pragmatic aspects of using language in social contexts. Finally, some children may not exhibit a conspicuous language disorder until it becomes apparent through reading difficulties, in which they fail to integrate and comprehend printed information.

Classifications of Language Disorders.   Language disorders exhibited by children are classified in various ways. Traditionally, the communication disorders (speech and language disorders) exhibited by children have been classified in either of two broad categories, organic or functional. **Organic language disorders** are associated with such etiologies as congenital hearing loss and cerebral palsy. The characteristics of the language disorders associated with organic causes will vary widely depending on the specifics of the conditions.

The factors associated with **functional language disorders** have been more difficult to isolate. In fact, for the most part, the *absence* of an identifiable organic cause is often the determining factor in classifying a language

organic language disorders Language disorders associated with physiological causes such as brain damage or hearing loss.

functional language disorders Language disorders that have no apparent organic basis.

disorder as functional. This is thought to represent the largest group of child language disorders. Accordingly, the features of these disorders have generally been found to be very diverse. Although, these children may vary greatly in their developmental and social histories, one factor is constant: they have not learned to communicate orally and experience significant failure in their interactions at home and in school. The term that is currently used for this category is **specific language impairment.**

A final category might be referred to as **mixed language disorders.** In some cases, a syndrome (e.g., Down syndrome, brain injury, or autism) can be identified. However, beyond this syndrome, a functional component such as ineffective parenting, physical and emotional neglect, or the absence of any intervention exacerbates the child's language disorder.

specific language impairment Language disorders that appear unrelated to organic causes or any other general disability.

mixed language disorder A language impairment resulting from both organic and environmental factors.

Evaluation of Language Disorders. The identification of language disorders is accomplished through various means. **Standardized assessment** includes formal test instruments that have been normed with a number of children at equivalent ages. The performances of children whose language development is a source for concern are compared to the performances of

 There are synonymous or related terms that students will find as they pursue their interest in language disorders. Some differentiate further between *language disorder* and *language delay*. Others may subsume all of these under *language impairment.*

these peers. Tests may be constructed to assess children's vocabulary and grammar skills at various levels in either comprehension or production. If their performance is statistically unexpected according to the norms, then it suggests the possibility of a language disorder. However, standardized assessments are notorious for confronting children with unnatural communication tasks and, therefore, should always be supplemented with more natural observations.

Nonstandardized assessments, by definition, assess language through more informal procedures that do not rely on the rigid tasks required for standardized tests. Natural language samples are a good example of a nonstandardized assessment. In this procedure, the professional will arrange a setting that prompts the child to interact as naturally as possible through play, storytelling, or conversation, depending on the child's overall level.

standardized assessment Evaluation of language abilities using formal test instruments.

Another scheme characterizes language disorders as disorders of form, content, or use (Bloom & Lahey, 1978). ∎

nonstandardized assessment Evaluation of language abilities through informal procedures.

Intervention for Language Disorders. When a professional assists those who interact with a child to facilitate language development, it is called **intervention.** Language intervention essentially consists of arranging the appropriate input in a setting that will encourage verbal responding and then ensuring that appropriate verbal behaviors result in natural communication. Depending on the level of the child, the input and consequences may be more structured to ensure that they are salient. Or, the setting may be less structured and more natural to build on the child's present level of skills.

Intervention should be a multifaceted process, involving the significant people in the settings where the child must communicate. Intervention

intervention Arranging treatment factors in an individual's environment to facilitate language learning.

speech-language pathologist Specialist trained in the identification, assessment, and treatment of human communication disorders.

audiologist Specialist trained in the identification, assessment, and treatment of hearing disorders.

otorhinolaryngologist Medical practitioner trained in diseases of the ear, nose, and throat.

neurologist Medical practitioner specializing in evaluating and treating brain function.

psychologists Professionals who evaluate and treat emotional disorders.

child development specialists Professionals specializing in evaluating child development and counseling parents.

should be a coordinated process of determining individualized goals for the specific needs of each child. Addressing those goals might require the involvement of different professionals who fill specific roles.

Often, several professions will be involved in providing language intervention to children with language disorders. **Speech-language pathologists** are specially trained in the identification, assessment, and treatment of disordered language. They have studied the normal processes and characteristics of language development extensively. Speech-language pathologists may frequently play a coordinating role in making appropriate referrals, collecting information, and developing goals and procedures with the other persons involved, both professionals and caregivers. **Audiologists** are specially trained professionals who evaluate hearing and assist in providing treatment for hearing losses.

If a child's hearing loss can be medically treated, an **otorhinolaryngologist,** a physician trained in diseases of the ear, nose, throat, would provide this service. **Neurologists** are physicians who specialize in evaluating brain function and, in cases where it is called for, may evaluate the extent of brain injury or the presence of seizures.

Some children may exhibit an emotional disorder, such as autism, in relation to their language disorder. **Psychologists** evaluate the presence of such conditions and provide recommendations for treating them in the context of the planned language intervention. When caregivers are in need of additional assistance in parenting, **child development specialists** will provide counseling and training for effective techniques.

The professionals involved in school settings will typically include psychometrists, who evaluate the child's cognitive and academic abilities, and classroom or special education teachers. The psychometric testing information will be combined with the teacher's observations of the child's classroom functioning and peer interactions when making decisions about placing the child in the optimal educational situation.

Summary

- Researchers have found individual variation in children's language development.

- Researchers and clinicians assessing children's language must determine how much variation constitutes a language disorder.

- Language disorders can result from organic factors, environmental factors, or a combination of both.

- Assessing children's language might involve standardized or nonstandardized procedures.

- Intervention will usually involve multiple professions and occur in interactions and settings that are as natural as possible.

I t has been observed that human languages are said to share certain fundamental similarities called *language universals.* However, language exists only as a result of human interaction. Human interaction and the cultures it forms have evolved over thousands of years, with a myriad of individual differences in the languages used in these cultures. This diversity in human language is called *language variations.*

Primary languages are those that serve as the predominate language for a population. In many societies, it is not uncommon for more than one language to be used. *Bilingual* speakers, capable of speaking two (or more) languages, are usually also able to *code switch* in order to communicate in either language. Within a language community, some groups of speakers share *dialects,* or identifiable variants of the primary language. Speakers who are capable of using both the standard dialect and their particular dialect are exhibiting *style shifting.*

Researchers have found that, although there are trends and patterns that define normal language development, there is still a good measure of individual variation. When an individual child's language development varies from normal to the extent that it interferes with overall development, that child exhibits a *language disorder.* Language disorders might be caused by *organic* etiologies, such as hearing impairment or brain injury. Those language disorders that cannot be attributed to a specific organic etiology might be classified as *functional. Specific language impairment* is the current term for the most commonly diagnosed functional language disorder. Determining whether or not a child is exhibiting a language disorder is accomplished through *standardized* and *nonstandardized assessment* procedures. *Language intervention* is a process that involves multiple professionals who collaborate to facilitate effective communication in the child's natural interactions.

Chapter Summary

1. What considerations would account for the similarities common to all human languages?

2. How has diversity evolved in the many different languages? Why do languages develop different words, grammatical structures, and so forth?

3. How many different major languages are spoken on the North American continent? How many bilingual combinations are possible from this collection of languages?

Review Questions

4. Compare the complications and advantages in becoming bilingual through simultaneous versus successive acquisition.

5. How are code switching and style shifting different?

6. How do the natural variations evident in language learning make the identification of language disorders more difficult?

Practice Questions

To the student: You are encouraged to use the following questions to prepare for multiple-choice examinations. This exercise is not intended to simply "provide the answers to questions." Instead, it is hoped that you will use the material to develop your ability to analyze questions and choices to identify correct answers based on a critical understanding of the distinctions among the answers. Use the answer key at the end of the book to prompt your analysis of each item and to confirm the correct answer. Remember that there is a difference between recognizing the correct answer and understanding why it is the correct one.

1. An individual who grew up in a family and country that speak Spanish and who later learns English while attending high school in an English-speaking community _____ .
   a. will never learn English
   b. will learn English easier than he or she would have in kindergarten
   c. will demonstrate "successive acquisition"
   d. will demonstrate "simultaneous acquisition"
   e. all of these are true

2. An individual who uses Black English with his friends in informal interactions, but speaks to his teachers, principal, and boss in a more formal manner using Standard American English _____ .
   a. would be considered to be bilingual
   b. would be demonstrating "code switching"
   c. would be demonstrating "style shifting"
   d. a and b
   e. a and c

3. Different dialects might be based on influences related to _____ .
   a. socioeconomic levels
   b. cultural differences
   c. geographic differences
   d. ethnic differences
   e. all of these

4. Which of the following general statements regarding dialects is true?
   a. dialects are based solely on phonological difference—when people's speech sounds different
   b. the use of a dialect always reflects that individuals are less educated
   c. dialects are aberrations of the primary language that reflect lower intelligence
   d. dialects typically have internal consistency in that the rules and patterns are logical, predictable, and complex—just like those found in primary languages.
   e. all of these statements are true

5. Variations that might be expected in Black English would include _____ .
   a. lack of rising intonation when producing questions
   b. reduced variety of vowels
   c. optional or reduced past tense inflection as part of consonant cluster
   d. dangling prepositional phrases
   e. all of these

6. Variations that might be expected in Hispanic English would include _____ .
   a. omission of noun-copula/auxiliary inversion in questions
   b. deletion of all initial consonants
   c. use of postnoun modifiers to mark possession
   d. a and b
   e. a and c

7. Variations that might be expected in Asian English would include _____ .
   a. omission of numerous final consonants
   b. omission of possessive inflections
   c. omission of plural inflections
   d. incorrect forms of comparative and superlative adjective inflections
   e. all of these

8. Language disorders can be indicated by delays in development of _____ .
   a. grammatical abilities
   b. semantic abilities
   c. pragmatic abilities
   d. expressive abilities or comprehension abilities
   e. any combination of these

9. Broad traditional classifications of language disorders based on their causes or etiologies include _____ .
   a. standardized language disorders and nonstandardized language disorders
   b. language disorders and language delays
   c. organic language disorders and functional language disorders
   d. style shifting and code switching
   e. none of these

10. The differences between standardized assessments and nonstandardized assessments include _____ .
    a. the use of norms to compare performances
    b. the use of uniform test materials
    c. the level of natural communication
    d. a and b
    e. a, b, and c

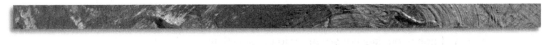

Suggested Readings

Backus, A. (1999). Mixed native language: A challenge to the monolithic view of language. *Topics in Language Disorders, 19*(4), 11–22.

Jia, G., Aaronson, D., & Wu, Y. (2002). Long-term language attainment of bilingual immigrants: Predictive variables and language group differences. *Applied Psycholinguistics, 23,* 599–621.

Peña, E., Bedore, L. M., & Rappazzo, D. (2003). Comparison of Spanish, English, and bilingual children's performance across semantic tasks. *Language, Speech, and Hearing Services in Schools, 34,* 5–16.

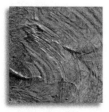

Answer Key and Analysis

Chapter 1

1. (Answer: e) The key word "speech" eliminates several choices. *Syntax* and *semantics* are aspects of language, not speech. *Phonology* is the study of meaningful speech sound patterns that occur in language. Vocal quality is an aspect of speech but reflects our perception of vocal fold activity. *Fluency* is an aspect of speech and refers to the rhythm and rate of speech produced by the speaker.

2. (Answer: b) The key term is "mental operations." *Paralinguistics* refers to production features we produce "parallel" to the units of language such as the intonation and stress we superimpose on our words and phrases. *Nonlinguistic* refers to cues such as gestures and facial expressions that only supplement the meaning of our utterances. *Sociolinguistics* emphasizes the influence of social contexts on language. In *metalinguistics* the prefix "meta" suggests the ability to consider language as an object. In *psycholinguistics,* the prefix "psycho" (as in "psyche") refers to the mind and suggests that the focus is on the mental operations involved in producing and understanding language.

3. (Answer: d) *Neuromuscular* refers to the connection between the nervous system and muscles that move the structures for speech. *Dynamic* is frequently used to suggest the active nature of producing speech sounds. Producing speech *sounds* is not necessary for language to occur, as in writing. *Resonance* refers to the way the spaces or cavities of the vocal tract (e.g., the nasal cavity) modify the sound of our voice. *Symbolic* relates to elements of language (e.g., spoken words, written words, sign language gestures) that can "stand for" an idea, object, event, or relationship.

4. (Answer: c) The key element in this question is represented by the phrase "while talking to you." The behaviors mentioned (lowering the head, raising an eyebrow, and squinting) do not represent linguistic symbols, so they would not be considered *sign language* or *gestural language.* The facial and postural behaviors in question are not *suprasegmental devices,* such as intonation, stress, and pauses. The remaining two answers—*nonlinguistic cues* and *nonverbal communication*—can be distinguished by their roles in communication. Behaviors that qualify as *nonverbal communication,* while not verbal or linguistic, still communicate (e.g., shaking your head for "no" communicates rejection without saying a word). However, when these behaviors accompany language, they instead take the role of *nonlinguistic cues* that supplement verbal communication (e.g., shaking your head "no" while rejecting an idea makes the rejection more emphatic).

5. (Answer: a) The concept of "implicit, idealized knowledge" is central to this question. *Linguistic performance* is the actual production of language, so it would be explicit, not implicit. *Prescriptive grammar* refers to the notion that there are "correct" forms of language that are prescribed and must be used in a language. *Descriptive grammar* is a set of rules that describes the patterns exhibited by speakers in a language. *Intelligence* refers to an individual's general ability to learn, recall, and reason. *Linguistic competence* refers to our ability to "instinctively" recognize when sentences may be grammatically incorrect, even though we may not be able to explain what is wrong.

423

6. (Answer: d) The component or aspect of language in which the two utterances contrast must be analyzed to determine how they differ. The two utterances seem to convey the same *semantic relationship*—they both negate the caregiver's proposition. Similarly, both seem to express the same communicative intention or pragmatic function—that of rejecting the caregiver's request. There are no *dialectal features* present in either utterance, so that leaves *grammatical structure*—a single word versus a complete sentence—as the main level of distinction.

7. (Answer: c) As we develop our understanding of the meanings of words, we combine our experience in circumstances involving that word and our understanding of the meanings of other words related to it. *Linguistic competence* relates to our implicit understanding of the grammatical rules of our language. *Metalinguistic ability* refers to our capacity to evaluate words as objects aside from their meanings. The concept of *generative grammar* addresses our ability to produce and understand an infinite number of acceptable sentences in spite of our limited intelligence and memory. The meanings of associated words and phrases that contribute to our understanding of a word represent our *semantic memory* for that word. It is the accumulated recall of experiences or episodes involving a word that is represented in our *episodic memory* for that word.

8. (Answer: d) The sense of this question is that we instinctively "know" whether the meanings of words can "go together." This suggests an aspect of semantics (or content). *Distinctive features* refer to the production features that differentiate one phoneme from another. *Prosodic features* refer to production effects that give speech its melodic character. *Morphology* is the study of the forms of words in a language, not their individual meanings. The different roles the nouns in a sentence take on in relationship to the verb are the *semantic relations;* although this is an aspect of semantics, this term does not refer to the concordance between word meanings. *Selection restrictions* pertain to the notion that the semantic features of words might conflict (e g , +*animate* in "mommy" and −*animate* in "brick") and prohibit them from occurring together.

9. (Answer: b) *Form* refers to the structure of language, including phonology and grammar (morphology and syntax). *Proxemics* is the study of interpersonal space in communication. *Pragmatics* is not a "contemporary" term; it is the traditional term for *use*. This leaves *content,* which conveys the notion that words contain features that confer meaning.

10. (Answer: c) Analyze the difference between the two "headlines" based on the major aspects of language. Because the question is based on the premise that they are both "headlines" announcing new information, these propositions would not differ based on *use* or *pragmatics.* (Remember that *use* and *pragmatics* refer to the same aspect of language.) The sounds present in both "headlines" are identical—just rearranged. Finally, the morphological forms (or words) in both "headlines" are also the same—again, just rearranged. This brings us to the fact that the "headlines" are the same except for the rearrangement of the words to convey different relationships—*syntax.*

Chapter 2

1. (Answer: d) The *cell body* responds by generating an impulse as a result of "processing" stimulation from surrounding neurons. *Axons* convey or transmit the impulses away from the cell body where they can be collected by the surrounding *dendrites.* Each neuron has numerous branching dendrites and one axon; therefore, dendrites do outnumber the axons. However, each neuron has one cell body and one axon so cell bodies cannot outnumber axons.

2. (Answer: d) The *visual system* tracks from the retina behind the eye through areas deep in the temporal lobe and back to the occipital lobe. Damage in the precentral gyrus would not be close to these areas. The precentral gyrus is the location of the primary motor strip. It exerts control over the opposite side of the body. Damage in the left hemisphere would be evidenced by *paralysis on the right side of the body.*

3. (Answer: d) The opening between the vocal folds is called the *glottis.* After the lungs have filled with air, if the vocal folds are closed or *adducted,* the air pressure *below* the glottis, or *subglottic*

pressure, increases. At that point, the air pressure above the vocal folds is relatively *less;* the vocal folds blow open to release a puff of air and then draw closed again. As this cycle rapidly repeats phonation occurs.

4. (Answer: e) *Broca's area* is located just anterior to the lower region of the primary motor cortex near the area that controls the structures for speech. The areas just ahead of the primary motor cortex seem to be involved in *planning and initiating* the movements executed by the motor cortex. Wernicke's area, located in the posterior region of the temporal lobe, appears to process the language we hear for comprehension. It also is involved in formulating and monitoring the speech and language units we use to express our ideas.

5. (Answer: a) The *cerebrum* includes the cortical regions that we call Broca's area and Wernicke's area—both intimately involved in speech and language. *Cranial nerves* are part of the peripheral nervous system. Some are motor nerves that control structures for speech. Some cranial nerves are sensory nerves; the vestibular acoustic or auditory nerve carries the sensation of sound to the brain where we hear speech and interpret language. The *cerebellum* is the structure primarily responsible for coordinating movements, including speech movements. *Spinal nerves* are the final pathway from the brain to the muscles, some of which execute the movements that support and produce speech. Finally, the *autonomic nerves,* while important for the regulation of life support systems, do not play a major direct role in speech and language.

6. (Answer: b) The first form in embryonic development is the *zygote.* The latest stage represented in the sequence is the *embryonic disc.* The zygote becomes the *morula,* and the morula develops into the *blastocyst,* which becomes the embryonic disc.

7. (Answer: e) The *embryonic period* includes the period from birth through the eighth week. The *fetal period* extends from the ninth week to birth. Because trimesters are based on 12-week periods and the fetal period begins in the ninth week, it includes some of all three trimesters.

8. (Answer: a) *Brain weight* increases dramatically in the first 2 years of life. *Dendritic interconnec-*

tions also expand significantly during the first 2 years. *Myelination,* the development of the myelin sheath that increases the conducting efficiency of nerves, occurs continuously throughout this period. At least partly as a result of the myelination, our ability to *inhibit* many *reflexes* is increased; therefore, voluntary movement, not reflexive movement, becomes more prominent.

9. (Answer: e) Infantile reflexes that affect a specific structure are called *specific activity reflexes;* those that have more widespread effects are called *mass activity reflexes.* Reflexes are considered to provide various *survival mechanisms;* for example, the sucking and rooting reflexes would be crucial to feeding behavior. With myelination and maturing nervous system, infantile reflexes are expected to *diminish* during the first 2 years of life. Many of the behaviors provided by infantile reflexes, such as the Palmar reflex, appear to evolve into useful voluntary behaviors such as grasping, which allows manipulating items of interest.

10. (Answer: b) Newborns' *vision* gives them visual acuity for a few inches at birth, so it is not the most ready sense. In addition, even children who are severely visually impaired develop language, albeit with some semantic deficits (e.g., color names). Infants' *olfactory* sense is developed sufficiently to allow them to identify their caregivers' scent very soon after birth; however, this is probably not the most significant sensory experience relevant to language development. Infants' *gustatory* sense is developed enough to distinguish between sweetness and saltiness at a very young age; however, this is still not the earliest developed sense nor is it the most significant to language development. The *tactile* sense in infants matures only with myelination, especially for sensory nerves from the periphery, including the fingers and hands. Even at that, language development would not seem to be strongly influenced by the textures and temperatures experienced by the infant. Because the cochlea and auditory nerve develop around the 24th week in utero, the sound of the caregivers' voices, especially the mother's, would be among the earliest sensory experiences. In addition to being the most ready at birth, caregivers' voices and speech patterns will frequently accompany

every activity following birth, laying the ground-work for language development.

Chapter 3

1. (Answer: c) The key word, of course, is *attachment*. For individuals to form an attachment with each other would mean that they must recognize each other. In addition, an attachment would suggest that the behavior of one influences the other and the individuals would therefore become dependent on each other. Although infants and their biological parents may bear even strong resemblances, this is not a requirement for attachment, as illustrated by millions of successful adoptions.

2. (Answer: d) The term *deictic gaze* indicates the notion of "pointing to." When infants seem to avoid eye contact, it has been called *gaze aversion*. Gazing into the caregiver's eyes likely represents *mutual gaze,* and the mother's use of shaking an item to draw attention to it is called *marking.* When an infant fixes his or her gaze on an item and that directs the caregiver's intention, whether intentionally or not, it is called a *deictic gaze.*

3. (Answer: e) The relationship being addressed is that between language and cognition—as in which one determines the other. The word sequence in the term *linguistic determinism* can be used as a mnemonic device to recall the answer—language determines or influences cognition. Additionally, an illustration of this would be when a group's view of the world is determined by or reflected in the words it has for certain aspects in their environment (e.g., colors, foods, weather, etc.).

4. (Answer: e) *Stimulus bound* indicates that the stimulus must be present for that level of processing to occur. *Abstraction, conceptualization, imagery,* and *symbolization* are all higher level processes that do not require the stimulus to be present. In contrast, *sensation* does not require recall or reasoning—there must simply be a stimulus that activates our touch, audition, vision, taste, or smell receptors. In addition, the process of *perception,* at the simplest level, involves determining whether a stimulus that is detected by our senses is novel or familiar.

5. (Answer: e) Infants are not recognized as having "intentions" and do not apparently react to the outside world with an "agenda." The earliest vocalizations are *reflexive* in nature, occur in response to internal *physiological stimuli* (hunger, thirst, cold, etc.), and, frequently, caregivers can *discriminate* or distinguish the source of the discomfort from the sound of the vocalizations.

6. (Answer: d) In motherese, it is observed that caregivers produce utterances that emphasize certain characteristics, seemingly to increase and maintain the infant's interest. These include *exaggerated prosody* to make the utterance more melodic, changes in *rate,* and *facial expressions* that coincide with these undulations. *Longer utterances* do not usually correlate with simpler utterances and are less likely to maintain the infant's interest.

7. (Answer: d) First, both terms are associated with operant conditioning; neither of these terms is associated with *classical conditioning.* When analyzing consequences such as reinforcement and punishment in an operant analysis, it is useful to contrast their definitions based on "effects" and "procedures." In terms of effects, *negative reinforcement* would increase the frequency or strength of a behavior; *Type II punishment* would decrease its frequency or strength. However, to achieve these effects, both procedures would involve *removing stimuli*—negative reinforcement would remove an aversive stimulus and Type II punishment would remove a reinforcing stimulus.

8. (Answer: c) *Assimilation* is one component of Piaget's cognitive process, *adaptation.* An analogy that might fit here is to think about immigrants who *assimilate* to a new country and culture. This usually means that it is the immigrant who tries to "fit in" with those around him in the existing culture. This is in contrast to the notion of a society modifying its ways to accept the different ways of each new immigrant (which in a pluralistic society can and should happen to some degree). According to Piaget, *assimilation* does not develop with the later period of formal operations; it is a lifelong component of adapting to new experiences. Finally, the ability to assume your listener's perspective would be related to what Piaget called *decentration.*

9. (Answer: e) This item is to be analyzed in the context of an *operant analysis. Unconditioned stimuli* (UCS) and *conditioned stimuli* (CS) are

associated with classical conditioning. This leaves *negative reinforcers* and *secondary reinforcers. Negative reinforcement* involves removing aversive stimuli, which is not suggested in this scenario. Instead, since the first moment, the caregiver's facial expressions, voice, physical contours, and physical smell have been associated with primary reinforcers (food, warmth, etc.), making them very powerful *secondary reinforcers.*

10. (Answer: b) *Symbolic play,* according to Piaget, emerges later in the first year during the sensorimotor period and refers to the ability to let one item stand represent other items. Mouthing a rattle is a simple act of exploration associated with the early sensorimotor period. Pushing a car back and forth represents functional play, in which the child plays with an item according to its assigned function. Although more later stages of babbling has been called *vocal play,* it is not symbolic. Rather, using a wood block as if it were a car, then a table, and then a building, would represent the flexible thought that Piaget would likely call *symbolic play.*

Chapter 4

1. (Answer: c) Based on its name, one knows that the transformational generative grammar model emphasizes grammar. Accordingly, the critical "data" or input the child receives will not be pragmatic in nature, as in *intentions* and *purposes.* Although the *output* or product of the LAD in TGG will eventually be a complete "idealized" TGG, that is not what constitutes the *input.* According to the TGG model, parents provide no input that is tutorial in nature—parents do not "teach" grammar and even the utterances they provide are far from perfect examples of the *standard grammar* for the language. Instead, the LAD receives input that consists of every utterance, however deficient or exemplary, that is within hearing distance.

2. (Answer: a) The answers indicate that understanding the nature of Skinner's primary verbal operants is necessary. The child's utterance ("cookie, cookie, cookie") could be taken to be just a label, which would be a *tact.* To be an *echoic,* the mother would have first had to produce a model of the word, which is not suggested

by the question. An *extended tact* would be based on stimulus generalization and refer to something other than the original stimulus (e.g., a cracker). *Intraverbals* involve speech that is strongly controlled by or associated with other responses that precede it (e.g., "Mary had a little _____"). A *mand,* based on the notion of *demand* or *command,* specifies its reinforcer, in this case, a cookie.

3. (Answer: c) According to Chomsky's transformational generative grammar, every sentence begins as a simple active declarative (SAD). If no transformations are applied, it will be produced as a SAD. One of these utterances is a yes-no question (a), another is a negative (b), and yet another is a passive (d) in which the subject of the sentence is passive. A fourth choice is not a sentence at all, at least in English (e). The remaining choice is a *simple* (one subject) *active* (the subject is active) *declarative* (it is not a question, negative, passive, or imperative form).

4. (Answer: c) Although all linguists would acknowledge that language is used in social contexts, only two models emphasize the underlying social nature as a dynamic force in language learning. *Chomsky* emphasized the *genetic predisposition* as the primary variable responsible for language development. *Fillmore* saw language as primarily serving to express the *semantic relationships* perceived by speakers. It was *Searle* and *Skinner* (and others who followed their thinking) who saw the dynamics of social interaction as the driving force behind language behavior.

5. (Answer: e) The choices represent semantic cases, which must be analyzed by determining the relationship between each noun and the verb in the sentence. In this sentence the Buick is not active and therefore cannot be in the *agentive* case. Bob did not build the Buick (General Motors should get credit for that) and, therefore, it is not in the *factitive* case. Bob is not sitting on the Buick and the Buick is not animate, eliminating the *locative* case and the *dative* case. Bob's polishing should change the appearance of the Buick and, therefore, as the inanimate affected by the action, it would be in the *objective* case.

6. (Answer: d) Speech acts theory provides the context for this question. Case relations do not have a role in speech acts theory. In speech acts theory,

the *locutionary* component refers to the words and phrases used in speech acts, and the *illocutionary* component refers to the intentions expressed in speech acts. The *perlocutionary* component refers to the listener's *interpretation* of the words and phrases as he or she attempts to determine the speaker's intention.

7. (Answer: c) Sociolinguists emphasize the influence of social context on language and the purposes it serves in social interaction. They would more likely see learning syntax as the product of these forces as children learn to communicate. Sociolinguists might concede that some form of a LAD might extract the grammatical rules of language, but they would not recognize it as the sole determinant or motivation in language development. Finally, although sociolinguists do not invoke the term "reinforcement," their model does emphasize the outcomes and feedback that occur as part of the natural consequences in human communication, which effectively is reinforcement.

8. (Answer: c) The term *phrase structure rule* refers to a key element in the transformational grammar model, and the term *suprasegmental* refers to characteristics of production. A key factor in the operant analysis of verbal behavior is the contingency that develops between responses and the situations in which they occur. If a response is effectively reinforced, that setting becomes a collection of discriminative stimuli or setting stimuli for that response. That is, they "set the occasion" for that behavior or similar behaviors to occur in the future.

9. (Answer: b) *Syntax* refers to the underlying mental rules for word order in language. Skinner did not address underlying mental rules, but rather overt behaviors. His model included primary verbal behaviors (e.g., *mands, tacts,* and *echoics*). He also addressed the concept that speakers exhibit *autoclitic behavior* that rearranges the orders of primary verbal behaviors that convey relationships among them in ways that correspond to their verbal community; in other words, *syntax.*

10. (Answer: e) The "semantic revolution" emphasized the primary role of children's understanding of meanings and relationships preliminary to learning how to express them. Their understanding of relationships is driven by their cognitive

development. As a result, they were viewed as doing more than learning syntactic word orders; they were learning word orders that conveyed the relationships they wanted to express. Overall, this relationship was expressed as "meaning precedes form."

Chapter 5

1. (Answer: e) The phenomenon in question relates to the observation that infants' babbling gradually includes more of the sounds heard in the speech that they are exposed to in their environment—their native tongue. This evolution is what some have called *phonetic drift.* The *discontinuity hypothesis,* by definition, contends that there is no continuum or connection between babbling and speech—that they are separate phenomena. In contrast, the *continuity hypothesis,* by definition, supports that a continuum or connection between babbling and speech does exist.

2. (Answer: c) Mowrer's Autism Theory addresses the influence of behavioral learning principles in infant sound productions. As such, it would not invoke a concept like the *LAD,* which was proposed by Chomsky as a mechanism for grammatical development. *Stimulus generalization, negative reinforcement,* and *punishment* are all behavioral learning principles but were not centrally involved in Mowrer's theory. The term *autism* in Mowrer's theory refers to events that are *self-reinforcing.* In this case, as the infant's sounds increasingly resemble the sounds produced by caregivers while providing primary reinforcers (food, warmth, etc.), they become self-reinforcing.

3. (Answer: b) Analyzing the term *prelinguistic* indicates that it refers to behaviors that occur prior to the onset of conventional language (i.e., the *first word*). The first word would constitute the onset of conventional language, whereas the other behaviors (*cooing, babbling, jargon,* and *vocal play*) predate the first word.

4. (Answer: a) A key consideration in this question is that the caregiver is addressing a 3-month-old infant. The stages refer to the components of communication according to the speech acts theory. This would eliminate the *phonological* stage and the *politeness* stage (although it is certainly important to model civility for children). The lo-

cutionary stage refers to the onset of words and phrases used in speech acts at about 1 year. The illocutionary stage is based on the onset of intentionality, which occurs after 6 months of age. Prior to the infants exhibiting their own intentions, caregivers speak to them in ways that project intentionality onto purely physiological behaviors (e.g., a burp).

5. (Answer: c) *Conversations* are based on alternating verbal exchanges between partners and the term *turn taking* refers to this pattern. *Gaze patterns* between infants and their caregivers exhibit analogous patterns of eye contact. The term *gaze coupling* refers to the alternating patterns of eye contact that occur between the infant and caregiver.

6. (Answer: c) Deixis can be interpreted as "pointing to" an item. Words such as "this" and "that" exhibit deixis by indicating items that are more or less proximal to the speaker. With infants, such words have no meaning, but caregivers can still reference or direct attention to an item through proximity by moving closer to it. (Infants are not capable of such mobility, so deixis for them is exhibited through eye gaze.)

7. (Answer: a) Analyzing the term *phonetically consistent forms* (PCFs) indicates that their phonetic composition or *sound is consistently similar.* They are used in a consistent manner, which suggests they relate to *consistent contexts.* As a result, they give the appearance of being a transition to *real* words, in the same way that jargon might be considered a predecessor to syntax. However, they do not represent attempts at real words.

8. (Answer: a) The key element in this question is the infant's desire to achieve some "goal" or result. Although no words are involved, the use of relatively conventional gestures (e.g., pointing, reaching) that can be correctly interpreted, not inferred, signals the onset of intentionality. Intentionality is the essential development of the illocutionary stage.

9. (Answer: b) This question reflects the chronology of infant vocal behavior milestones. The earliest vocal behavior is *reflexive cries,* followed by *cooing, marginal babbling,* and *vocal play. Jargon,* which mimics the syllable strings and intonational contours of adult speech, is the latest developing of these infant prelinguistic behaviors.

10. (Answer: e) When infants and their caregivers engage in game playing, there is a distinct pattern in their behaviors. There is first a *greeting* phase, in which they recognize and acknowledge each other's presence. The game is initiated in what is called the *engagement* phase. Finally, at the end of each episode of a game, there will be a *pause* phase that follows one game and precedes the next episode, if there is to be one. Finally, games such as "pat-a-cake" are clear examples of *joint action* between infants and caregivers.

Chapter 6

1. (Answer: b) No one has proposed (at least recently) that any words are genetically imprinted. Otherwise, the key phrase in Clark's hypothesis is "semantic feature." The *uses or actions* associated with items would usually constitute their *functions;* this would relate to Nelson's functional core hypothesis. The first experience of a word and its referent could be called a *prototype,* as in Bowerman's prototypic complex hypothesis. Semantic features would refer to *perceptual features* (size, shape, etc.), which were the defining aspects for words according to Clark's semantic feature hypothesis.

2. (Answer: e) Classically, in terms of grammatical categories, children's earliest words are assumed to be nouns. However, according to Bloom and Lahey, the early words also represent basic semantic roles within the larger category of *reflexive* relations. Although nouns label objects, words used in *reflexive* relations relate the object to itself in some way. These roles include *existence, nonexistence, disappearance,* and *recurrence.* In fulfilling these roles, Bloom and Lahey also noted that children might use words other than nouns, as in *dis* (this), *dat* (that), *allgone,* and *more.*

3. (Answer: b) Early true single words and successive single-word utterances are produced similarly. In both, the words are produced individually, under separate intonational contours; each sounds like a series of individual words. Distinguishing among them requires analyzing their referents and contexts. True single words occur in response to separate, isolated referents—each additional word, produced one after the other, could be considered a listing of

separate items. In contrast, each word in successive single-word utterances relates to the *same* context.

4. (Answer: e) Most researchers have long agreed that imitation is necessary for learning vocabulary. Caregivers teach many new words daily with the phrase "Can you say _____?" The role of imitation in learning grammar has been more controversial, but it is now generally agreed that children *selectively imitate* those structures they are trying to learn.

5. (Answer: e) Overextensions have been described as words used with *broad reference*. They often can be traced to some physical or functional *similarity*. Overextensions are *more common* than underextensions. And they are based on *stimulus generalization* usually tied to the physical or functional similarities.

6. (Answer: c) Most adults would not respond with more information than a child can understand or confirm (a). Occasionally, a busy, distracted adult responds in a way that fails to acknowledge the child's utterance (b). Some adult responses serve simply to affirm the child's utterance (d). Rarely would adult responses attempt to specifically teach grammar or the technical terms of grammar (e). When adults expand children's utterances, they repeat the utterance and insert one or two additional grammatical structures.

7. (Answer: a) As children develop vocabulary, they exhibit different behaviors that evoke responses from adults. In a present context, they may simply *imitate* the adult's model. Later, if uncertain, they may use the word affirmatively, with the expectation that this *evocative utterance* will evoke a confirmation or correction. On the other hand, if they do not have an available response, they may simply produce an *interrogative utterance,* such as "Wassat?" to ask for a name. Finally, when children have a word available, but are uncertain that it applies, they may engage in *hypothesis testing* by producing the word with a rising intonation.

8. (Answer: c) Caregivers have been observed to produce *imitations* of children's early utterances, seemingly to confirm when they are grammatically well formed. They tend to produce *expansions,* adding one or two grammatical structures, in response to their children's grammatically deficient utterances. When caregivers produce ex-

tensions, they address the topic mentioned by the child while adding relevant semantic information. If the assumption is that, as children's utterances become longer they are becoming grammatically more mature, it becomes less likely that caregivers will need to engage in teaching grammatical structure as MLU increases and more likely that they will engage in exchanging additional semantic information.

9. (Answer: c) Focus operations (and substitution operations) are forms of *selective imitation* that appear to be grammatically progress. In focus operations, children focus on two key elements (words) in the adult's model to imitate. In this instance, the child's response that includes two key elements from the adult utterance demonstrates a *focus operation.*

10. (Answer: a) There are no attributes (pretty, dirty, etc.) being mentioned with regard to either the leaves or Daddy. The child does not appear to be indicating that the leaves "belong to" Daddy (although Mommy would probably see it that way). Neither does the child seem to be addressing the location of the leaves (although the neighbors would be sure to clarify that, if necessary). Nor is the child addressing the location of Daddy; he is not lying down in the leaves (although the "little boy" in Daddy might be tempted). In the child's utterance, Daddy is acting on the leaves and, conversely, the leaves are being affected by Daddy's action.

Chapter 7

1. (Answer: c) *Functional stimuli* include those stimuli that have become capable of *influencing* an individual's behavior. The types of stimuli that would qualify in that way would be discriminative stimuli that set the occasion for certain responses, reinforcing stimuli that increase the likelihood of certain responses, and even eliciting stimuli that have become classically conditioned to be associated with certain autonomic responses (e.g., hunger, anxiety, etc.)

2. (Answer: d) Children learn dimensional words in distinct patterns in which they tend to first apply the term for the "positive" end or presence of the dimension overall. This is the *unmarked* word. They also tend to learn terms that refer to more general dimensions. In other words, for the size

continuum, they will tend to first use "big" to describe any size dimensions; big signals the "presence" of size. Additionally, they will tend to learn the "big-little" dimension, which applies to a broad array of contexts, before they learn the "shallow-deep" dimension, which applies to a very limited set of contexts.

3. (Answer: b) Primitive narratives are an early form of storytelling and are not relevant to this question. Parallel play is described as children playing separately alongside each other—nearby one another with each one "doing his or her own thing." In terms of socialized speech, *monologue* and *affect expressive monologue* would be analogous to solitary play, and *associated monologue* would be relatively analogous to *cooperative play*. A *collective monologue* would occur when several children are near each other, each one narrating his or her play activities without regard for anyone else.

4. (Answer: c) The order of learning in relational words generally follows a sequence from broader contexts and simpler discriminations to more limited contexts and more complex discriminations. In the choices provided, *in* and *on* are simpler than *in front* and *behind, big* and *little* are broader in application than *deep* and *shallow, mother* and *father* are simpler, more familiar relationships than *grandfather* and *grandmother,* and the colors *blue* and *green* are more commonplace than *chartreuse* and *taupe.* However, the concept of separate but simultaneous events encoded by *while* and *at the same time* is more abstract than the concept of sequential events as in *before* and *after.*

5. (Answer: b) The types of stimuli that contribute to settings can be categorized by the nature of the sensations. *Physical stimuli* are items with a physical or tangible existence. *Organismic stimuli* are those sensations that originate from within the individual. *Social stimuli* relate to interactions with other individuals. *Chemical stimuli* emanate from the environment and relate to the nature of substances, gases, solutions, and so forth, such as the chemicals carried into the air from cooking spinach.

6. (Answer: d) *Fast mapping* and *extended mapping* both relate to how children learn words. *Fast mapping* refers to the child's first exposure to a word and precedes *extended mapping* in which

the child gradually expands and modifies his or her understanding of the word's meaning—similar to your first impression of someone and what you learn about the person as the relationship continues.

7. (Answer: b) One of the earliest narrative forms, *eventcasts,* exhibited by children relate primarily to social roles in playing. *Heaps* are stories that, much like their name suggests, consist of story elements that are "piled up" and not clearly related by topic or chronology. Of the remaining types, *centering* might involve a chronology but primarily focuses on relating story elements to a central theme (e.g., goodness, anger, loneliness). In addition, it develops later than *chaining,* which is primarily based on linking the elements of a story together in a temporal sequence.

8. (Answer: a) Mastering locational terms is influenced by the complexity of the discriminations that must be made. For example, judging *in front* and *behind* might be based on whether an item is between the speaker and the referent (*The chair is in front of the table*) or the referent is between the item and the speaker (*The chair is behind the table*). In addition, these terms might also be based on whether the referent has an inherent front and back, such as a TV, in which case the speaker's perspective does not matter. In contrast, locational terms such as *in* and *on* are determined directly.

9. (Answer: e) *Topic maintenance* occurs when alternating utterances between partners address the same topic. *Turn taking* refers to the alternating utterances by partners in a conversation. *Presupposition* relates to the ability of speakers to understand their listener's abilities and knowledge about the topic. These elements all contribute to the *cohesion* or relatedness between utterances in *discourse.*

10. (Answer: e) Language that is contextualized refers to utterances that relate to the immediate surroundings; their meanings are closely tied to the immediate context. This is typical of younger children who tend to talk about "the here-and-now." *Decontextualized language* refers to language that is based on objects, people, and events in remote contexts and is associated with the development of narratives in which children begin to "tell stories."

Chapter 8

1. (Answer: c) Brown was interested in whether there was any uniformity in the children's development of the 14 grammatical morphemes. He found that Eve was precocious in her rate of development and Adam was generally a little later. The three children developed the 14 grammatical morphemes in relatively similar sequences.

2. (Answer: c) Punctuation concerns only apply in written forms, and production effects such as pauses or a confident tone have nothing to do with this grammatical distinction. Clauses by definition have to contain more than one word; similarly, sentences may consist of only two words but may contain more than that. Clauses consist of groups of words that contain a subject and a predicate. Sentences are also groups of words that contain a subject and a predicate. However, a clause is not grammatically complete, whereas a sentence is grammatically complete.

3. (Answer: b) Brown was interested in determining if any particular measure could be predictive of development, at least within the grammatical morphemes he studied. He correlated several measures with the development of the grammatical morphemes. It has not been indicated anywhere that he even recorded the children's height. It is possible that he indexed the average number of syllables, but this has not been widely reported. Two of the choices, birth date and chronological age would be equivalent; more importantly, chronological age was not found to be as predictive of the grammatical morphemes' development as the average number of morphemes per utterance, or "mean length of utterance in morphemes" (MLU).

4. (Answer: e) The distinction being posed for analysis is between the auxiliary and copula forms. In this case, the form "was" has been *transposed* to form a yes-no question. It may help to place it back in its original position between the subject and complement, resulting in the simple active declarative form, "He was at the house." The first decision is based on determining whether "was" is a helping verb (auxiliary) or the main verb (copula). The next decision is to decide if it is contractible without losing any of its sense of past tense.

5. (Answer: a) The earliest questions of young children will be based on the semantic relationships they recognize and respond to cognitively. Young preschoolers do not yet have a mature sense of *causality*. The younger they are, the more they tend to "operate in the here-and-now" as opposed to thinking about *future events*. Similarly, they are less concerned with the role of items as *instruments* or *ownership* of objects beyond mere association. However, younger children are very eager to learn the *labels for objects and actions*.

6. (Answer: b) Presentence negation indicates that the negative form (no, not, don't, etc.) precedes the entire sentence construction. Prepredicate negation indicates that the negative form is placed in front of the predicate or verb in the sentence.

7. (Answer: e) Pronominal, or pronouns, represent a very complex set of forms with many variations. As a result, mastering the pronominal system varies across children. As with many other forms of language, children tend to first learn the forms that have the broadest application and do not vary for gender or person, as in "it" and "that." In addition, younger children, still in Piaget's egocentric period, see the world from a point of view that requires forms like "I" and "me."

8. (Answer: d) Modal auxiliaries are forms that convey a sense of mood or attitude regarding the verb. Forms such as *should, could, must, can, may, might,* and *will* indicate various attitudes toward the verbs they precede. Forms like *have been* consist of multiple auxiliaries.

9. (Answer: e) The reversible and plausible distinctions refer to factors that influence children's interpretation of roles within sentences, especially when trying to comprehend active form versus passive form. A *reversible* sentence carries the possibility of reversing the nouns—"Tom kissed Mary" ("Mary kissed Tom") versus "Tom kissed the trophy" ("The trophy kissed Tom"). The feature of *plausibility* is a secondary consideration with sentences that are reversible. The reverse versions may be more or less likely—"Tom kissed the kitty" is technically reversible, but the reverse version ("The kitty kissed Tom") is less *plausible,* unless licking can be equated to kissing.

10. (Answer: c) *Order of mention* refers to the sequential relationship among the events in compound sentences based on temporal conjunctions

(*before, after, until, while, since*). Perhaps due to the prevalence of simple active declarative forms in our language, children come to rely more on the left-to-right order of events as reflecting their sequence. In that case, a child would interpret the sentence posed in this question based on the order of events mentioned—painted the house, had some lunch—without regard for the temporal conjunction, *before.*

Chapter 9

1. (Answer: d) Various forms qualify as figurative language by the fact that their interpretation is based on stimulus generalization—a figurative as opposed to a literal interpretation. *Idioms* are short expressions of analogous relationships ("Don't let the cat out of the bag"). *Metaphoric transparency* refers to the directness of the analogy in resembling the actual relationship described. For example, although most of us understand the idiom "He kicked the bucket," it does not directly suggest its meaning the way "He spilled the beans" does. *Metalinguistics* is the ability to evaluate the significance of language elements apart from their usual referents or contexts; metalinguistic ability is basic to appreciating the symbolic nature of figurative language and the nature of *humor. Embedding* is strictly a grammatical process in which one independent clause is grammatically inserted into another.

2. (Answer: a) The shift from *syntagmatic* to *paradigmatic* word associations is reflected in a child's changing from associations based on a possible syntactic relationship (e.g., between "car" and "drive" as a noun and verb) to a more semantically based relationship (e.g., "car" and "truck" as members of a category).

3. (Answer: d) Figurative language is a later developing ability in which children can interpret and use *idioms, metaphors,* and *proverbs* appropriately and *creatively.* Although grammatical inflections for nouns and verbs might coincide with this development, their mastery is not directly related.

4. (Answer: e) *Humor* is a complex, multifaceted phenomenon. It involves *metalinguistics* in that one must recognize that words can be objects of

analysis. Analyzing words in a given context might reveal *ambiguity,* and, further, that one of the possible meanings is unexpected and therefore funny. Finally, the ambiguity can be introduced at various levels—*phonological, lexical, surface structure,* and *deep structure.*

5. (Answer: c) The structures that tend to be mastered later by children are those that are less commonly used and also have varied forms that require multiple discriminations. Of the choices presented, the *present progressive inflection* "ing," the "be" verbs is and *are,* prepositions *in* and *on,* and *personal pronouns,* are mastered earlier. The *reflexive pronouns,* such as *myself, yourself,* and *himself,* are used less commonly and are mastered later.

6. (Answer: c) *Horizontal development* refers to learning additional features that are associated with a word. Recognizing that words rhyme is related to *metalinguistic ability.* Learning the rules for spelling is related to development of *literacy. Vertical development* in vocabulary involves learning that a word can have multiple meanings and they might exist at different levels of association.

7. (Answer: b) The relationship indicated by the child's statement reflects *superordinate-subordinate categories* and a shift from *thematic-taxonomic organization* of vocabulary, which occur at a *later stage of vocabulary development* associated with exposure to *school* and academic settings. It is not likely that the word "furniture" would be learned before the word "table," and, even so, there is no set order of vocabulary development.

8. (Answer: b) The patterns indicated in the answers reflect *expository style* and *textbook grammar.* Some words or phrases (*refers to, similar to*) used in textbooks represent *description patterns,* which obviously refer to words that describe something. There are words (*first, next*) that signal a sequence pattern. Some words (*including, such as*) indicate a *collection pattern,* in which examples will follow. Other words (*because, consequently*) signal a *cause-effect pattern.* Finally, other words (*similarly, although,* or *conversely*) signal that comparisons will be made.

9. (Answer: d) *Jargon* can refer to the strings of nonsense syllable produced by infants as well as

technical terms associated with a specialized area that sound nonsensical to those who are not familiar with them. *Genderlect,* as the stem word "gender" suggests, refers to language styles that are distinct to the two genders. Although the term *dialect* might be remotely related to differences in how we speak to people representing different social roles, it is not as specific as the term *register. Illocutions* would relate only to the intentions that might be involved (e.g., getting a raise) as opposed to the language style or *register* we might invoke in attempting to convey them (when asking for a raise).

10. (Answer: c) To the extent someone has spent time with elderly person, it would be recognized that most do not experience dramatic changes in *grammatical ability, comprehension, abstract reasoning,* or their *sense of humor.* However, *word finding* is occasionally more difficult for many elderly.

Chapter 10

1. (Answer: c) The situation described proposes nothing that would preclude someone from learning English, especially if the native language had been learned without difficulty. Learning new languages appears to be easier for younger individuals, especially prior to adolescence. When an individual grows up with exposure to two or more languages and learns them concurrently, it is called *simultaneous acquisition.* The scenario described in this question relates to what is described as *successive acquisition,* in which one language is learned first followed by learning another language.

2. (Answer: c) The term *bilingual* indicates that an individual speaks two languages. Because languages are defined as *codes,* changing from one language to the other is called *code switching.* In contrast, when an individual is capable of changing the manner of speaking between the devices and styles associated with a dialect and the standard form of a language, it is called *style shifting.*

3. (Answer: e) Dialects have been found to evidence differences related to *socioeconomic* levels, *cultural* differences, *geographic* influences, and *ethnic* origins.

4. (Answer: d) Dialects can be evident in changes affecting aspects beyond the phonological component, including lexical items and grammatical patterns. Although some dialects reflect differences due to socioeconomic level, which can be a reflection of education, there is not a direct connection between dialects and education or intelligence. Dialects are based on systematic differences in rules that have their own internal consistency.

5. (Answer: c) Many changes in Black English are related to reducing consonant clusters, including those related to past tense inflections, especially when the context provides additional necessary information. However, normal intonation is maintained and there is no reduction in the variety of vowels used in speakers of Black English. Dangling prepositional phrases is a pattern in north central regions of the country, but it is not characteristic of Black English.

6. (Answer: e) In the case of Hispanic English (or any language), the deletion of all initial consonants would render speech almost unintelligible. On the other hand, many speakers of Hispanic English customarily omit the inversion of the noun-copula in auxiliary inversion questions ("Bill is coming?") or use postnoun modifiers to mark possession ("Find the book of Billy's, please").

7. (Answer: e) All of the changes indicated as answers to the question are possible in Asian English.

8. (Answer: e) The term *language disorders* can refer to disruptions in the learning of language in a multifaceted manner. Development of the abilities related to *grammar, semantics,* and *pragmatics* can be affected in an isolated or combined manner in a language disorder. In addition, some children may exhibit disturbances in their expressive abilities or receptive abilities, or both.

9. (Answer: c) The terms *standardized* and *nonstandardized* apply to testing or assessment procedures but have not been used to describe language disorders. *Language disorders* and *language delays* have traditionally been more descriptive than etiological in nature. *Style shifting* and *code shifting* might be considered evidence of language differences, but not language disorders. With re-

gard to etiology, the terms *organic* and *functional* have traditionally been used to distinguish between language disorders with physical causes (hearing loss, brain damage, etc.) versus those due to faulty learning or deficient models.

10. (Answer: e) There are several distinctions implied by the terms *standardized* and *nonstandardized* as applied to assessment. *Standardized* can refer to the use of norms based on peer performances as the standard or measure of normal. It can also mean "to make uniform," as in the use of materials and procedures that are uniform whenever a test is administered. Finally, *nonstandardized* can suggest the other end of the continuum, in which procedures are less uniform and more natural, as in language sampling.

Major Communication Milestones

Age	Communication Milestones	Prompts for Eliciting Behavioral Observations
Birth–4 months	Exhibits startle response (Moro reflex) to sudden, loud noises.	What does your child do when a door slams or someone shouts unexpectedly?
	Localizes to sound, especially the human voice.	What does your child do when a new sound occurs in the room or when someone begins talking?
	Produces differentiated cries (different cries for hunger, pain, etc.) within a few weeks following birth.	Does your child's cry sound different at times?
	Produces cooing (primarily vowel-like) sounds during comfortable states.	What does your child do when he or she is alone, comfortable, and awake?
4–6 months	Exhibits social smile in response to familiar faces.	How does your child react when he or she sees a familiar face?
	Quiets and attends when adult voice is heard or person enters his or her visual field.	What does your child do when someone enters the room or begins talking?
	Takes turns in mutual gaze and vocalization patterns with adult partner.	How does your child react when you make eye contact and speak softly to him or her?
	Produces babbling that is redundant in syllable structure—*dada, baba.*	What kinds of sounds and syllables does your child produce when playing or resting alone?
6–9 months	Recognizes others' emotions through their facial expressions and vocal tones.	How does your child respond to you when you are happy? How does he or she respond when firmly told, for example, "No, don't touch"?
	Responds to routinized words and phrases (e.g., "hi," "bye-bye") and gestures ("peek-a-boo" and "please-thank you games").	How does your child respond to people coming and going? How do you and your child play games?
	Exhibits babbling that is increasingly varied in sounds and syllable structure.	How varied are the sounds and syllables your child produces?
	Recognizes own name when spoken to him or her.	What does your child do if you call him or her by name?

(continued)

Age	Communication Milestones	Prompts for Eliciting Behavioral Observations
9–12 months	Expresses intentions to obtain objects (protoimperatives) or attention (protodeclaratives) through characteristic gestures and vocalizations.	How does your child obtain objects he or she desires or direct your attention?
	Searches for family members or favorite objects when named.	What does your child do when a favorite toy or a family member's name is mentioned?
	Exhibits vocal play and jargon with adultlike syllable strings and intonation.	What does your child do that appears as though he or she is trying to talk more?
	Names or requests objects with phonetically consistent forms.	How does your child indicate he or she desires a favorite toy or ask for a favorite food?
12–18 months	Produces first true word (i.e., approximation of a conventional adult word).	What does your child say to familiar people arriving or leaving? How does he or she ask for items that they want?
	Points to one to three body parts when named.	What does your child do if you ask him or her to find their tummy? Nose? Eyes?
	Imitates individual words frequently.	How does your child indicate that he or she hears words you use when talking to him or her?
	Learns new words quickly, accumulating approximately 50 words by 18 months.	How many different words does your child use regularly to name things and talk to people?
18–24 months	Listens as pictures are named or stories are read and indicates those that are "favorites."	How much does your child like picture books or story books?
	Produces frequent two-word phrases with noun-verb (agent-action) and adjective-noun (attribute-entity).	How does your child describe objects or others' activities?
	Understands basic categories such as toys, foods, clothes.	What does your child do when asked to "find a toy"?
	Achieves vocabulary of 200–300 words by 24 months; frequently requests labels for unfamiliar objects ("Watdis?").	What does your child do when he or she does not know the name for something?
24–30 months	Produces two- and three-word utterances and simple sentences with increasing frequency.	How complete are your child's sentences when he or she talks about things?
	Executes two-part commands.	How many simple tasks can your child be asked to do at once?
	Gives simple answers to certain wh-questions involving location ("where"), action ("what doing"), and functions ("what for").	How does your child respond when asked where things are, what someone is doing, or what things are for?
	Includes early grammatical morphemes (articles, progressive inflection, plural inflection) in simple sentences.	How many word endings does your child include in his or her sentences?

Age	Communication Milestones	Prompts for Eliciting Behavioral Observations
30–36 months	Achieves a vocabulary of 800–900 words; asks and answers a variety of simple wh-questions (who, what doing, what, where).	How does your child learn about the people, things, and events around him or her?
	Uses short simple sentences, typically three to four words in length with additional grammatical words and word endings (copula/auxiliary verbs, past tense inflections, personal pronouns).	How complete are your child's sentences?
	Understands basic concepts of color, shape, size, location.	How much detail does your child give when describing things to you?
	Maintains topic over several conversational turns when sharing a book or telling a story about a topic related to the immediate context.	Describe a conversation you have had with your child while looking at a book or talking about something you're doing.
3–4 years	Produces predominantly four- or five-word sentences and an increasing number of compound or complex sentences.	How does your child make his or her sentences longer to combine several ideas into one sentence?
	Reaches peak of question-asking phase with frequent wh-questions—Why? How? Where? When?	How does your child exhibit his or her curiosity?
	Includes plurals, possessives, and multiple adjectives in sentences when appropriate.	How does your child indicate that he or she wants more than one snack? That something belongs to him or her? Or, which of several similar items is the one he or she wants?
	Maintains longer, detailed conversations or narratives about topics that are present, remote, and imaginary.	What kinds of "stories" does your child tell when you are having a long conversation?
4–5 years	Understands 10,000-plus words, including words for relative concepts of time (before/after, yesterday/tomorrow) and quantity (more/less, most/least).	How does your child tell you about past and upcoming events? How does he or she describe amounts when trying to share candies or cookies?
	Produces five- to eight-word sentences with few grammatical errors, primarily in irregular forms (e.g., children), reflexive pronouns (e.g., himself), adverbial suffixes (e.g., quick*ly*), and comparative/superlative inflections (-er/-est).	How much do your child's sentences sound similar to or different from your own?

(continued)

Age	Communication Milestones	Prompts for Eliciting Behavioral Observations
	Uses indirect requests, requests clarifications, and adjusts speaking styles for listeners of different ages or roles.	How much does your child's language reflect that he or she is aware of who they are talking to (e.g., little brothers versus teachers) when trying to achieve some goal?
	Tells relatively detailed narratives about own experiences, in both the recent and remote past.	How much detail does your child include when telling about his or her past experiences?
Lower Grades	Demonstrates vocabulary for almost everything in daily experiences with definitions based on the functions of things.	Are there any items that your child frequently interacts with that he or she cannot name? How would your child define the word *car* . . .?
	Evidences syntagmatic-paradigmatic shift while beginning to organize words according to hierarchical categories.	How does your child indicate that some things "go together" (as in "conceptual families")?
	Applies verbal strategies in describing ideas and reasoning about relationships.	How does your child develop new ideas or analyze problems by talking about them?
	Exhibits understanding of figurative language and ambiguous meanings.	How has your child used "a figure of speech" (idioms or metaphors) to describe people or events? How does your child show his or her sense of humor?
Upper Grades	Exhibits general mastery of remaining grammatical features, including irregular nouns and verbs, comparatives and superlatives, and adverbial suffixes.	What kinds of grammatical errors are you aware of in your child's speech?
	Expands vocabulary skills, including use of definitions based on categorical or taxonomic style.	How would your child define the word *car* . . .?
	Exhibits flexibility and creativity in using multiple word meanings.	How creative is your child in describing something or making a point during a discussion?
	Exhibits emerging formal expository writing skills.	How does your child construct a class term paper on a topic assigned by a teacher?
Adult years	Develops specialized vocabulary according to vocation or profession.	What new skills or information have you acquired as part of your training/education?
	Uses expository language to effectively alter others' opinions or actions.	How would you convince a police officer that you really weren't speeding, or ask a waitress to make substitutions from the menu?
	Exhibits genderlect in talking to persons of the different sexes.	How do you talk differently to your spouse as opposed to your best friends?
	Exhibits speech registers based on social roles and contexts.	How would you ask for a glass of water from your boss? Your neighbor? Your wife?

Age	Communication Milestones	Prompts for Eliciting Behavioral Observations
Senior years	Exhibits increasing difficulty related to hearing and discriminating the speech of those around them, especially in noisy situations.	How often does your spouse ask others to repeat themselves? When does this seem to happen most often?
	Exhibits changes in vocal quality, breath groups, and fragmentation behaviors related to word-finding.	How has the sound and flow of your spouse's speech changed since he or she retired?
	Exhibits increased difficulty in using precise vocabulary—the names and terms—for people and things.	How much difficulty does your spouse have naming the people and things he or she talks about?

NOTE. Adapted from *Terminology of Communication Disorders: Speech—Language—Hearing* (5th ed.), by L. Nicolosi, E. Harryman, and J. Kresheck, 2003, Baltimore: Williams & Wilkins; *Language Development: An Introduction* (5th ed.), by R. E. Owens, 2005, Boston: Allyn & Bacon; *The Dynamics of Communicative Development,* by V. W. Lane and D. Molyneaux, 1992, Englewood Cliffs, NJ: Prentice-Hall.

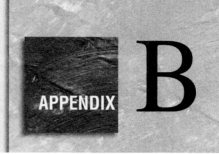

Language and Literacy Expectations by School Grade

B-1 Kindergarten through Fourth Grade

(Skills are presented cumulatively; that is, those expected in earlier grades would be expected in subsequent grades also.)

Language Skills

Listening

The student will listen for information and for pleasure.

Kindergarten

1. Hear and repeat sounds in a sequence.
2. Listen with interest to stories read aloud.
3. Follow one- and two-step directions.

First Grade

1. Listen attentively and ask questions for clarification and understanding.
2. Give, restate, and follow simple two-step directions.

Second Grade

1. Give, restate, and follow simple two- and three-step directions.

Third Grade

1. Listen critically for information and incorporate the information into other activities.
2. Listen actively for pleasure and respond appropriately.

Fourth Grade

1. Listen to directions and questions and respond appropriately.
2. Listen critically and respond appropriately to oral communication.
3. Listen and respond to teacher-read stories.

Speaking

The student will express ideas or opinions in group or individual settings.

Kindergarten

1. Share information and ideas, speaking in clear, complete, coherent sentences.
2. Recite short poems, rhymes, and songs.

First Grade

1. Stay on topic when speaking.
2. Use descriptive words when speaking about people, places, things, and events.
3. Retell stories using basic story grammar and relating the sequence of story events by answering who, what, when, where, why, and how questions.
4. Relate an important life event or personal experience in a simple sequence.
5. Provide descriptions with careful attention to sensory detail.
6. Use visual aids such as pictures and objects to present oral information.

Second Grade

1. Speak articulately and audibly using appropriate language, correct usage, enunciation, and volume.
2. Provide descriptions using correct sequence of events and details.
3. Use verbal and nonverbal communication in effective ways, such as making announcements, giving directions, or making instructions.

Third Grade

1. Make brief narrative (story) presentations that:
   a. Provide a context for an event that is the subject of the presentation.
   b. Provide insight into why the selected event should be of interest to the audience.
   c. Include well-chosen details to develop characters, a setting, and a plot.

3. Plan and present dramatic interpretations of experiences, stories, poems, or plays.

4. Organize ideas chronologically (in the order they happened) or around major points of information.

5. Use clear and specific vocabulary to communicate ideas and establish the tone of the message.

6. Provide a clear beginning, middle, and end when making oral presentations and include details that develop a central idea.

Fourth Grade

1. Use traditional structures for conveying information, including cause and effect, similarity and difference, and posing and answering a question.

2. Emphasize points in ways that help the listener or viewer to follow important ideas and concepts (e.g., pausing, hand gestures, inflection volume, body language).

Literacy Skills

Print Awareness

The student will understand the characteristics of written language.

Kindergarten

1. Demonstrate correct book orientation by holding the book correctly (right side up) and indicating where to begin (e.g., front to back, top to bottom, left to right).

2. Identify the front cover, back cover, and title page of a book and title and author.

3. Follow words from left to right and from top to bottom on the printed page.

4. Understand that printed materials provide information.

5. Recognize that sentences in print are made up of separate words.

6. Distinguish letters from words.

7. Recognize and name all capital and lowercase letters of the alphabet.

First Grade

1. Read from left to right, top to bottom.

2. Match spoken word to print.

3. Recognize the difference among letters, words, and sentences.

Phonological/Phonemic Awareness

The student will demonstrate the ability to hear, identify, and manipulate large parts of spoken language (e.g., words, syllables, onsets, and rhymes) and individual sounds (phonemes) in spoken words.

Kindergarten

1. Identify and produce simple rhyming pairs.
2. Identify and count syllables in spoken words.
3. Distinguish onset (beginning sound[s]) and rhymes in one-syllable words.
4. Recognize ending sounds in spoken words.
5. Recognize the same sounds in different words.
6. Begin to blend phonemes to form a word.
7. Begin to segment phonemes of one-syllable words.

First Grade

1. Create and state groups of rhyming words.
2. Identify onsets and rhymes.
3. Segment and blend the phonemes of one-syllable words.
4. Isolate phonemes within words by identifying the beginning, middle, and ending sounds in one-syllable words.
5. Add or delete a phoneme to change a word.

Second Grade

1. Demonstrate an awareness of the sounds that are made by different letters by distinguishing beginning, middle, and ending sounds in words, rhyming words, and clearly pronouncing blends and vowel sounds.
   a. Segment and blend the phonemes of one- and two-syllable words.
   b. Substitute a phoneme change to create a different word.

Phonics/Decoding

The student will demonstrate the ability to apply sound/symbol relationships.

Kindergarten

1. Identify the alphabet by name.
2. Identify the alphabet by sound.

First Grade

1. Phonetic Analysis—Apply phonics knowledge to decode one-syllable words.
   a. Use short and long vowel patterns.
   b. Use r-controlled vowel patterns.
   c. Use blends (e.g., fl, tr), digraphs (e.g., sh, th), and diphthongs (e.g., oi, ow).
2. Structural Analysis—Apply knowledge of structural analysis to decode words using strategies such as inflectional endings, contractions and compound words, and possessives.

Second Grade

1. Phonetic Analysis
   a. Use consonant sounds in beginning, medial, and final positions.
   b. Use short, long, and r-controlled vowel sounds.
2. Structural Analysis
   a. Build and understand compound words, contractions, and base words using prefixes and suffixes.
   b. Apply knowledge of basic syllabication rules to decode words in text.

Third Grade

1. Phonetic Analysis—Apply knowledge of phonetic analysis to decode unknown words (e.g., common letter/sound relationships, consonants, blends, digraphs, vowels, and diphthongs).
2. Structural Analysis—Apply knowledge of structural analysis to decode unknown words (e.g., syllabication rules, affixes, root words, compound words, spelling patterns, contractions, final stable syllables).
3. Apply knowledge of sentence structures and semantics in conjunction with phonics and structural analysis to decode unknown words.

Vocabulary

The student will develop and expand knowledge of words and word meanings to increase vocabulary.

Kindergarten

1. Use new vocabulary and language in own speech.
2. Use new vocabulary and language in own writing.

First Grade

1. Increase personal vocabulary by listening to and reading a variety of literature.
2. Discuss unfamiliar oral and/or written vocabulary after listening to or reading texts.
3. Use new vocabulary and language in own speech and writing.
4. Classify categories of words.

Second Grade

1. Words in Context—Expand vocabulary in language and writing by reading and listening to a variety of texts.
2. Synonyms, Antonyms, and Homonyms—Understand and explain common antonyms (words with opposite meanings), synonyms (words with the same meanings), and homonyms (words with the same sound and spelling but different meanings).
3. Affixes—Know the meaning of simple prefixes and suffixes.

Third Grade

1. Words in Context—Use context clues (the meaning of the text around the word) to determine the meaning of grade-level appropriate words.
2. Affixes—Use prefixes (for example, un-, pre-, bi-, mis-, dis-, en-, in-, im-, ir-), suffixes (for example, -er, -est, -ful, -ness, -ing, -ish, -less), and roots to determine the meaning of words.
3. Synonyms, Antonyms, and Homonyms—Determine the meanings of words using knowledge of synonyms, antonyms, homonyms, and multiple-meaning words.
4. Using Resource Materials—Use word reference materials (glossary, dictionary, thesaurus) to determine the meaning and pronunciation of unknown words.

Fourth Grade

1. Words in Context—Use context clues (the meaning of the text around a word) to distinguish and interpret the meaning of multiple-meaning words a well as other unfamiliar words.
2. Affixes, Roots, and Derivatives
    a. Interpret new words by analyzing the meaning of prefixes and suffixes.
    b. Use knowledge of root words (e.g., snow, snowbound, snowdrift) and word parts (therm = heat) derived from Greek and Latin to analyze the meaning of complex words (thermometer).

3. Synonyms, Antonyms, and Homonyms—Apply knowledge of fourth-grade-level synonyms, antonyms, homonyms, multiple-meaning words, and idioms to determine the meanings of words and phrases.

4. Using Resource Materials
   a. Use a thesaurus to determine related words and concepts.
   b. Determine the meanings and pronunciations of unknown words by using a glossary and/or dictionary.

Fluency

The student will demonstrate the ability to identify words in text.

Kindergarten

1. "Read" familiar texts emergently, not necessarily verbatim from the print alone.
2. Recognize some words by sight, including a few very common ones (e.g., a, the, I, my, you, is, are).

First Grade

1. Read regularly in independent-level text (text in which no more than 1 in 20 words is difficult for the reader) effortlessly and with expression.
2. Read regularly in instructional-level text (text in which no more than 1 in 10 words is difficult for the reader; a "typical" first grader reads approximately 60 words per minute).
3. Engage in repeated readings of the same text to increase fluency.
4. Recognize 100–200 high-frequency and/or common irregularly spelled words in text. (e.g., have, to, was, where, said).
5. Use punctuation cues (e.g., periods, commas, question marks) in text as a guide to understand meaning.

Second Grade

1. Read regularly in independent-level text (text in which no more than 1 in 20 words is difficult for the reader) effortlessly and with expression.
2. Read regularly in instructional-level text that is challenging yet manageable (texts in which no more than 1 in 10 words is difficult for the reader; a "typical" second grader reads approximately 75 words per minute).
3. Accurately and fluently read 200–300 high-frequency and/or irregularly spelled words in meaningful text.

Third Grade

1. Read regularly in independent-level texts (texts in which no more than 1 in 20 words is difficult for the reader) fluently and accurately, and with appropriate rate, change in voice, and expression.
2. Read regularly in instructional-level texts that are challenging yet manageable (texts in which no more than 1 in 10 words is difficult for the reader; a "typical" third grader reads approximately 85 words per minute).
3. Accurately and fluently read 300–400 high-frequency and/or irregularly spelled words in meaningful texts.

Fourth Grade

1. Read aloud regularly in independent-level texts (texts in which no more than 1 in 20 words is difficult for the reader) fluently and accurately, and with appropriate rate, change in voice, and expression.
2. Read aloud regularly in instructional-level texts that are challenging yet manageable (texts in which no more than 1 in 10 words is difficult for the reader; a "typical" fourth grader reads approximately 95 words per minute).
3. Increase silent reading speed through daily independent reading.

Comprehension/Critical Literacy

The student will interact with the words and concepts in a text to construct an appropriate meaning.

Kindergarten

1. Use prereading skills (e.g., connecting prior knowledge to text, making predictions about text and using picture clues).
2. Retell, reenact, or dramatize a story read to the student or by the student.
3. Make predictions and confirm after reading or listening to text.
4. Tell what is happening in a picture.

First Grade

1. Literal Understanding
   a. Read and comprehend both fiction and nonfiction that is appropriately designed for the second half of first grade.
   b. Use prereading strategies such as previewing, using prior knowledge, predicting, and establishing a purpose for reading.
   c. Respond to questions designed to aid general comprehension.

2. Inferences and Interpretations—Make simple inferences based on what is stated in text.

3. Summary and Generalization
   a. Retell or act out stories and events using beginning, middle, and ending.
   b. Respond to who, what, when, where, why, and how questions and discuss the main idea of what is read.
   c. Draw and discuss visual images based on text information.

4. Analysis and Evaluation
   a. Identify simple cause-and-effect relationships.
   b. Mark favorite passages.

5. Monitoring and Correction Strategies—Apply a basic use of semantics, syntax, and graphophonic cues (e.g., Semantics—Does it make sense? Syntax—Does it sound right? Graphophonic—Does it look right?).

Second Grade

1. Literal Understanding
   a. Read and comprehend both fiction and nonfiction that is appropriately designed for the second half of second grade.
   b. Use prereading strategies to preview, activate prior knowledge, make predictions, use picture clues, and establish the purpose for reading (i.e., graphic organizers).
   c. Ask and respond to questions to aid comprehension about important elements of fiction and nonfiction.

2. Inferences and Interpretation
   a. Make inferences about events, characters, and ideas in fictional texts by connecting knowledge and experience to the story.
   b. Support interpretations or conclusions with examples taken from the text.

3. Summary and Generalization
   a. Retell or act out narrative text by identifying story elements and sequencing the events.
   b. Produce oral or written summaries of text selections by discussing who, what, when, where, why, and how to identify the main idea and significant supporting details of a text.

4. Analysis and Evaluation
   a. Identify cause-and-effect relationships in a text.
   b. Make comparisons and draw conclusions based on what is read.
   c. Describe character traits, changes, and relationships.

5. Monitoring and Correction Strategies—Integrate the use of semantics, syntax, and graphophonic cues to gain meaning from the text. (e.g., Semantics—Does it make sense? Syntax—Does it sound right? Graphophonic—Does it look right?)

Third Grade

1. Literal Understanding
   a. Read and comprehend poetry, fiction, and nonfiction that is appropriately designed for the second half of third grade.
   b. Use prereading strategies independently to preview, activate prior knowledge, predict content of text, and establish a purpose for reading.
   c. Recall major points in a text and revise predictions about what is read.
   d. Show understanding by asking questions and supporting answers with literal information from the text.

2. Inferences and Interpretation
   a. Make inferences by connecting prior knowledge and experience with information from the text.
   b. Interpret text, including lessons or morals depicted in fairytales, fables, and so forth, and draw conclusions from evidence presented in the text.
   c. Participate in creative response to text (e.g., art, drama, and oral presentations).

3. Summary and Generalization
   a. Summarize by recognizing main ideas, key concepts, key actions, and supporting details in fiction and nonfiction.
   b. Make generalizations about a text (e.g., theme of a story or main idea of an informational text).

4. Analysis and Evaluation
   a. Analyze characters, including their traits, relationships, feelings, and changes in text.
   b. Distinguish between fact and opinion in nonfiction text.
   c. Analyze the causes, motivations, sequences, and results of events from a text.

5. Monitoring and Correction Strategies
   a. Monitor own reading and modify strategies as needed (e.g., recognize when he or she is confused by a section of text, questions whether the text makes sense)
   b. Predict, monitor, and cross-check using semantic, syntactic, and graphophonic cues.
   c. Clarify meaning by rereading, questioning, and modifying predictions.

Fourth Grade

1. Literal Understanding
   a. Use prereading strategies independently to preview, activate prior knowledge, predict content of text, formulate questions that might

be answered in the text, establish and adjust purposes for reading (e.g., to find out, to understand, to enjoy, to solve problems).

2. Inferences and Interpretation
   a. Use prior knowledge and experience to make inferences and support them with information presented in text.
   b. Make interpretations and draw conclusions from fiction and nonfiction text beyond personal experience.
   c. Make inferences and draw conclusions about characters' qualities and actions (i.e., based on knowledge of plot, setting, characters' motives, characters' appearances, and other characters' responses to a character).
   d. Participate in creative responses to text (i.e., art, drama, and oral presentation).

3. Summary and Generalization
   a. Paraphrase by recognizing main ideas, key concepts, key actions, and supporting details in fiction and nonfiction to recall, inform, or organize ideas.
   b. Support ideas, arguments, and generalizations by reference to evidence in the text.
   c. Represent text information in different ways such as in outline, time line, or graphic organizer.

4. Analysis and Evaluation
   a. Evaluate new information and hypotheses by testing them against known information and ideas.
   b. Compare and contrast information on the same topic after reading several passages or articles.

Writing Process

The student will use the writing process to write coherently.

Kindergarten

1. Participate in frequent writing opportunities; for example, modeled writing, shared writing, journal writing, and interactive writing.
2. Dictate a story about an event or experience.
3. Read his or her own writing to the group, teacher, and/or parent.

First Grade

1. Participate in prewriting activities such as brainstorming, discussion, webbing, or story starters.
2. Write first drafts.
3. Be introduced to proofreading and editing.

4. Publish and share writing with various audiences, such as peers or adults.

Second Grade

1. Create a list of topic ideas for writing.
2. Use a process approach to write coherently, using developmentally appropriate steps of the writing process: prewriting, drafting, revising, editing or proofreading, and publishing or sharing.
3. Organize related ideas together to maintain a consistent focus by establishing a beginning, middle, and ending.

Third Grade

1. Use a variety of prewriting activities such as brainstorming, clustering, illustrating, and webbing.
2. Compose first drafts.
3. Revise selected drafts, changing or adding details and vivid words.
4. Proofread or edit writing with peers or teacher.
5. Share writing with peers or adults.

Fourth Grade

1. Use a variety of prewriting activities such as brainstorming, clustering, illustrating, webbing, and graphic organizers.
2. Select a focus and an organizational structure based on purpose, audience, length, and required format, and write one or more drafts by categorizing ideas, organizing them into paragraphs, and blending paragraphs into longer text.
3. Revise selected drafts by adding, elaborating, deleting, combining, and rearranging text.
4. Edit drafts to ensure standard usage, mechanics, spelling, and varied sentence structure.
5. Share writing with peers and adults.
6. Use common organizational structures for providing information in writing, such as chronological order (beginning, middle, and end), cause and effect, or similarity and difference, and posing and answering questions.

Grammar/Usage and Mechanics

The student will demonstrate appropriate practices in writing by applying Standard English conventions to the revising and editing stages of writing.

Kindergarten

1. Spelling: Demonstrate the process of representing language by means of a writing system.
   a. Recognize that letters have different sounds.
   b. Recognize and record some beginning and ending sounds in words.
   c. Generate temporary spelling using letters, particularly to represent initial and ending consonant sounds.

2. Handwriting: Demonstrate appropriate handwriting in the writing process.
   a. Trace, copy, and generate letters. Children may still be reversing some letters.
   b. Print his or her first and last names.

First Grade

1. Grammar/Usage: Students are beginning to recognize and use appropriate nouns, verbs, and adjectives in their writing.
   a. Singular and plural nouns
   b. Singular possessive pronouns
   c. Present and past tense verbs
   d. Contractions
   e. Adjectives

2. Mechanics: Students are expected to demonstrate appropriate language mechanics in writing; for example, capitalize the first word of a sentence, names of people, places, major holidays, days of the week, months of the year, and the pronoun "I."

3. Punctuation: Students are expected to demonstrate appropriate punctuation in writing; for example, correctly use periods, exclamation points, and question marks at the end of sentences.

4. Sentence Structure: The student will demonstrate appropriate sentence structure in writing; for example, write in complete sentences using a noun and verb in each sentence.

5. Spelling: Students are expected to demonstrate appropriate application of spelling knowledge to the revising and editing stages of writing.
   a. Spell correctly three- and four-letter words, and grade-level-appropriate sight words.
   b. Use a picture dictionary to gain information.

Second Grade

1. Grammar/Usage: Students are expected to recognize and use correctly nouns, verbs, contractions, and adjectives in their writing.
   a. Common and proper nouns
   b. Pronouns

c. Subjects (naming part) and predicates (action part)

d. Helping "auxiliary" verbs

2. Mechanics: Students are expected to demonstrate appropriate language mechanics in writing.

   a. Capitalize all proper nouns (names of specific people or things, such as Mike, Indian, Jeep), greetings, months and days of the week, titles (Dr., Mr., Mrs., and Miss), and initials of people.

   b. Capitalize correctly the first word in a sentence and the pronoun "I."

3. Punctuation: Students are expected to demonstrate appropriate punctuation in writing.

   a. Correctly use end punctuation.

   b. Use commas correctly in dates.

   c. Use apostrophes correctly in contractions.

   d. Use quotation marks to show that someone is speaking.

   e. Use period in common abbreviations.

4. Sentence Structure: The student will demonstrate appropriate sentence structure in writing.

5. Spelling: Students are expected to demonstrate appropriate application of spelling knowledge to the revising and editing stages of writing.

   a. Spell correctly words with short and long vowel sounds, r-controlled vowels, and consonant vowel patterns.

   b. Spell frequently used words with irregular spelling patterns.

   c. Spell prefixes and suffixes correctly.

   d. Recognize the use of homophones/ homonyms in spelling.

Third Grade

1. Grammar/Usage: Students are expected to recognize and use nouns, pronouns, verbs, adjectives, adverbs, and conjunctions correctly in their writing.

   a. Singular and plural possessive nouns

   b. Subject, object, and possessive pronouns

   c. Present, past, and future tense verbs

   d. Regular, irregular, and helping verbs

   e. Past participle of verbs

   f. Subject-verb agreement

   g. Descriptive, comparative, and superlative adjective

2. Mechanics: Students are expected to demonstrate appropriate language mechanics in writing; for example, capitalize correctly geographical names, holidays, dates, proper nouns, book titles, titles of respect, sentences, and quotations.

3. Punctuation: Students are expected to demonstrate appropriate punctuation in writing.

    a. Periods in abbreviations and sentence endings

    b. Question marks

    c. Commas in dates, addresses, locations, quotes, introductory words, words in a series, greetings, and closings in a letter

    d. Apostrophes in contractions and possessives

    e. Colon in notation of time, formal letter writing, and the introduction of words or concepts in a series (e.g., bring the following supplies: glue, paper, scissors)

    f. Quotation marks around direct quotations, titles of individual poems, and short stories

4. Sentence Structure: The student will demonstrate appropriate sentence structure in writing; for example: Write correctly the four basic kinds of sentences (declarative, exclamatory, imperative, and interrogative) with final punctuation.

5. Spelling: Students are expected to demonstrate appropriate application of spelling knowledge to the revising and editing stages of writing.

    a. Demonstrate recall of spelling patterns (e.g., grapheme or blend), consonant doubling (e.g., bat + ed = batted), changing the ending of a word from -y to –ies when forming the plural (e.g., carry = carries), and common homophones (e.g., hair/hare).

    b. Spell phonetically regular multisyllabic words, contractions, and compounds.

    c. Increase the number of high-frequency words spelled correctly.

    d. Spell words ending in -tion and -sion correctly.

    e. Use various sources of materials to check and correct spelling.

Fourth Grade

1. Grammar/Usage: Students are expected to recognize and use nouns, pronouns, verbs, adjectives, adverbs, and conjunctions correctly in their writing.

    a. Subject, object, reflexive, and possessive pronouns

    b. Subject, direct object, and object of prepositions

    c. Present, past, future, and present perfect verbs tense

    d. Regular, irregular, and helping verbs

    e. Descriptive, comparative, superlative, and demonstrative adjectives

    f. Time, place, and manner adverbs

    g. Comparative forms of adverbs

2. Mechanics: Students are expected to demonstrate appropriate language mechanics in writing.

    a. Capitalize correctly geographical names, holidays, dates, proper nouns, book titles, titles of respect, sentences, and quotations.

    b. Capitalize correctly familial relations, proper adjectives, and conventions of letter writing.

    c. Indent correctly at the beginning of each paragraph.

    d. Observe left-hand and right-hand margins.

3. Punctuation: Students are expected to demonstrate appropriate punctuation in writing.

    a. Parentheses

    b. Quotation marks

    c. Terminal punctuation

    d. Apostrophes in contractions and possessives

    e. Commas

    f. Colons and semicolons

4. Sentence Structure: The student will demonstrate appropriate sentence structure in writing.

    a. Use simple, compound, and complex sentences appropriately in writing.

    b. Create interesting sentences using words that describe, explain, or provide additional details and connections, such as adjectives, adverbs, appositives, participial phrases, prepositional phrases, and conjunctions.

    c. Correct sentence fragments and run-ons.

5. Spelling: Students are expected to demonstrate appropriate application of spelling knowledge to the revising and editing stages of writing.

    a. Spell correctly roots, inflections (e.g., -s/es, -ing, -ly, -er), suffixes (e.g., -ment, -ness, -able, -sion, -tion), and prefixes (e.g., dis-, in-, un-, re-, mis-, pre-).

    b. Spell homophones correctly according to usage (e.g., to, too, two; there, their, they're).

    c. Use more complex patterns in producing conventional spellings (e.g., ought = brought, fought; urse = nurse, purse).

    d. Use word reference materials, including a glossary, a dictionary, and technology to check correct spelling.

Note. Adapted from *Priority Academic Student Skills (PASS),* by the Oklahoma State Department of Education, July 2002.

B-2 Grades 5 through 8

(Skills are presented cumulatively; that is, those expected in earlier grades would be expected in subsequent grades also.)

Language Skills

Listening

The student will listen for information and for pleasure.

Fifth Grade

1. Interpret a speaker's verbal and nonverbal message, purpose, and perspective.

2. Listen critically and respond appropriately to oral communication to seek information not already discussed.

Sixth Grade

1. Identify the major ideas and supporting evidence in informative and persuasive messages.

2. Determine the purpose for listening (i.e., gaining information, solving problems; or for enjoying, appreciating, recalling, interpreting, applying, analyzing, evaluating, receiving directions, or learning concepts).

3. Recognize and understand barriers to effective listening (i.e., internal and external distractions, personal biases, and conflicting demands).

4. Evaluate the spoken message in terms of content, credibility, and delivery.

Seventh and Eighth Grades

1. Identify the major ideas and supporting evidence in informative and persuasive messages.

2. Listen in order to identify and discuss topic, purpose, and perspective.

3. Recognize and understand barriers to effective listening (i.e., internal and external distractions, personal biases, and conflicting demands).

4. Evaluate the spoken message in terms of content, credibility, and delivery.

Speaking

The student will express ideas and opinions in group or individual situations.

Fifth Grade

1. Speak articulately and audibly before a group using appropriate delivery (enunciation, volume, timing, and gestures) and language skills (pronunciation, word choice, and usage).

2. Present effective introductions and conclusions that guide and inform the listeners' understanding of important ideas and details by clarifying and supporting spoken ideas with evidence and examples.

3. Use traditional structures for conveying information, including cause and effect, similarity and difference, and posing and answering a question.

4. Engage the audience with appropriate words, phrasing, facial expressions, and gestures.

5. Deliver narrative (story) presentations that establish a situation, develop a plot, point of view, and setting with descriptive words and phrases.

6. Deliver informative presentations about an important topic, issue, or event that frames a question to guide the investigation, establishes a central idea or topic, and develops that topic appropriately.

7. Deliver oral responses to literature that summarizes important events and details, demonstrate an understanding of several ideas communicated in the work, and use examples from the literature to support conclusions.

Sixth Grade

1. Analyze purpose, audience, and occasion and consider this information in planning an effective presentation or response.

2. Compose a presentation with a well-organized introduction, body, and conclusion that is appropriate for different purposes, audiences, and occasions.

3. Communicate using appropriate delivery (volume, rate, enunciation, and movement).

Seventh and Eighth Grades

1. Analyze purpose, audience, and occasion and consider this information in planning an effective presentation or response.

2. Use level-appropriate vocabulary in speech (e.g., metaphorical language, sensory details, or specialized vocabulary).

3. Adjust message wording and delivery according to particular audience and purpose.

Literacy Skills

Vocabulary

The student will develop and expand the knowledge of words and word meanings to increase vocabulary.

Fifth Grade

1. Words in Context
   a. Use knowledge of word parts and word relationships, as well as context clues (the meaning of the text around a word), to determine

the meaning of specialized vocabulary and to understand the precise meaning of grade-level appropriate words.

b. Use prior experience and context to understand and explain the figurative use of words and similes (comparisons that use *like* or *as: His feet were as big as boats*), and metaphors (implied comparisons: *The giants' steps were thunderous*).

2. Affixes, Roots, and Stems

a. Interpret new words by analyzing the meaning of prefixes and suffixes.

b. Apply knowledge of root words to determine the meaning of unknown words within a passage.

c. Use word origins, including knowledge of less-common roots (*graph = writing, terras = earth*) and word parts (*hemi = half, bio = life*) from Greek and Latin to analyze the meaning of complex words (*terrain, hemisphere, biography*).

3. Synonyms, Antonyms, and Homonyms—Apply knowledge of fifth-grade-level synonyms, antonyms, homonyms, and multiple-meaning words to determine the meaning of words and phrases.

4. Using Resource Materials and Aids

a. Use a thesaurus to determine related words and concepts.

b. Determine the meanings, pronunciation, and derivations of unknown words by using a glossary and/or dictionary.

Sixth Grade

1. Words in Context

2. Word Origins

a. Recognize the origins and meanings of foreign words frequently used in English.

b. Apply knowledge of root words to determine the meaning of unknown words within a passage.

c. Use word origins, including knowledge of less-common roots (*graph = writing, logos = the study of*) and word parts (*auto = self, bio = life*) from Greek and Latin to analyze the meaning of complex words (*autograph, autobiography, biology*).

3. Using Resource Materials and Aids

a. Relate dictionary definitions to context of the reading in order to aid understanding.

Seventh Grade

1. Words in Context—Verify the meaning of a word in its context, even when its meaning is not directly stated, through the use of definitions, restatement, example, comparison, or contrast.

2. Word Origins
   a. Identify the origins and meanings of foreign words frequently used in English and use these words accurately in speaking and writing.

3. Idioms and Comparisons—Identify and explain idioms and comparisons, such as analogies, metaphors, and similes, to infer the literal and figurative meanings of phrases.
   a. Idioms: expressions that cannot be understood just by knowing the meanings of the words in the expression, such as *the apple of his eye* or *beat around the bush.*
   b. Analogies: comparisons of the similar aspects of two different things.
   c. Metaphors: implies comparisons, such as *The street light was my security guard.*
   d. Similes: comparisons that use *like* or *as,* such as *A gentle summer breeze feels like a soft cotton sheet.*

Eighth Grade

1. Words in Context—Verify the meaning of a word in its context, even when its meaning is not directly stated, through the use of definitions, restatement, example, comparison, or contrast.

2. Word Origins—Recognize and analyze the influence of historical events on English word meaning and vocabulary expansion.

Fluency

The student will identify words rapidly so that attention is directed at the meaning of the text.

Fifth, Sixth, Seventh, and Eighth Grades

1. Read regularly in independent-level texts (texts in which no more than approximately 1 in 20 words is difficult for the reader) fluently and accurately, and with appropriate timing, change in voice, and expression.

2. Read regularly in instructional-level texts (texts in which no more than approximately 1 in 10 words is difficult for the reader). A "typical" fifth grader reads approximately 105 words per minute; a "typical" sixth grader reads approximately 120 words per minute; a "typical" seventh grader reads 135 words per minute; a "typical" eighth grader reads 150 words per minute.

3. Read silently for increased periods of time.

4. Increase silent reading speed through daily independent reading.

Comprehension/Critical Literacy

The student will interact with the words and concepts in the text to construct an appropriate meaning.

Fifth and Sixth Grades

1. Literal Understanding
   a. Use prereading strategies independently (to preview, activate prior knowledge, predict content of text, formulate questions that might be answered by the text, and establish purpose for reading).
   b. Read and comprehend both fiction and nonfiction that are appropriately designed for fifth grade.
   c. Recognize main ideas presented in a particular segment of text; identify and assess evidence that supports those ideas.
   d. Use the text's structure or progression of ideas, such as cause and effect or chronology, to organize or recall information.

2. Inferences and Interpretation
   a. Apply prior knowledge and experience to make inferences and respond to new information presented in text.
   b. Draw inferences and conclusions about the text and support them with textual evidence and prior knowledge.
   c. Describe elements of character development in written works (e.g., differences between main and minor characters; stereotypical characters as opposed to fully developed characters; changes that characters undergo; the importance of a character's actions, motives, and appearance to the plot and theme).
   d. Make inferences or draw conclusions about characters' qualities and actions (e.g., based on knowledge of plot, setting, characters' motives, characters' appearances, other characters' responses to a character).
   e. Participate in creative response to text (e.g., art, drama, and oral presentation).

3. Summary and Generalization
   a. Summarize and paraphrase information from the entire reading selection, including the main idea and significant supporting details.
   b. Make generalizations with information gleaned from text.
   c. Support ideas and arguments by reference to relevant aspects of text and issues across texts.
   d. Organize text information in different ways (e.g., time line, outline, graphic organizer) to support and explain ideas.

4. Analysis and Evaluation
   a. Identify and analyze the characteristics of poetry, drama, fiction, and nonfiction, and explain the appropriateness of the literary form chosen by an author for a specific purpose.

b. Identify the main problem or conflict of the plot and explain how it is resolved.

c. Contrast the actions, motives, and appearances of characters in a work of fiction and discuss the importance of the contrasts to the plot or theme.

d. Make observations and connections, react, speculate, interpret, and raise questions in analysis of texts.

e. Recognize structural patterns found in information text (e.g., cause/effect, problem/solution, sequential order).

f. Distinguish among facts and inferences supported by evidence and opinions in text.

5. Monitoring and Correction Strategies
   a. Monitor own reading and modify strategies as needed when understanding breaks down (e.g., rereading a portion aloud, using reference aids, searching for clues, and asking questions).
   b. Predict, monitor, and cross-check using semantic, syntactic, and graphophonic cues.
   c. Monitor and adjust the reading rate according to the purpose for reading and the difficulty of the text.

Seventh and Eighth Grades

1. Literal Understanding
   a. Apply prereading strategies when reading both fiction and nonfiction that are appropriately designed for grade level.
   b. Determine the purpose for reading such as to be informed, entertained, or persuaded.
   c. Preview the material and use prior knowledge to make connections between text and personal experience.
   d. Recognize transition words to guide understanding of the text (e.g., as a result, first of all, furthermore).
   e. Show understanding by asking questions and supporting answers with literal information from text.

2. Inference and Interpretation
   a. Make inferences and draw conclusions with evidence drawn from the text and/or student experiences.
   b. Make inferences supported by a character's thoughts, words, and actions or the narrator's description.

3. Summary and Generalization
   a. Summarize the main idea and how it is supported with specific details.
   b. Recall major points in the text and make and revise predictions
   c. Recognize the importance and relevance of details on the development of the plot.

    d. Support reasonable statements by reference to relevant aspects of text and examples.

    e. Determine the main (or major) idea and how those ideas are supported with specific details.

    f. Paraphrase and summarize text to recall, inform, or organize ideas.

4. Analysis and Evaluation

    a. Distinguish among stated fact, reasoned judgment, and opinion in various texts.

    b. Use the text's structure or progression of ideas, such as cause and effect or chronology (sequential order).

    c. Compare/contrast to determine similarities and differences in treatment, scope, or organization.

    d. Problem/solution—offer observations, make connections, react, speculate, interpret, and raise questions in response to text.

    e. Analyze character traits, conflicts, motivations, points of view, and changes that occur within the story.

    f. Analyze the structural elements of the plot, subplot, and climax and explain the way in which conflicts are or are not resolved.

    g. Distinguish among stated fact, reasoned judgment, and opinion in text.

5. Monitoring and Correction Strategies

    a. Monitor the understanding of text and use correcting strategies, such as rereading a portion, using reference aids, or searching for content when needed.

    b. Make, confirm, and revise predictions when reading.

    c. Adjust the reading rate and determine appropriate strategies to match the purpose, difficulty, and characteristics of the text.

Writing Process

The student will use the writing process to write coherently.

Fifth Grade

1. Use the writing process to develop, extend, and refine composition skills, for example, use a variety of prewriting activities, such as brainstorming, clustering, illustrating, webbing, using graphic organizers, notes, and logs.

2. Select a focus and an organizational structure based on purpose, audience, length, and required format and write one or more drafts by categorizing ideas, organizing them into paragraphs, and blending paragraphs into longer compositions.

3. Use common organizational structures for providing information in writing, such as chronological order, cause and effect, or similarity and difference, and posing and answering questions.

4. Edit drafts to ensure standard usage, mechanics, spelling, and varied sentence structure to improve meaning and clarity.
   a. Proofread to edit one's own writing, as well as that of others, using an editing checklist or set of rules, with specific examples of corrections of specific errors.
5. Review, evaluate, and revise selected drafts by adding, elaborating, deleting, combining, and rearranging text for meaning and clarity.
6. Publish and share writing with peers and adults.

Sixth, Seventh, and Eighth Grades

1. Use a writing process to develop composition skills. Students are expected to use prewriting strategies, write and revise multiple drafts, edit, and share their compositions.
2. Use details, examples, reasons, and evidence to develop an idea.
3. Use spatial, chronological, and climactic organizational patterns as appropriate to the purpose.
4. Use precise word choices, including figurative language, that convey specific meaning and tone.
5. Use a variety of sentence structures, types, and lengths to contribute to fluency and interest.
6. Edit for errors in Standard English usage, sentence structure, mechanics, and spelling.

Grammar/Usage and Mechanics

The student will demonstrate appropriate practices in writing by applying Standard English conventions to the revising and editing stages of writing.

Fifth, Sixth, Seventh, and Eighth Grades

1. Standard English Usage—Demonstrate the correct use of Standard English in speaking and writing.
   a. Use the principal parts of verbs and progressive verb forms.
   b. Make subjects and verbs agree.
   c. Use nominative, objective, and possessive pronouns correctly.
   d. Make pronouns agree with their antecedents.
   e. Use correct pronoun reference.
   f. Correctly form and use the comparative and superlative forms of adjectives.
   g. Identify and use appositives and appositive phrases.
   h. Use infinitives, gerunds, and participles to vary sentence structure in writing.
   i. Correctly use conjunctions for coordination and subordination.

    j. Distinguish commonly confused words (e.g., there, their, they're; two, to, too; accept, except; affect, effect).

2. Mechanics and Spelling—Demonstrate appropriate language mechanics in writing.
    a. Apply the capitalization rules appropriately in writing.
    b. Punctuate correctly in writing, including:
        i. Commas
        ii. Quotation marks
        iii. Apostrophes
        iv. Colons
        v. Conventions of letter writing
    c. Distinguish the correct spelling of commonly misspelled words and homonyms.

3. Sentence Structure—Demonstrate appropriate sentence structure in writing.
    a. Correct sentence run-ons and fragments.
    b. Correct dangling and misplaced modifiers.
    c. Differentiate between dependent clauses and independent clauses.
    d. Write simple, compound, complex, and compound-complex sentences.

Note. Adapted from *Priority Academic Student Skills (PASS),* by the Oklahoma State Department of Education, July 2002.

B-3 Grades 9 through 12

(Skills are presented cumulatively; that is, those expected in earlier grades would be expected in subsequent grades also.)

Language Skills

Listening

The student will listen for information and for pleasure.

Ninth Grade

1. Focus attention on the speaker's message.
2. Use knowledge of language and develop vocabulary to accurately interpret the speaker's message.
3. Listen and respond appropriately to presentations and performances of peers or published works such as original essays or narratives, interpretations of poetry, and individual or group performances.

4. Monitor the speaker's message and clarity and understanding to formulate and provide effective verbal and nonverbal feedback.

5. Use feedback to evaluate own effectiveness and set goals for future presentations.

Tenth Grade

1. Engage in critical, empathetic, appreciative, and reflective listening to interpret, respond, and evaluate the speaker's messages.

2. Evaluate informative and persuasive presentations of peers, public figures, and media presentations.

Eleventh and Twelfth Grades

1. Demonstrate proficiency in critical, empathetic, appreciative, and reflective listening to interpret, respond, and evaluate the speaker's messages.

2. Use effective strategies for listening that identifies the types of listening and adopts appropriate strategies.

3. Use effective strategies to evaluate own listening, such as asking questions for clarification, comparing and contrasting interpretations with others, and researching points of interest or contention.

4. Use effective listening to provide appropriate feedback in a variety of situations, such as conversations and discussions and informative, persuasive, or artistic presentations.

5. Demonstrate proficiency in critical, empathetic, appreciative, and reflective listening to interpret, respond and evaluate the speaker's messages.

Speaking

The student will express ideas and opinions in group or individual situations.

Ninth and Tenth Grades

1. Use formal, informal, standard, and technical language effectively to meet the needs of purpose, audience, occasion, and task.

2. Prepare, organize, and present a variety of informative messages effectively.

3. Analyze purpose, audience, and occasion to choose effective verbal and nonverbal strategies such as pitch and tone of voice, posture, and eye contact.

4. Use a variety of verbal and nonverbal techniques in presenting oral messages, and demonstrate poise and control while presenting.

Eleventh and Twelfth Grades

1. Use a variety of verbal and nonverbal techniques in presenting oral messages such as pitch and tone of voice, posture, and eye contact, and demonstrate poise and control while presenting.

2. Use logical, ethical, and emotional appeals that enhance a specific tone and purpose.

3. Evaluate when to use different kinds of effects (including visuals, music, sound, and graphics) to create effective presentations.

4. Ask clear questions for a variety of purposes and respond appropriately to the questions of others.

5. Use effective and interesting language, including informal expressions for effect, Standard English for clarity, and technical language for specificity.

Literacy Skills

Vocabulary

The student will expand vocabulary through word study, literature, and class discussion.

Ninth and Tenth Grades

1. Apply a knowledge of Greek (e.g., tele/phone. micro/phone), Latin (e.g., flex/ible), and Anglo-Saxon (e.g., un/friend/ly) roots, prefixes, and suffixes to determine word meanings.

2. Use word meanings within the appropriate context and verify those meanings by definition, restatement, example, and analogy.

3. Expand vocabulary through wide reading, listening, and discussing.

4. Use reference materials such as a glossary, a dictionary, a thesaurus, and available technology to determine precise meaning and usage.

5. Identify the relation of word meanings in analogies, homonyms, synonyms/antonyms, and connotations and denotations.

6. Research word origins as an aid to understanding meaning, derivations, and spelling as well as influences on the English language.

7. Discriminate between connotative meanings and denotative meanings, and interpret the connotative power of words.

Eleventh and Twelfth Grades

1. Analyze the meaning of analogies encountered, analyzing specific comparisons as well as relationships and inferences.

2. Rely on context to determine meanings of words and phrases such as figurative language, connotations and denotations of words, analogies, idioms, and technical vocabulary.

3. Use word meanings within the appropriate context and verify these meanings by definition, restatement, example, and analogy.

Comprehension

The student will interact with the words to construct an appropriate meaning.

Ninth Grade

1. Literal Understanding
   a. Examine the structures and format of functional workplace documents, including graphics and headers, and explain how authors use the features to achieve their purpose.
   b. Draw on own background to provide connections to text.
   c. Monitor reading strategies and modify them when understanding breaks down such as rereading, using resources, and questioning.
   d. Recognize text structures such as compare and contrast, cause and effect, and chronological ordering.
   e. Use study strategies such as skimming and scanning, note taking, outlining, and using study guide questions to better understand texts.

2. Inferences and Interpretation
   a. Analyze characteristics of text, including its structure, word choice, and intended audience.
   b. Draw inferences such as conclusions, generalizations, and predictions, and support them with text evidence and personal experience.
   c. Recognize influences on a reader's response to a text (e.g., personal experience and values; perspective shapes by age, gender, class, or nationality).

3. Summary and Generalization
   a. Identify the main idea and supporting details by producing summaries of text.
   b. Use text features and elements to support inferences and generalizations about information.
   c. Summarize and paraphrase complex, implicit hierarchic structures in informational texts, including relationships among concepts and details in those structures.

4. Analysis and Evaluation
   a. Discriminate between fact and opinion and fiction and nonfiction.
   b. Recognize deceptive and/or faulty arguments in persuasive texts.

    c. Analyze the structure and format of informational and literary documents and explain how authors use the features to achieve their purposes.

    d. Identify techniques (e.g., language, organization, tone, context) used to convey point of view or impressions.

Tenth Grade

1. Literal Understanding
    a. Identify the structures and format of various informational documents and explain how authors use the features to achieve their purpose.
    b. Understand specific devices an author uses to accomplish purpose (persuasive techniques, style, literary forms or genre, portrayal of themes, language).
    c. Use a range of automatic monitoring and self-correcting methods (e.g., rereading, slowing down, subvocalizing, consulting resources, questioning).
    d. Recognize signal/transitional words and phrases and their contributions to the meaning of the text (e.g., however, in spite of, for example, consequently).
2. Inferences and Interpretation
    a. Use elements of the text to defend responses and interpretations.
3. Summary and Generalization
    a. Determine the main idea and locate and interpret minor or subtly stated details in complex passages.

Eleventh and Twelfth Grades

1. Literal Understanding
    a. Use study strategies such as note taking, outlining, and using study guide questions to better understand texts.
    b. Construct images such as graphic organizers based on text descriptions and text structures.
2. Inferences and Interpretation
    a. Interpret the possible inferences of the historical context on literary works.
    b. Describe the development of plot and identify conflict and how they are addressed and resolved.
    c. Make reasonable assertions about an author's arguments by using elements of the text to defend and clarify interpretations.
    d. Identify influences on a reader's response to a text (e.g., personal experience and values; perspectives shapes by age, gender, class, or nationality).

3. Summary and Generalization
   a. Summarize and paraphrase complex, implicit hierarchic structures in informational texts, including relationships among concepts and details in those structures.

4. Analysis and Evaluation
   a. Compare and contrast aspects of texts such as themes, conflicts, and allusions both within and across texts.
   b. Analyze the structure and format of informational and literary documents and explain how authors use the features to achieve their purposes.
   c. Examine the way in which clarity of meaning is affected by the patterns of organization, repetition of the main ideas, organization of language, and word choice in the text.
   d. Analyze the way in which authors have used archetypes (universal modes or patterns) drawn from myth and tradition in literature, film, political speeches, and religious writings.
   e. Investigate both the features and the rhetorical (communication) devices of different types of public documents, such as policy statements, speeches, or debates, and the ways in which authors use those features and devices.
   f. Evaluate the credibility of information sources, including how the writer's motivation may affect that credibility.

Writing Process

The student will use the writing process to write coherently.

Ninth, Tenth, Eleventh, and Twelfth Grades

1. Use a writing process to develop and refine composition skills. Students are expected to:
   a. Use prewriting strategies to generate ideas such as brainstorming, using graphic organizers, keeping notes and logs.
   b. Develop multiple drafts both alone and collaboratively to categorize ideas, organizing them into paragraphs and blending paragraphs into larger text.
   c. Organize and reorganize drafts and refine style to suit the occasion, audience, and purpose.
   d. Proofread writing for appropriateness of organization, content, and style.
   e. Edit for specific purposes to ensure standard usage, varied sentence structure, appropriate word choice, mechanics, and spelling.
   f. Refine selected pieces frequently to publish for general and specific audiences.

2. Use extension and elaboration to develop an idea.

3. Demonstrate organization, unity, and coherence by using transitions and sequencing.

4. Use precise word choices, including figurative language, that convey specific meaning and tone.

5. Use a variety of sentence structures, types, and lengths to contribute to fluency and interest.

6. Evaluate own writing and others' writing (e.g., determine the best features of a piece of writing, determine how own writing achieves its purpose, ask for feedback, respond to classmates' writing).

7. Demonstrate an understanding of the elements of discourse, such as purpose, speaker, audience, and form when completing narrative expository, persuasive, or descriptive writing assignments.

8. Use language in creative and vivid ways to establish a specific tone.

9. Use point of view, characterization, style, and related elements for specific rhetorical (communication) and aesthetic (artistic) purposes.

10. Structure ideas and arguments in a sustained and persuasive way and support them with precise and relevant examples.

11. Evaluate own writing and others' writing to highlight the individual voice, improve sentence variety and style, and enhance subtlety of meaning and tone in ways that are consistent with the purpose, audience, and form of writing.

12. Enhance meaning by using rhetorical devices, including the extended use of parallelism, repetition, and analogy and the issuance of a call for action.

13. Use point of view, characterization, style, and related elements for specific rhetorical (communication) and aesthetic (artistic) purposes.

14. Structure ideas and arguments in a sustained and persuasive way and support them with precise and relevant examples.

15. Evaluate own writing and others' writing to highlight the individual voice, improve sentence variety and style, and enhance subtlety of meaning and tone in ways that are consistent with the purpose, audience, and form of writing.

16. Further develop a unique writing style and voice, improve sentence variety, and enhance subtlety of meaning and tone in ways that are consistent with the purpose, audience, and form of writing.

Grammar/Usage and Mechanics

The student will demonstrate appropriate practices in writing by applying grammatical knowledge to the revising and editing stages of writing.

Ninth, Tenth, Eleventh, and Twelfth Grades

1. Standard English Usage—Demonstrate correct use of Standard English in speaking and writing.

a. Distinguish commonly confused words (e.g., there, their, they're; two, too, to; accept, except; affect, effect).
b. Use correct verb forms and tenses.
c. Use correct subject-verb agreement.
d. Use active and passive voice.
e. Correct pronoun/antecedent agreement and clear pronoun reference.
f. Use correct forms of comparative and superlative adjectives.

2. Mechanics and Spelling—Demonstrate appropriate language mechanics in writing.
   a. Demonstrate correct use of capitals.
   b. Use correct formation of plurals.
   c. Demonstrate correct use of punctuation and recognize its effect on sentence structure.
   d. Distinguish correct spelling of commonly misspelled words and homonyms.

3. Sentence Structure—Demonstrate appropriate sentence structure in writing.
   a. Use parallel structure.
   b. Correct dangling and misplaced modifiers.
   c. Correct run-on sentences.
   d. Correct fragments.

Note. Adapted from *Priority Academic Student Skills (PASS),* by the Oklahoma State Department of Education, July 2002.

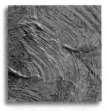

Glossary

abstraction The ability to perceive relationships among isolated aspects of objects, events, or persons.

accommodation A process of cognitive adaptation that modifies an existing scheme in response to new experiences.

account A type of narrative in which the speaker evaluates and interprets the significance of events.

acoustic nerve (or **cranial nerve VIII**) The eighth cranial nerve important for transmitting sound and balance sensation from the inner ear to the brain.

action relational words Early relational words that refer to actions associated with an object of interest.

action verbs Words that refer to activity that is observable.

adaptation The cognitive process of organizing new experiences to achieve equilibrium in one's understanding of the world.

affect expressive monologues Instances in which preschoolers' talk to themselves as they reflect on their emotions.

afferent roots The peripheral nerve bundles carrying sensory information to the ventral horns of the spinal cord.

agenda The speaker's overall goal, including the steps that proceed toward that goal.

allophones The individual sound variations that are still heard as a class of sounds.

alternation The variations in linguistic structure and speaking style in response to the roles and audience in a setting.

ambiguity The observation that a sentence has more than one interpretation.

anaphoric reference The linguistic effect in which pronouns replace nouns or noun phrases and refer to their occurrence earlier in the context.

antonyms Two words whose meanings contrast due to opposite values in a single semantic feature, as in *hot* and *cold.*

arbitrary The capricious connection between words and their meanings.

arcuate fasciculus The primary association fiber tract within each hemisphere; connects Wernicke's area in the temporal lobe with Broca's area in the frontal lobe of the language dominant hemisphere.

articulation The modification of the vocal tone and airstream into distinctive sounds through movements of oral structures.

assimilation A process of cognitive adaptation in which new experiences are organized into existing schemes.

associated monologue A mode of play behavior in which children playing together contribute individual monologues related to the same topic.

association fibers Cerebral nerve fibers that interconnect areas within a hemisphere.

attachment The development of recognition and expectations for interaction between caregivers and infants.

attribution relational words Early relational words that refer to the attributes or characteristics of objects.

audience Persons whose presence may set the occasion for an address or naming response, influence whether an utterance occurs, or influence the form of the utterances that do occur.

audiologist   Specialist trained in the identification, assessment, and treatment of hearing disorders.

auditory association area   Cortical area surrounding the primary auditory cortex in the temporal lobe; responsible for interpreting the significance of sounds.

auricle (also **pinna**)   The outermost, visible, cartilaginous portion of the ear.

autoclitic   A secondary verbal operant in which a conventional form (a tag, word, or order) comments on the relationships among the primary verbal operants; the behavioral equivalent to syntax and grammar.

autoclitic frames   Skinner's concept of certain orders in verbal responses that express relationships among stimuli.

autonomic nerves   A portion of the nervous system responsible for regulating involuntary life support systems.

auxiliary verb   Grammatical verbs that serve as helping verbs by conveying number and tense.

axon   The single longer filament of a neuron that carries the neural impulse away from the cell body.

baby talk   Characteristic speech patterns, including shorter phrases and exaggerated intonation, used when talking to infants.

basal ganglia   A group of large cell bodies located deep within the cerebral hemispheres whose interconnections regulate automatic background adjustments in movement.

basilar membrane   A membrane within the inner ear that supports the sensory end organ for hearing, the organ of Corti, along the length of the cochlea.

behaviorism   A philosophical perspective on learning and behavior that emphasizes observable behaviors and their effects.

bilingualism   The ability to speak two languages.

blastocyst   A fluid-filled sphere containing embryonic cells, formed by the end of the first week following conception.

bound morpheme   A subclass of morphemes that are meaningless unless attached to a free morpheme; includes **derivational** and **inflectional morphemes.**

bottom-up model   The model that proposes reading proceeds from interpreting phonemes to words to phrases to sentences, and so forth.

Broca's area   The motor speech area located in the lower region of the frontal lobe in the language dominant hemisphere.

case frames   Brown's concept of the early consistent word orders used by children to express semantic relationships.

case grammar   A generative grammar that emphasizes the cases or semantic roles assumed by nouns in relationship to the verb of a sentence.

cataphoric reference   The linguistic effect in which pronouns replace nouns or noun phrases and refer to their occurrence later in the context.

categorical perception   The observation that listeners hear classes of similar sounds within a continuous range of sounds.

caudate nucleus   A major deep brain cell body that is part of the basal ganglia.

cause-effect pattern   Syntactic devices in text grammar that signal a cause-effect relationship is being proposed.

central nervous system   The portion of the nervous system composed of the brain and spinal cord.

cerebellum   The lower, hindmost portion of the brain primarily responsible for coordination and balance.

cerebral hemispheres   The two halves of the cerebrum defined by the longitudinal fissure.

cerebrum   The larger, most visible portion of the brain consisting of two hemispheres.

chained associations   Phenomenon in conceptual development in which a word occurs in successive contexts that are linked by one feature from the preceding situation.

chaining   A behavioral process in which responses are learned as fixed sequences in which each response leads to a subsequent response.

child development specialists   Professionals specializing in evaluating child development and counseling parents.

child-directed speech (CDS) (also **motherese** or **parentese**)   Characteristic speech directed to toddlers and preschoolers by caregivers.

classical (or **respondent**) **conditioning**   A model of learning in which a neutral stimulus (e.g., a bell) associated with an unconditioned stimulus (e.g., food) subsequently elicits conditioned responses similar to the unconditioned response (e.g., salivation).

clause   A group of words that includes a subject and a predicate but is not necessarily grammatically complete.

cochlea   The portion of the inner ear that contains the sensory end organ for hearing, the organ of Corti.

code   The systematic, orderly nature of language that allows speakers and listeners to express and comprehend meanings.

code switching   A phenomenon in bilingualism in which speakers unknowingly include elements of one language in the other.

cognition   The mental processes related to organizing and understanding experience.

cognitive determinism   A philosophy that emphasizes the primary role played by cognition in determining the acquisition of language.

cohesion   The relatedness of successive utterances in discourse.

collection patterns   Syntactic devices associated with text grammar that indicate a listing of items.

collective monologue   A phenomenon in which children playing in proximity of each other talk simultaneously but not necessarily to each other.

colliculi   Four paired bodies on the brain stem important for regulating visual and auditory reflexes.

commissural fibers   Neural fibers that transmit information between the cerebral hemispheres.

communication   The process of sharing ideas involving a sender who encodes a message and a receiver who decodes the message.

communicative competence   The ability of speakers to adjust their messages to effectively influence their listeners.

communicative functions   Halliday's classification of intentions exhibited by infants and toddlers.

comparative   Adjective form that expresses the relative degree of an attribute in comparing two items (e.g., *big* vs. *bigger*).

comparative linguistics   A branch of linguistics that analyzes the differences and similarities between languages.

comparison patterns   Syntactic devices associated with text grammar signaling that similarities or differences are being noted.

complete narrative   Story that includes all of the required elements of mature narratives.

complex narrative   Mature narratives that include subplots that are related to each other and an overall plot.

complex sentence   A sentence composed of a main clause with an embedded subordinate clause.

compound sentence   A sentence composed of two independent clauses joined by a conjunction.

compounding strategy   Comprehension strategy in which all actions in a sentence are attributed to the first noun mentioned in the sentence.

comprehension   Understanding or decoding the meaning of an utterance.

conceptual behavior   Responding to a variety of items that are related by some feature defining them as a class.

conceptualization   The perceptual level at which stimuli are responded to as a class or concept based on some similarity.

conditioned reinforcers   Stimuli that take on reinforcing properties as a result of their association with a known reinforcer.

confirmational yes/no question   A caregiver prompt that requires a simple *yes* or *no* response.

conjoining   The linguistic process of linking two independent clauses into a single sentence structure.

constituent equivalence   The status pronouns assume with regard to the nouns or noun phrases they replace.

constituent structures   The morphemes, words, and phrases that contribute to an overall sentence structure.

contextualized language   Utterances that relate to the context in which they occur.

contingent   A conditional or interdependent relationship between stimuli.

contingent queries   A conversational device used to prompt for specific information that maintains the conversational flow.

continuity hypothesis   The phonological theory that the sounds of babbling evolve into the sounds of speech.

contralateral   The relationship in which cortical areas responsible for motor control and sensory reception are opposite from the body areas affected.

control   A scientific goal in which scientists seek to influence whether or not a phenomenon occurs.

conventional   The notion that language must be based on shared, customary, or implicitly agreed-on patterns of behavior.

convergent semantic production   The ability to identify a topic based on inferences from associated words.

conversational acts   Dore's classification of functions served by utterances within discourse.

conversational repairs   Devices used by individuals to clarify messages within a conversation.

cooing   Infant sound productions in the first few months that are vowel-like and associated with comfortable states.

cooperative play   Play behavior in which children interact in organized goal-directed ways.

coordinating conjunction   A connecting word that links two structures into one sentence.

copula verb   A grammatical verb that serves to link or equate its subject to a noun phrase, adjective, or prepositional phrase.

corpus callosum   A major bundle of commissural fibers forming an arched body beneath the longitudinal fissure and connecting the cerebral hemispheres.

cortex   Outer convoluted layers of dense neurons covering the cerebral hemispheres; responsible for high mental functions.

count noun   Nouns that represent items that can be counted as individual units (e.g., pennies, forks); compare **mass noun.**

cranial nerves   Twelve paired bundles of peripheral nerve bundles that exit the CNS at the level of the brain stem.

cross-sectional research design   Research design in which groups of subjects at different ages are used to simulate changes related to chronological development.

declarative   A major sentence type that makes a statement.

decontextualized language   Utterances that refer to objects, people, events, and relationships outside the immediate context.

deep structure   The underlying structure of a sentence generated by the phrase structure rules.

deictic gaze   A gaze pattern in which visual focus on an object directs a partner's attention to that object.

deixis   The ability of words and gaze patterns to "point to" objects being referenced.

dendrites   Branched nerve fibers that conduct impulses toward the cell body of a neuron.

derivational morpheme   A type of bound morpheme that changes the grammatical class of the free morpheme to which it is attached (e.g., teach*er*).

derivational noun suffix   A type of derivational morpheme in the form of a suffix (-er) that derives a noun from a verb (e.g., the noun *runner* derives from the verb *run*).

descriptive grammar   A set of linguistic rules that describes the regularities present in a set of utterances.

descriptive linguistics   That branch of linguistics that analyzes and describes languages.

descriptive patterns   Syntactic devices found in text grammar that signal a topic is being described.

determiners   Words, including articles, adjectives, and demonstratives, that modify the noun with which they are associated; traditionally called modifiers.

developmental linguistics   The branch of linguistics that studies the linguistic aspects of children's developing language.

dialect   A collection of consistent or systematic variations in a major language that occur in an identifiable subgroup.

dialogue   A series of related verbal exchanges between at least two persons.

dimensional words   Word pairs that refer to the physical dimensions of objects.

direct speech act   A speech act in which the intention is expressed directly in the grammatical form of the utterance.

disappearance   Early reflexive relation in which children's words indicates that an object has left their immediate experience.

discontinuity hypothesis   The phonological theory that the sounds in babbling and eventual speech are unrelated.

discourse   A series of verbal interchanges between speakers on a shared topic.

discriminative stimulus (S^D)   A stimulus that has been often present when a response has been reinforced and comes to influence the likelihood of that response occurring.

distinctive features   The individual acoustic or articulatory characteristics that distinguish one class of phonemes from another.

divergent semantic production   The ability to produce a diverse collection of words based on their association with a topic.

dorsal horns   The posterior areas of the spinal cord containing nuclei for relaying incoming sensory information up the spinal cord.

D-structures   A component within government-binding theory that contains the sentence structure rules and the lexicon.

dummy forms   Utterances consisting of a true word combined with an additional sound or syllable that give the appearance of approximating multiword utterances.

dyad   Two individuals interacting as a unit; for example, a caregiver and child.

ear canal (also **external auditory meatus**)   Funnel-shaped tube that conducts sound waves from the opening in the pinna to the tympanic membrane.

echoic   A primary verbal operant whose reinforcement is contingent on reproducing the acoustic characteristics of others' speech; the behavioral equivalent of imitation.

echolalia   Infants' sound production that appears to immediately imitate the speech around them.

ectoderm   The outermost embryonic germ layer that contributes to various organs, including the nervous system and skin.

efferent roots   Nerve fiber bundles carrying motor impulses away from the spinal cord.

elementary operations   Transformational rules that are applied to a single deep structure, such as addition, deletion, transposition, and substitution.

elicited imitation   Imitation by the child specifically prompted by the caregiver.

embedding   The linguistic process of inserting a subordinate clause into an independent main clause.

embryo   The fertilized egg during the first 8 weeks of development.

embryoblast   The blastocyst's inner cell mass that will develop into the embryo.

embryonic disc   A cluster of cells in embryonic development at about 2 weeks following conception.

embryonic period   The period from conception through the eighth week following conception.

empiricism   The philosophical view that experience is the source of learning and knowledge.

empty forms   Forms that are consistent but do not represent conventional words are combined with a true word and appear to approximate multiword utterances.

endoderm   The innermost embryonic germ layer that contributes to various organs, including the digestive tract and lungs.

episode   A part of a narrative that relates a series of events as part of the overall plot.

episodic memory   The cumulative set of experiences that make up an individual's understanding of a concept or event.

equilibrium   The goal of adaptive processes in cognition in which new information is assimilated or accommodated.

eventcast   A type of narrative that relates the characters, roles, and relationships related to a situation.

event knowledge   The child's accumulation of experiences in familiar routines.

evocative utterances   Assertions by toddlers that appear to anticipate affirmation or feedback from the caregiver.

executive function   The ability to review, evaluate, proofread, and edit one's own writing.

existence   Early reflexive relation in which a word denotes that an object is present.

expansions   Caregiver utterances that reproduce the child's utterance and include additional grammatical elements. Also, preschoolers' inclusion of additional elements in the noun phrase, which expands the length of their utterances.

expiratory cycle   The phase of respiration in which air is exhaled from the lungs.

expository style   The structured and formal style of tutorial language in classrooms and textbooks.

expressive words   Early words whose apparent purpose is to engage others in social exchanges.

extended mapping   The more prolonged process of modifying word meanings with additional experiences following their initial fast mapping.

extended tact   A primary verbal operant in which responses to stimuli other than the original stimuli occur due to stimulus generalization; the behavioral equivalent of figurative language.

extension   Caregiver utterances that follow their child's preceding utterance and include additional related semantic information.

extralinguistic aspects   The nonlinguistic elements of communication (gestures, intonation, etc.) that supplement or alter the message expressed by the words and phrases.

extrapyramidal system   A hypothetical system of multiple cerebral interconnections involving the basal ganglia, cortical areas, and cerebellum, which integrate background adjustments and purposeful movements.

fast mapping   The hypothetical process in which children form initial associations when first exposed to a new word.

fetus   The developing unborn child from the 10th week of gestation until birth.

figurative language   Language that conveys meaning through analogy based on stimulus generalization rather than through literal interpretation of the words and phrases.

fill-in   A device used by caregivers to allow their child to complete a statement by supplying the correct word or label.

fissure   A deep furrow or valley in the convoluted surface of the cortex.

fluency   The flow of speech that is free of abnormal interruptions or disfluencies.

focused chains   Narratives that organize a sequence of events around a character but omit reasons for the character's actions.

foramen magnum   The large opening in the base of the skull through which the spinal cord passes to lower areas of the body.

formal grammar   The collective set of written rules that describe the conventional regularities in a language.

free morphemes   Morphemes that can occur independently and still carry meaning.

frequency of occurrence   The relative number of occurrences of a structure in a language sample.

fully resonant nuclei   Infant sound productions that more closely approximate mature vowels.

functional analysis   The process of experimentally determining which variables influence the occurrence or nonoccurrence of a behavior.

functional language disorders   Language disorders that have no apparent organic basis.

functional stimulus   A stimulus that is causally related to the occurrence of a behavior.

functions   The pragmatic or practical purposes served by utterances.

gaze coupling   A gaze pattern in which caregivers and infants maintain eye contact in long, alternating intervals.

generalized conditioned reinforcer   Stimulus that obtains its reinforcing potential from association with a variety of other reinforcing stimuli.

generalized operations   Transformational rules that are applied across more than one deep structure to create complex or compound sentences.

generative grammar   A grammar composed of a limited number of rules capable of generating an unlimited number of acceptable sentences in a language.

genderlect   The communication styles that appear to be characteristic of each gender.

genres   Styles of classifications of discourse that occur in different circumstances.

gestation   The period of embryological and fetal development from conception to birth.

glial cells   Cells that support and nourish other nerve cells in the central nervous system.

glottis   The source of laryngeal sound production, including the true vocal folds and the space between them.

grammar   The collection of rules that characterize the regularities or patterns of a language.

grammatical complexity   The number of transformational rules related to the production or comprehension of a grammatical structure.

grammatical ellipsis   Linguistic device in which speakers eliminate information apparent to listeners from the context.

grammatical verbs   Verbs that play a grammatical role without conveying specific actions; compare **lexical verbs.**

graphemes   Letters or letter combinations that represent the phonemes of a language.

groping patterns   Early attempts at true two-word utterances produced with effort and hesitation.

gyrus (pl., **gyri**)   The ridges or convolutions on the cortical surface of the brain.

heaps An early form of children's narrative in which unrelated elements are told in unorganized collections.

hierarchical structure The levels of constituent structures that relate the words and phrases of a sentence to its underlying structure.

historical linguistics The branch of linguistics that studies the changes that occur in languages over time.

horizontal development The process of adding associated features that expand the meaning of a word; compare **vertical development.**

hypernasality Excess resonance in the nasal cavities during production of nonnasal speech sounds.

hyponymy The semantic relationship in which the meaning of one word, the hyponym (e.g., *chair*), contains the meaning of another word, the superordinate (e.g., *furniture*).

hypothesis testing Utterances by toddlers produced with rising intonation as an apparent request for confirmation or feedback from the caregiver.

idiolect Language variations unique to an individual speaker.

idiom Figurative language that expresses ideas through analogy (e.g., *Don't let the cat out of the bag*).

illocutionary The component of a speech act that includes the outcome or effect intended by a speaker.

illocutionary force Speakers' dispositions or attitudes toward their utterances.

illocutionary stage The stage in communication development beginning at approximately 6 months when the infant begins to signal intentions through gesture and vocalization.

imagery A perceptual level in which at least part of a stimulus is recalled.

imitation The relatively immediate reproduction of a significant portion of someone's preceding behavior.

imperative A major sentence type that expresses a command while omitting the sentence subject.

incus The middle bone in the ossicular chain in the middle ear.

indicating Caregivers' use of their infants' line of sight to locate the object of their current interest.

indirect speech act A speech act in which the speaker's intention is implied rather than expressed.

infinitive A phrase in the form of *to verb* that serves as a noun, adjective, or adverb (e.g., *To err* is human . . .).

inflectional morpheme A type of bound morpheme that inflects the word it is attached to for tense (play*ed*), plurality (cat*s*), possession (John*'s*), and degree (green*er*).

information processing The hypothetical concept of mental stages or processes that organize and access information.

inspiratory cycle The respiratory phase in which air is inhaled into the lungs.

intention The effects speakers expect to follow their utterances.

intentionality Behavior that exhibits the conscious attempt to achieve some goal through influencing others' behavior.

interactionism A philosophical perspective that emphasizes the mutual influence of cognitive processes or social contexts on language development.

interference The observation that features or rules of one language conflict with learning another language.

interlocking verbal behavior paradigm Skinner's model illustrating the interactive nature of verbal exchanges between speaking partners.

International Phonetic Alphabet An alphabet designed to provide universal symbols to represent all the known speech sounds used in human languages.

interrogative A major sentence type that asks a question.

interrogative utterances Toddler utterances that directly request information or labels.

intervention Arranging treatment factors in an individual's environment to facilitate language learning.

intransitive verb Lexical verbs that are incapable of carrying a grammatical object; compare **transitive verb.**

intraverbal A primary verbal operant in which a speaker's verbal behavior is influenced by his or her own prior verbal behavior; the behavioral equivalent of chains as in recitation, alliteration, tongue twisters, and clichés.

intuitive grammar Speakers' implicit, underlying knowledge of the acceptable patterns and regularities in their language.

jargon Infant sound production consisting of syllable strings produced with adultlike intonation.

joint actions Actions shared by partners that result in their mutual or shared attention.

joint attention Shared attention on a context by partners.

joint reference Establishing an object as the shared topic of communication.

language The system of arbitrary verbal symbols arranged in a conventional code that evolved as a social tool to communicate ideas and influence the behavior of others.

language acquisition device The hypothetical innate mental structure that allows the child to process incoming language and derive a generative grammar.

language disorder Language behaviors that exhibit slower than expected development or variations in development that significantly interfere with an individual's communication abilities.

language families Groups of languages that share historical roots.

language universals Those features that are considered to be part of every human language.

language variations Structural or phonological differences in individuals' or subgroups' production of a major language.

larynx Cartilaginous and muscular framework that supports and regulates the vocal folds for phonation.

lenticular nucleus A cell body in the basal ganglia.

lexical verbs Verbs that express a specific activity.

lexicon The total collection of words and morphemes in a language.

linear syntactic relationships A description of children's early grammar that described the additive meanings of words combined in utterances.

linguistic aspects The dimensions of grammar, semantics, and pragmatics relating to the structure, meaning, and use of language.

linguistic competence Speakers' underlying, idealized knowledge of their language system.

linguistic context The utterances that precede and contribute to the setting responded to by a speaker.

linguistic performance Speakers' actualized production of sentences, potentially affected by memory, fatigue, and distraction.

literacy The ability to communicate through written language.

literacy artifacts Items that commonly display stimuli associated with literacy such as books, news-papers, nursery rhyme characters, t-shirts with slogans, logo adorned ball caps, and so forth.

literacy events Interactions or behaviors related to literacy, including storytelling, book reading, letter writing, and so forth.

literacy knowledge Familiarity with the various aspects of literacy, including print awareness, book orientation, typeface styles, genres, and styles.

literate language The style of formal written language that is structured and organized in distinctive ways.

location relational words Early relational words that refer to the location of items of interest.

locative action relations Spatial relationships or location of actions.

locative state relations Spatial relationships between entities.

locutionary The component of speech acts that includes the words and propositional content used by speakers to convey their intentions.

locutionary stage The stage in communication development beginning when the first words are used to convey intentions.

logical form rules The component of government-binding theory dealing with the logical aspect of sentences.

longitudinal research design Research design that follows the continuous development of its subjects.

malleus The largest, outermost bone in the ossicular chain of the middle ear and attached to the tympanic membrane.

mand A primary verbal operant that occurs in response to a deprivation state or aversive stimulus and specifies its reinforcer; the behavioral equivalent of commanding, demanding, or requesting.

marginal babbling Infant sound productions with a variety of vowels and consonant-like productions that approximate syllables.

marked Semantic aspect of words that refers to the negative end of a dimension or continuum (e.g., length); compare **unmarked.**

marking Caregivers' means of attracting attention to an object by moving or shaking it in their infants' field of view.

mass activity reflex A reflex in which the response is evidenced by the entire body.

mass noun   Nouns that express items perceived as integral wholes that cannot be divided (e.g., milk and sand); compare **count noun.**

mean length of utterance (MLU)   Measure of language development based on average number of morphemes per utterance.

means-end   Cognitive ability to apply a scheme or behavior pattern to achieve a desired goal.

medulla oblongata   Lower portion of brain stem whose fibers are continuous with the spinal cord.

mentalism   A philosophical perspective that emphasizes that knowledge derives from the organization of the mind.

mesoderm   The middle embryonic germ layer that contributes to bones, cartilage, muscles, and blood.

metalinguistic ability   Speakers' ability to consciously evaluate their language behavior.

metaphor   Figurative language that implies an analogous relationship (e.g., *He's an ox!*); compare **simile.**

metaphoric transparency   The extent of similarity between a figurative expression and its literal referent.

method of rich interpretation   Process of analyzing children's utterances while considering the linguistic and nonlinguistic context.

midbrain   The uppermost portion of the brain stem.

minimal distance principle   Comprehension strategy in which the noun closest to the verb is assumed to be the agent.

mitotic division   The cell division that follows conception.

mixed language disorder   A language impairment resulting from both organic and environmental factors.

modal auxiliary verbs   Auxiliary verbs that express the speaker's attitude or mood regarding the main verb.

modality   The component of deep structure in case grammar that carries the tense and sentence type.

model   Any behavior that is produced within the awareness of a child and presents an opportunity to be imitated.

monologue   An instance of private speech in which children talk to themselves during play or to reflect on their emotional state.

morpheme   The minimal, meaningful units of language.

morphology   The study of morphemes.

morula   Cluster of cells formed by the fourth or fifth day following conception.

motherese (also **parentese** or **child-directed speech**)   Distinctive style of talking exhibited by caregivers when speaking with their toddlers.

multiple causation   The concept that many variables are capable of simultaneously influencing a speaker's behavior.

mutual gaze   Shared eye contact with a partner to signal attention.

naming   Caregivers' use of label to direct their infants' attention.

narratives   A series of utterances that relates an event or idea.

nasality   Resonation of the vocal tone through the nasal cavities.

nativism   The philosophical perspective that certain knowledge and abilities are innate.

negative   A major sentence type that expresses denial, rejection, or nonexistence.

negative reinforcement   A procedure that increases the frequency of a behavior by removing an aversive stimulus contingent on each occurrence.

neural folds   The embryonic predecessor to the neural groove.

neural groove   The embryonic predecessor to the neural tube.

neural tube   The embryonic predecessor to the spinal cord.

neurologist   Medical practitioner specializing in evaluating and treating brain function.

neuron   Basic unit of the nervous system consisting of a cell body, an axon, and dendrites.

nonexistence   Early reflexive relation in which a word indicates an object is not present where it would be expected.

nonlinguistic cues   Nonspeech behaviors that accompany the speaker's words and transmit certain cues through facial expressions, eye contact, gestures, body language, or proxemics.

nonreduplicated babbling (also **variegated babbling**)   Babbling that consists of strings of varied syllables.

nonstandard dialect   Variations of the major language spoken by the overall population.

nonstandardized assessment   Evaluation of language abilities through informal procedures.

nonverbal communication   Conveying attitudes or ideas through gesture, facial expression, proxemics, without the use of words, whether spoken, written, or gestured.

noun-verb-noun strategy   Comprehension strategy that relies strictly on word order.

nucleus   Central element in a cell body.

object noun phrase complements   Clauses introduced by *that* which serve as object phrases and complete a sentence (e.g., *I see that he is here*).

onomatopoeia   Words that mimic the sounds associated with the objects or events they represent, such as *zip, splash,* or *sizzle.*

open-ended question   A caregiver prompt that allows for a variety of information to be included in the child's response.

operant   A group of behaviors that operate on the environment and are affected by the consequences that follow their occurrence.

operant behavior   Behavior that is influenced by the consequences it produces.

operant (or **instrumental**) **conditioning**   A learning model in which behaviors that act on the environment are affected by the consequences that follow their occurrence.

order of mention strategy   Comprehension strategy that assumes the first event mentioned occurred earlier than events in the remainder of the sentence.

organ of Corti   The sense organ for hearing contained in the cochlea of the inner ear.

organic language disorders   Language disorders associated with physiological causes such as brain damage or hearing loss.

organization   The cognitive process of structuring patterns of interaction to deal more effectively with the environment.

ossicles   The three tiny bones of the middle ear that transmit energy from the tympanic membrane to the cochlea.

otorhinolaryngologist   Medical practitioner trained in diseases of the ear, nose, and throat.

oval window   The resting place for the footplate of the stapes where movements of the ossicular chain are transmitted to the cochlea.

overextensions   Words that overgeneralize to items that do not represent the conventional referents for the word.

paralinguistic codes   Production aspects such as prosody, intonation, rate, rhythm, and stress that accompany the spoken message to express attitude or emotion.

parallel play   Instances in which children engage in similar play activity in proximity to one another but do not actually interact.

parasympathetic division   The division of the autonomic nervous system that quiets and normalizes bodily functions.

parentese (also **motherese** or **child directed speech**)   Gender neutral term for the distinctive style of speech exhibited by caregivers with their toddlers.

passive   A major sentence type in which the grammatical subject of the sentence is the passive recipient of the action in the verb.

perception   Process of attending to, identifying, and interpreting stimuli.

performatives   A speech act in which the utterance itself performs the intended act, such as promising, teasing, and apologizing.

peripheral nervous system   That part of the nervous system that conducts sensory and motor impulses between the body and the CNS.

perlocutionary   The component of speech consisting of the listener's interpretation.

perlocutionary stage   The stage of communication development from birth to approximately 6 months in which caregivers infer intentions on the part of infants.

pharynx   Tubular cavity extending from the larynx to the oral and nasal cavities.

phonation   The production of vocal tone in the physiological process of setting the approximated vocal folds into vibration with exhaled air.

phone   An individual instance of a speech sound production notated within brackets (i.e., [ ]).

phoneme A conceptual family of sounds whose acoustic features are similar enough to be heard as the same speech sound; notated within slashes (i.e., / /).

phonetically consistent form (PCF) Infant sound productions that are stable in form and seemingly refer to certain objects, but do not resemble conventional words for them.

phonetic form rules A component of government-binding theory that generates an abstract characterization of sounds.

phonological awareness An aspect of metalinguistic abilities in which the child becomes conscious of the sounds of language in words, as evidenced by skills such as syllabification, segmentation, rhyming, alliteration, and blending.

phonology The study of the speech sounds of languages.

phrase Groups of words that are structurally related but do not comprise a clause or sentence.

phrase structure rules The underlying universal rules that generate the basic syntactic relationships in the deep structure of a sentence.

pivot grammar A description of children's early grammar that described a limited number of words (pivots) occurring only in certain positions and a larger set of words (open) combined with them.

placental barrier The membranous structure that allows nourishment and oxygen to pass between the mother and the embryo or fetus.

plausibility The notion that a relationship expressed in a sentence is a likelihood.

plausible event strategy Comprehension strategy that relies on determining the most probable state of affairs.

plot The central theme that provides the focus for story elements.

pons The middle portion of the brain stem that connects the midbrain and medulla.

positive reinforcer A stimulus that when presented contingent on a response increases the likelihood of that response; compare **negative reinforcement.**

possession The semantic case signaling that an entity is associated with, held, or owned by a possessor.

pragmatics The practical aspects of language used as a social tool, including the functions and alternations observed in social contexts.

prediction The scientific goal of identifying the variables that reliably precede a phenomenon.

presbycusis Hearing loss associated with aging.

prescriptive grammar A collection of rules that purports to dictate correct grammatical structures to the speakers of a language.

presupposition Speakers' ability to adjust their message based on their listeners' abilities and knowledge of the topic.

primary auditory cortex Cortical area in the temporal lobe where the sensation of sound is received.

primary language The major language spoken and understood by a population.

primary motor cortex Cortical area in the precentral gyrus responsible for initiating specific, voluntary movements.

primary reinforcers Stimuli that have reinforcing potential due to their survival value.

primary sensory cortex Cortical area in the postcentral gyrus responsible for receiving somesthetic sensations from the body.

primary visual cortex Cortical area in the occipital lobe where visual sensation is received.

primitive narratives (or **centering**) Narratives in which story elements are related in a conceptual way, but otherwise unorganized.

primitive speech acts Dore's classification of intentions expressed by infants and toddlers through characteristic gestures and vocalizations.

primitive streak A feature of the embryonic disc that generates the mesoderm, endoderm and ectoderm.

print awareness The recognition of print and its distinctive patterns (left-to-right flow, character orientation, etc.) as meaningful symbols related to reading and writing.

probability A behavioral concept indicating response strength.

process verbs Words that refer to unobservable activity or gradual changes.

production The expression or encoding of an idea in an utterance.

projection fibers   Neural fibers that transmit motor and sensory fibers between the cortical areas and peripheral nerves.

prompts   Caregiver utterances that stimulate responses from their children to continue their verbal exchange.

pronominalization   The process of replacing a noun or noun phrase with a pronoun form (or pronominal).

pronoun   Words that can replace a noun or noun phrase through anaphoric or cataphoric reference; also called pronominals.

proposition   The set of semantic relations that specify the relationships between the nouns of the sentence and its verb.

propositional force   The linguistic meanings expressed by the words and phrases of a speech act.

proprioception   The sense of body position and orientation.

prosody   Production features of speech, such as intonation, stress, rate, and rhythm, that provide its melodic character.

protoconversations   Early interactions between caregivers and infants that include aspects such as turn taking.

protodeclaratives   Early infant vocal and gestural behaviors that appear to note an object for the purpose of gaining the caregiver's attention.

protoimperatives   Early infant vocal and gestural behaviors that suggest commanding or requesting action on the part of the infant.

protonarratives (or **prenarratives**)   The earliest forms of children's stories.

proverbs   Figurative language that expresses truths or gives advice through analogy (e.g., *Look before you leap!*).

proxemics   The study of personal space in social interactions, including interpersonal communication.

pseudophrase   Early approximation of multi-word utterances through production of conventional two-word phrases (e.g., *allgone, nomore*) in which the individual elements do not occur elsewhere independently.

psycholinguistics   The branch of linguistics concerned with studying the mental operations related to language.

psychologists   Professionals who evaluate and treat emotional disorders.

punishment   The contingent presentation of an aversive stimulus that results in a decrease in the probability of a response.

pyramidal tract   The tract of nerve fibers carrying motor impulses from the cortex to various levels of the spinal cord.

quasi-resonant nuclei   Early infant oral sounds that are not as resonant as mature vowel sounds.

recognition   The perceptual process of identifying a stimulus as having been experienced previously; the ability of individuals to attend to and identify a particular person's presence.

recombinations   The developmental process of combining two shorter language constructions into a longer construction.

recounts   A type of narrative that relates a series of events.

recurrence   An early reflexive relation in which a word indicates that an object or its duplicate has reappeared.

reduplicated babbling   Babbling in which a syllable is repeated in strings, as in *dadada*.

reduplication   An early approximation of a multi-word utterance through repeating a conventional word within the same intonational contour.

referential   Behaving in ways that identify a stimulus as the topic for communication.

referential words   Early words whose primary purpose is to refer to objects.

reflexes   Preprogrammed neuromuscular responses to stimuli.

reflexive cry   Infant cry behavior in response to physiologic stimuli.

reflexive relations   Ways in which objects relate to themselves, including existence, nonexistence, disappearance, and recurrence.

reflexive smile   Infant smile behavior that is in apparent response to internal physiologic stimuli.

registers   Speaking styles that are characteristic of certain roles of social contexts.

reinforcement   Procedures that result in increased response strength through contingent presentation or withdrawal of stimuli.

reinforcer Any stimulus presented contingently that increases the frequency or strength of a response.

relational words Words that refer to abstract relationships between objects.

relative pronoun Pronouns that introduce relative clauses, which act as adjectives for the noun they follow (e.g., *The boy who came thanked me*).

resonation The modification of the vocal tone produced through changing the shape and size of the spaces in the vocal tract.

respiration The physiologic process of ventilating the body to inhale fresh air and exhale used air.

response A reaction to a stimulus.

response induction The behavioral process in which there is a tendency for responses different from the original to occur.

response strength Indicated through the frequency, probability, or intensity of responses.

reversibility The possibility that the subject and object phrase nouns could logically change places.

scheme Organized patterns of responding to stimuli.

science A body of principles and attitudes that attempts to objectively understand natural phenomena.

scientific determinism The belief that all events have causes.

scientific elegance The belief that the best scientific explanation is the most economical explanation.

scientific explanation Identification and verification of the variables that cause an event to occur.

scientific objectivity The belief that data and evidence are more important than authorities or opinions.

scientific restraint The willingness to wait for objective, scientifically supported explanations.

scripts Familiar structured interactions associated with a routine.

secondary reinforcers Stimuli that obtain their reinforcing potential through association with primary reinforcers.

segmentation The ability to analyze the stream of speech into units such as phonemes, syllables, and words.

selection restrictions Constraints on the words that can occur together because of the semantic features carried by each.

selective imitation Children's partial imitations of adult utterances.

semantic complexity Measures the complexity of a linguistic structure by gauging the number of semantic relationships that must be discriminated to use it correctly.

semantic features The perceptual features such as size, shape, color, and so on, that define a conceptual class.

semantic memory An individual's understanding of a word's meaning, including the words and concepts they associate with that word.

semantic network The pattern of associated words and concepts that evolve out of experiencing a word.

semantic (or case) relations The relationships between objects, persons, and events expressed through language.

semantics The study of meaning in language.

semantic-syntactic rules Describes children's early grammar emphasizing that expressing meaning provides the motivation for attempting to learn correct forms.

semicircular canals Three fluid-filled bony loops in the inner ear that contain fluid and contribute to maintaining balance.

sensation The initial stage of perception in which sense organs are affected by a physical stimulus.

sensorineural Hearing loss due to damage nerve endings.

sensory association area The cortical areas just posterior to the sensory strip that assist in interpreting sensations.

sentence A group of words that includes a subject and a predicate and is structurally complete.

sequence pattern Syntactic devices associated with text grammar that signal the description of a sequence of events or steps.

sequences (or chaining) Early narratives that relate heaps of elements that are related to a central topic.

setting The characters, location, and circumstances for a narrative.

setting events The collection of stimuli present in a setting that are capable of influencing behavior.

shaping   The gradual modification of a behavior as reinforcement follows variations that progressively approximate a final form of the behavior.

simile   Figurative language that directly states an analogous relationship (e.g., *He's as clumsy as an ox!*).

simultaneous acquisition   Learning two languages at the same time.

single-subject experimental designs   Research design in which an individual subject serves as his or her own control.

social context   The nature of a setting and the status, roles, and agendas of the speakers in that setting.

social interaction   Successive interchanges between at least two persons in which the behavior of one affects the other.

socialized speech   Speech that is addressed to others and acknowledges their needs and interests.

social smile   A smile in response to another person's presence or behavior.

sociolinguistics   The branch of linguistics studying the influence of social context on language.

solitary play   Play behavior in which a child plays independent of others, even those in close proximity.

specific activity reflex   A reflex that affects an individual body part.

specific language impairment   Language disorders that appear unrelated to organic causes or any other general disability.

speech   The dynamic production of speech sounds through the processes of respiration, phonation, resonation, and articulation for communication.

speech act   The concept of a unit of communication involving a speaker's intention, the linguistic form of the message conveying the intention, and the listener's interpretation of the message.

speech discrimination   The ability to distinguish meaningful differences between speech sounds.

speech-language pathologist   Specialist trained in the identification, assessment, and treatment of human communication disorders.

speech mechanism   The anatomical structures for the production of speech sounds.

spinal cord   The part of the CNS that extends below the brain stem.

spinal nerves   The peripheral nerves that exit the spinal cord.

S-structures   A component of government-binding theory that occurs just prior to the production of the surface structure.

stacked repair sequences   Successive attempts to clarify an utterance in which additional elements are included in each subsequent attempt.

standard dialect   The generally accepted version of the primary language used in a group.

standardized assessment   Evaluation of language abilities using formal test instruments.

standard language   The primary language expected by most speakers in formal contexts.

stapes   The smallest and innermost ossicle in the middle ear; its contact with the oval window transmits movements to the cochlea.

state relations   Several relationships regarding the status of objects such as location, possession, and attribution.

state verbs   Words that link a subject to a stable or unchanging condition or attribute.

stimulus generalization   The behavioral process in which old responses occur to new stimuli.

stories   Typically fictitious narratives that exhibit discernible organization and structure.

structuralism   A philosophical perspective that emphasizes that the structure and organization of language reflects the inherent nature of the mind.

style shifting   Modifications in style speakers make in response to social contexts or the status of their listeners.

subglottic pressure   The air pressure that occurs below the vocal folds.

subordinate category   Subgroup of objects defined by a greater number of specific features than those defining the overall or superordinate category.

subordinate clause   An embedded clause that supplements the main clause in a complex sentence.

subordinating conjunction   A conjunction that introduces a clause that acts as an adverb to describe time, location, cause, or conditions related to the main clause.

substantive words Classification of early words that occur in response to objects and classes of objects.

successive acquisition Learning a second language following establishment of a first language.

successive single-word utterance Utterance composed of two words spoken separately, where both words are related to the same context; taken by some as evidence of successive approximation of grammar.

sulcus (pl., **sulci**) The narrower, more shallow grooves that occur on the convoluted cortical surface of the brain.

superlative Adjective form that expresses relative degree of an attribute when comparing more than two items (e.g. *big* vs. *bigger* vs. *biggest*).

superordinate category The highest conceptual level in a hierarchical classification of meanings, which includes all of the subgroups or subordinate categories in a given class.

suprasegmental devices Speech production effects, including intonation, stress, and rhythm, superimposed across the linguistic segments (i.e., words and phrases) to modify their meaning.

supplementary variables Those stimuli, such as audiences, that additionally influence the likelihood of certain verbal behaviors.

surface structure The actualized production of a sentence by a speaker.

symbol Something (e.g., the word *chair*, whether spoken or written) that stands for or represents something else without bearing physical resemblance to it.

symbolic function The cognitive process of using symbols to represent actual objects or events.

symbolic play Play behavior in which one item is used to represent another.

symbolization The perceptual ability to identify the symbolic representation of objects or events with words.

sympathetic division The division of the autonomic nervous system that stimulates the body's "fight or flight" responses.

synapse The junction or gap where neural impulses jump from the axon of one neuron to the dendrite of another.

synonym A word that shares the majority of its semantic features with another word having similar meaning.

syntagmatic-paradigmatic shift A transition in which word associations shift from a syntactic to semantic basis.

syntax The linguistic rules that describe the relationship between word orders and the meanings they express.

systematic The regularities exhibited by speakers of a language that make occurrences in the language predictable.

tacts A primary verbal operant that occurs in response to an object, event, or relationship and the form of the response exhibits a conventional correspondence to others' responses; the behavioral equivalent of naming, describing, or labeling.

taxonomic organization Associating words based on hierarchical categories.

technical application The goal of applied science in which knowledge results in technology that is helpful to society.

telegraphic speech A traditional concept of children's grammar that viewed their utterances as reduced forms of adult grammar.

temporal words Words that relate events in time.

text grammar Characteristic styles associated with language found in textbooks.

textual A primary verbal operant that occurs in response to written, printed, or graphic stimuli; the behavioral equivalent of reading.

thematic organization Associating words based on their relationship to a theme or context.

thyroarytenoid muscle (also **vocalis**) The paired muscles that contribute the bulk of the vocal folds.

top-down model The model that proposes reading progresses from confirming ideas about overall content as additional written material is decoded.

topic initiation Introducing a topic in discourse.

topic maintenance The continuation of a topic in discourse through successive utterances related to that topic.

topic shading Subtle shifts in the conversational topic through addressing an isolated aspect of a previous utterance.

transformational generative grammar A linguistic theory proposing that universal rules generate underlying structures that may be transformed by rules to derive the specific sentence forms of each language.

transformational rules   The linguistic rules applied in each language to transform underlying sentence structure into the varying surface structures produced in each language.

transitional utterances   Any of several utterance types that appear to represent a progression from single-word utterances to multiword utterances reflecting syntactic order.

transitive verb   Lexical verbs capable of carrying a grammatical object affected by the action of the verb; compare **intransitive verb.**

trimesters   Three equal intervals of approximately 3 months each in a typical pregnancy.

turnabouts   Comments and replies used by caregivers to maintain the momentum in a conversation and shift the turn back to the child.

trophoblast   The outermost cells in the blastocyst that attach the embryo to the uterine wall and serve as the pathway for nutrients.

turn taking   The alternation of speaking and listening behaviors in a conversation.

tympanic membrane (or **eardrum**)   The membrane that divides the outer and middle ear and receives sound waves from the environment.

Type I punishment   The procedure of delivering a stimulus contingent on a behavior that results in its decrease.

Type II punishment   The procedure of removing a stimulus contingent on a behavior that results in its decrease.

uncertainty behaviors (or **verbal fragmentations**)   Excessive interjections and filler sometimes noted in utterances of aging individuals.

underextension   A word that is excessively discriminated in that it occurs only in response to a specific stimulus or context; compare **overextension.**

understanding   The process of decoding meaning from an encoded message, as in comprehending the significance of words and sentences.

unfocused chains   Narratives based on elements linked together logically but in an unorganized manner.

unmarked   Semantic aspect of words that refer to the presence of a dimension, including the positive end of that dimension (e.g., length); compare **marked.**

vegetative sounds   Infant oral sounds (e.g., clicks, burps) associated with feeding and digestion.

ventral horns   The anterior areas of the spinal cord containing nuclei for relaying outgoing motor impulses to the body.

verbal communication   The use of symbols (i.e., words), whether spoken, written, or gestured by a speaker to express ideas.

verbal operant   A group of responses that share a history of occurring under similar circumstances and resulting in similar consequences.

vertical development   The process of associating additional meanings and contexts with a word; compare **horizontal development.**

visual association area   The cortical area surrounding the primary visual cortex and responsible for interpreting the significance of visual stimuli.

vocabulary   A speaker's total accumulation of words understood or used in the language.

vocal play   Infant sound productions exhibiting longer strings of varied syllables.

vocal tract   The cavities and structures above the vocal folds capable of modifying the vocal tone and airflow into distinctive speech sounds.

voice   The tone produced by vibration of the vocal folds and modified by the resonating cavities of the vocal tract.

Wernicke's area   Cortical area in the posterior temporal lobe primarily responsible for interpreting oral language.

wh-constituent question   A caregiver prompt used to evoke specific information in a child's response (e.g., *where* questions to evoke locational information).

wholistic associations   Extension of a word to items sharing a number of features with the original referent for that word.

word awareness   The conscious awareness that words are objects with phonetic structure and can have multiple meanings.

world knowledge   An individual's understanding of the world based on his or her accumulated experiences and memory.

zygote   The single cell formed at conception containing the genetic codes of both the father and mother.

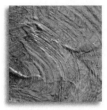

References

Akhtar, N., Dunham, F., & Dunham, P. J. (1991). Directive interactions and early vocabulary development: The role of joint attentional focus. *Journal of Child Language, 18,* 41–49.

Allen, H. B. (1996). Language. In *Compton's Interactive Encyclopedia.* Cambridge, MA: Compton's NewMedia.

American Heritage Dictionary. (1970). New York: American Heritage Publishing.

Anselmi, D., Tomasello, M., & Acunzo, M. (1986). Young children's responses to neutral and specific contingent queries. *Journal of Child Language, 13,* 135–144.

Applebee, A. N. (1978). The child's concept of story. Chicago: University of Chicago Press.

Atchley, R. C. (1987). *Aging: Continuity and change* (2nd ed.). Belmont, CA: Wadsworth.

Atherton, S., & Hegde, M. N. (1996, April). *Experimental enrichment of language in toddlers.* Paper presented at the Third Treatment Research in Communication Disorders, Chicago, IL.

Austin, J. (1962). *How to do things with words.* London: Oxford University Press.

Axtell, R. E. (1991). *Gestures: The DO's and TABOOS of body language around the world.* New York: John Wiley & Sons.

Bachrach, A. J. (1972). *Psychological research: An introduction* (3rd ed.). New York: Random House.

Barret-Goldfarb, M. S., & Whitehurst, G. J. (1973). Infant vocalizations as a function of parental voice selection. *Developmental Psychology, 8,* 273–276.

Bates, E. (1976). *Language and context: The acquisition of pragmatics.* New York: Academic Press.

Bates, E., Bretherton, I., & Snyder, L. (1988). *From first words to grammar: Individual differences and dissociable mechanisms.* New York: Cambridge University Press.

Bateson, M. (1971). The interpersonal context of infant vocalizations. *Quarterly Progress Report, Research Laboratory of Electronics, MIT, 100,* 170–176.

Bateson, M. (1975). Mother-infant exchanges: The epigenesis of conversational interaction. *Annals of the New York Academy of Sciences, 263,* 101–113.

Bellugi, U. (1967). *The acquisition of negation.* Unpublished doctoral dissertation. Harvard University, Cambridge, MA.

Benedict, H. (1979). Early lexical development: Comprehension and production. *Journal of Child Language, 6,* 183–200.

Benson, D. F., & Ardilla, A. (1996). *Aphasia: A clinical perspective.* New York: Oxford University Press.

Berko Gleason, J. (2001). *The development of language (5th edition).* Needham Heights, MA: Allyn & Bacon.

Bhatnagar, S. C., & Andy, O. J. (1995). *Neuroscience for the study of communicative disorders.* Baltimore: Williams & Wilkins.

Bijou, S. W., & Baer, D. M. (1961). *Child development I: A systematic and empirical theory.* Englewood Cliffs, NJ: Prentice-Hall.

Bijou, S. W., & Baer, D. M. (1965). *Child development II: Universal stage of infancy.* Englewood Cliffs, NJ: Prentice-Hall.

Bijou, S. W., & Baer, D. M. (1978). *Behavior analysis of child development.* Englewood Cliffs, NJ: Prentice-Hall.

Bloom, L. (1970). *Language development: Form and function of emerging grammars.* Cambridge: MIT Press.

Bloom, L. (1973). *One word at a time: The use of single-word utterances before syntax*. The Hague: Mouton.

Bloom, L., Hood, L., & Lightbown, P. (1974). Imitation in language development: If, when and why. *Cognitive Psychology, 6,* 380–420.

Bloom, L., & Lahey, M. (1978). *Language development and language disorders*. New York: John Wiley & Sons.

Bloom, L., Lahey, M., Hood, L., Lifter, K., & Feiss, K. (1980). Complex sentences: Acquisition of syntactic connections and the semantic relations they encode. *Journal of Child Language, 7,* 235–261.

Bloom, L., Lightbown, P., & Hood, L. (1975). Structure and variation in child language. *Monographs of the Society for Research in Child Development, 40.*

Bloom, L., Miller, P., & Hood, L. (1975). Variation and reduction as aspects of competence in language development. In A. Pick (Ed.), *Minnesota Symposia on Child Psychology* (Vol. 9, pp. 3–55). Minneapolis: University of Minnesota Press.

Bloom, L., Rocissano, L., & Hood, L. (1976). Adult-child discourse: Developmental interaction between information processing and linguistic interaction. *Cognitive Psychology, 8,* 521–552.

Bohannon, J. N., & Stanowicz, L. (1988). Adult responses to children's language errors: The issue of negative evidence. *Developmental Psychology, 24,* 684–689.

Bohannon, J. N., & Warren-Luebecker, A. (1985). Theoretical approaches to language acquisition. In J. Berko Gleason (Ed.), *The development of language* (pp. 173–226). Columbus, OH: Merrill.

Bornstein, M. (1985). On the development of color naming in young children: Data and theory. *Brain and Language, 26,* 72–93.

Bowerman, M. (1973). *Early syntactic development: A cross-linguistic study with special reference to Finnish*. Cambridge: Cambridge University Press.

Bowerman, M. (1978). The acquisition of word meaning: An investigation in some current conflicts. In N. Waterson & C. Snow (Eds.), *The development of communication* (pp. 263–287). New York: John Wiley.

Braine, M. D. S. (1963). The ontogeny of English phrase structure: The first phase. *Language, 39,* 1–14.

Braine, M. D. S. (1976). Children's first word combinations. *Monographs of the Society for Research in Child Development, 41.*

Breitmayer, B. J., & Ricciuti, H. N. (1988). The effect of neonatal temperament on caregiver behavior in the newborn nursery. *Infant Mental Health Journal, 9,* 158–172.

Brinton, B., & Fujiki, M. (1984). Development of topic manipulation skills in discourse. *Journal of Speech and Hearing Research, 27,* 350–358.

Brinton, B., Fujiki, M., Loeb, D., & Winkler, E. (1986). Development of conversational repair strategies in response to requests for clarification. *Journal of Speech and Hearing Research, 29,* 75–81.

Brown, R. (1958). *Words and things*. New York: Free Press.

Brown, R. (1973). *A first language: The early stages*. Cambridge, MA: Harvard University Press.

Brown, R., & Fraser, C. (1963). The acquisition of syntax. In C. N. Cofer & B. Musgrave (Eds.), *Verbal behavior and learning: Problems and processes* (pp. 158–201). New York: McGraw-Hill.

Brown, R., & Hanlon, C. (1970). Derivational complexity and order of acquisition in child speech. In J. R. Hayes (Ed.), *Cognition and the development of language* (pp. 155–207). New York: John Wiley.

Bruner, J. (1977). Early social interaction and language acquisition. In R. Schaffer (Ed.), *Studies in mother-infant interaction* (pp. 271–289). New York: Academic Press.

Cairns, H. S. (1996). *The acquisition of language* (2nd ed.). Austin, TX: Pro-Ed.

Capelli, R. (1985). *An experimental analysis of morphologic acquisition*. Unpublished master's thesis, California State University, Fresno.

Carey, S. (1978). The child as word learner. In M. Halle, J. Bresnan, & G. Miller (Eds.), *Linguistic theory and psychological reality* (pp. 264–293). Cambridge, MA: MIT Press.

Carey, S., & Bartlett, E. (1978). Acquiring a single new word. *Papers and Reports on Child Language Development, 15,* 17–29.

Casby, M. W. (2003). The development of play in infants, toddlers, and young children. *Communication Disorders Quarterly, 24*(4), 163–173.

Chafe, W. (1970). *Meaning and the structure of language*. Chicago: University of Chicago Press.

Chall, J. S. (1983). *Stages of reading development*. New York: McGraw-Hill.

Chapman, R. S. (1981). Mother-child interaction in the second year of life. In R. L. Schiefelbusch &

D. D. Bricker (Eds.), *Early language: Acquisition and intervention.* Baltimore: University Park Press.

Chapman, R., Streim, N. W., Crais, E. R., Salmon, D., Strand, E. A., & Negri, N. A. (1992). Child talk: Assumptions of a developmental process model for early language learning. In R. Chapman (Ed.), *Processes in language acquisition and disorders* (pp. 3–19). St. Louis, MO: Mosby-Year Book.

Cheng, L. (1987). Cross-cultural and linguistic considerations in working with Asian populations. *ASHA, 29*(6), 33–38.

Chomsky, N. (1957). *Syntactic structures.* The Hague: Mouton.

Chomsky, N. (1959). A review of Skinner's Verbal Behavior. *Language, 35,* 26–58.

Chomsky, N. (1965). *Aspects of the theory of syntax.* Cambridge, MA: MIT Press.

Chomsky, N. (1968). *Language and mind.* New York: Harcourt, Brace & World.

Chomsky, N. (1981). *Lectures on government and binding.* Dordrecht, The Netherlands: Foris.

Chomsky, N., & Halle, M. (1968). *The sound pattern of English.* New York: Harper & Row.

Clark, E., & Sengul, C. (1978). Strategies in the acquisition of deixis. *Journal of Child Language, 5,* 457–475.

Clark, E. V. (1973a). Non-linguistic strategies and the acquisition of word meanings. *Cognition, 2,* 161–182.

Clark, E. V. (1973b). What's in a word? On the child's acquisition of semantics in his first language. In T. E. Moore (Ed.), *Cognitive development and the acquisition of language* (pp. 65–110). New York: Academic Press.

Clark, E. V. (1980). Here's the top: Non-linguistic strategies in the acquisition of orientational terms. *Child Development, 51,* 329–338.

Collis, G. M., & Schaffer, H. R. (1975). Synchronization of visual attention in mother-infant pairs. *Journal of Child Psychology and Psychiatry, 16,* 315–320.

Cox, M. V., & Richardson, J. R. (1985). How do children describe spatial relationships? *Journal of Child Language, 12,* 611–620.

Crais, E. R. (1992). Fast mapping: A new look at word learning. In R. S. Chapman (Ed.), *Processes in language acquisition and disorders* (pp. 159–185). St. Louis, MO: Mosby.

Cromer, R. F. (1981). Reconceptualizing language acquisition and cognitive development. In R. L.

Schiefelbusch & D. D. Bricker (Eds.), *Early language: Acquisition and intervention* (pp. 51–137). Baltimore: University Park Press.

Cruttendon, A. (1970). A phonetic study of babbling. *British Journal of Psychology, 61,* 397–408.

Darley, F., & Winitz, H. (1961). Age of the first word: Review of the research. *Journal of Speech and Hearing Disorders, 26,* 271–290.

de Vries, J. P., Visser, G. H. A., & Prechtl, H. F. R. (1982). The emergence of fetal behavior. I. Qualitative aspects. *Early Human Development, 7,* 301–322.

deBoysson-Bardies, B., Sagart, L., & Durand, C. (1984). Discernible differences in the babbling of infants according to target language. *Journal of Child Language, 11,* 1–15.

DeCasper, A., & Fifer, W. P. (1980). On human bonding: Newborns prefer their mothers' voices. *Science, 208,* 1174–1176.

DeCesari, R. (1985). *Experimental training of grammatic morphemes: Effects on the order of acquisition.* Unpublished master's thesis, University of California, Fresno.

Dever, R. (1978). *Talk: Teaching the American language to kids.* Columbus, OH: Merrill.

deVilliers, J., & deVilliers, P. (1973). A cross-sectional study of the acquisition of grammatical morphemes. *Journal of Psycholinguistic Research, 2,* 267–278.

Dore, J. (1974). A pragmatic description of early language development. *Journal of Psycholinguistic Research, 3,* 343–350.

Dore, J. (1975). Holophrases, speech acts, and language universals. *Journal of Child Language, 2,* 21–40.

Dore, J. (1978). Variation in preschool children's conversational performances. In K. Nelson (Ed.), *Children's language* (Vol. 1, pp. 397–444). New York: Gardner Press.

Dore, J. (1986). The development of conversational competence. In R. Schiefelbusch (Ed.), *Language competence: Assessment and intervention* (pp. 3–60). San Diego, CA: College-Hill Press.

Dore, J., Franklin, M., Miller, R., & Ramer, A. (1976). Transitional phenomena in early language acquisition. *Journal of Child Language, 3,* 13–28.

Ehri, L. (1991). Development of the ability to read words. In R. Barr, M. Kamil, P. Mosenthal, & P. Pearson (Eds.), *Handbook of reading research* (Vol. 2, pp. 383–417). White Plains, NY: Longman.

Ehri, L., & McCormick, S. (1998). Phases of word learning: Implications for instruction with delayed and disabled readers. *Reading and Writing Quarterly, 14,* 135–164.

Eilers, R. E., & Minifie, F. D. (1975). Fricative discrimination in early infancy. *Journal of Speech and Hearing Research, 18,* 158–167.

Eimas, P. D. (1974). Linguistic processing of speech by young infants. In R. L. Schiefelbusch & L. L. Lloyd (Eds.), *Language perspectives—acquisition, retardation, and intervention* (pp. 55–73). Baltimore: University Park Press.

Einstein, A. (1949). Quoted in: News Chronicle (14 March 1949). *The Columbia Dictionary of Quotations.* New York: Columbia University Press.

Ely, R. (1997). Language and literacy in the school years. In J. B. Gleason (Ed.), *The development of language* (4th ed., pp. 398–439). Boston: Allyn & Bacon.

Erickson, J. G. (1985). How many languages do you speak? An overview of bilingual education. *Topics in Language Disorders, 5,* 1–14.

Ervin-Tripp, S. (1964). Imitation and structural change in children's language. In E. Lenneberg (Ed.), *New directions in the study of language* (pp. 163–189). Cambridge, MA: MIT Press.

Ervin-Tripp, S., & Mitchell-Kernan, C. (1977). Introduction. In S. Ervin-Tripp & C. Mitchell-Kernan (Eds.), *Child discourse* (pp. 1–23). New York: Academic Press.

Farrar, J. (1992). Negative evidence and grammatical morpheme acquisition. *Developmental Psychology, 28,* 90–98.

Ferguson, C., & Farwell, C. (1975). Words and sounds in early language acquisition: English initial consonants in the first fifty words. *Language, 51,* 419–439.

Ferguson, C. A. (1964). Baby talk in six languages. *American Anthropologist, 66,* 103–114.

Fernald, A. (1985). Four-month-old infants prefer to listen to motherese. *Infant Behavior and Development, 8,* 181–195.

Fernald, A., Taeschner, T., Dunn, J., Papousek, M., deBoysson-Bardies, B., & Fukui, I. (1989). A cross-language study of prosody modifications in mothers' and fathers' speech to preverbal infants. *Journal of Child Language, 16,* 477–401.

Field, T. M., Cohen, D., Garcia, R., & Greenberg, R. (1984). Mother-stranger face discrimination by the newborn. *Infant Behavior and Development, 7,* 19–25.

Fillmore, C. (1968). The case for case. In E. Bach & R. Harms (Eds.), *Universals in linguistic theory* (pp. 1–88). New York: Holt, Rinehart & Winston.

Fitzgerald, J., & Shanahan, T. (2000). Reading and writing relations and their development. *Educational Psychologist, 35*(1), 39–50.

Formby, D. (1967). Maternal recognition of infant's cry. *Developmental Medicine and Child Neurology, 9,* 293–298.

Fulghum, R. (1986). *All I really need to know I learned in kindergarten.* New York: Ballantine.

Gallagher, T. (1981). Contingent query sequences within adult-child discourse. *Journal of Child Language, 8,* 51–62.

Garvey, C., & Hogan, R. (1973). Social speech and social interaction: Egocentrism revisited. *Child Development, 44,* 562–568.

Geller, E. (1989). The assessment of perspective taking skills. *Seminars in Speech and Language, 10,* 28–41.

Gentry, J. R., & Gillet, J. W. (1993). *Teaching kids to spell.* Portsmouth, NH: Heinemann.

Gibbs, R. (1987). Linguistic factors in children's understanding of idioms. *Journal of Child Language, 14,* 569–586.

Gilger, J. W. (1995). Behavioral genetics: Concepts for research and practice in language development and disorders. *Journal of Speech and Hearing Research, 38,* 1126–1142.

Gillon, G. (2004). *Phonological awareness: From research to practice.* New York: Guilford Press.

Ginsburg, H., & Opper, S. (1969). *Piaget's theory of intellectual development: An introduction.* Englewood Cliffs, NJ: Prentice-Hall.

Goldfield, B. A. (1993). Noun bias in maternal speech to one-year-olds. *Journal of Child Language, 20,* 85–99.

Gordon, P. (1988). Count/mass category acquisition: Distributional distinctions in children's speech. *Journal of Child Language, 15,* 109–128.

Greenfield, P., & Smith, J. (1976). *The structure of communication in early language development.* New York: Academic Press.

Grice, H. P. (1975). Logic and conversation. In P. Cole & J. L. Morgan (Eds.), *Syntax and semantics 3: Speech acts* (pp. 41–58). New York: Academic Press.

Grosjean, F. (1982). *Life with two languages.* Cambridge, MA: Harvard University Press.

Guilford, J. P., & Hoepfner, R. (1971). *The analysis of intelligence.* New York: McGraw-Hill.

Haith, M. M., Bergman, T., & Moore, M. (1977). Eye contact and face scanning in early infancy. *Science, 198,* 853–855.

Halliday, M. A. K. (1967). Notes on transitivity and theme in English, part 2. *Journal of Linguistics, 3,* 199–244.

Halliday, M. A. K. (1975). *Learning how to mean: Explorations in the development of language.* New York: Arnold.

Haynes, H., White, B. L., & Held, R. (1965). Visual accommodation in human infants. *Science, 148,* 528–538.

Haynes, W. O. (1994a). Caretaker-child interactions. In W. O. Haynes & B. B. Shulman (Eds.), *Communication development: Foundations, processes, and clinical applications* (pp. 82–113). Englewood Cliffs, NJ: Prentice-Hall.

Haynes, W. O. (1994b). Concepts in neurolinguistics and information processing. In W. O. Haynes & B. B. Shulman (Eds.), *Communication development: Foundations, processes, and clinical applications* (pp. 29–54). Englewood Cliffs, NJ: Prentice-Hall.

Haynes, W. O. (1994c). Individual differences in the acquisition of communication and directions for future research. In W. O. Haynes & B. B. Shulman (Eds.), *Communication development: Foundations, processes, and clinical applications* (pp. 412–432). Englewood Cliffs, NJ: Prentice-Hall.

Haynes, W. O. (1994d). Single-word communication: A period of transitions. In W. O. Haynes & B. B. Shulman (Eds.), *Communication development: Foundations, processes, and clinical applications* (pp. 230–256). Englewood Cliffs, NJ: Prentice-Hall.

Haynes, W. O., & Shulman, B. B. (1994). Ethnic and cultural differences in communication development. In W. O. Haynes & B. B. Shulman (Eds.), *Communication development: Foundations, processes, and clinical applications* (pp. 387–411). Englewood Cliffs, NJ: Prentice-Hall.

Heath, S. B. (1986). Taking a cross-cultural look at narratives. *Topics in Language Disorders, 7,* 84–95.

Hegde, M. N. (1980). Issues in the study and explanation of language behavior. *Journal of Psycholinguistic Research, 9,* 1–22.

Hegde, M. N. (1996). *Clinical research in communicative disorders: Principles and strategies* (2nd ed.). San Diego, CA: Singular.

Heidinger, V. A. (1984). *Analyzing syntax and semantics: A self-instructional approach for teachers and clinicians.* Washington, DC: Gallaudet College Press.

Highnam, C. L. (1994). Cognitive aspects of communication development. In W. O. Haynes & B. B. Shulman (Eds.), *Communication development: Foundations, processes, and clinical applications* (pp. 165–198). Englewood Cliffs, NJ: Prentice-Hall.

Hockett, C. (1960). The origin of speech. *Scientific American, 203,* 89–96.

Hooper, S. R., Swartz, C. W., Wakely, M. B., de Kruif, R. E. L., & Montgomery, J. W. (2002). Executive functions in elementary school children with and without problems in expression. *Journal of Learning Disabilities, 35*(1), 57–68.

Horgan, D. (1978). The development of the full passive. *Journal of Child Language, 5,* 65–80.

Hymes, D. (1972). Introduction. In C. Cazden, V. John, & D. Hymes (Eds.), *Functions of language in the classroom* (pp. i–xii). New York: Teachers College, Columbia University.

Ingram, D. (1974). The relationship between comprehension and production. In R. Schiefelbusch & L. Lloyd (Eds.), *Language perspectives—acquisition, retardation, and intervention* (pp. 313–334). Baltimore: University Park Press.

Ingram, D. (1976). *Phonological disability in children.* London: Arnold.

Irwin, O. C. (1947). Infant speech: Consonant sounds according to place of articulation. *Journal of Speech Disorders, 12,* 397–401.

Irwin, O. C. (1948). Infant speech: The effect of family occupational status and of age on use of sound types. *Journal of Speech and Hearing Disorders, 13,* 224–226.

Irwin, O. C. (1952). Speech development in the young child. 2. Some factors related to the speech development of the infant and the young child. *Journal of Speech and Hearing Disorders, 17,* 269–279.

Jakobson, R. (1968). *Child language, aphasia, and phonological universals.* The Hague: Mouton. (Original copyright, 1941)

James, S. L. (1990). *Normal language acquisition.* Austin, TX: Pro-Ed.

Jusczyk, P. W. (1992). Developing phonological categories for the speech signal. In C. A. Ferguson, L. Menn, & C. Stoel-Gammon, (Eds.), *Phonological development: Models, research, implications.* Parkston, MD: York Press.

Kamhi, A. G. (1992). Three perspectives on language processing: Interactionism, modularity, and holism. In R. Chapman (Ed.), *Processes in language acquisition and disorders* (pp. 45–64). St. Louis, MO: Mosby-Year Book.

Kamhi, A. G., & Catts, H. W. (2005). Reading development. In H. W. Catts & A. G. Kamhi (Eds.), *Language and reading disabilities* (2nd ed.). Boston: Allyn & Bacon.

Kantor, J. R. (1959a). *Interbehavioral psychology* (Rev. ed.). Bloomington, IN: Principia.

Kantor, J. R. (1959b). Evolution and the science of psychology. *Psychological Record, 9,* 131–142.

Katz, J., & Fodor, J. (1963). The structure of a semantic theory. *Language, 39,* 170–210.

Kaye, K., & Charney, R. (1981). Conversational asymmetry between mothers and children. *Journal of Child Language, 8,* 35–49.

Kent R. D. (1997). *The speech sciences.* San Diego, CA: Singular.

Kent, R. D., & Bauer, H. R. (1985). Vocalizations of one-year-olds. *Journal of Child Language, 12,* 491–526.

Klaus, M. H., & Kennell, J. H. (1976). *Maternal-infant bonding.* St. Louis, MO: C. V. Mosby.

Klima E., & Bellugi, U. (1966). Syntactic regularities in the speech of children. In J. Lyons & R. Wales (Eds.), *Psycholinguistic papers* (pp. 183–208). Edinburgh: Edinburgh University Press.

Kuhl, P. K. (1989). On babies, birds, modules, and mechanisms: A comparative approach to the acquisition of vocal communication. In R. J. Dooling & S. H. Hulse (Eds.), *The comparative psychology of audition: Perceiving complex sounds* (pp. 379–419). Hillsdale, NJ: Lawrence Erlbaum.

Kuhl, P. K. (1991). Perception, cognition, and the ontogenetic and phylogenetic emergence of speech. In S. E. Brauth, W. S. Hall, & R. J. Dooling (Eds.), *Plasticity of development* (pp. 73–106). Cambridge, MA: MIT Press.

Kuhl, P. K. & Meltzoff, A. N. (1982). The bimodal perception of speech in infancy. *Science, 218,* 1138–1141.

Kuhl, P., & Miller, J. D. (1975). Speech perception by the chinchilla: Voiced-voiceless distinction in alveolar-plosive consonants. *Science, 190,* 69–72.

Labov, W. (1972). *Language in the inner city: Studies in the black English vernacular.* Philadelphia: University of Pennsylvania Press.

Lane, V. W., & Molyneaux, D. (1992). *The dynamics of communicative development.* Englewood Cliffs, NJ: Prentice-Hall.

Lenneberg, E. (1967). *Biological foundations of language.* New York: John Wiley.

Leonard, L., & Loeb, D. (1988). Government-binding theory and some of its applications: A tutorial. *Journal of Speech and Hearing Research, 31,* 515–524.

Lieberman, P. (1967). *Intonation, perception, and language.* Cambridge, MA: MIT Press.

Limber, J. (1973). The genesis of complex sentences. In T. Moore (Ed.), *Cognitive development and the acquisition of language* (pp. 169–185). New York: Academic Press.

Locke, J. L. (1983). *Phonological acquisition and change.* New York: Academic Press.

Locke, J. L. (1993). *The child's path to spoken language.* Cambridge, MA: Harvard University Press.

Love, R. J., & Webb, W. G. (2001). *Neurology for the speech-language pathologist* (4th ed.). Stoneham, MA: Butterworth-Heinemann.

Lund, N. J., & Duchan, J. F. (1993). *Assessing children's language in naturalistic contexts* (3rd ed.). Englewood Cliffs, NJ: Prentice-Hall.

MacCorquodale, K. (1969). B. F. Skinner's *Verbal Behavior:* A retrospective appreciation. *Journal of Experimental Analysis of Behavior, 12,* 831–841.

MacCorquodale, K. (1970). On Chomsky's review of Skinner's *Verbal Behavior. Journal of Experimental Analysis of Behavior, 13,* 83–99.

Martin, G. B., & Clark, R. D. (1982). Distress crying in neonates: Species and peer specificity. *Developmental Psychology, 18,* 3–9.

Masur, E. F. (1983). Gestural development, dual-directional signaling, and the transition to words. *Journal of Psycholinguistic Research, 12,* 93–109.

May, F. B. (1990). *Reading as communication: An interactive approach.* Columbus, OH: Merrill.

McLaughlin, S. F., & Cullinan, W. L. (1981). An empirical perspective on language development and language training. In N. J. Lass (Ed.), *Speech and language: Advances in basic research and practice* (Vol. 5, pp. 249–310). New York: Academic Press.

McNeill, D. (1970). *The acquisition of language.* New York: Harper & Row.

Meltzoff, A., & Moore, M. (1977). Imitation of facial and manual gestures by human neonates. *Science, 198,* 75–78.

Menyuk, P. (1977). *Language and maturation.* Cambridge: MIT Press.

Miller, P., & Sperry, L. (1988). Early talk about the past: The origins of conversational stories of personal experiences. *Journal of Child Language, 15,* 293–315.

Milosky, L. M. (1990). The role of world knowledge in language comprehension and language intervention. *Topics in Language Disorders, 10,* 1–13.

Moerk, E. L. (1977). Processes and products of imitation: Additional evidence that imitation is progressive. *Journal of Psycholinguistic Research, 6,* 187–202.

Moerk, E. L. (1983). *The mother of Eve—as a first language teacher.* Norwood, NJ: Ablex.

Moerk, E. L. (1991). Positive evidence for negative evidence. *First Language, 11,* 219–251.

Moerk, E. L. (1992a). *A first langauge taught and learned.* Baltimore: Paul H. Brookes.

Moerk, E. L. (1992b). The clash of giants over terminological differences. *Behavior and Social Issues, 2,* 1–26.

Moerk, E. L. (1994). Corrections in first language acquisition: Theoretical controversies and factual evidence. *International Journal of Psycholinguistic Research, 10,* 33–58.

Morgan, J., & Travis, L. (1989). Limits on negative information in language input. *Journal of Child Language, 16,* 531–552.

Morris, C. (1958). Verbal behavior, by B. F. Skinner. *Contemporary Psychology, 3,* 212–214.

Morse, P. A., & Snowden, C. T. (1975). An investigation of categorical speech discrimination by rhesus monkeys. *Perception and Psychophysics, 17,* 9–16.

Mowrer, O. (1960). *Learning theory and symbolic processes.* New York: John Wiley & Sons.

Mowrer, O. H. (1952). Speech development in the young child: 1. The autism theory of speech development and some clinical applications. *Journal of Speech and Hearing Disorders, 17,* 263–268.

Murray, A., Johnson, J., & Peters, J. (1990). Fine-tuning of utterance length to preverbal infants: Effects on later language development. *Journal of Child Language, 17,* 511–525.

Myklebust, H. R. (1964). *The psychology of deafness* (2nd ed.). New York: Grune & Stratton.

Nakazima, S. A. (1962). A comparative study of the speech developments of Japanese and American English in childhood (1): A comparison of the developments of voices at the prelinguistic period. *Studia Phonologica, 2,* 27–46.

Nelson, K. (1973a). Some evidence for the cognitive primacy of categorization and its functional basis. *Merrill-Palmer Quarterly, 19,* 21–39.

Nelson, K. (1973b). Structure and strategy in learning to talk. *Monographs of the Society for Research in Child Development, 38* (Serial No. 149).

Nelson, K. (1974). Concept, word, and sentence: Interrelations in acquisition and development. *Psychological Review, 81,* 11–56.

Nelson, N. W. (1984). Beyond information processing: The language of teachers and textbooks. In G. P. Wallach & K. G. Butler (Eds.), *Language learning disabilities in school-age children.* Baltimore: Williams & Wilkins.

Nelson, N. W. (1993). *Childhood language disorders in context: Infancy through adolescence.* New York: Macmillan.

Nicolosi, L., Harryman, E., & Kresheck, J. (2003). *Terminology of communication disorders: Speech—language—hearing* (5th ed.). Baltimore: Williams & Wilkins.

Nippold, M., & Erkine, B. (1988). Proverb comprehension in context: A developmental study with children and adolescents. *Journal of Speech and Hearing Research, 31,* 19–28.

Nippold, M., & Martin, S. (1989). Idiom interpretation in isolation versus context: A developmental study with adolescents. *Journal of Speech and Hearing Research, 32,* 59–66.

Nippold, M. A., & Haq, F. S. (1996). Proverb comprehension in youth: The role of concreteness and familiarity. *Journal of Speech and Hearing Research, 39,* 166–176.

Nippold, M. A., & Rudzinksi, M. (1993). Familiarity and transparency in idiom explanation: A developmental study of children and adolescents. *Journal of Speech and Hearing Research, 36,* 728–737.

Nippold, M. A., Schwarz, I. E., & Undlin, R. A. (1992). Use and understanding of adverbial conjuncts: A developmental study of adolescents and young adults. *Journal of Speech and Hearing Research, 35,* 108–118.

Norris J., & Brunig, R. (1988). Cohesion in the narratives of good and poor readers. *Journal of Speech and Hearing Disorders, 53,* 416–423.

Ohala, J. J. (1980, November). *The acoustic origin of the smile.* Paper delivered to the Acoustical Society of America, Los Angeles, CA.

Oklahoma State Department of Education. (2002, July). *Priority academic student skills (PASS)*: Author.

Oller, D. (1978). Infant vocalizations and the development of speech. *Allied Health and Behavior Sciences, 1,* 523–549.

Oller, D., Eilers, R., Bull, D., & Carney, A. (1985). Prespeech vocalizations of a deaf infant: A comparison with normal metaphonological development. *Journal of Speech and Hearing Research, 28,* 47–62.

Oller, D. K., & Eilers, R. E. (1982). Similarity of babbling in Spanish- and English-learning babies. *Journal of Child Language, 9,* 565–577.

Oller, D. K., Wieman, L. A., Doyle, W. J., & Ross, C. (1976). Infant babbling and speech. *Journal of Child Language, 3,* 1–11.

Owens, R. E. (2005). *Language development: An introduction* (6th ed.). Boston: Allyn & Bacon.

Oyama, S. (1976). A sensitive period for the acquisition of a non-native phonological system. *Journal of Psycholinguistic Research, 5,* 261–285.

Palermo, D. (1982). Theoretical issues in semantic development. In S. Kuczaj (Ed.), *Language development: Vol. I. Syntax and semantics.* Hillsdale, NJ: Lawrence Erlbaum.

Parker, F., & Riley, K. (2004). *Linguistics for nonlinguiste: A primer with exercises* (4th ed.). Boston: Allyn & Bacon.

Patterson, J. L., & Westby, C. E. (1994). The development of play. In W. O. Haynes & B. B. Shulman (Eds.), *Communication development: Foundations, processes, and clinical applications* (pp. 135–164). Englewood Cliffs, NJ: Prentice-Hall.

Pease, D., & Berko Gleason, J. (1985). Gaining meaning: Semantic development. In J. Berko Gleason, (Ed.), *The development of language.* Columbus, OH: Merrill.

Petrovich-Bartell, N., Cowan, N., & Morse, P. A. (1982). Mothers' perceptions of infant distress vocalizations. *Journal of Speech and Hearing Research, 25,* 371–376.

Porter, R. H., Boyle, C., Hardister, T., & Balogh, R. D. (1989). Salience of neonates' facial features for recognition by family members. *Ethology and Sociobiology, 10,* 325–330.

Ramer, A. L. H. (1976). The function of imitation in child language. *Journal of Speech and Language Research, 19,* 700–717.

Ratner, N. K., & Bruner, J. S. (1978). Games, social exchange and the acquisition of language. *Journal of Child Language, 5,* 391–401.

Reich, P. A. (1986). *Language development.* Englewood Cliffs, NJ: Prentice-Hall.

Retherford, K. S. (1993). *Guide to analysis of language transcripts* (2nd ed.). Eau Claire, WI: Thinking Publications.

Rheingold, H., Gewirtz, J., & Ross, H. (1959). Social conditioning of vocalizations in the infant. *Journal of Comparative and Physiological Psychology, 52,* 68–73.

Ricillo, S. C., & Watterson, T. (1984). The suppression of crying in the human neonate: Response to human vocal tract stimuli. *Brain and Language, 23,* 34–42.

Routh, D. K. (1969). Conditioning of vocal response differentiation in infants. *Developmental Psychology, 1,* 219–226.

Sachs, J. (1985). Prelinguistic development. In J. Berko Gleason (Ed.), *The development of language* (pp. 37–60). Columbus, OH: Merrill.

Sawyer, D. J. (1991). Whole language in context: Insights into the current great debate. *Topics in Language Disorders, 11,* 1–13.

Scott, C. (1988). The development of complex sentences. *Topics in Language Disorders, 8,* 44–62.

Searle, J. R. (1969). *Speech acts.* Cambridge, England: Cambridge University Press.

Searle, J. R. (1975). Indirect speech acts. In P. Cole & J. L. Morgan (Eds.), *Syntax and semantics 3: Speech acts* (pp. 59–82). New York: Academic Press.

Segal, E. V. (1975). Psycholinguistics discovers the operant: A review of *Roger Brown's A first language: The early stages. Journal of Experimental Analysis of Behavior, 23,* 149–158.

Segal, E. V. (1977). Toward a coherent psychology of language. In W. K. Honig & J. E. R. Staddon (Eds.), *Handbook of operant conditioning* (pp. 628–653). Englewood Cliffs, NJ: Prentice-Hall.

Shadden, B. (1997). Language and communication changes with aging. In B. B. Shadden & M. A. Toner (Eds.), *Aging and communication.* Austin, TX: Pro-Ed.

Shorr, D., & Dale, P. (1981). Prepositional marking of source-goal structure and children's comprehension of English passives. *Journal of Speech and Hearing Research, 24,* 179–184.

Shulman, B. B. (1994). Child development. In W. O. Haynes & B. B. Shulman (Eds.), *Communication* development: Foundations, processes, and clinical applications* (pp. 63–81). Englewood Cliffs, NJ: Prentice-Hall.

Silliman, E. R., Jimerson, T. L., & Wilkinson, L. C. (2000). A dynamic systems approach to writing assessment in student with language learning problems. *Topics in Language Disorders, 20*(4), 45–64.

Simonds, R. J., & Scheibel, A. B. (1989). The postnatal development of the motor speech area: A preliminary study. *Brain and Language, 37,* 42–58.

Skinner, B. F. (1938). *The behavior of organisms.* Englewood Cliffs, NJ: Prentice-Hall.

Skinner, B. F. (1953). *Science and human behavior.* New York: Macmillan.

Skinner, B. F. (1957). *Verbal behavior.* New York: Appleton-Century-Crofts.

Skinner, B. F. (1969). *Contingencies of reinforcement: A theoretical analysis.* Englewood Cliffs, NJ: Prentice-Hall.

Skinner, B. F. (1974). *About behaviorism.* New York: Alfred A. Knopf.

Skinner, B. F. (1986). The evolution of verbal behavior. *Journal of the Experimental Analysis of Behavior, 45,* 115–122.

Skinner, B. F. (1990). Can psychology be a science of mind? *American Psychologist, 45,* 1206–1210.

Slobin, D. I. (Ed.). (1985). *The cross-linguistic study of language acquisition: Vol. I. The data.* Hillsdale, NJ: Lawrence Erlbaum.

Snow, C. (1977a). The development of conversation between mothers and babies. *Journal of Child Language, 4,* 1–22.

Snow, C. E. (1977b). Mothers' speech research: From input to acquisition. In C. E. Snow & C. A. Ferguson (Eds.), *Talking to children: Language input and acquisition* (pp. 31–49). Cambridge: Cambridge University Press.

Snow, C. E., Scarborough, H. S., & Burns, M. S. (1999). What speech-language pathologists need to know about early reading. *Topics in Language Disorders, 20*(1), 48–58.

Snyder-McLean, L., & McLean, J. (1978). Verbal information gathering strategies: The child's use of language to acquire language. *Journal of Speech and Hearing Disorders, 43,* 306–325.

Spelke, E. S., & Owsley, C. J. (1979). Intermodal exploration and knowledge in infancy. *Infant Behavior and Development, 2,* 13–24.

Stark, R. E., Bernstein, L. E., & Demorest, M. E. (1993). Vocal communication in the first 18 months of life. *Journal of Speech and Hearing Research, 36,* 548–558.

Stern, D. (1977). *The first relationship.* Cambridge, MA: Harvard University Press.

Stockman, I. J., Woods, D. R., & Tishman, A. (1981). Listener agreement on phonetic segments in early infant vocalization. *Journal of Psycholinguistic Research, 10,* 593–617.

Stoel-Gammon, C., & Otomo, K. (1986). Babbling development of hearing-impaired and normally hearing subjects. *Journal of Speech and Hearing Disorders, 51,* 33–41.

Tannen, D. (1990). *You just don't understand: Men and women in conversation.* New York: William Morrow.

Taylor, O. (Ed.). (1986). *Nature of communication disorders in culturally and linguistically diverse populations.* San Diego: College-Hill Press.

Templin, M. (1957). *Certain language skills in children: Their development and interrelationship.* Minneapolis: University of Minnesota Press.

Terrell, S. L., & Terrell, F. (1993). African-American cultures. In D. E. Battle (Ed.), *Communication disorders in multicultural populations* (pp. 3–37). Boston: Andover Medical.

Todd, G., & Palmer, B. (1968). Social reinforcement of infant babbling. *Child Development, 39,* 591–596.

Tomasello, M. (1988). The role of joint attentional processes in early language development. *Language Sciences, 10,* 69–88.

Tomasello, M., Conti-Ramsden, G., & Ewert, B. (1990). Young children's conversations with their mothers and fathers: Differences in breakdown and repair. *Journal of Child Language, 17,* 115–130.

Tomasello, M., & Kruger, A. C. (1992). Joint attention on actions: Acquiring verbs in ostensive and non-ostensive contexts. *Journal of Child Language, 19,* 311–333.

Tomblin, B., & Buckwalter, P. (1994). Studies of genetics of specific language impairments. In R. Watkins & M. Rice (Eds.), *Specific language impairments in children* (pp. 17–34). Baltimore: Paul Brookes.

Trehub, S. E. (1973). Infant's sensitivity to vowel and tonal contrasts. *Developmental Psychology, 9,* 91–96.

Trehub, S. E. (1976). The discrimination of foreign speech contrasts by infants and adults. *Child Development, 47,* 466–472.

van Kleeck, A. (1984). Metalinguistic skills: Cutting across spoken and written language and problem-solving abilities. In G. P. Wallach & K. G. Butler (Eds.), *Language learning disabilities in school-age children.* Baltimore: Williams & Wilkins.

van Kleeck, A. (1995). Emphasizing form and meaning separately in prereading and early reading instruction. *Topics in Language Disorders, 16*(1), 27–49.

van Kleeck, A., & Schuele, C. (1987). Precursors to literacy: Normal development. *Topics in Language Disorders, 7*(2), 13–31.

Volterra, V., & Taeschner, T. (1978). The acquisition and development of language by bilingual children. *Journal of Child Language, 5,* 311–326.

Vygotsky, L. (1962). *Thought and language.* Cambridge, MA : MIT Press. (Original work published in 1934.)

Wagner, K. (1985). How much do children say in a day? *Journal of Child Language, 12,* 475–487.

Wahler, R. G. (1969). Infant social development: Some experimental analyses of an infant-mother interaction during the first year of life. *Journal of Experimental Child Psychology, 7,* 101–113.

Wallach, G. P. (1984). Later language learning: Syntactic structures and strategies. In G. P. Wallach & K. G. Butler (Eds.), *Language learning disabilities in school-age children* (pp. 82–102). Baltimore: Williams & Wilkins.

Wallach, G. P., & Miller, L. (1988). *Language intervention and academic success.* Boston: College-Hill Press.

Warren-Leubecker, A., & Bohannon, J. N., III. (1985). Language in society: Variation and adaptation. In J. B. Gleason (Ed.), *The development of language* (pp. 331–367). Columbus, OH: Merrill.

Washburn, S. L. (1960). Tools and human evolution. *Scientific American, 203,* 63–75.

Waters, R. S., & Wilson, W. A., Jr. (1976). Speech perception by rhesus monkeys: The voicing distinction in synthesized labial and velar stop consonants. *Perception and Psychophysics, 19,* 285–289.

Webb, P., & Abrahmson, A. (1976). Stages of egocentrism in children's use of "this" and "that": A different point of view. *Journal of Child Language, 3,* 349–367.

Webster's Word Histories. (1991). Springfield, MA: Merriam-Webster.

Weisberg, P. (1963). Social and nonsocial conditioning of infant vocalization. *Child Development, 39,* 377–388.

Wells, G. (1985). *Language development in the preschool years.* New York: Cambridge University Press.

Westby, C. E. (1984). Development of narrative language abilities. In G. P. Wallach & K. G. Butler (Eds.), *Language learning disabilities in school-age children* (pp. 103–127). Baltimore: Williams & Wilkins.

Westby, C. E. (1994a). Communication refinement in school age and adolescence. In W. O. Haynes & B. B. Shulman (Eds.), *Communication development: Foundations, processes, and clinical applications* (pp. 341–383). Englewood Cliffs, NJ: Prentice-Hall.

Westby, C. E. (1994b). Sociocommunicative bases of communication development. In W. O. Haynes & B. B. Shulman (Eds.), *Communication development: Foundations, processes, and clinical applications* (pp. 199–229). Englewood Cliffs, NJ: Prentice-Hall.

Whorf, B. (1956). *Language, thought, and reality.* New York: John Wiley.

Winitz, H. (1969). *Articulatory acquisition and behavior.* New York: Appleton-Century-Crofts.

Winokur, S. (1976). *A primer of verbal behavior: An operant view.* Englewood Cliffs, NJ: Prentice-Hall.

Wolff, P. (1966). The causes, controls and organization of behavior in the neonate. *Psychological Issues, 5,* 1–19.

Wolff, P. H. (1963). Observations on the early development of smiling. In B. M. Foss (Ed.), *Determinants of infant behaviour II* (pp. 113–138). London: Metheun.

Wolff, P. H. (1969). The natural history of crying and other vocalizations in early infancy. In B. M. Foss (Ed.), *Determinants of infant behaviour IV* (pp. 81–109). London: Metheun.

Wood, W. S. (1986). Bertrand Russell's review of *The Meaning of Meaning. Journal of the Experimental Analysis of Behavior, 45,* 107–113.

Zeskind, P., & Lester, B. (1978). Acoustic features and auditory perception of the cries of newborns with prenatal and perinatal complications. *Child Development, 49,* 580–589.

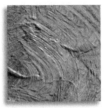

Index

Intentionality, 205–206
Intentions, 225–226
Interactionism, 129, 130
Interference, 405
Interlocking verbal behavior paradigm, 133
International Phonetic Alphabet (IPA), 15, 16
Interrogative sentences, 28, 330–333
Interrogative utterances, 252
Intervention, 417
Intransitive verbs, 327
Intraverbal, 138
Intuitive grammar, 30
Irwin, Orvis C., 185

J

Jargon, 184
Joint actions, 90, 200–201
Joint attention, 89, 200–202
Joint reference, 89, 200–201

K

Kinship words, 293–294

L

Language, 19–37, 127–167. *See also* Literacy
  changes during life span, 390–394
  changes in during aging, 393–394
  Child Talk model, 165–166
  and cognition, 100–103
  defining, 22
  expressive *vs.* receptive, 21
  and infant communication, 177–178
  linguistic aspects of, 24–31
  for literacy, 379–389
  metalinguistics, 366–373
  operant model, 129–144
  oral skills, 382–383
  pragmatic aspect of, 35–37
  pragmatic model, 161–167
  pragmatics, 373–379
  prelinguistic foundations for, 178–189
  and the school years, 349–394
  semantic aspect of, 32–35
  semantic model, 155–161
  structural model, 144–155
  study of, 22–23
  vs. dialect, 20–21
  vs. speech, 20
Language acquisition device (LAD), 146
Language development
  and infants, 173–212
  and preschoolers, 265–295
  science and research in, 125–127
  and toddlers, 217–259
Language disorders, 401, 415–418
Language diversity, 401–415
  bilingualism, 403–406
  cross-linguistic differences, 401–403

dialects, 407
  regional dialects, 407–415
Language expectations
  and preschoolers, 268
  in the school years, 352–353
Language families, 402
Language universals, 400
Language variations, 400
Larynx, 55
Learning
  cognitive principles of, 92–103
  social principles of, 81–92
Lenticular nucleus, 50, 51
Lexical verbs, 327
Lexicon, 33
  first, 231–233
Linear syntactic relationships, 247–248
Linguistic aspects, 10
Linguistic competence, 31
Linguistic context, 36
Linguistic performance, 31
Literacy, 379–389. *See also* Language
  emerging, 211–212, 297–298, 380–381
  language differences, 381–382
  and the school years, 349–394
Literacy artifacts, 211
Literacy events, 212
Literacy knowledge, 212
Literate language, 382
Location relational words, 238
Locative action relations, 250
Locative state relations, 250
Locutionary, 163
Locutionary stage, of communication, 192, 221–226
Logical form rules, 152
Logographic stage, 297
Longitudinal research design, 190

M

Malleus, 60
Mand, 135
Marginal babbling, 182–183
Marked, 292
Marking, 201
Mass activity reflexes, 70
Mass noun, 358, 359
Mean length of utterance (MLU), 307–309, 343
Means-end schemata, 97–98
Mentalism, 128
Mesoderm, 63
Metalinguistic ability, 366–372
Metalinguistics, 366–373
Metaphoric transparency, 371
Metaphors, 370
Method of rich interpretation, 160
Midbrain, 50, 52
Minimal distance principle, 341–342
Mitotic division, 62
Mixed language disorder, 417
Modal auxiliary verbs, 328